AGE-RELATED
MACULAR
DEGENERATION

AGE-RELATED MACULAR DEGENERATION

Third Edition

Edited by
Jennifer I. Lim, MD

*Professor of Ophthalmology, Marion H. Schenk, Esq., Chair in Ophthalmology
for Research of the Aging Eye, Director of the Retina Service, University of Illinois at Chicago,
Illinois Eye and Ear Infirmary, Chicago, IL, USA*

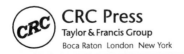

CRC Press
Taylor & Francis Group
Boca Raton London New York

CRC Press is an imprint of the
Taylor & Francis Group, an **informa** business

CRC Press
Taylor & Francis Group
6000 Broken Sound Parkway NW, Suite 300
Boca Raton, FL 33487-2742, USA

First issued in paperback 2019

Fifth edition © 2013 by Taylor & Francis Group, LLC
CRC Press is an imprint of Taylor & Francis Group, an Informa business

No claim to original U.S. Government works

Typeset by Exeter Premedia Services Pvt Ltd., Chennai, India

ISBN-13: 978-1-84184-949-2 (hbk)
ISBN-13: 978-0-367-38066-3 (pbk)

Visit the Taylor & Francis website at
http://www.taylorandfrancis.com

and the CRC Press website at
http://www.crcpress.com

I dedicate this book to:

my students, whose interest in AMD (age-related macular degeneration) spark new research ideas and studies;

my colleagues, whose collaborations enable clinical trials and research to proceed and thus bring new treatments to our AMD patients;

my patients who inspire me to continue to search for better treatments for AMD;

my parents, Dr. Diosdado Lim and Dr. Amada Lim, who first sparked my interest in science and whose unconditional support led me to become the person that I am today;

my own family, John and Bernadette Miao, for their daily, unconditional support of my career and their understanding and value of vision.

Contents

Contributors

Irene A. Barbazetto Vitreous Retina Macula Consultants of New York, New York, NY, USA

Neelakshi Bhagat Director, Vitreoretinal Surgery, Associate Professor of Ophthalmology, Institute of Ophthalmology and Visual Science, New Jersey Medical School, Newark, NJ, USA

Milam A. Brantley Jr Assistant Professor of Ophthalmology and Visual Sciences, Vanderbilt Eye Institute, Nashville, TN, USA

Kelly M. Bui Resident, University of Illinois at Chicago, Department of Ophthalmology and Visual Sciences, Illinois Eye and Ear Infirmary, Chicago, IL, USA

Jennifer R. Chao Assistant Professor of Ophthalmology, Department of Ophthalmology, University of Washington, Seattle, WA, USA

Felix Y. Chau Assistant Professor of Ophthalmology, University of Illinois at Chicago, Department of Ophthalmology and Visual Sciences, Illinois Eye and Ear Infirmary, Chicago, IL, USA

Emily Y. Chew Deputy Director of Division of Epidemiology and Clinical Applications, Chief of Clinical Trials Branch, National Eye Institute/National Institutes of Health, Bethesda, MD, USA

Clement C. Chow Retina Fellow, University of Illinois School of Medicine, Department of Ophthalmology, Eye and Ear Infirmary, Chicago, IL, USA

Karl G. Csaky T. Boone Pickens Senior Scientist, Retina Foundation of the Southwest, Dallas, TX, USA

Scott W. Cousins Robert Machemer, M.D. Professor of Ophthalmology, Professor of Immunology, Vice Chair for Research, Department of Ophthalmology, Director, Duke Center for Macular Diseases, and Medical Director, Hospital-Based Injections and Procedures, Department of Ophthalmology, Duke University School of Medicine, Durham, NC, USA

Catherine A. Cukras Staff Clinician, Division of Epidemiology and Clinical Applications, National Eye Institute/National Institutes of Health, Bethesda, MD, USA

Anthony B. Daniels Department of Ophthalmology, Massachusetts Eye and Ear Infirmary and Harvard Medical School, Boston, MA, USA

Francis Char DeCroos Retina Fellow, Wills Eye Institute/Mid Atlantic Retina, Philadelphia, PA, USA

Lucian V. Del Priore Pierre G. Jenkins Professor and Chairman, Department of Ophthalmology, Charleston, SC, USA, Director, Albert Florens Storm Eye Institute, Medical University of South Carolina, Charleston, SC, USA

Bruno Diniz Research Associate, Doheny Eye Institute and Department of Ophthalmology, Keck School of Medicine of the University of Southern California, Los Angeles, CA, USA

Pravin U. Dugel Retinal Consultants of Arizona, Phoenix, AZ, USA

Paul T. Finger Clinical Professor of Ophthalmology, New York University School of Medicine, and Director of Ocular Tumor Services, The New York Eye Cancer Center, The New York Eye and Ear Infirmary, New York University School of Medicine, New York, NY, USA

Christina Flaxel Professor of Ophthalmology, Casey Eye Institute, Oregon Health and Science University, Portland, OR, USA

Robert W. Flower Professor of Ophthalmology, New York University School of Medicine, New York, NY, USA and Associate Professor of Ophthalmology, University of Maryland School of Medicine, Baltimore, MD, USA

Francisco A. Folgar   Resident, Department of Ophthalmology, Duke University, Durham, NC, USA

K. Bailey Freund   Vitreous Retina Macula Consultants of New York, Clinical Associate Professor of Ophthalmology, Department of Ophthalmology, New York University, Edward S. Harkness Eye Institute, Columbia University College of Physicians and Surgeons, New York, NY, USA

Cheryl Frueh   Clinical Consultant, Director of Low Vision Services, VisionCare Ophthalmic Technologies, Saratoga, CA, USA

Adrian T. Fung   Retina Fellow, Vitreous Retina Macula Consultants of New York, LuEsther T. Mertz Retinal Research Center, Manhattan Eye, Ear, and Throat Institute, New York, NY, USA

Bianca S. Gerendas   Supervisor, Research & Development, Vienna Reading Center, Department of Ophthalmology, Medical University of Vienna, Vienna, Austria

Darin R. Goldman   Retinal Fellow, Ophthalmic Consultants of Boston, New England Eye Center at Tufts Medical Center, Boston, MA, USA

Hans E. Grossniklaus   F. Phinzy Calhoun Jr Professor of Ophthalmology, Director of L. F. Montgomery Pathology Laboratory, Director of Ocular Oncology and Pathology, Department of Ophthalmology, Emory University School of Medicine, Atlanta, GA, USA

Divakar Gupta   Department of Ophthalmology, University of Washington, Seattle, WA, USA

Julia A. Haller   Ophthalmologist-in-Chief, The William Tasman MD Endowed Chair in Ophthalmology, Professor and Chair, Department of Ophthalmology, Jefferson Medical College, Philadelphia, PA, USA

Jeffrey S. Heier   Director of Vitreoretinal Research, Ophthalmic Consultants of Boston, Assistant Professor of Ophthalmology, Tufts University School of Medicine, Boston, MA, USA

Quan V. Hoang   Vitreous Retina Macula Consultants of New York, Department of Ophthalmology, New York University, Edward S. Harkness Eye Institute, Assistant Professor of Ophthalmology, Columbia University College of Physicians and Surgeons, New York, NY, USA

Mark S. Humayun   Cornelius Pings Professor of Biomedical Sciences, Professor of Ophthalmology, Biomedical Engineering and Cell & Neurobiology, Doheny Eye Institute, Department of Ophthalmology, Keck School of Medicine, University of Southern California, Los Angeles, CA, USA

Jesse J. Jung   New York School of Medicine, Department of Ophthalmology, New York, NY, USA

Peter Kaiser   Chaney Family Endowed Chair in Ophthalmology Research, Professor of Ophthalmology, Cleveland Clinic Lerner College of Medicine, Director, Digital Optical Coherence Tomography Reading Center, Cleveland, OH, USA

Shin J. Kang   L.F. Montgomery Ophthalmic Pathology Laboratory, Emory Eye Center, Emory University School of Medicine, Atlanta, GA, USA

Henry J. Kaplan   Evans Professor of Ophthalmology, Chairman, Department of Ophthalmology and Visual Sciences, Louisville, KY, USA, Director, Kentucky Lions Eye Center, Louisville, KY, USA

Pearse A. Keane   NIHR Biomedical Research Centre for Ophthalmology, Moorfields Eye Hospital NHS Foundation Trust, UCL Institute of Ophthalmology, London, UK

Ivana K. Kim   Assistant Professor of Ophthalmology, Department of Ophthalmology, Massachusetts Eye and Ear Infirmary and Harvard Medical School, Boston, MA, USA

Judy E. Kim   Professor of Ophthalmology, Vitreoretinal Section, Medical College of Wisconsin, Milwaukee, WI, USA

Todd R. Klesert   Acting Assistant Professor, University of Washington Eye Institute, Seattle, WA, USA

Madhavi Kurli   Retinal Consultants of Arizona, Phoenix, AZ, USA

Yannek Leiderman   Assistant Professor of Ophthalmology, University of Illinois at Chicago, Department of Ophthalmology and Visual Sciences, Illinois Eye and Ear Infirmary, Chicago, IL, USA

Jennifer I. Lim   Professor of Ophthalmology, Marion H. Schenk, Esq., Chair in Ophthalmology for Research of the Aging Eye, Director of the Retina Service, University of Illinois at Chicago, Department of Ophthalmology and Visual Sciences, Illinois Eye and Ear Infirmary, Chicago, IL, USA

Anat Loewenstein   Chairman of Ophthalmology, Tel Aviv Medical Center, and Professor of Ophthalmology, Sackler Faculty of Medicine, Tel Aviv University, Tel-Aviv, Israel

George N. Magrath   Department of Ophthalmology, Albert Florens Storm Eye Institute, Medical University of South Carolina, Charleston, SC, USA

Priyatham S. Mettu   Assistant Professor of Ophthalmology, Duke Center for Macular Diseases, Duke Eye Center, Durham, NC, USA

Joan W. Miller   Henry Willard Williams Professor of Ophthalmology, Chair, Department of Ophthalmology, Massachusetts Eye and Ear Infirmary, Harvard Medical School, Boston, MA, USA

Dimple Modi   Retina Fellow, Bascom Palmer Eye Institute, University of Miami Miller School of Medicine, Miami, FL, USA

Benjamin P. Nicholson   Fellow, National Eye Institute, National Institutes of Health, The Division of Epidemiology and Clinical Applications, Clinical Trials Branch, Bethesda, MD, USA

Oded Ohana   Professor of Ophthalmology, Tel Aviv Medical Center, Sackler Faculty of Medicine, Tel Aviv University, Tel-Aviv, Israel

Melissa P. Osborn   Vanderbilt Eye Institute, Nashville, TN, USA

Susan A. Primo   Director, Vision and Optical Services, Emory Eye Center, Professor, Department of Ophthalmology, Emory University School of Medicine, Atlanta, GA, USA

Rajiv Rathod   Retina Fellow, University of Illinois at Chicago, Department of Ophthalmology and Visual Sciences, Illinois Eye and Ear Infirmary, Chicago, IL, USA

Caio V. Regatieri   Assistant Professor, New England Eye Center, Tufts Medical Center, and Adjunct Professor, Department of Ophthalmology, Universidade Federal de São Paulo, São Paulo, Brazil

Elias Reichel   Professor and Vice Chair, Director, Vitreoretinal Service, New England Eye Center, Tufts University School of Medicine, Boston, MA, USA

Markus Ritter   Vienna Reading Center, Department of Ophthalmology, Medical University of Vienna, Vienna, Austria

Philip J. Rosenfeld   Professor of Ophthalmology, Bascom Palmer Eye Institute, University of Miami Miller School of Medicine, Miami, FL, USA

Srinivas R. Sadda   Associate Professor of Ophthalmology and Director, Medical Retina Unit, Ophthalmic Imaging Unit, Doheny Image Reading Center, Doheny Eye Institute, Keck School of Medicine, University of Southern California, Los Angeles, CA, USA

Ursula Schmidt-Erfurth   Professor and Chair of the Department of Ophthalmology, Medical University of Vienna, Vienna, Austria

Chirag P. Shah   Ophthalmic Consultants of Boston, and Assistant Professor, Tufts School of Medicine, Boston, MA, USA Boston, MA, USA

Ravi S. J. Singh   Retina Fellow, Medical College of Wisconsin, Milwaukee, WI, USA

Rishi P. Singh   Assistant Professor of Ophthalmology, Cleveland Clinic Lerner College of Medicine, Cole Eye Institute, Cleveland Clinic Foundation, Cleveland, OH, USA

Jason S. Slakter   Clinical Professor of Ophthalmology, New York University School of Medicine and Vitreous Retina Macula Consultants of New York, New York, NY, USA

Sharon D. Solomon   Katharine M. Graham Professorship, Associate Professor of Ophthalmology, Wilmer Eye Institute, Johns Hopkins University School of Medicine, Baltimore, MD, USA

Richard F. Spaide Clinical Assistant Professor, New York Medical College, and Vitreous, Retina, Macula Consultants of New York, New York, NY, USA

Paul Sternberg Jr G. W. Hale Professor and Chairman, Vanderbilt Eye Institute, Associate Dean for Clinical Affairs, Vanderbilt School of Medicine, Chief Medical Officer, Vanderbilt Medical Group, Assistant Vice Chancellor for Adult Health Affairs, Nashville, TN, USA

Janet S. Sunness Professor of Ophthalmology and Medical Director of The Richard E. Hoover Services for Low Vision and Blindness, Greater Baltimore Medical Center, Baltimore, MD, USA

Tongalp H. Tezel Associate Professor of Ophthalmology, Kentucky Lions Endowed Chair, Department of Ophthalmology and Visual Sciences, and Director of Fellowship Program in Vitreoretinal Diseases and Surgery, University of Louisville, Louisville, KY, USA

Cynthia A. Toth Professor of Ophthalmology and Biomedical Engineering, Duke University, Durham, NC, USA

Demetrios G. Vavvas Department of Ophthalmology, Massachusetts Assistant Professor of Ophthalmology, J. W. Miller Scholar in Retina Research, Eye and Ear Infirmary and Harvard Medical School, Boston, MA, USA

Robin Vora New England Eye Center, Tufts Medical Center, Boston Retina Fellow, MA, USA

Sebastian M. Waldstein Vienna Reading Center, Department of Ophthalmology, Medical University of Vienna, Vienna, Austria

James D. Weiland Associate Professor of Ophthalmology and Biomedical Engineering, Doheny Eye Institute and Department of Ophthalmology, Keck School of Medicine of the University of Southern California, Los Angeles, CA, USA

Alex Yuan Staff physician, Cole Eye Institute, Cleveland Clinic Foundation, Cleveland, OH, USA

Lawrence A. Yannuzzi Vice–Chairman and Director, LuEsther T. Mertz Retinal Research Center, Manhattan Eye, Ear & Throat Hospital, and Professor of Clinical Ophthalmology, Columbia University Medical School, New York, NY, USA

Dinah Zur Department of Ophthalmology, Tel Aviv Sourasky Medical Center, Tel-Aviv, Israel

A. Frances Walonker Doheny Eye Institute and Department of Ophthalmology, Keck School of Medicine, University of Southern California, Los Angeles, California, U.S.A

Kenneth R. Diddie Retinal Consultants of Southern California, Westlake Village, California, U.S.A.

Marcia Niec Department of Ophthalmology and Visual Sciences, Eye and Ear Infirmary, Lions of Illinois Eye Research Institute, University of Illinois at Chicago, Chicago, IL, USA

Foreword

In this timely Third Edition of *Age-Related Macular Degeneration*, Professor Jennifer Lim and her colleagues provide highly useful information on an important group of macular diseases, namely, "Age-Related Macular Degeneration." As noted in the first edition in 2002 and again in the second edition in 2007, there has been a major accretion of new knowledge since the prior publication. Hence, the need for this excellent new volume.

The value of *Age-Related Macular Degeneration* has clearly stood the test of time, but progress in both basic and clinical ophthalmology has been relentless, thereby mandating the need for an updated book. The physicians, scientists, and patients who read this Third Edition will be reassured that this markedly enhanced edition has met the challenge of providing new information that is both intellectually and clinically valuable. Dr Lim has again chosen expert authors for the important topics in this stimulating compendium.

Chapters are devoted to the following: pathophysiology and epidemiology of age-related macular degeneration (AMD); clinical features of AMD; imaging techniques; and medical therapy for both non-neovascular AMD and neovascular AMD. Both clinically validated and experimental therapies are well described, including rehabilitation technology (a highly important topic that is often overlooked in the management of patients with AMD).

New chapters now constitute almost half of the total number. They describe and discuss the following: the pathologic biology of AMD; the importance of evidence-based therapy; new imaging techniques that can guide decisions for treatment; and comprehensive analyses of AMD variants.

No doubt, some very important questions remain: for example, what are the precise etiologies and the various aspects of pathophysiology of AMD? What are the best diagnostic tests available now, and which ones are likely to be supplanted (and by what?)? What is the actual evidence for the most successful new therapies or combinations of therapies? What are the best dosing schedules? What are the most promising new delivery systems, including intraocular implants, etc.? Importantly, how soon can we expect validated therapies for the currently unsuccessful treatment of non-neovascular AMD? And what are these new therapies likely to be?

Again, Professor Lim has brought us up to the moment. We owe her and her collaborators a vote of thanks and a vote of confidence. Hopefully, the march of time, with its inexorable acquisition of new knowledge, will mandate the need for yet another edition. For the time being, however, this Third Edition of *Age-Related Macular Degeneration* does its job commendably and effectively.

Morton F. Goldberg, MD
Director Emeritus
The Wilmer Eye Institute
Johns Hopkins Hospital
Baltimore, MD, USA

Preface

Novel and myriad advancements are accelerating in our field of age-related macular degeneration (AMD). These discoveries about the mechanisms of disease and novel treatments for AMD inspire and warrant the creation of this Third Edition of *Age-Related Macular Degeneration*. A little over a decade ago, the first edition of *Age-Related Macular Degeneration* was created to capture and collate the existing knowledge gleaned from advances in the field of AMD research. At that time photodynamic therapy was heralded as a major advancement in the treatment of AMD. Then, six years later, the Second Edition was published in response to groundbreaking therapeutic advances, such as anti-angiogenesis therapy, which revolutionized the care of AMD patients and offered them the real possibility of improved visual acuity and function. Fortunately, we have again reached another threshold which includes the understanding of the pathophysiology of AMD, better imaging techniques, and novel therapeutic options. Throughout this edition, these advancements are highlighted. Emphasis remains on evidence-based data and applications to clinical practice as in prior editions.

The first section of this third edition captures knowledge about the pathophysiology and epidemiology of both non-neovascular and neovascular AMD. Experts in the field describe and discuss different mechanisms of disease pathobiology. Histopathology, immunology, genetics, VEGF pathways, oxidative stress and clinical risk factors are discussed in detail by experts in the field.

The second section emphasizes the clinical features of AMD. Many new images have been added to the chapters on diagnosis and treatment of AMD. In addition, this new edition captures advancements in ocular imaging. Spectral domain optical coherence tomography (SD-OCT), fundus autofluorescence, and microperimetry as applied to AMD evaluation and management are presented with numerous examples within those chapters. Of course, the classic findings of fluorescein angiography remain with examples given for the various disease states.

The next major section presents the current and experimental treatments for AMD. The findings of numerous clinical trials on AMD are discussed in detail, in almost all cases, by the leaders of those clinical trials. These trials encompass non-neovascular as well as neovascular AMD. The past few years witnessed a profusion of AMD clinical trials. The latest clinical trial results have been included with an emphasis on the clinical usefulness of the data in treating the AMD patient.

Several new chapters have been added to ensure that this edition contains the latest information. New chapters include oxidative stress in the pathophysiology of AMD, polypoidal choroidal vasculopathy, retinal angiomatous proliferation, SD-OCT guided therapy for AMD, non-VEGF related anti-angiogenesis pathways for treatment of AMD, Age-Related Eye Disease Study results, visual cycle modulation, stem cell therapy, and surgery for AMD. The existing chapters have undergone extensive revision to ensure timeliness of the information.

It is my hope that this third edition will serve as a valuable resource for the care of AMD patients. I hope that it will serve as a resource for students interested in basic mechanisms of AMD as well as a reference for practicing clinicians interested in new treatment modalities and clinical trial results. The future of AMD care remains bright, with major advancements in the field occurring within a few years. It is inspiring to know that translational research has led to visual acuity sparing and vision-improving therapies. I hope that the information presented herein will spark new ideas and research that will eventually result in a cure for AMD.

I acknowledge all authors for their outstanding contributions to this book and offer my sincere gratitude to them. Their expertise, collegiality, and scholarship made my job as editor of this book enjoyable, educational, and satisfying. I also thank my administrative assistant, Vee, and my Informa Editor, Parita, for their invaluable assistance in the creation of this book. Lastly, I thank once again my family for their support, interest, and understanding during the writing and editing of this book.

I hope the third edition of *Age-Related Macular Degeneration* is as educational and enjoyable as our previous ones.

Jennifer I. Lim, MD

Histopathology of age-related macular degeneration

Shin J. Kang and Hans E. Grossniklaus

INTRODUCTION

Pathological changes in age-related macular degeneration (AMD) occur in the various structures in the posterior pole, such as the outer retina, the retinal pigment epithelium (RPE), Bruch's membrane, and the choriocapillaris (1,2). Early lesions of AMD are located either between the RPE and its basement membrane [e.g., basal laminar deposits (BLamD)] or between the basement membrane of the RPE and the remainder of Bruch's membrane [e.g., basal linear deposits (BLinD)] (2–5). Focal and diffuse deposition between the RPE and Bruch's membrane is called drusen. Alterations of RPE such as hypopigmentation, depigmentation, or atrophy and attenuation of photoreceptor cells are also observed. This form of macular degeneration is known as dry AMD (non-neovascular AMD), whereas choroidal neovascularization (CNV) is the main feature of wet AMD (neovascular AMD), which ultimately results in a disciform scar in end stage AMD.

HISTOPATHOLOGY OF NON-NEOVASCULAR (DRY) AMD
Changes in Bruch's Membrane

Bruch's membrane increases in thickness with age (6,7). The pathological changes in AMD first appear in the inner collagenous zone and generally extend into central elastic zone and outer collagenous zone and the intercapillary connective tissue during later stages of the disease (8). Drusen and BLinD contribute to a diffuse thickening of the inner aspect of Bruch's membrane (Fig. 1.1A) (1,6,9–14). With a change in the pH of the collagenous fibers and the deposition of calcium salts in the elastic tissue, Bruch's membrane shows increased basophilia. Accumulation of lipid substance from the RPE also results in sudanophilia (12,14–16). The lipid deposition in the Bruch's membrane begins by the fourth decade of life, and extends inward to form a "lipid wall" between the inner collagenous layer and the basal lamina of Bruch's membrane (17). Thickening and hyalinization of Bruch's membrane in the macular area has also been found in the outer collagenous zone (5,18), presumably due to the accumulation of cellular waste products (12,19).

Ultrastructural examination of Bruch's membrane in elderly humans typically shows focal areas of wide-spaced banded collagen, membrane-bounded bodies, tube-like structures of degenerated collagen fibers, electron dense granular material surrounded by a double membrane, and electron lucent droplets (3,6,14). These findings may be accompanied by an increase in native

collagen within the central elastic layer (type IV collagen), the inner and outer collagenous zone (type I and III collagen) and in the intercapillary connective tissue (6,20). Focal thinning and disruption of Bruch's membrane are also found to be associated with an increased cellular activity (e.g., macrophage-derived hematopoietic cells, leukocytes) on both sides of the membrane (Fig. 1.1A). The close relationship between inflammatory cell component and breaks in Bruch's membrane suggests that these cells might be involved in the focal destruction of Bruch's membrane (Fig. 1.1B) (5,19).

Spraul and Grossniklaus showed that the degree of calcification as well as the number of fragmentations in Bruch's membrane correlated with the presence of non-neovascular and neovascular AMD (Fig. 1.1C) (10). Eyes with neovascular AMD demonstrated a higher degree of calcification and fragmentation of Bruch's membrane in the macular area compared with the extramacular regions than eyes with non-neovascular AMD. A correlation was also found between the degree of calcification, ranging from focal patches to long continuous areas, and the number of breaks in Bruch's membrane (10).

Changes in Retinal Pigment Epithelium

RPE cells with AMD have cytoplasmic "lipofuscin" granules, as a result of incompletely digested photoreceptor outer segments. Accumulation of lipofuscin granules increases in the cytoplasm of RPE. Eyes with early AMD show a decreased number and density of RPE cells in the macula, resulting in RPE mottling (21). These changes include pleomorphism, enlargement, depigmentation, hypertrophy, hyperplasia, and atrophy of the RPE cells (1,9).

Another clinical finding called non-geographic RPE atrophy is related to moderate RPE hypopigmentation and atrophy in areas overlying diffuse BLamD and BLinD (Fig. 1.2) (9). Hypopigmentation, attenuation, or atrophy of the RPE may also be accompanied by soft drusen, RPE detachment, and geographic atrophy (2,9,22,23). Lipoidal degeneration of individual RPE cells which are characterized by foamy cytoplasm may be found in eyes with nodular drusen.

Changes in Choriocapillaris

The choriocapillaris in eyes with AMD is usually thinned and sclerosed with a thickening of the intercapillary septae (24). Capillaries between hyalinized pillars of Bruch's membrane are occasionally more widely spaced than in age-matched control eyes (14). The choroidal arteries are

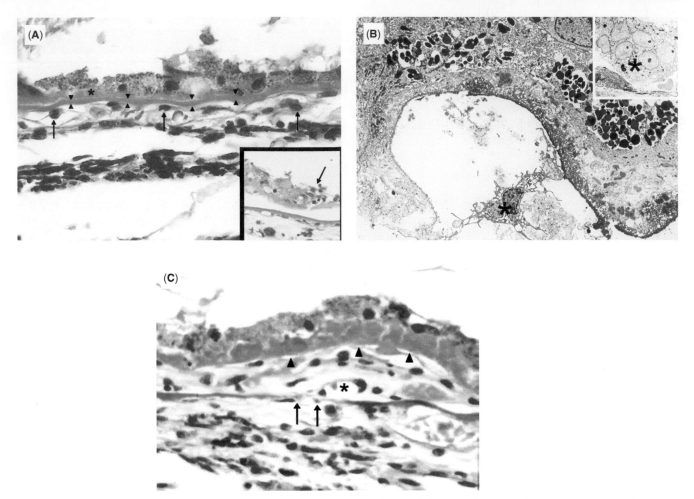

Figure 1.1 (**A**) Diffuse thickening of Bruch's membrane (arrowheads) is associated with increased deposits (asterisk) under the retinal pigment epithelium (RPE). Macrophage-derived inflammatory cells (arrows) are present at the outer aspect of Bruch's membrane as well as at the inner aspect of Bruch's membrane (arrow, inset) (**B**) Transmission electron microscopy shows macrophages and multinucleated giant cells (asterisks) digesting basal laminar deposits overlying Bruch's membrane. (**C**) Focal disruption of Bruch's membrane (arrows) with ingrowths of new vessels (asterisks) in the space between the inner aspect (arrowheads) and the remainder of Bruch's membrane in an eye with choroidal neovascularization.

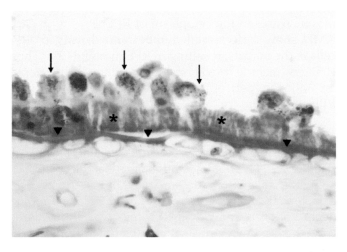

Figure 1.2 Histopathology of retinal pigment epithelium (RPE) and Bruch's membrane in an eye with non-neovascular age-related macular degeneration. The RPE cell monolayer (arrows) is diminished and exhibits hypopigmentation associated with areas of scattered prominent pigment granules. A thick layer of basal laminar deposit (asterisks) is located between the plasma membrane and basal lamina of the RPE. The remaining Bruch's membrane is also thickened (arrowheads).

usually shrunken and show replacement of the muscular media by fibrillar fibrous tissue with retention of wide vascular lumens. Occasionally, remains of occluded vessels with collapsed fibrous walls may be present (2). The number of ghost vessels is positively associated with sub-RPE deposit density (25). However, it is unclear whether these observed changes in the choriocapillaris in AMD are secondary to changes in the overlying RPE, or are primary changes directly from the disease (26,27).

Changes in Neurosensory Retina

Aging changes of the neurosensory retina occur in Müller cells and axons of ganglion cells including hypertrophy, lipid accumulation or decrease, and replacement by connective tissue (28). While rods gradually disappear with aging even without evidence of overt RPE disease, cones only begin to degenerate by advanced stages of non-neovascular AMD (29,30). Red-green cones seem to be more resistant than blue cones to aging and may also increase in size in AMD (4,30,31). The greatest photoreceptor cell loss is located in the parafovea (1.5–10°) and may finally result in disappearance of all photoreceptors

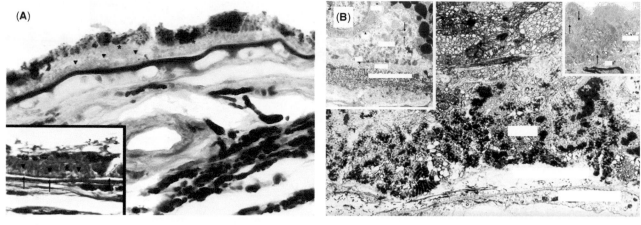

Figure 1.3 (**A**) A prominent layer of basal laminar deposit (BLamD, asterisks) and basal linear deposits (BLinD, arrowheads) is located between the retinal pigment epithelium (RPE) and Bruch's membrane. Artifactual spaces are present between the inner collagenous zone and the remaining layers of Bruch's membrane (inset, arrows). (**B**) BLamDs are composed of wide-spaced collagen (insets, arrows), electron dense material, and membrane bounded vacuoles. They are located between the plasma membrane (pm) and the basal lamina (bm) of the RPE. Ultrastructure of the BLinD shows abundant coated vesicles and electron dense granules.

in the presence of geographic atrophy or disciform degeneration (4,30). A recent study with three-dimensional optical coherence tomography shows that retinal thickness is reduced in early AMD (32).

Basal Deposits
Accumulation of waste material between the RPE and Bruch's membrane (Fig. 1.3A) is termed "basal deposit," one of the earliest pathological features of AMD. Green and Enger have defined two distinct types of basal deposit(s): basal laminar and basal linear deposits (1–3,9,12,33).

Basal Laminar Deposit
BLamD is composed of granular material with much wide-spaced collagen located between the plasma and basement membranes of the RPE. BLamD stains light red with Mallory staining, and light blue with Masson's trichrome (Fig. 1.3A). Electron microscopic examination shows that BLamD is composed of long-spacing collagen with a periodicity of 120 nm, membrane-bounded vacuoles and minor deposits of granular electron-dense material (Fig. 1.3B) (1). Studies have shown that BLamD is composed of collagen (type IV), laminin, glycoproteins, glycosaminoglycans (chondroitin-, heparin-sulfate), carbohydrates (N-acetylgalactosamine), cholesterol (unesterified, esterified), and apolipoproteins B and E (34–36).

Basal Linear Deposit
BLinD is located external to the RPE basement membrane (e.g., in the inner collagenous zone of Bruch's membrane) (Fig. 1.3A, inset). Electron microscopy shows that BLinD is primarily composed of an electron dense, lipid-rich material with coated and non-coated vesicles and granules that result in diffuse thickening of the inner aspect of Bruch's membrane (Fig. 1.3B, inset top left). BLinD may represent an extension or

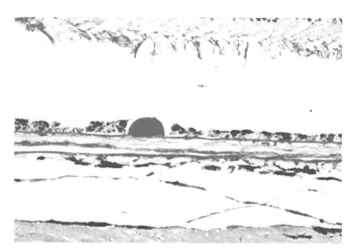

Figure 1.4 Photomicrograph shows a nodular druse with loss of the overlying retinal pigment epithelium.

progression of BLamD and is found in association with soft drusen and small detachments of the RPE. BLinD appears to be a more specific marker than BLamD for AMD, particularly for progression to late stage disease, whereas the amount of BLamD seems to be a more reliable indicator of the degree of RPE atrophy and photoreceptor degeneration (2,5,13).

Drusen
Drusen are important features of AMD, which can be ophthalmoscopically observed as small yellowish white lesions located deep to the retina in the posterior pole.

Nodular (Hard) Drusen
Nodular (hard) drusen are smooth surfaced, dome-shaped structures between the RPE and Bruch's membrane (Fig. 1.4). They consist of hyaline material and stain positively with periodic acid-Schiff (1). Nodular drusen often contain multiple globular calcifications,

mucopolysaccharides, and lipids (37). The latter supports the possibility of lipoidal degeneration of individual RPE cells (21,38,39). Ultrastructurally, nodular drusen are composed of finely granular or amorphous material, which has the same electron density as the basement membrane of the RPE. Variable numbers of pale and bristle-coated vesicles, tubular structures, curly membranes, and occasionally abnormal collagen may be also found within these drusen (22,34,40). The RPE overlying the drusen is often attenuated and hypopigmented, while the cells located at the lateral border demonstrate a hyperpigmented and hypertrophic appearance (41).

Drusen are primarily located in the inner collagenous zone of Bruch's membrane, but may extend to the outer collagenous zone and to the intercapillary pillars if discontinuities of the central elastic layer occur (14,42).

Immunohistochemical studies have shown that drusen are composed of acute phase proteins (e.g., vitronectin, a1-antichymotrypsin, CRP, amyloid P component, and fibrinogen), complement components (e.g., C3C5 and C5b-9 complex), complement inhibitors (e.g., clusterin), apolipoproteins (B, E), tissue metalloproteinase inhibitor 3, crystalline, serum albumin, fibronectin, mucopolysaccharides (e.g., sialomucin), lipids (e.g., cerebroside), mannose, sialic acid, N-acetylglucosamine, β-galactose, and immunoreactive factors like immunoglobulin G, immunoglobulin light chains, Factor X, and other components, termed drusen-associated molecules (DRAMs) (37,43–46). Amyloid beta (Aβ) peptide, a major component of senile plaque in Alzheimer disease (AD), is identified within drusen, and mice lacking the Aβ–degrading enzyme develop RPE degeneration and sub-RPE deposits similar to those of AMD in humans. These findings imply that there may be some similarities in the pathogenic mechanism between AMD and AD (47,48).

Soft Drusen

Cleavage in BLamD and BLinD may occur with the formation of a localized detachment (soft drusen). Soft drusen may become confluent with diameters larger than 63 μm and are then termed "large drusen." Soft drusen formation may result in a diffuse thickening of the inner aspect of Bruch's membrane with separation of the overlying RPE basement membrane from the remaining Bruch's membrane (Fig. 1.5) (9,22).

At least three types of soft drusen can be differentiated by light microscopic examination: (i) a localized detachment of the RPE with BLamD in eyes with diffuse BLamD, (ii) a localized detachment of RPE by BLinD in eyes with diffuse BLamD and BLinD; or (iii) a localized detachment due to the localized accumulation of BLinD in eyes with diffuse BLamD but in absence of diffuse BLinD (9). All subtypes may appear as large drusen with sloping edges. The hydrophobic space between these types of soft drusen and Bruch's membrane is a potential space for CNV (10). Soft drusen seem to be often empty or to contain pale staining amorphous membranous or fibrillar material (49). The overlying RPE may be attenuated, diminished, or atrophic. In late stages, geographic atrophies may occur (1).

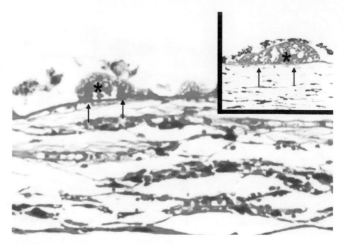

Figure 1.5 Photomicrograph shows soft drusen formation (asterisks) consisting of lightly staining proteinaceous material between the basement membrane of the retinal pigment epithelium (RPE) and the inner aspect of Bruch's membrane (arrows). The overlying RPE is partially lost or hypertrophic.

Electron microscopy shows that soft drusen are composed of double-layered coiled membranes with amorphous material and calcification (19). BLamD overlying the soft drusen has been found in many eyes with AMD (22).

A variant of soft drusen is more clearly studied with the help of spectral domain optical coherence tomography. Reticular pseudodrusen, a type of soft drusen best visible with blue light, is more accurately described as "subretinal drusenoid deposits." The subretinal drusenoid deposits are composed of membranous debris, cholesterol, cholesterol esters, and positive staining for complement, which is similar to the composition of soft drusen (50,51). Both soft drusen and subretinal drusenoid deposits are significantly associated with late AMD (52).

Diffuse Drusen

Diffuse drusen is a diffuse thickening of the inner aspect of Bruch's membrane (22,24). This term also includes basal laminar (cuticular) drusen, which are characterized by an internal nodularity (1,33). Electron microscopy shows that diffuse drusen have revealed the presence of vesicles, electron-dense particles, and fibrils between the thickened basement membrane of the RPE and the inner collagenous layer of Bruch's membrane (22,24).

Geographic Atrophy

Geographic atrophy, which is characterized by the areas of well-demarcated atrophy of RPE, represents the classic clinical picture of end-stage non-neovascular AMD. Although drusen are apparently central direct factors for initiation of RPE cell loss, they may disappear over time, especially when geographic atrophy occurs (2).

Histological studies have shown that the loss of RPE is usually accompanied by a gradual degeneration of the outer layers of the neurosensory retina (photoreceptors, outer nuclear layer, and external limiting membrane),

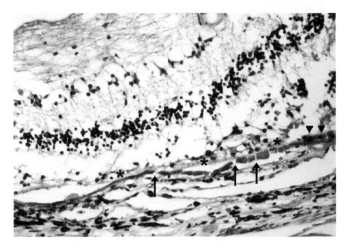

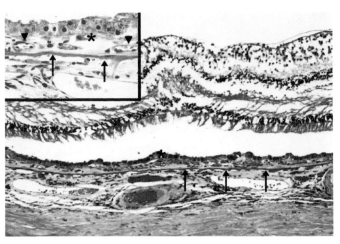

Figure 1.6 Photomicrograph shows a section of an eye with geographic atrophy of the retinal pigment epithelium (RPE). The photoreceptor cell layer is atrophic and the RPE is largely absent (arrowheads). A thin fibrotic scar (asterisks) associated with mononuclear inflammatory cells is covering the inner aspect of Bruch's membrane. Bruch's membrane is focally disrupted (arrows).

Figure 1.7 Photomicrographs of an eye with neovascular age-related macular degeneration. A choroidal neovascular membrane (asterisk) with prominent vessels (inset, arrowheads) grows between Bruch's membrane (arrows) and the overlying retinal pigment epithelium.

marked atrophy and sclerosis of the choriocapillaris, without breaks in Bruch's membrane (Fig. 1.6) (2,22,23,53). Areas of geographic atrophy also are commonly characterized by residual pigmented material and a closely related monolayer of macrophages, which develop between the basement membrane of the RPE and the inner collagenous layer of Bruch's membrane (23). Occasionally accompanying the macrophages are other cell types like melanocytes, fibroblasts, and detached RPE cells in the subretinal space (23). The edges adjacent to areas of geographic atrophy, also termed junctional zones, are usually hyperpigmented and characterized by the presence of hypertrophic RPE cells and multinucleated giant cells which contain RPE–derived pigment in association with secondary lysosomes (23,34).

HISTOPATHOLOGY OF NEOVASCULAR (WET) AMD
Choroidal Neovascularization

The hallmark of neovascular (wet type) AMD is the development of CNV. CNV represents new blood vessel formation typically from the choroid (21).

Changes in Bruch's membrane such as calcification and focal breaks correlate with the presence of neovascular AMD (10). Decreased thickness and disruption of the elastic lamina of Bruch's membrane in the macula may also be a prerequisite for invasion of CNV into the space underneath the RPE (54). Vascular channels supplied by the choroid begin as a capillary-like structure and evolve into arterioles and venules (1,21,24,55,56). Most of the vessels arise from the choroid, although a retinal vessel contribution has been observed in about 6% of CNV in AMD (1). These choroidal vessels traverse the defects in the Bruch's membrane and grow into the plane between the RPE and Bruch's membrane (sub-RPE CNV: type 1 growth pattern), between the retina and RPE (subretinal CNV: type 2 growth pattern), or in the combination of both patterns(combined growth

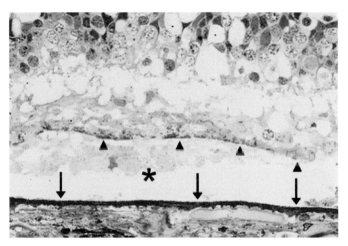

Figure 1.8 Separation of the basal laminar deposits (BLamD, arrowheads) and the remainder of Bruch's membrane (arrows). The space between the BLamD and Bruch's membrane acts as a natural cleavage plane facilitating vessel ingrowth (asterisk).

pattern) (56,57). The latter appears to arise from the type 1 growth pattern.

Subretinal Pigment Epithelium CNV
(Type 1 Growth Pattern)
In type 1 pattern, CNV originates with multiple ingrowth sites, ranging 1–12, from the choriocapillaris (Fig. 1.7). After breaking through Bruch's membrane, CNV tufts extend laterally and merge in a horizontal fashion under the RPE. This is facilitated by a natural cleavage plane in the space between BLamD and Bruch's membrane that has accumulated lipids with aging (Fig. 1.8) (1,2,49,56–61). The CNV growth recapitulates the embryological development of the choriocapillaris, presumably in an attempt to provide nutrients and oxygen to ischemic RPE and photoreceptors. The relationship

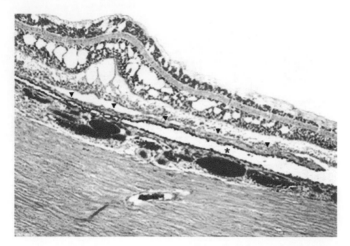

Figure 1.9 Choroidal neovascular membrane with a type II growth pattern (arrowheads) between the retinal pigment epithelium (RPE) and the outer segments of the photoreceptor cell layer. A reflected layer of RPE (asterisk) and atrophy of photoreceptors are present.

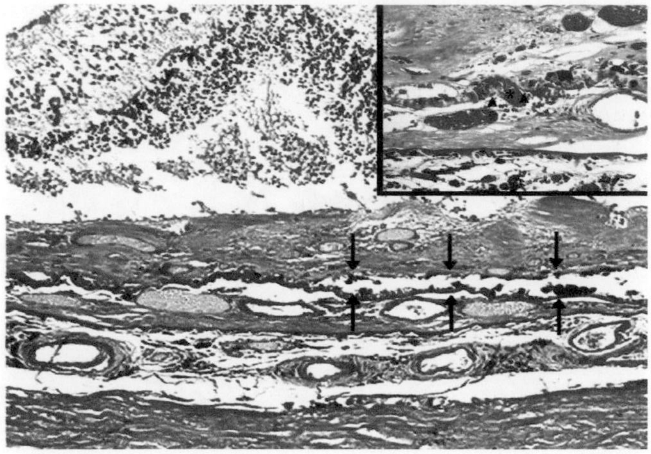

Figure 1.10 Photomicrographs demonstrates a combined growth pattern of a choroidal neovascularization with a reflected layer of retinal pigment epithelium (arrows). Inset: A new vessel (asterisk) extends through a break in the basal laminar deposits (arrowheads).

between the CNV and BLamD is similar to that between the choriocapillaris and Bruch's membrane.

Patients with type 1 CNV have relatively intact retina and few visual symptoms. This growth pattern likely corresponds to the "occult" type of angiographic appearance of CNV (57). Secondary changes can be noted in the surrounding retina such as serous or hemorrhagic detachment of the RPE and overlying retina, RPE tears, and lipid exudation (21,62). In histopathological studies of surgically excised CNV, type 1 membranes are firmly attached to the overlying native RPE as well as the underlying Bruch's membrane. Therefore, it is difficult to surgically remove type 1 membrane without damaging the surrounding tissue (56).

Subretinal CNV (Type 2 Growth Pattern)

The type 2 (subretinal) growth pattern demonstrates single or few ingrowth sites with a focal defect in Bruch's membrane (Fig. 1.9). There is a reflected layer of RPE on the outer surface of the CNV and little or no RPE on its inner surface. Since there is no support from the RPE, the overlying outer layers of retina become atrophic. Angiographically, type II CNV membranes leak under the RPE and in the outer retina. This growth pattern correlates with the "classic" angiographic appearance (57,63). In the study of surgically excised CNV, there is a reflected layer of RPE lined on the outer surface of type 2 CNV by a monolayer of inverted proliferating RPE cells and the native RPE (Figs. 1.10, 1.11) (56). The overlying photoreceptors are atrophic.

Combined Growth Pattern CNV

There are many theoretical variations leading to a combined pattern of CNV growth. A progression from the type 1 to the type 2 growth pattern as well as temporal development of the type 2 growth prior to the type 1 growth have been discussed (Fig. 1.10) (57). These growth patterns correspond to angiographic "minimally classic" and "predominantly classic" appearances.

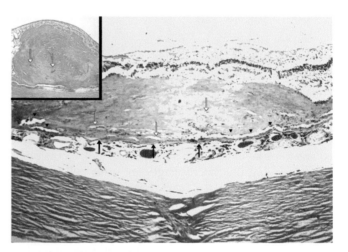

Figure 1.11 Late stage of age-related macular degeneration with the formation of a disciform scar between Bruch's membrane (black arrows) and the photoreceptor outer segments. Prominent vessels (white arrows) and a reflected layer of the retinal pigment epithelium (arrowheads) are present in the scar.

Histopathology of CNV

The cellular and extracellular components of CNV include RPE, vascular endothelium, fibrocytes, macrophages, photoreceptors, erythrocytes, lymphocytes, myofibroblasts, collagen, fibrin, and BLamD (56,64). These components are similar regardless of the underlying disease including AMD, ocular histoplasmosis syndrome, myopia, idiopathic, and pattern dystrophy. The only exception is BLamD, which is seen almost exclusively in AMD. These findings suggest that CNV represents a nonspecific wound repair response to a specific stimulus, similar to fibrovascular granulation tissue proliferation (56,62,64,65).

Disciform Scar

Disciform scar represents the end stage of the neovascular form of AMD. Disciform scars are usually vascularized, but predominantly composed of fibrotic scar tissue

(Fig. 1.11). The vascular supply is provided from the choroid (96%), retina (2.5%), or both (0.6%) (1,62). A disciform scar is generally associated with the loss of neural tissue. Photoreceptor loss increases as the diameter and thickness of the disciform scar increase. In a morphometric analysis, eyes with disciform scars due to AMD showed severe reduction in the number of outer nuclear layer cells, but good preservation of cells in the inner nuclear layer and ganglion cell layer (66). Despite massive photoreceptor loss in neovascular AMD, ganglion cell neurons are known to survive in relatively large numbers (67).

SUMMARY POINTS

- Pathological changes with AMD first appear in the inner collagenous zone and generally extend into the central elastic zone and outer collagenous zone and the intercapillary connective tissue during later stages of the disease.
- RPE cells with AMD have cytoplasmic "lipofuscin" granules due to incompletely digested photoreceptor outer segments.
- Although rods gradually disappear with age, cones begin to degenerate only with advanced stages of non-neovascular AMD.
- Early lesions of AMD are located either between the RPE and its basement membrane (e.g., BLamD) or between the basement membrane of the RPE and the remainder of Bruch's membrane (e.g., BLinD).
- Focal and diffuse deposits between the RPE and Bruch's membrane are called drusen.
- Immunohistochemical studies have shown that drusen are composed of acute phase proteins, complement components, complement inhibitors, apolipoproteins, tissue metalloproteinase inhibitor 3, crystalline, serum albumin, fibronectin, mucopolysaccharides, lipids, mannose, sialic acid, N-acetylglucosamine, β-galactose, and immunoreactive factors like IgG, immunoglobulin light chains, Factor X, and other components termed DRAMs.
- CNV has two patterns: sub-RPE associated with "occult" CNV and subretinal associated with "classic CNV."

REFERENCES

1. Green WR, Enger C. Age-related macular degeneration histopathologic studies: the 1992 Lorenz E. Zimmerman lecture. Ophthalmology 1993; 100: 1519–39.
2. Sarks SH. Ageing and degeneration in macular region: a clinicopathological study. Br J Ophthalmol 1976; 60: 324–41.
3. Löffler KU, Lee WR. Basal linear deposits in the human macula. Graefes Arch Clin Exp Ophthalmol 1986; 224: 493–501.
4. Sarks JP, Sarks SH, Killingsworth MC. Evolution of geographic atrophy of the retinal pigment epithelium. Eye 1988; 2: 552–77.
5. van der Schaft TL, de Bruijn WC, Mooy CM, et al. Histologic features of the early stages of age-related macular degeneration: a statistical analysis. Ophthalmology 1992; 99: 278–86.
6. Hogan M, Alvarado J. Studies on the human macula: IV. Aging changes in Bruch's membrane. Arch Ophthalmol 1967; 77: 410–20.
7. Ramrattan RS, van der Schaft TL, Mooy CM, et al. Morphometric analysis of bruch's membrane, the choriocapillaris and the choroid in aging. Invest Ophthalmol Vis Sci 1994; 35: 2857–64.
8. Hogan MJ, Alvarado J, Weddell JE. Histology of the Human Eye. Philadelphia: Saunders, 1971: 344.
9. Bressler NM, Silva JC, Bressler SB, et al. Clinicopathologic correlation of drusen and retinal pigment abnormalities in age-related macular degeneration. Retina 1994; 14: 130–42.
10. Spraul CW, Grossniklaus HE. Characteristics of drusen and Bruch's membrane in post-mortem eyes with age-related macular degeneration. Arch Ophthalmol 1997; 115: 267–73.
11. Grindle CFJ, Marshall J. Ageing changes in bruch's membrane and their functional implications. Trans Ophthalmol Soc UK 1978; 98: 172–5.
12. Feeney-Burns L, Ellersieck M. Age-related changes in the ultrastructure of Bruch's membrane. Am J Ophthalmol 1985; 100: 686–97.
13. Curcio CA, Millican CL. Basal linear deposit and large drusen are specific for early age-related maculopathy. Arch Ophthalmol 1999; 117: 329–39.
14. Sarks SH, Arnold JJ, Killingsworth MC, et al. Early drusen formation in the normal and aging eye and their relation to age-related maculopathy: a clinicopathological study. Br J Ophthalmol 1999; 83: 358–68.
15. Spencer WH. Macular disease; pathogenesis: light microscopy (Symposium). Trans Am Acad Ophthalmol Otolaryngol 1965; 69: 662–7.
16. Holz FG, Sheraidah G, Pauleikhoff D, et al. Analysis of lipid deposits extracted from human macular and peripheral bruch's membrane. Arch Ophthalmol 1994; 112: 402–6.
17. Curcio CA, Johnson M, Rudolf M, et al. The oil spill in ageing bruch membrane. Br J Ophthalmol 2011; 95: 1638–45.
18. Killingsworth MC. Age-related components of bruch's membrane in the human eye. Graefes Arch Clin Exp Ophthalmol 1987; 225: 406–12.
19. Killingsworth MC, Sarks JP, Sarks SH. Macrophages related to bruch's membrane in age-related macular degeneration. Eye 1990; 4: 613–21.
20. Das A, Frank RN, Zhang NL, et al. Ultrastructural localization of extracellular matrix components in the human retinal vessels and bruch's membrane. Arch Ophthalmol 1990; 108: 421–9.
21. Green WR. Histopathology of age-related macular degeneration. Mol Vis 1999; 5: 27–36.
22. Green WR, McDonnell PH, Yeo JH. Pathologic features of senile macular degeneration. Ophthalmology 1985; 92: 615–27.
23. Penfold PL, Killingsworth MC, Sarks SH. Senile macular degeneration. Invest Ophthalmol Vis Sci 1986; 27: 364–71.
24. Green WR, Key SN. Senile macular degeneration: a histopathologic study. Trans Am Ophthalmol Soc 1977; 75: 180–254.

25. Mullins RF, Johnson MN, Faidley EA, et al. Choriocapillaris vascular dropout related to density of drusen in human eyes with early age-related macular degeneration. Invest Ophthalmol Vis Sci 2011; 52: 1606–12.

26. Tso MOM, Friedman E. The retinal pigment epithelium: I. comparative histology. Arch Ophthalmol 1967; 78: 641–9.

27. Delaney WV, Oates RP. Senile macular degeneration: a preliminary study. Ann Ophthalmol 1982; 14: 21–4.

28. Sharma RK, Ehinger BEJ. Development and structure of the retina. In: Kaufman PL, Alm A, eds. Adler's Physiology of the Eye, 10th edn. St. Louis: Mosby, 2003: 319–47.

29. Curcio CA, Millican CL, Allen KA, et al. Aging of the human photoreceptor mosaic: evidence for selective vulnerability of rods in the central retina. Invest Ophthalmol Vis Sci 1993; 34: 3278–96.

30. Curcio CA, Medeiros NE, Millican LC. Photoreceptor loss in age-related macular degeneration. Invest Ophthalmol Vis Sci 1996; 37: 1236–49.

31. Eisner A, Klien ML, Zilis JD, et al. Visual function and the subsequent development of exudative age-related macular degeneration. Invest Ophthalmol Vis Sci 1992; 33: 3091–102.

32. Wood A, Binns A, Margrain T, et al. Retinal and choroidal thickness in early age-related macular degeneration. Am J Ophthalmol 2011; 152: 1030–8.

33. van der Schaft TL, de Bruijn WC, Mooy CM, et al. Is basal laminar deposit unique for age-related macular degeneration? Arch Ophthalmol 1991; 109: 420–5.

34. Kliffen M, van der Schaft TL, Mooy CM, et al. Morphologic changes in age-related maculopathy. Microsc Res Tech 1997; 36: 106–22.

35. van der Schaft TL, Mooy CM, de Bruijn WC, et al. Immunohistochemical light and electron microscopy of basal laminar deposit. Graefes Arch Clin Ophthalmol 1994; 232: 40–6.

36. Malek G, Li CM, Guidry C, et al. Apolipoprotein B in cholesterol-containing drusen and basal deposits of human eyes with age-related maculopathy. Am J Pathol 2003; 162: 413–25.

37. Farkas TG, Sylvester V, Archer D, et al. The histochemistry of drusen. Am J Ophthalmol 1971; 71: 1206–15.

38. El Baba F, Green WR, Fleischmann J, et al. Clinicopathologic correlation of lipidization and detachment of the retinal pigment epithelium. Am J Ophthalmol 1986; 101: 576–83.

39. Fine BS. Lipoidal degeneration of the retinal pigment epithelium. Am J Ophthalmol 1981; 91: 469–73.

40. Hogan MJ. Role of the retinal pigment epithelium in macular disease. Trans Am Acad Ophthalmol Otolaryngol 1972; 76: 64–80.

41. Burns RP, Feeney-Burns L. Clinico-morphologic correlations of drusen of bruch's membrane. Trans Am Ophthalmol Soc 1980; 78: 206–25.

42. Farkas TG, Sylvester V, Archer D. The ultrastructure of drusen. Am J Ophthalmol 1971; 71: 1196–205.

43. Hageman G, Mullins R, Russel S, et al. Vibronectin is a constituent of ocular drusen and the vitronectin gene is expressed in human retinal pigment epithelial cells. FASEB J 1999; 13: 477–84.

44. Mullins RF, Russel SR, Anderson DH, et al. Drusen associated with aging and age-related degeneration contain proteins common to extracellular deposits associated with atherosclerosis, elastosis, amyloidosis, and dense deposit disease. FASEB J 2000; 14: 835–46.

45. Crabb JW, Miyagi M, Gu X, et al. Drusen proteome analysis: an approach to the etiology of age-related macular degeneration. Proc Natl Acad Sci USA 2002; 99: 14682–7.

46. Anderson DH, Johnson LV, Schneider BL, et al. Age-related maculopathy: a model of drusen biogenesis. Invest Ophthalmol Vis Sci 1999; 40: S922.

47. Johnson LV, Leitner WP, Rivest AJ, et al. The alzheimer's A beta-peptide is deposited at sites of complement activation in pathologic deposits associated with aging and age-related macular degeneration. Proc Natl Acad Sci USA 2002; 99: 11830–5.

48. Ohno-Matsui K. Parallel findings in age-related macular degeneration and alzheimer's disease. Prog Retin Eye Res 2011; 30: 217–30.

49. Sarks SH. Drusen and their relationship to senile macular degeneration. Aust J Ophthalmol 1980; 8: 117–30.

50. Zweifel SA, Spaide RF, Curcio CA, et al. Reticular pseudodrusen are subretinal drusenoid deposits. Ophthalmology 2010; 117: 303–12.

51. Rudolf M, Malek G, Messinger JD, et al. Sub-retinal drusenoid deposits in human retina: organization and composition. Exp Eye Res 2008; 87: 402–8.

52. Zweifel SA, Imamura Y, Spaide TC, et al. Prevalence and significance of subretinal drusenoid deposits (reticular pseudodrusen) in age-related macular degeneration. Ophthalmology 2010; 117: 1775–81.

53. Bressler NM, Bressler B, Fine SL. Age-related macular degeneration. Surv Ophthalmol 1988; 32: 375–413.

54. Chong NHV, Keonin J, Luthert PJ, et al. Decreased thickness and integrity of the macular elastic layer of bruch's membrane correspond to the distribution of lesions associated with age-related macular degeneration. Am J Pathol 2005; 16: 241–51.

55. Schneider S, Greven CM, Green WR. Photocoagulation of well-defined choroidal neovascularization in age-related macular degeneration: clinicopathologic correlation. Retina 1998; 18: 242–50.

56. Grossniklaus HE, Gass JDM. Clinicopathologic correlation of surgically excised type 1 and type 2 submacular choroidal neovascular membranes. Am J Ophthalmol 1998; 126: 59–69.

57. Grossniklaus HE, Green WR. Choroidal neovascularization. Am J Ophthalmol 2004; 137: 496–503.

58. Gass JDM. Biomicroscopic and histopathologic consideration regarding the feasibility of surgical excision of subfoveal neovascular membranes. Am J Ophthalmol 1994; 118: 285–98.

59. Gass JDM. Stereoscopic Atlas of Macular Diseases: Diagrams and Treatment, 4th edn. Vol 1. St. Louis: Mosby, 1997: 26–37.

60. Gass JDM. Pathogenesis of disciform detachment of the neuroepithelium: III. senile disciform degeneration. Am J Ophthalmol 1967; 63: 617–44.

61. Sarks SH. New vessel formation beneath the retinal pigment epithelium in senile eyes. Br J Ophthalmol 1973; 57: 951–65.

62. Ambati J, Ambati BK, Yoo SH, et al. Age-related macular degeneration: etiology, pathogenesis, and therapeutic strategies. Surv Ophthalmol 2003; 48: 257–93.

63. LaFaut BA, Bartz-Schmidt KU, van den Broecke C, et al. Clinicopathologic correlation in exudative age-related macular degeneration: histological differentiation between

classic and occult neovascularization. Br J Ophthalmol 2000; 84: 239–43.

64. Grossniklaus HE, Martinez JA, Brown VB, et al. Immuno-histochemical and histochemical properties of surgically excised subretinal neovascular membranes in age-related macular degeneration. Am J Ophthalmol 1992; 114: 464–72.

65. Frank RN, Amin RH, Eliott D, et al. Basic fibroblast growth factor and vascular endothelial growth factor are present in epiretinal and choroidal neovascular membranes. Am J Ophthalmol 1996; 122: 393–403.

66. Kim SY, Sadda S, Pearlman J, et al. Morphometric analysis of the macula in eyes with disciform age-related macular degeneration. Retina 2002; 22: 471–7.

67. Medeiros NE, Curcio CA. Preservation of ganglion cell layer neurons in age-related macular degeneration. Invest Ophthalmol Vis Sci 2001; 42: 795–803.

2

Immunology of age-related macular degeneration

Karl G. Csaky, Priyatham S. Mettu, and Scott W. Cousins

INTRODUCTION

Traditionally, immune and inflammatory mechanisms of disease pathogenesis were applied only to disorders characterized by acute onset and progression associated with obvious clinical signs of inflammation. However, it has become clear that many chronic degenerative diseases associated with aging demonstrate important immune and inflammatory components. Increasing evidence points to a pivotal connection between immune mechanisms of disease and age-related macular degeneration (AMD).

In this chapter we attempt to achieve three goals. First, we will provide a brief overview of the biology of the low-grade inflammatory mechanisms relevant to chronic degenerative diseases of aging, excluding the mechanisms associated with acute severe inflammation. Innate immunity, antigen-specific immunity, and amplification systems will be defined and explored. Second, we will explore the role of inflammation in two other age-related degenerative diseases with immunologic features, atherosclerosis, and renal glomerular diseases that share epidemiologic, genetic, and physiological associations with AMD. Finally, this chapter will introduce the paradigm of "response to injury" as a model for AMD pathogenesis. This paradigm proposes that immune mechanisms as well as amplifiers (e.g., oxidants) not only participate in the initiation of injury, but also contribute to abnormal reparative responses that result in disease pathogenesis and subsequent complications. The response to injury paradigm provides a connection between immunologic mechanisms of disease and the biology of tissue injury and repair in chronic degenerative disorders such as AMD.

OVERVIEW OF BIOLOGY OF IMMUNOLOGY RELEVANT TO AMD
Innate Versus Antigen-Specific Immunity

In general, an immune response is a sequence of cellular and molecular events designed to rid the host off an offending stimulus, which usually represents a pathogenic organism, toxic substance, cellular debris, neoplastic cell, or other similar signals. Two broad categories of immune responses have been recognized: innate immunity and antigen-specific immunity (1–3).

Innate Immunity

Innate immunity (also called "natural" immunity) is a pattern recognition response by certain cells of the immune system, typically macrophages and neutrophils, to identify broad groups of offensive stimuli, especially infectious agents, toxins, or cellular debris resulting from injury (4–6). Additionally, many stimuli of innate immunity can directly interact with parenchymal cells of tissues (e.g., the retinal pigment epithelium (RPE) to initiate a response. Innate immunity is triggered by a preprogrammed, antigen-independent cellular response, determined by the pre-existence of receptors for a category of stimuli, leading to generation of biochemical mediators that recruit additional inflammatory cells. These cells remove the offending stimulus in a nonspecific manner via phagocytosis or enzymatic degradation. The key concept is that the stimuli of innate immunity interact with receptors on monocytes, neutrophils, or parenchymal cells that have been genetically predetermined by evolution to recognize and respond to conserved molecular patterns or "motifs" on different triggering stimuli. These motifs often include specific amino acid sequences, certain lipoproteins, certain phospholipids, or other specific molecular patterns. Different stimuli often trigger the same stereotyped program. Thus, the receptors of innate immunity are identical among all individuals within a species in the same way that receptors for neurotransmitters or hormones are genetically identical within a species.

The classic example of the innate immune response is the immune response to acute infection. For example, in endophthalmitis, bacteria-derived toxins or host cell debris stimulates the recruitment of neutrophils and monocytes, leading to the production of inflammatory mediators and phagocytosis of the bacteria. Bacterial toxins can also directly activate receptors on retinal neurons, leading to injury. The triggering mechanisms and subsequent effector responses to bacteria such as *Staphylococcus* are nearly identical to those of other organisms, determined by nonspecific receptors recognizing families of related toxins or molecules in the environment.

Antigen-Specific Immunity

Antigen-specific immunity (also called "adaptive" or "acquired" immunity) is an acquired host response, which is generated in reaction to exposure to a specific "antigenic" molecule, and is not a genetically predetermined response to a broad category of stimuli (1–3). The response is initially triggered by the "recognition" of a unique foreign "antigenic" substance as distinguished from "self" by cells of the immune system (and not by non-immune parenchymal cells). Recognition is followed by subsequent "processing" of the unique antigen by specialized cells of the immune system. The response results in the production of unique antigen-specific immunologic effector cells (T and B lymphocytes) and unique antigen-specific soluble effector molecules (antibodies), the aim of which is to remove the specific stimulating antigenic substance from the organism, and to ignore the presence of other irrelevant antigenic stimuli. The key concept is that an antigen (usually) represents a foreign substance against which specific cells of immune system must generate, *de novo*, a specific receptor, which, in turn, must recognize a unique molecular structure in the antigen for which no pre-existing gene was present. Thus, the antigen-specific immune system has evolved a mechanism whereby an individual's B and T lymphocytes continually generate new antigen receptor genes through recombination, rearrangement, and mutation of the germline genetic structure. This results in a "repertoire" of novel antigen receptor molecules that vary tremendously in the spectrum of recognition among individuals within a species.

The classic example of acquired immunity is the immune response to a mutated virus. Viruses (e.g.,adenovirus found in epidemic keratoconjunctivitis) are continuously evolving or mutating new "antigenic" structures. The susceptible host could not have possibly evolved receptors for recognition to these new viral mutations. However, these new mutations do serve as "antigens" that stimulate an adaptive antigen-specific immune response by the host to the virus. The antigen-specific response recognizes the virus in question and not other viruses (e.g.,poliovirus).

Amplification Mechanisms for Both Forms of Immunity

Although innate or antigen-specific immunity may directly induce injury or inflammation, in most cases, these effectors initiate a process that must be amplified in order to produce overt clinical manifestations. Molecules generated within tissues that amplify immunity are termed "mediators," of which there are several categories: (i) plasma-derived enzyme systems, which include complement, kinins, and fibrin; (ii) cytokines (growth factors, angiogenic factors, others); (iii) oxidants (free radicals and reactive nitrogen); (iv) vasoactive amines (histamine and serotonin); (v) lipid mediators (prostaglandins, leukotrienes, other eicosanoids and platelet activating factors); (vi) neutrophil-derived granule products. This chapter will focus on complement, cytokines, and oxidants as modulators of the immune response in AMD.

Complement

Components and fragments of the complement cascade are present in the plasma at a concentration of $3\,g/L$, which represent almost 30% of the total serum protein content. These proteins, comprising over 30 different protein molecules, represent important endogenous amplifiers of innate and antigen-specific immunity as well as mediators of injury responses (7–9). All complement factors are synthesized by the liver and released into blood. However, some specific factors can also be synthesized locally within tissues, including within cornea, sclera and retina (8). Indeed a recent work has indicated that the RPE is a capable of synthesizing various complement related proteins including C3, factors B, H, H-like 1, CD46, CD55, CD59, and clusterin (10).

Upon activation, the various proteins of the complement system interact in a sequential amplifying cascade to produce varying cellular effects. Three specific pathways have been identified to activate the complement cascade: classical pathway, alternative pathway, and the lectin pathway (Fig. 2.1).

Antigen-specific immunity typically activates complement via the classical pathway with antigen/antibody (immune) complexes, referred to as pentraxins, especially those formed by IgM, IgG1 and IgG3 (7–9). However, some innate stimuli, such as DNA, RNA, insoluble deposits of abnormal proteins (e.g., amyloid P) or apoptotic cells can also trigger the classical pathway (11–14).

The lectin pathway utilizes pattern-recognition receptors, found within the mannose-binding lectin (MBL), to identify previously hidden regions on apoptotic cells referred to as damage-associated molecular patterns or in other cases highly conserved structures on microorganisms known as pathogen-associated molecular patterns (15). While MBL does not normally recognize the body's own tissue, oxidant injury, as can occur in AMD, may alter surface protein expression and glycosylation, leading to MBL deposition and complement activation (16–19).

And finally, innate immunity can activate complement, primarily by activating C3 via the alternative pathway, through recognition of certain chemical moieties on the cell wall of microorganisms (e.g., LPS) or activated surfaces (e.g., implanted medical devices) (11). Photo-oxidative products of A2E, a bis-retinoid pigment that may accumulate in the RPE in AMD, have been shown to convert C3 into C3b and C3a (20).

Each activation pathway results in the generation of the same complement by-products that amplify injury or inflammation by at least three distinct mechanisms: (i) a specific fragment of the third component, C3b, can coat antigenic or pathogenic surfaces, a process known as opsonization, to enhance phagocytosis by macrophages or neutrophils; (ii) activation of terminal complement components C5–9, called the membrane attack complex (MAC), forms transmembrane channels that disrupt cell membrane of target cells, leading to loss of cytoplasm or lysis, and death; (iii) generation of small proinflammatory polypeptides, called anaphylatoxins (C3a, C4a and C5a), induces many inflammatory mediators and leads to the recruitment of inflammatory cells (Fig. 2.3). The activation of complement is tightly regulated by inhibitors, such as decay accelerating factor (CD55), CD46, complement factor H (CFH), complement receptor 1 (CR1), and others that serve to block,

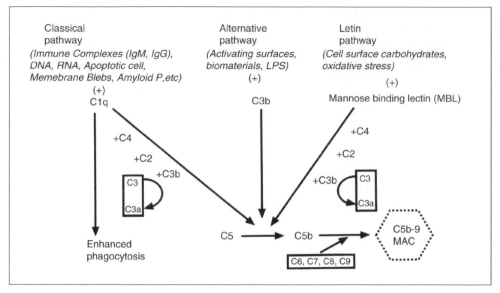

Figure 2.1 Schematic representation of the components and fragments of the complement cascade indicating three primary sources of activation via the classical, alternative or lectin pathway.

resist, or modulate the induction of various activation pathways especially in degrading the C5b–9 MAC. As will be discussed below, the role of CFH in particular may have critical relevance for AMD (7–9).

As mentioned above, local production of complement components by the RPE has been demonstrated. C3 and other complement proteins can be cleaved into biologically activated fragments by various enzyme systems, in the absence of the entire cascade, to activate certain specific cellular functions (21,22). Further, complement activation inhibitors can be produced by cells within tissues, including the RPE, serving as local protective mechanism against complement-mediated injury (23).

Cytokines

Cytokine is a generic term for any soluble polypeptide mediator (i.e., protein) synthesized and released by cells for the purposes of intercellular signaling and communication. Cytokines can be released to signal neighboring cells at the site (paracrine action), to stimulate a receptor on its own surface (autocrine action) or in some cases, released into the blood to act upon a distant site (hormonal action). Traditionally, investigators have used terms like "growth factors," "angiogenic factors," "interleukins," "lymphokines," "interferons," "monokines," "chemokines," etc. to subdivide cytokines into families with related activities, sources, and targets. Nevertheless, research has demonstrated that although some cytokines are cell-type specific, most cytokines have multiplicity and redundancy of source, function, and target such that excessive focus on specific terminology is neither clinically nor physiologically meaningful. As will be discussed, cells of the immune system can produce a variety of cytokines, including TNF-a, vascular endothelial growth factor (VEGF), platelet-derived growth factor (PDGF), transforming growth factor-β (TGF-β), and many others, which mediate a spectrum of

effects depending on the target cell and tissue. In response to nonimmune and immune injury, the RPE is capable of producing a host of cytokines relevant to AMD pathobiology, some of which may facilitate tissue repair or modulate inflammatory response.

Oxidants

Under certain conditions, oxygen-containing molecules can accept an electron from various substrates to become highly reactive products with the potential to damage cellular molecules and inhibit functional properties in pathogens or host cells. Four of the most important oxidants are singlet oxygen, superoxide anion, hydrogen peroxide, and the hydroxyl radical. In addition, various nitrogen oxides, certain metal ions, and other molecules can become reactive oxidants or participate in oxidizing reactions.

Oxidants are continuously generated as a consequence of normal noninflammatory cellular biochemical processes, including electron transport during mitochondrial respiration, auto-oxidation of catecholamines, cellular interactions with environmental light or radiation, or prostaglandin metabolism within cell membranes. During immune responses, however, oxidants are typically produced by neutrophils and macrophages by various enzyme-dependent oxidase systems (24). Some of these enzymes are bound to the inner cell membrane (e.g., NADPH oxidase) and catalyze the intracellular transfer of electrons from specific substrates (like NADPH) to oxygen or hydrogen peroxide to form highly chemically reactive compounds meant to destroy internalized, phagocytosed pathogens (25). Other oxidases, like myeloperoxidase, can be secreted extracellularly or released into phagocytic vesicles to catalyze oxidant reactions between hydrogen peroxide and chloride to form extremely toxic products that are highly damaging to bacteria, cell surfaces, and extracellular matrix molecules (26). Finally, several important oxidant reactions involve the formation of reactive nitrogen species (5).

Oxidants can interact with several cellular targets to cause injury. Among the most important are damage to proteins (i.e., enzymes, receptors) by crosslinking of sulfhydryl groups or other chemical modifications, damage to the cell membrane by lipid peroxidation of fatty acids in the phospholipid bilayers, depletion of ATP by loss of integrity of the inner membrane of the mitochondria, and breaks or crosslinks in DNA due to chemical alterations of nucleotides (1,27). Not surprisingly, nature has developed many protective antioxidant systems including soluble intracellular antioxidants (i.e., glutathione or vitamin C), cell membrane–bound lipid soluble antioxidants (i.e., vitamin E), and extracellular antioxidants (1,27). More information on oxidative stress mechanisms in AMD can be found in chapter 6.

Cells of the Immune Response

Both innate and antigen-specific immune systems use leukocytes as cellular mediators to effect and amplify the response (i.e., immune effectors). In general, leukocyte subsets include lymphocytes (T cells and B cells), monocytes (macrophages, microglia, dendritic cells), and granulocytes (neutrophils, eosinophils, and basophils). A complete overview is beyond the scope of this chapter, especially as no evidence exists that all of these cellular effectors participate in AMD. Thus, this section will focus only upon leukocyte subsets potentially relevant to AMD, including monocytes, basophils/mast cells, and B lymphocytes/antibodies.

Monocytes and Macrophages

The monocyte (the circulating cell) and the macrophage (the tissue-infiltrating equivalent) are important effectors in all forms of immunity and inflammation (4). Monocytes are relatively large cells (12–20 μm in suspension, but up to 40 μm in tissues) and traffic through many normal sites. Most normal tissues have at least two identifiable macrophage populations: tissue-resident macrophages and blood-derived macrophages. Although many exceptions exist, in general, tissue-resident macrophages represent monocytes that have migrated into a tissue weeks or months previously, or even during embryologic development of the tissue, thereby acquiring tissue-specific properties and specific cellular markers. In many tissues, resident macrophages have been given tissue-specific names (e.g., microglia in the brain and retina, Kupffer cells in the liver, alveolar macrophages in the lungs, etc.) (28–30). In contrast, blood-derived macrophages usually represent monocytes that have recently migrated from the blood into a fully developed tissue site, usually within a few days, still maintaining many generic properties of the circulating cell.

Macrophages serve three primary functions: as scavengers to clear cell debris and pathogens without tissue damage, as antigen-presenting cells for T lymphocytes, and as inflammatory effector cells. Conceptually, macrophages exist in different levels or stages of metabolic and functional activity, each representing different "programs" of gene activation and mediator synthesis. Three different stages are often described: (i) *M0*, scavenging (sometimes considered immature) macrophages; (ii) *M1*, (classically activated) inflammatory macrophages; and (iii) *M2*, (alternatively activated) reparative macrophages. M1 macrophages often undergo a morphologic change in size and histologic features into a cell called an epithelioid cell. Epithelioid cells can fuse into multinucleated giant cells. Only upon full activation are macrophages most efficient at synthesis and release of mediators to amplify inflammation and to kill pathogens. Typical activational stimuli include bacterial toxins (such as lipopolysaccharides), antibody-coated pathogens, complement-coated debris, or certain cytokines (Fig. 2.2) (31–33).

M2, or reparative, macrophages, considered by some investigators to have partial or intermediate level of activation (34–37), can mediate chronic injury in the absence of inflammatory cell infiltration or widespread tissue destruction. For example, M2 reparative macrophages contribute to physiologic processes such as fibrosis, wound repair, extracellular matrix turnover, and angiogenesis (38–46). M2 macrophages play important roles in the pathogenesis of atherosclerosis, glomerulosclerosis, osteoarthritis, keloid formation, pulmonary fibrosis, and other noninflammatory disorders, indicating that the "repair" process is not always beneficial to tissues with complex morphologies with precise structure–function requirements. In eyes with AMD, choroidal macrophages and occasionally choroidal epithelioid cells have been observed underlying the areas of drusen, geographic atrophy, and choroidal neovascularization (CNV) (47–51). Also, cell culture data suggest that blood monocytes from patients with AMD can assume an M2

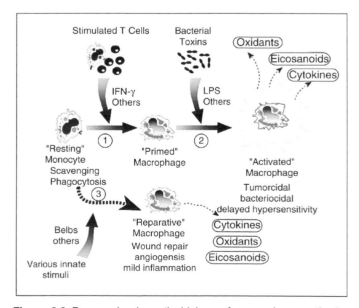

Figure 2.2 Proposed schematic biology of macrophage activation indicating process to M1 macrophage (step 1) by IFN-γ and subsequent activation through the exposure to LPS (step 2). Alternatively, via scavenging and phagocytosis (step 3), macrophages can become "reparative" or M2, resulting in local tissue rearrangement.

phenotype upon exposure to growth factors and debris released by oxidant-injured RPE (52).

Dendritic Cells

Dendritic cells (DCs) are terminally differentiated bone-marrow derived circulating mononuclear cells distinct from the macrophage–monocyte lineage and comprise approximately 0.1–1.0% of blood mononuclear cells (53). However, in tissue sites, DCs become large (15–30 µm) with cytoplasmic veils which form extensions two to three times the diameter of the cell, resembling the dendritic structure of neurons. In many non-lymphoid and lymphoid organs, DCs become a system of antigen-presenting cells. These sites recruit DCs by defined migration pathways, and in each site, DCs share features of structure and function. DCs function as accessory cells, which play an important role in the processing and presentation of antigens to T cells, and their distinctive role is to initiate responses in naïve lymphocytes. Thus, DCs serve as the most potent leukocytes for activating T-cell dependent immune responses. However, DCs do not seem to serve as phagocytic scavengers nor are they effectors of repair or inflammation. Both the retina and the choroid contain high density of DCs (54,55).

Basophils and Mast Cells

Basophils are the blood-borne equivalent of the tissue-bound mast cell. Mast cells exist in two major subtypes, connective tissue versus mucosal types, both of which can release preformed granules and synthesize certain mediators de novo (56,57). Connective tissue mast cells contain abundant granules with histamine and heparin, and synthesize prostaglandin D2 upon stimulation. In contrast, mucosal mast cells require T-cell cytokine's help for granule formation, and therefore normally contain low levels of histamine. Also, mucosal mast cells synthesize mostly leukotrienes after stimulation. Importantly, the granule type and functional activity can be altered by the tissue location, but the regulation of these important differences is not well understood. Basophils and mast cells differ from other granulocytes in several important ways. The granule contents are different from those of polymorphonuclear neutrophils or eosinophils, and mast cells express high-affinity Fc receptors for IgE. They act as the major effector cells in IgE-mediated immune responses, especially with allergy or immediate hypersensitivity. Mast cells also participate in the induction of cell-mediated immunity, wound healing, and other functions not directly related to IgE-mediated degranulation (58,59). Other stimuli, such as complement or certain cytokines, may also trigger degranulation (60). Mast cells are also capable of inducing cell injury or death through their release of TNF-a. For example, mast cells have been associated with neuronal degeneration and death in thiamine deficiency and toxic metabolic diseases. Reports in the past have demonstrated the presence of mast cells in atherosclerotic lesions and the co-localization of mast cells with the angiogenic protein, platelet-derived endothelial growth factor (60–66).

Mast cells are widely distributed in the connective tissue and are frequently found in close proximity to blood vessels and are in present in abundance in the choroid (54,67). Mast cells may play important roles in the pathogenesis of AMD since they have an ability to induce angiogenesis and are mediators of cell injury. Mast cells have also been shown to accumulate at sites of angiogenesis and have been demonstrated to be present around Bruch's membrane during both the early and late stages of CNV in AMD (48). Mast cells can interact with endothelial cells and induce their proliferation through the release of heparin, metalloproteinases, and VEGF (68–70). Interestingly, oral tranilast, an antiallergic drug that inhibits the release of chemical mediators from mast cells has been shown to suppress laser-induced CNV in the rat (71). 4. T Lymphocytes.

Lymphocytes are small (10–20 um) cells with large dense nuclei also derived from stem cell precursors within the bone marrow (3,72,73). However, unlike other leukocytes, lymphocytes require subsequent maturation in peripheral lymphoid organs. Originally characterized and differentiated based upon a series of ingenious but esoteric laboratory tests, lymphocytes can now be subdivided based upon detection of specific cell surface proteins (i.e., surface markers). These "markers" are in turn related to functional and molecular activities of individual subsets. Three broad categories of lymphocytes have been determined: B cells, T cells, and non-T and non-B lymphocytes.

Thymus-derived lymphocytes (or T cells) exist in several subsets (74,75). Helper T cells function to assist in antigen processing for antigen-specific immunity within lymph nodes, especially in helping B cells to produce antibody and effector T cells to become sensitized. Effector T lymphocyte subsets function as effector cells to mediate antigen-specific inflammation and immune responses. Effector T cells can be distinguished into two main types. CD8 T cells (often called cytotoxic T lymphocytes) serve as effector cells for killing tumors or virally infected host cells via release of cytotoxic cytokines or specialized pore forming molecules. It is possible but unlikely that these cells play a major role in AMD.

CD4 T cells (often called delayed-hypersensitivity T cells) effect responses by the release of specific cytokines such as interferon-γ and TNF-β (76). They function by homing into a tissue, recognizing antigen and antigen-presenting cells (APCs), and becoming fully activated, releasing cytokines and mediators, which then amplify the inflammatory reaction. Occasionally, CD4 T cells can also become activated in an antigen-independent manner, called bystander activation (77–79), a process that may explain the presence of T lymphocytes identified in CNV specimens surgically excised from AMD eyes.

B Lymphocytes and Antibody

B-lymphocytes mature in the bone marrow and are responsible for the production of antibodies. Antibodies (or immunoglobulins) are soluble antigen-specific effector molecules of antigen-specific immunity (3,72,73). After appropriate antigenic stimulation with T cell help, B cells secrete IgM antibodies, and later other isotypes, into the efferent lymph fluid draining into the venous circulation. Antibodies then mediate a variety of immune effector activities by binding to antigen in the blood or in tissues.

Antibodies serve as effectors of tissue-specific immune responses by four main mechanisms. Intravascular circulating antibodies can bind antigen in the blood, thereby form circulating immune complexes. Then the entire complex of antigen plus antibody can deposit into tissues. Alternatively, circulating B cells can infiltrate into a tissue and secrete antibody locally to form an immune complex. Third, antibody can bind to an effector cell (especially mast cell, macrophage, or neutrophil) by the Fc portion of the molecule to produce a combined antibody and cellular effector mechanism. It is unlikely that any of these mechanisms play a major role in AMD.

However, one possible antibody-dependent mechanism relevant to AMD is the capacity for circulating antibodies, usually of the IgG subclasses previously formed in lymph nodes or in other tissue sites, to passively leak into a tissue with fenestrated capillaries (like the choriocapillaris). Then, these antibodies form an immune complex with antigens present in the substratum or on the cells of the tissue, to initiate one of the following effectors (Fig. 2.3) (3,72,73,80–83).

Immune Complexes with Extracellular Matrix-Bound Antigens

When free antibody passively leaks from the serum into a tissue, it can combine with tissue-bound antigens (i.e., antigen trapped in the extracellular matrix). These *in situ*, or locally formed, complexes can in some instances activate the complement pathway to produce complement fragments called anaphylatoxins. This mechanism should be differentiated from the deposition of circulating immune complexes, which are preformed in the blood.

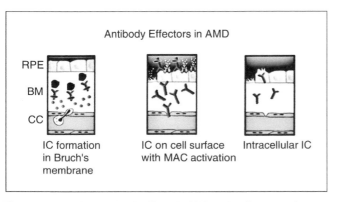

Figure 2.3 Possible antibody effects in AMD with subsequent immune complex (IC) formation at variation locations in the subretinal space, on or within the retinal pigment epithelium. Abbreviations: AMD, age-related macular degeneration; BM, Bruch's membrane; CC, choroidal capillaries; MAC, membrane attack complex; RPE, retinal pigment epithelium.

Typically, the histology is dominated by neutrophils and monocytes, but at low level of activation, minimal cellular infiltration may be observed. Many types of glomerulonephritis and vasculitis are thought to represent this mechanism.

Immune Complexes with Cell-Surface Antigen

If an antigen is associated with the external surface of the plasma membrane, antibody binding might activate the terminal complement cascade to induce cell injury via formation of the MAC. Hemolytic anemia of the newborn due to Rh incompatibility is the classic example of this process. Hashimoto's thyroiditis, nephritis of Goodpasture's syndrome, and autoimmune thrombocytopenia are other examples.

Immune Complex with Intracellular Antigen, a Novel Mechanism

Circulating antibodies can cause tissue injury by mechanisms different from complement activation, using pathogenic mechanisms not yet clearly elucidated (82,83). For example, some autoantibodies in systemic lupus erythematosus appear to be internalized by renal cells independent of antigen binding; these autoantibodies then combine with intracellular nuclear or ribosomal antigens to alter cellular metabolism and signaling pathways. This novel pathway of intracellular antibody/antigen complex formation may cause some cases of nephritis in the absence of complement activation. This pathway has also been implicated in paraneoplastic syndromes, most notably cancer-associated retinopathy, in which autoantibodies to intracellular photoreceptor-associated antigens may mediate rod or cone degeneration (84).

Mechanisms for the Activation of the Immune Responses in Degenerative Diseases
Activation of Innate Immunity
Cellular Injury as a Trigger of Innate Immunity

Not only can immune responses cause cellular injury, but cellular responses to nonimmune injury are also common initiators of innate immunity (3,72,73,85–87). Injury can be defined as tissue exposure to any physical and/or biochemical stimulus that alters pre-existing homeostasis to produce a physiological cellular response. In addition to injury stimuli produced by the immune effector and amplification systems described earlier, nonimmune injurious stimuli include physical injury (heat, light, and mechanical) or biochemical stimulation (hypoxia, pH change, oxidants, chemical mediators, and cytokines) (87). Typical cellular reactions to injury include a wide spectrum of responses, including changes in intracellular metabolism, plasma membrane alterations, cytokine production and gene upregulation, morphological changes, cellular migration, proliferation, or even death. Some of these cellular responses, in turn, can result in the recruitment and activation of macrophages or activation of amplification systems, especially if they include upregulation of cell adhesion molecules, production of macrophage chemotactic factors, or release of activational stimuli.

Two important injury responses relevant to AMD that commonly activate innate immunity include vascular injury and extracellular deposit accumulation (87,88). Vascular injury induced by physical stimuli (i.e., mechanical stretch of capillaries or arterioles by hydrostatic expansion induced by hypertension or thermal injury from laser) or biochemical stimuli (i.e., hormones associated with hypertension and aging) can upregulate cell adhesion molecules and chemotactic factors that lead to macrophage recruitment into various vascularized tissues. Extracellular deposit accumulation can also contribute to activation of innate immunity by serving as a substrate for scavenging and phagocytosis, especially if the deposits are chemically modified by oxidation or other processes (see atherosclerosis section).

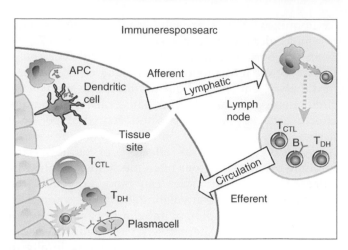

Figure 2.4 The immune response arc indicating the cross-talk between the tissue site, where antigen recognition and effector processes take place and the lymph node, the site of antigen processing.

Infection as a Trigger of Innate Immunity

Infection can also activate innate immunity, usually by the release of toxic molecules (i.e., endotoxins, exotoxins, and cell wall components) that directly interact with receptors on macrophages, on neutrophils or, in some cases, on parenchymal cells. Active infection is differentiated from harmless colonization by the presence of invasion and replication of the infectious agent (89). However, active infections do not always trigger innate immunity; this is illustrated by some retinal parasitic infections in which inflammation occurs only when the parasite dies.

Over the past couple decades, there has been growing interest in the idea that certain kinds of chronic infections might cause (or at least contribute to) degenerative diseases that are not considered to be truly inflammatory (86–89). One of the most dramatic examples is peptic ulcer disease, which was recognized to be caused by infection of the gastric subepithelial mucosa with a Gram-positive bacterium called *Helicobacter pylori* (90). Accordingly, ulcer disease is now treated using antibiotics and not with diet or surgery. Chronic bacterial or viral infection of vascular endothelial cells has been suggested as an etiology for coronary artery atherosclerosis, and infection with an unusual agent called a prion has been shown as a cause of certain neurodegenerative diseases. Evidence for a causative role for infection in AMD is lacking, though several studies have found an association between AMD and latent cytomegalovirus (CMV) infection as well as with *Chlamydia pneumoniae* infection (76,91–93). The mechanisms whereby infection might trigger disease onset or influence disease severity are currently under investigation (94).

Activation of Normal and Aberrant Antigen-Specific Immunity
Activation of Antigen-Specific Immunity

Often expressed as the idea of the "immune response arc," this idea proposes that interaction between antigen and the antigen-specific immune system at a peripheral site (such as the skin) can conceptually be subdivided

into three phases: afferent (at the site), processing (within the immune system), and effector (at the original site, completing the arc) (Fig. 2.4) (3,72,73). Antigen within the skin or any other site is recognized by the afferent phase of the immune response, which conveys the antigenic information to the lymph node in one of two forms. APCs, typically DCs, can take up antigen (almost always in the form of a protein) at a site, digest the antigen into fragments, and carry the digested fragments to the lymph node to interact with T cells (74,75,95). Alternatively, the natural, intact antigen can directly flow into the node via lymphatics where it interacts with B cells (3,72,73).

In the lymph node, processing of the antigenic signal occurs where antigen, APCs, T cells, and B cells interact to activate the immune response. For tissues without draining lymph nodes (such as the retina and choroid), the spleen is often a major site of processing. Immunologic processing has been the topic of extensive research and the details are beyond the scope of this chapter. Processing results in release of immune effectors (antibodies, B cells, and T cells) into efferent lymphatics and venous circulation which conveys the intent of the immune system back to the original site where an effector response occurs (i.e., immune complex formation or delayed hypersensitivity reaction). Compared with that of the skin, the immune response arc of the retina and choroid express many similarities as well as important differences (i.e., immune privilege, anatomy), which are discussed in relevant reviews (96,97).

Aberrant Activation of Antigen-Specific Immunity

The inappropriate activation of antigen-specific immunity may play a role in the pathogenesis of chronic degenerative diseases. Autoimmunity is the activation of antigen-specific immunity to normal self-antigens, and two different mechanisms of autoimmunity may be relevant to AMD: molecular mimicry and desequestration. Additionally, immune responses directed at "neoantigens" or foreign antigens inappropriately trapped within normal tissues may also play a role in AMD.

Molecular mimicry is the immunologic cross-reaction between antigenic regions (epitopes) of an unrelated foreign molecule and self-antigens with similar structures (98). For example, immune system exposure to foreign antigens, such as those present within yeast, viruses, or bacteria, can induce an appropriate afferent, processing, and effector immune response to the organism. However, antimicrobial antibodies or effector lymphocytes generated to the organism can inappropriately cross-react with similar antigenic regions of a self-antigen. A dynamic process would then be initiated, causing tissue injury by an autoimmune response that would induce additional lymphocyte responses directed at other self-antigens. Thus, the process would not require the ongoing replication of a pathogen or the continuous presence of the inciting antigen. Molecular mimicry against antigens from a wide range of organisms, including streptococcus, yeast, *E. Coli*, and various viruses, has been shown to be a potential mechanism for antiretinal autoimmunity (99).

A second mechanism for aberrant autoimmunity is desequestration (100–102). For most self-antigens, the immune system is actively "tolerized" to the antigen by various mechanisms, preventing the activation of antigen-specific immune effector responses even when the self-antigen is fully exposed to the immune system. For some other antigens, however, the immune system relies on sequestration of the antigen within cellular compartments that are isolated from antigen-presenting cells and effector mechanisms. If the sequestered molecules are allowed to escape their protective isolation, they can become recognized as foreign, thereby initiating an autoimmune reaction. For example, certain nuclear or ribosomal-associated enzymes are apparently sequestered, and if organelles become extruded into a location with exposure to DCs or macrophages, an immune response can be triggered against these antigens (101). Accordingly, some RPE and retina-associated peptides appear to be sequestered from the immune system and could potentially serve as antigens if RPE injury or death leads to their release into the choroid (96,102).

Another mechanism for aberrant activation of antigen-specific immunity is the formation of "neoantigens" secondary to chemical modification of normal self-proteins trapped or deposited within tissues (103). For example, oxidation or acetylation of peptides in apolipoproteins trapped within atherosclerotic plaques can induce new antigenic properties resulting in specific T cell and antibodies immunized to the modified protein.

A final mechanism for aberrant antigen-specific immunity is antigen trapping (104). Antigen trapping is the immunologic reaction to circulating foreign antigens inappropriately trapped within the extracellular matrix of a normal tissue site containing fenestrated capillaries. Typically occurring after invasive infection or iatrogenically administered drugs, this mechanism may be very

important in glomerular diseases (104) and has been postulated to induce ocular inflammation (105,106). Physical size and charge of the antigen are important. For example, antigen trapping within the choriocapillaris may contribute to ocular histoplasmosis syndrome (106).

EXAMPLES OF IMMUNE AND INFLAMMATORY MECHANISMS OF NONOCULAR DEGENERATIVE DISEASES

Immune Mechanisms in Atherosclerosis

Myocardial infarction due to thrombosis of atherosclerotic coronary arteries is the major cause of death in western countries, and epidemiologic studies suggest a possible association with AMD (107,108). The pathology of atherosclerosis suggests a spectrum of changes whose pathogenesis may be relevant to the understanding of AMD (109,110). The fatty streak, representing the earliest phase of atherosclerosis, is characterized by lipid deposition and macrophage infiltration within the vessel wall (103,110,111). Some investigators have suggested similarities in pathogenesis between fatty streak formation and early AMD (112). The fatty streak can progress into the fibrous plaque, characterized by the proliferation of smooth muscle cells, increasing inflammation, and formation of connective tissue with neovascularization within the vessel wall. The fibrous plaque predisposes to the complications of atherosclerosis such as thrombosis, dissection, or plaque ulceration (103,110,111). The pathogenesis of the fibrous plaque may share similarity with mechanisms for the late complications of AMD, including formation of CNV and disciform scars (Fig. 2.5).

Many mechanisms contribute to the pathogenesis of atherosclerosis, including genetic predisposition and physiological risk factors like high blood cholesterol, smoking, diabetes, and hypertension. However, most authorities now believe that chronic low-grade inflammation, induced by a wide variety of injury stimuli, followed by a fibroproliferative (wound healing) response within the vessel wall is central to the pathogenesis of atherosclerosis. Thus, various immune mechanisms implicated in atherosclerosis might be relevant to AMD.

Innate Mechanisms

Injury and Atherosclerosis

The "response to injury" hypothesis for the initiation and progression of atherosclerosis has been supported by numerous investigators who cite many different participating injury stimuli (103,110,111). For example, hemodynamic injury by blood flow turbulence can directly injury endothelial cells at bifurcations of major vessels (113). Biochemical injury secondary to exposure to polypeptide mediators associated with hypertension (i.e., angiotensin II or endothelin-1) can stimulate the endothelial and smooth muscle responses. Oxidized LDL cholesterol particles in the blood, advanced glycosylation end products in diabetes, or toxic chemicals secondary to smoking are other potential sources of injury (114).

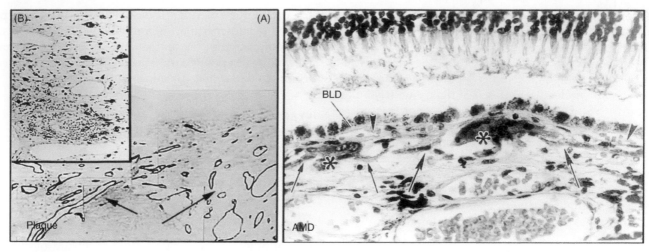

Figure 2.5 Micrographs of an atheromatous plaque (left) and a choroidal neovascular membrane (right) indicating similar histologic components of intrastromal neovascularization (arrows) and macrophages (left - B) and (right - *asterisk*). BLD = basal linear deposit. *Source*: From Refs. 266 (left) and 267 (right).

Macrophages in Atherosclerosis

Blood-derived macrophages are major contributors to the pathogenesis of atherosclerosis (103,110,115). In the fatty streak phase of atherosclerosis, lipids accumulate in the subendothelial vascular wall at sites of vascular injury. Injury results in the oxidation of lipids or endothelial production of specific macrophage chemotactic signals, such as macrophage chemotactic protein-1, recruiting circulating monocytes to sites of endothelial injury. There, they migrate into the subendothelial extracellular matrix to scavenge the extracellular lipid-rich deposits (i.e., scavenging macrophages). Macrophages may also contribute to the solubilization of lipid deposits by the release of apolipoprotein E (ApoE), which may facilitate uptake and scavenging of lipids. Genetic polymorphisms of ApoE have been associated with variations in the severity of atherosclerosis and AMD (116).

Foam cells and macrophages are very numerous in fibrous plaques and probably play a major role in lesion progression. Although overly simplistic, experimental data suggest that scavenging macrophages can become activated into reparative (M2) "foam" cells by numerous stimuli, including by phagocytosis of oxidized lipoproteins (115,116). These M2 macrophages secrete amplifying mediators, including PDGF, VEGF, TGF-β, matrix metalloproteinases, or others, which contribute to fibrosis, smooth muscle proliferation, or vascularization of the plaque (117–120).

Infectious Etiology of Atherosclerosis

Although numerous risk factors are associated with the initiation and progression of atherosclerosis, an infectious etiology has been suggested by de Boer et al. Many patients with atherosclerosis exhibit signs of mild systemic inflammation, especially elevated serum C-reactive protein and erythrocyte sedimentation rate (121). Statistical evidence has been generated to suggest that infection with various infectious agents, especially *C. pneumoniae* or MV, might initiate vascular injury and explain the systemic inflammatory signs (122–125).

Numerous epidemiologic studies have revealed a statistical correlation between atherosclerosis and serologic evidence of infection with *C. pneumoniae* (122). Follow-up studies have demonstrated the presence of *C. pneumoniae* by histochemical methods within atherosclerotic plaques and organisms have been cultured from the lesions (125). Additionally, pilot studies using appropriate antibiotic therapy have demonstrated a beneficial effect in patients with severe atherosclerosis (123,124). Several proposed mechanisms for the role of *C. pneumoniae* in atherosclerosis may be relevant to AMD. Chronic infection of vascular endothelial cells may upregulate cell surface molecules that recruit macrophages or alter responses to injury. For instance, *C. pneumoniae* endothelial infection can enhance endotoxin binding to LDL particles that might induce various inflammatory cascades at the site of uptake (126). Additionally, chlamydial heat shock proteins (HSPs) can directly stimulate macrophages and other cellular amplification systems (127). Also, antigen-specific immune responses directed against chlamydial HSPs may cross-react with host cellular HSPs including those expressed in the retina (128).

Similar but less extensive data have been generated to support a role for CMV infection in atherosclerosis (129–131). Cytomegalovirus infects 60–70% of adults in the United States. Several studies have linked serologic evidence of prior CMV infection to atherosclerosis. Although the association is mild, studies have elucidated possible mechanisms for this association such as enhanced scavenging of LDL particles by virally infected endothelial cells.

Antigen-Specific Immunity

The potential importance of antigen-specific immune mechanisms in atherosclerosis is illustrated by the observation of accelerated atherosclerosis in heart transplant patients who experience vascular injury associated with mild, chronic allograft rejection (95). In normal patients with atherosclerosis, T lymphocytes are numerous in fibrous plaques and a role for lymphocyte-mediated, antigen-specific immunity has been proposed for progression of atherosclerotic fibrous plaques (103). Experimental data suggest that oxidized lipoproteins can become neoantigens to activate an immune response arc (132). Scavenging macrophages may become antigen-presenting cells at the site of plaque formation, serving to restimulate recruited T cells and thereby activating the effector phase of the immune response. Immune responses to bacterial or viral antigens, especially chlamydial HSPs, trapped in tissues after occult infection, may also stimulate antigen-specific immunity, or autoimmunity by cross-reactive molecular mimicry (133). Alternatively, T cells may be recruited by innate responses and become activated by antigen-independent bystander mechanisms. Interestingly, vaccination against oxidized LDL produces antibodies seems to prevent or reduce formation of atherosclerotic plaques (20).

Nonspecific Amplification Cascades
Complement Activation in Atherosclerosis
In atherosclerotic lesions, several complement components and inhibitory proteins have been detected including MAC complexes (134–136). Cholesterol is also a potent activator of the complement system in vitro. Alternatively, MAC complex concentration has been shown to induce production of macrophage chemotactic factors in smooth muscle cells, and studies have shown MAC deposition in the arterial wall prior to monocyte infiltration and foam cell formation. Furthermore, the complement precursor protein C1q is deposited on apoptotic cells. Cell debris and cell membrane blebs that form because of injury can enhance phagocytosis by C1q receptor-bearing macrophages and thus may play a role in tissue repair.

Oxidants and Cytokines in Atherosclerosis
Oxidation is considered a major injury stimulus in the initiation and progression of atherosclerosis. The role of oxidized lipoproteins in circulating LDL cholesterol as an initiating injury stimulus as well as oxidation of lipid deposits within vessel walls as an amplifier of foam cell activation has been discussed above (114,115,137). Numerous cytokines, especially PDGF and TGF-β have also been implicated as major mediators of atherosclerosis progression (117–120).

Immune Mechanisms in Glomerular Diseases
Glomerular diseases account for 70% of chronic renal failure in the United States. Many glomerular diseases are primarily mediated by inflammatory mechanisms and are usually classified as glomerulonephritis. Other glomerular diseases are mediated by a mixture of degenerative and inflammatory mechanisms, and these are often classified as glomerulosclerosis (138,139). Genetic and systemic health factors contribute to the pathogenesis of both groups (138–141).

The glomerulus shares some anatomic similarities with the outer retina and inner choroid, so that the analysis of the mechanism of deposit formation and extracellular matrix changes of glomerular disorders might be informative in terms of AMD (138). For instance, both the glomerulus and inner choroid/outer retina can be described as containing capillary lobules with endothelium on one side of an extracellular matrix and epithelium on the other. In the glomerulus, endothelial cells (conceptually corresponding to the choriocapillaris) cover the internal surface of an extracellular matrix, whose external surface is covered by an epithelial layer (the podocyte). External to the podocyte is Bowman's capsule (conceptually corresponding to the subretinal space). Smooth muscle cells located internally to the endothelium, called mesangial cells, are responsible for regulating contractility and maintaining the glomerular matrix. These cells may share analogies with choroidal pericytes underlying and surrounding the choriocapillaris.

Innate Immunity in Glomerular Diseases
Chronic Injury
As is the case for atherosclerosis, a "response to injury" hypothesis has been substantiated for glomerulosclerosis due to aging, hypertension, or diabetes (138–145). Glomerulosclerosis is characterized by progressive thickening of the glomerular extracellular matrix, ultimately associated with loss of glomerular capillaries and epithelial cells. If enough glomeruli are involved, renal impairment occurs. In some ways, glomerulosclerosis resembles geographic atrophy in AMD (Fig. 2.6).

The response to injury hypothesis has been thoroughly evaluated for renal hypertension, a major cause of glomerulosclerosis (141–146). The hemodynamic injury hypothesis proposes that glomerular capillary hypertension causes excessive flow through the glomerulus or hydraulic stretching of the capillary wall to activate injury responses in glomerular cells. The humoral hypothesis proposes that hypertension-associated hormones or cytokines associated with low-grade

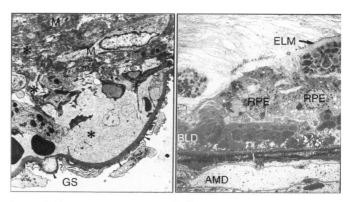

Figure 2.6 Electron micrographs from glomerulosclerosis (GS) and geographic atrophy from age-related macular degeneration (AMD) showing the appearance of excessive extracellular material and cellular loss. In glomerulosclerosis, there is accumulation of glomerular extracellular material (*asterisks*) and loss of cellular structure (M) in GS while in AMD there is accumulation of blood (BLD) and loss of retinal pigment epithelium (RPE)cells under the external limiting membrane (ELM). *Source*: From Refs. 268 (left) and 269 (right).

systemic inflammation induced by hypertensive vascular injury activate cellular injury responses. In either case, the injured endothelium, podocytes, and mesangial cells demonstrate abnormal production and turnover of collagen and other matrix molecules, leading to collagenous thickening of the matrix with degeneration of the glomerulus (146–148). Genetic background and gender can influence the rate of progression. Since hypertension is a risk factor associated with AMD and glomerular disease, hypertension-associated inflammation may also injure the choriocapillaris endothelium or RPE in an analogous fashion.

Macrophage-Mediated Injury

Macrophages contribute significantly to glomerular damage in renal diseases (149–159). Not surprisingly, infiltration with activated inflammatory macrophages is a significant histologic feature in inflammatory glomerulonephritis caused by antigen-specific immune mechanisms (i.e., immune complex disease or allograft rejection)(159), and blockade of macrophage infiltration or function ameliorates glomerular damage (153). Perhaps of more relevance to AMD is the contribution of M2 macrophages to glomerulosclerosis. Recruitment of blood-derived M2 macrophages develops early in the course of glomerulosclerosis in proportion to the severity of the injury (149,150). Various innate injury stimuli, including renal hypertension, hyperlipidemia, and glomerular capillary endothelial injury by oxidized LDL, can upregulate macrophage chemotactic factors and adhesion molecules in the capillaries to induce macrophage recruitment (154–156). Experimental data suggest that M2 macrophages release mediators that induce mesangial cell proliferation, amplify the accumulation of extracellular matrix, and may promote endothelial cell death.

Antigen-Specific Immunity in Glomerular Diseases

Antigen-specific immunity contributes significantly to inflammatory glomerular disorders. Lymphocyte-mediated immunity clearly contributes to glomerulonephritis, especially in renal allograft rejection (159). However, the relevance of this mechanism to AMD is probably minimal. Many forms of chronic glomerulonephritis are caused by antibody-dependent mechanisms, and some of these disorders are characterized by subendothelial or subepithelial deposit formation (104,160–162). Direct deposition of circulating antibodies targeted at antigens uniformly expressed within the glomerular matrix is a well-defined but rare form of glomerulonephritis, especially in Goodpasture's syndrome. Deposition of preformed circulating antigen/antibody complexes in the blood has been proposed as another major mechanism in many types of glomerulonephritis associated with deposit formation. Nevertheless, it is unlikely that deposition of either antibasement membrane antibodies or circulating immune complexes plays an important role in AMD.

However, another interpretation of the clinical and experimental data is that some forms of glomerulonephritis may actually represent antigen trapped or "planted" within the glomerular matrix, followed by the subsequent formation of *in situ* immune complexes. This alternative explanation is probably especially relevant to glomerulonephritis associated with subepithelial deposits rather than subendothelial deposits (since it is unlikely that large immune complexes would be able to filter through the matrix). For example, glomerulonephritis that occurs 10–20 days after streptococcal pharyngitis or streptococcal skin infections is characterized by subepithelial deposits (similar to homogenous basal laminar deposits). These do not stain for immune complexes (163).

Nonspecific Amplification Cascades in Glomerular Diseases

Complement deposition plays a major primary role in many glomerular diseases associated with deposits, especially those mediated by antigen-specific immune complexes. In these disorders, various fragments of the complement cascade, including C3, C5, and others are usually identified within extracellular deposits in association with immunoglobulin and acute cellular inflammation (164–166).

Complement seems to participate as a secondary amplification mechanism in some glomerular diseases. Type II membranoproliferative glomerulonephritis (or dense deposit disease), is especially relevant to AMD since these patients also develop drusen-like changes in the retina (166–169). Clinically, the retina demonstrates whitish drusen-like changes, and some eyes develop CNV. Histologically, the subretinal deposits appear to be localized between the RPE and its basement membrane (similar to basal laminar deposits) (Fig. 2.7). The glomerular deposits are characterized as electron dense linear deposits within the glomerular extracellular matrix, occasionally demonstrating dome-shaped subepithelial "humps" under the podocyte. C3 is present within the

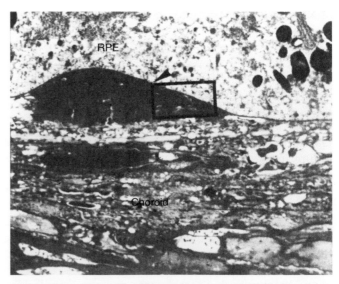

Figure 2.7 Electron micrograph of dense deposit disease of the retina demonstrating subretinal deposit (box) located between the retinal pigment epithelium and its basement membrane. *Source*: From Ref. 270.

deposits, but the presence of other complement proteins, immunoglobulins, and fibronectin is highly variable. Systemic complement is usually normal. The source of complement (i.e., locally synthesized or blood-derived) as well as the mechanisms for activation (typical cascades versus enzymatic cleavage) remain unknown. Finally, oxidants have been implicated as important mediators and amplifiers in progression of renal disease (170).

EVIDENCE FOR IMMUNE AND INFLAMMATORY MECHANISMS IN AMD

The accumulation of specific lipid- and protein-rich sub-RPE deposits, clinically characterized as drusen, remains the pathologic hallmark of AMD. While extensive histopathologic evidence suggests that inflammation plays an important role in AMD, direct evidence of the precise mechanisms by which immune cells and components contribute to disease pathogenesis is scant. Several reports have identified immunoglobulins and immune complexes in association with drusen, but their pathogenic role has not been defined (171–174). Additionally, it remains uncertain whether T cells observed within some CNV (50) are responding to specific antigens or have been recruited as part of bystander activation, and it is also unclear whether DCs play any role through sampling of deposit-associated antigens and subsequent interaction with T cells. Thus, the subsequent discussion will focus on potential roles for (A) monocytes/macrophages and microglia; (B) complement system; and (C) oxidant injury, in the onset and progression of AMD.

Monocytes/Macrophages and Microglia

There are now significant data from histopathology, preclinical in vivo and in vitro studies, and pilot clinical studies that support a key role for macrophage-mediated innate immunity in AMD (47–55,172). Investigators have observed that choroidal macrophages appear to be important in the pathogenesis of both early and late AMD. However, macrophage involvement is clearly different from their participation in overt inflammatory disorders characterized by widespread cellular infiltration. In early AMD, macrophages have been detected along the choriocapillaris side of Bruch's membrane underlying the areas of thick deposits, and a low-grade monocyte infiltration within the choriocapillaris is often present underlying the areas of deposits (173,175,176). Processes from choroidal monocytes have been noted to insert into Bruch's membrane deposits, presumably for the purpose of scavenging debris. In late AMD, macrophages and giant cells have been observed around CNV and are numerous in excised CNV, suggesting a role in promoting choroidal angiogenesis (47,50,177). Also, macrophages are present underlying zones of geographic atrophy, suggesting a role in RPE or endothelial death (49). While these data do not provide a self-evident mechanistic hypothesis for the contributions of monocytes/macrophages in AMD pathogenesis, they do suggest that monocytes/macrophages may be responding to sub-RPE deposits as an inflammatory stimulus (172).

There are, however, multiple hypotheses on whether the contributions of monocytes/macrophages are harmful or beneficial in the development of AMD. In the murine model of laser-induced CNV, pharmacologic depletion of macrophages prior to injury has been shown to diminish the CNV size and severity; upon laser induction of CNV, and blood-derived macrophages infiltrate the retina and appear to promote Muller cell activation (178–180). These data, as well as data in other murine models (181), suggest that macrophages could contribute to CNV formation in AMD. However, using a murine knockout model for IL-10, a cytokine thought to regulate macrophage activity, other investigators have demonstrated increased infiltration of macrophages, and these macrophages appear to inhibit pathologic CNV formation (182). While these studies appear to have contradictory data, the activation state of the macrophage may determine its functional contribution to disease. M0 macrophages may scavenge RPE cellular debris and sub-RPE deposits without damage and promote healthy repair of Bruch's membrane, serving a protective function. However, M1 and M2 macrophages may promote complications, including injury to Bruch's membrane, RPE, and choriocapillaris, with subsequent development of either RPE death/atrophy or CNV. M1 macrophages may mediate this through release of proinflammatory cytokines and recruitment of other effector cells. M2 macrophages may promote wound repair, angiogenesis, and matrix turnover. This therefore suggests a nuanced role for macrophages, and moreover, that the specific disease phenotype may reflect the types of cytokines, chemical mediators, MMPs, mitogens, or angiogenic factors released by infiltrating choroidal macrophages (183).

In support of this concept, numerous investigators have demonstrated that TNF-α induce major functional and morphological changes in RPE cells (184–188), and we have found that patients who have blood monocytes expressing high TNF-a levels demonstrated nearly a fivefold increased odds ratio for the presence of neovascular AMD(189). In the same study, we also observed that blood monocytes from some patients with AMD could assume an activated phenotype after exposure to RPE–derived cell debris and membrane blebs (189). While nonspecific therapy with intravitreal corticosteroids has met with variable success in the clinic for neovascular AMD treatment (190,191), therapeutic agents directed against macrophage-derived cytokines perhaps hold promise. Systemic administration of the anti-TNF-a agent, infliximab, reduced laser-induced CNV in a murine model (192), and pilot phase I/II study data of systemic immunosuppression in combination with intravitreal anti-VEGF suggested a possible therapeutic benefit for immune-modulating therapy (193). More intriguingly, intravitreal administration of the anti-TNF-a agent, infliximab, has been shown to be effective for cases of persistent disease activity after anti-VEGF therapy, though a high rate of concurrent ocular inflammation, related to either the drug or vehicle, has thus far limited its evaluation and clinical use (194–196).

Therapeutic strategies targeting macrophage-mediated mechanisms of RPE cellular injury, vascular maturation, and neurosensory retinal dysfunction represent promising avenues for expanding visual benefit to more patients with AMD (197).

Microglia represent the tissue-resident macrophages (as opposed to blood-derived monocyte) of the retina and CNS that perform dynamic immune surveillance in the inner retina and are not typically found in the outer retina (198). However, activated microglia have been found in the subretinal space in AMD eyes and have been found in close proximity to RPE cells overlying drusen, suggesting a response to injury (199). These observations suggest that microglia may respond to injury through interactions with the RPE (200). Importantly, microglia activated by injury or inflammation also interact with Muller cells; the complex interaction signaling and structural interaction of these cells may coordinate the response of neurosensory retina to inflammatory stimuli and may be important for maintenance of photoreceptor integrity (201,202). The contribution of microglia to AMD pathogenesis relative to blood-derived macrophages is uncertain. In the murine model of laser CNV, microglia density was not altered after injury and microglia appeared to play a less prominent role in retinal inflammation and Muller cell activation, than blood-derived macrophages (179). Nevertheless, the recognition of specific alterations of microglia distribution in AMD and the identification of specific molecular modulators of microglial activity, such as PPAR-γ, suggest that microglia may be a plausible cellular target for therapeutic intervention in AMD, once its functions in disease are better characterized (203).

Complement System

Extensive genetic and histopathologic data have implicated an important role for the complement system in AMD. In 2005, four separate research groups independently identified a single nucleotide polymorphism in CFH in association with AMD (204–207). Specifically, they found that individuals with an SNP resulting in a tyrosine to histidine substitution at amino acid 402 were at increased risk for both early and late forms of AMD and that this mutation may explain up to 40% of the genetic risk of the disease. CFH is a primary regulator of the alternative pathway and therefore controls the downstream activation of C3b. CFH competes with complement factor B for the binding of C3b on the surface of various tissues within the retina, thereby potentially acting as a protective mechanism (208). At present, the region of interest affected by the SNP on the CFH gene does not appear to be directly involved in complement activation but rather may affect binding to glycosaminoglycans in extracellular sites (209). Importantly, mutations in other pro-complement proteins such as C2 and complement factor B may positively influence complement activation (210) while mutations in negative regulators, such as CFH-related genes CFHR3 and CFHR1 may also be involved in complement deposition within the retina and/or drusen (211).

Further genetic studies are also focused on how paralogs to CFH and other genes might either directly or indirectly modulate the specific risk association of CFH with AMD (212,213).

There is also now abundant evidence that drusen in association with AMD contain many proteins of the complement system (214,215). Late-stage complement proteins such as C5, C6, C7, C8, C9 and the MAC have been demonstrated by immunohistochemistry to be present within drusen. Interestingly, proteins belonging to all of the activation pathways such as the mannose binding factor, C1q, and CFH as well as C3 and its fragments have also been demonstrated within drusen. And finally many proteins such as vitronectin, clusterin, and other potential activators of the complement pathway, such as amyloid beta and C reactive protein, appear to be found within drusen (173,216–218). Importantly, amyloid beta may play a major role in low-level deposition of complement by inhibiting complement factor I , a major inhibitor of C3 activation (218–220).

Subsequently, there has been significant interest in how complement activation might play a role in the development of sub-RPE deposits and the subsequent inflammatory response, (20,221–224) and in how negative regulation of the complement system by CFH may be protective in AMD pathogenesis (225). Preclinical models of complement dysregulation have raised many unanswered questions about the specific mechanism by which the complement system contributes to disease. The CFH (-/-) knockout mouse does not develop sub-RPE deposits but rather develops thinning of Bruch's membrane and unusual outer retinal pathology (226). However, a double ApoE4(-/-) CFH (-/-) knockout mouse fed a high fat cholesterol-enriched diet develops sub-RPE deposits with significant RPE damage and altered retinal function as measured by ERG (227). Interestingly aged chimeric transgenic mice expressing either 402Y or 402H CFH appeared to demonstrate sub-RPE deposits, accumulation of macrophage/microglia cells in the subretinal space, and increased C3d deposition under the RPE (228). These suggest that specific alterations of the complement system, possibly in combination with a second injury, are necessary to produce the disease phenotype. The RPE expresses specific and nonspecific complement inhibitors such as decay accelerating factor and vitronectin to suggest intrinsic defense mechanisms to prevent against complement-mediated injury (229).What proportion of the complement system components produced by the RPE versus systemically derived is unclear; there is clinical evidence suggesting high levels of complement proteins in the serum of patients with AMD (230). Nevertheless, further study is necessary to determine whether complement-mediated direct cell injury via MAC assembly plays a role in AMD, and a clear mechanism must be established to link this injury stimulus to relevant cellular responses involved in deposit formation.

Although the role of complement in AMD remains to be understood completely, novel therapeutics targeting the complement system are under evaluation in phase I and II clinical trials (231). Intravenous eculizumab, a systemic inhibitor of C5, was recently tested in two separate phase I/II studies on patients with early AMD (drusen) and advanced dry AMD (geographic atrophy), known collectively as the COMPLETE study. The treatment failed to reach its primary end point in either study (reduction in drusen volume in early AMD and reduction in the area of atrophic progression in geographic atrophy) (232,233).

Oxidants

As discussed previously, immune and nonimmune derived oxidants serve as potential injury stimuli and powerful amplifiers of the inflammatory response. While a complete review of oxidant injury is beyond the scope of this chapter, we will review how oxidants may mediate inflammatory injury in AMD. (Detailed discussion of oxidative injury and AMD is found in Chapter 6.) In the retina, oxidant-mediated effects at the RPE and photoreceptors have been proposed as major causes of nonimmune injury (234–237). Noninflammatory biochemical sources of oxidants in AMD include chronic exposure of the photoreceptors and RPE to blue light, dysfunctional lysosome metabolism in the RPE (resulting in accumulation of lipofuscin and other lipid- and protein-rich aggregates), prostaglandin biosynthesis, and environmental toxicants such as those found in cigarette smoke, like hydroquinone (238). Electron transfer to oxygen-containing molecules can then produce oxidant species, such as singlet oxygen, superoxide anion, hydrogen peroxide, and the hydroxyl radical, which perpetuate cellular damage. Several molecular targets are susceptible to damage from oxidant reactions, including DNA, carbohydrates, cellular proteins, and cell membranes; oxidative modifications in these key cellular molecules can often produce a cytotoxic chain reaction that contributes to the pathogenesis of many diseases, including atherosclerosis, diabetic retinopathy, and others (239–241). Damage to the cell membrane and proteins are of particular significance in AMD (242,243).

RPE cell membranes are highly susceptible to lipid peroxidation. As is the case for all cells, RPE cell membranes are comprised of a phospholipid bilayer, and each phospholipid molecule consists of a pair of fatty acids and a polar head group attached to a glycerol backbone (244). Phospholipids in RPE and photoreceptor membranes are especially rich in polyunsaturated fatty acid (PUFAs), including the ω-3 fatty acid docosahexanoic acid and the ω-6 fatty acid arachadonic acid. The presence of both types of PUFAs in phagocytosed photoreceptor outer segments renders the RPE cell membrane especially susceptible to lipid peroxidation (245,246).

Products of PUFA lipid peroxidation are potentially toxic molecules that can alter cellular metabolism and cell membrane properties. Cellular proteins are also important targets of oxidant-induced modification. Typical chemical modifications include breakdown of disulfide bonds, tyrosylation, acetylation and many other biochemical changes that can alter function of the molecule (247). Although any cellular protein is potentially susceptible, the actin cytoskeleton is especially vulnerable to oxidant-induced damage, and chronic damage to the RPE cell actin cytoskeleton may be associated with deposit formation (248–251). The mitochondria are another important site of injury. Using the environmental toxicant hydroquinone, we have observed that oxidant injury diminishes mitochondrial membrane potential in RPE cells in vitro by creating an electron leak from the mitochondria (Cousins SW, personal communication). Besides impairing cellular respiration, this produces additional oxidant species by perpetuation of aberrant electron transfer and subsequent cellular damage.

Given the ubiquitous nature of oxidant generation, the cell has several well-described pathways, including ubiquitin-proteasome and autophagy, to remove damaged biomolecules (252). Additionally, the cellular antioxidant response is critical for protection against oxidant-mediated injury; it has been found to be upregulated in RPE extracted from human donor eyes with AMD (253).

Many investigators hypothesize that inefficient or overwhelmed cellular antioxidant systems contribute to the development of pathology in AMD. In the Nrf2-deficient mice studied by Zhao et al., increased burden of oxidant species in the absence of key Nrf2-regualted antioxidant genes produced excessive organelle and protein damage, overwhelmed autophagy, and increased exocytosis. The disease phenotype manifested as accumulation of lipofuscin and drusen-like deposits in the retina (254). Knockout mice for superoxide dismutase 1 (SOD1) and SOD2 (enzymes that handle superoxide anion) demonstrate drusen-like deposits and thickened Bruch's membrane (SOD1); and increased accumulation of the bis-retinoid A2E as well as retinal/RPE degeneration (SOD2) (255).

Oxidant-damaged molecules as well as cellular debris and deposits produced because of nonimmune injury can serve as a powerful stimulus for macrophage infiltration and activation. Additionally, oxidants can serve as effective triggers of the complement cascade and subsequent deposition of complement fragments. However, macrophage-mediated innate immunity itself serves as a source of oxidants, through enzyme-dependent oxidase systems (24), both intracellular (NADPH oxidase) and extracellular (myeloperoxidase). These systems, which can generate powerful oxidants such as hydroxyl radicals, hydroperoxides, hypochlorous acid, and tyrosyl radicals, are used in response to encountered pathogens. However, in aberrant low-grade inflammatory response characterizing AMD, these systems may only exacerbate tissue injury and promote complications of the disease.

"RESPONSE TO INJURY": AN INTEGRATED HYPOTHESIS FOR THE PATHOBIOLOGY OF AMD

In AMD, response to injury is implicit in pathogenic models that propose a role for various injurious stimuli, such as oxidants, blue light exposure, and lipofuscin cytotoxicity, or systemic factors such as hyperlipidemia, oxidized lipoproteins, and hormonal changes associated with aging or hypertension (238,256). Both genetic determinants and environmental exposures can influence the individual's response to injury.

Within this conceptual framework, photoreceptors, RPE, choriocapillaris endothelium, and/or choroidal pericytes may all be relevant targets of injurious stimuli and/or the response to injury. RPE can react to nonlethal injury by many responses relevant to deposit formation in AMD, including blebbing, the process by which a cell can pinch off part of its plasma membrane and cytosol in an attempt to discard damaged cellular organelles, molecules, and lipid membranes. Nonlethal blebbing is a nonspecific response of the cell to a variety of injurious stimuli (oxidant injury in particular, but including any of those previously discussed) characterized by the formation of "focal adhesions" (membrane plaques of Hsp25/27, actin, and other proteins) and aggregates of cytoplasmic actin filaments and stress fibers (257–259). For example, RPE can undergo significant blebbing of cell membrane (Fig. 2.8), cytosol and organelles (but without activation of programmed cell death or nuclear fragmentation) after macrophage-derived, myeloperoxidase-mediated lipid peroxidation of the cell membrane.

Irrespective of the stimulus, accumulation of blebs and the concurrent response of the oxidant-injured RPE to alter synthesis of collagen, matrix metalloproteinases and other matrix molecules, lead to deposit formation which can in turn activate an immune response that interferes with healthy repair (260,261). In addition to innate immunity, blebbing might cause desequestration of intracellular antigens to provide a target for antigen-specific immunity or blebs might provide a substrate for nonspecific activation of complement or other amplification systems.

Importantly, response to injury may be critical not only for disease onset but also for disease progression, as with the development of CNV. All blood vessels, including the choriocapillaris, must continuously repair endothelial and vessel wall damage following injury. Increasing evidence suggests that aging is associated with dysregulated vascular repair after injury (113,262,263). For example, abnormal and exaggerated repair following acute vascular injury is a well-defined mechanism for accelerated re-stenosis after coronary artery angioplasty in older patients (262). A similar phenomenon may exist in the choroid in terms of CNV. Aging mice exposed to laser injury of the choroid develop much larger CNV than younger animals, as do mice exposed to toxicants such as nicotine and cigarette smoke (264,265). How alterations in immune and reparative responses determines increased disease severity of neovascular disease remains to be determined.

CONCLUSIONS

The response to injury hypothesis has been proposed for the pathogenesis of numerous diseases, and growing evidence suggests that this paradigm is central to AMD as well. This chapter has explored innate immunity, antigen-specific immunity, and immune amplification systems, and has examined how each might trigger injury and modulate abnormal repair in AMD and other diseases. The response to injury paradigm proposes that the interaction of these immune mechanisms with nonimmune cells and factors generates exaggerated or abnormal reparative responses to chronic, recurrent injurious stimuli, ultimately resulting in the pathological features of disease. Identifying which immune mechanisms make the greatest contribution to AMD pathogenesis may allow earlier diagnosis and effective therapies for those afflicted with this vision-threatening disease.

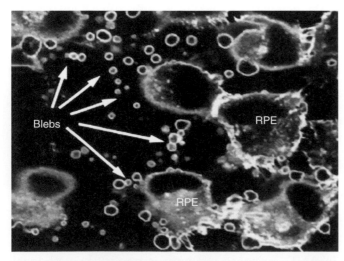

Figure 2.8 Image of retinal pigment epithelial cells in-culture exhibiting extensive cell membrane blebbing following sublethal oxidative injury.

SUMMARY POINTS

- Biology of the immune response in age-related macular degeneration (AMD)
- Innate immunity may be activated by retinal or choroidal injury or infection
- Antigen-specific immunity may be activated
  ° Normally by foreign antigens
  ° Aberrantly in AMD by molecular mimicry, antigen desequestration, neoantigen formation, or antigen trapping
- Amplification mechanisms involved in the immunology of AMD include complement, cytokines, oxidants, and others
- Immune cells that participate in the immunology of AMD include monocytes/ macrophages, dendritic cells, mast cells, and lymphocytes
- Innate immunity, antigen-specific immunity, and amplification cascades contribute to the pathogenesis of atherosclerosis and glomerular diseases which have parallels to AMD
- Evidence supports contributions of innate immunity (macrophages and microglia), complement, and oxidants to the pathobiology of AMD

REFERENCES

1. Halliwell B, Gutteridge JMC. Free Radicals in Biology and Medicine. Oxford: Clarendon Press, 1999.
2. Oppenheim JJ, Feldman M. Cytokine Reference: A Compendium of Cytokines and Other Mediators of Host Defense. London: Academic Press, 2000.
3. Male D, Male, D., Cooke A, Cooke, A., Owen M, Owen, M., Trowsdale J, Trowsdale, J., Champion B. Champion, B. Advanced Immunology. London: Mosby, 1996.
4. Gordon S. Macrophages and the Immune Response. Philadelphia: Lippencott-Raven Publishers, 1999.
5. Moilanen W, Whittle B, Moncada S. Nitric oxide as a factor in inflammation. In: Gallin JI, Synderman R, eds. Inflammation: Basic Principles and Clinical Correlates, 3rd edn. Philadelphia: Lippincott Williams and Wilkins, 1999.
6. Hamrick TS, Havell EA, Horton JR, Orndorff PE. Host and bacterial factors involved in the innate ability of mouse macrophages to eliminate internalized unopsonized Escherichia coli. Infect Immun 2000; 68: 125–32.
7. Cooper NR. Biology of complement. In: Gallin JI, Synderman R, eds. Inflammation: Basic Principles and Clinical Correlates, 3rd edn. Philadelphia: Lippincott Williams and Wilkins, 1999.
8. Prodinger WM, Wurzner R, Erdei A, Dietrich MP. Complement. In: Paul WE, ed. Fundamental Immunology, 4th edn. Philadelphia: Lippencott-Raven Publishers, 1999.
9. Gasque P, Dean YD, McGreal EP, VanBeek J, Morgan BP. Complement components of the innate immune system in health and disease in the CNS. Immunopharmacology 2000; 49: 171–86.
10. Juel HB, Kaestel C, Folkersen L, et al. Retinal pigment epithelial cells upregulate expression of complement factors after co-culture with activated T cells. Exp Eye Res 2011; 92: 180–8.
11. Gewurz H, Ying SC, Jiang H, Lint TF. Nonimmune activation of the classical complement pathway. Behring Inst Mitt 1993;138–47.
12. Preissner KT, Seiffert D. Role of vitronectin and its receptors in haemostasis and vascular remodeling. Thromb Res 1998; 89: 1–21.
13. Hogasen K, Mollnes TE, Harboe M. Heparin-binding properties of vitronectin are linked to complex formation as illustrated by in vitro polymerization and binding to the terminal complement complex. J Biol Chem 1992; 267: 23076–82.
14. Sorensen IJ, Nielsen EH, Andersen O, Danielsen B, Svehag SE. Binding of complement proteins C1q and C4bp to serum amyloid P component (SAP) in solid contra liquid phase. Scand J Immunol 1996; 44: 401–7.
15. Boldt AB, Goeldner I, de Messias-Reason IJ. Relevance of the lectin pathway of complement in rheumatic diseases. Adv Clin Chem 2012; 56: 105–53.
16. Ogawa S, Clauss M, Kuwabara K, et al. Hypoxia induces endothelial cell synthesis of membrane-associated proteins. Proc Natl Acad Sci USA 1991; 88: 9897–901.
17. Weinhouse GL, Belloni PN, Farber HW. Effect of hypoxia on endothelial cell surface glycoprotein expression: modulation of glycoprotein IIIa and other specific surface glycoproteins. Exp Cell Res 1993; 208: 465–78.
18. Collard CD, Lekowski R, Jordan JE, Agah A, Stahl GL. Complement activation following oxidative stress. Mol Immunol 1999; 36: 941–8.
19. Collard CD, Vakeva A, Morrissey MA, et al. Complement activation after oxidative stress: role of the lectin complement pathway. Am J Pathol 2000; 156: 1549–56.
20. Zhou J, Jang YP, Kim SR, Sparrow JR. Complement activation by photooxidation products of A2E, a lipofuscin constituent of the retinal pigment epithelium. Proc Natl Acad Sci USA 2006; 103: 16182–7.
21. Bardenstein DS, Cheyer C, Okada N, Morgan BP, Medof ME. Cell surface regulators of complement, 5I2 antigen, and CD59, in the rat eye and adnexal tissues. Invest Ophthalmol Vis Sci 1999; 40: 519–24.
22. Lass JH, Walter EI, Burris TE, et al. Expression of two molecular forms of the complement decay-accelerating factor in the eye and lacrimal gland. Invest Ophthalmol Vis Sci 1990; 31: 1136–48.
23. Wasmuth S, Lueck K, Baehler H, Lommatzsch A, Pauleikhoff D. Increased vitronectin production by complement-stimulated human retinal pigment epithelial cells. Invest Ophthalmol Vis Sci 2009; 50: 5304–9.
24. Khodr B, Khalil Z. Modulation of inflammation by reactive oxygen species: implications for aging and tissue repair. Free Radic Biol Med 2001; 30: 1–8.
25. Leto TS. Respiratory burst oxidase. In: Gallin JI, Synderman R, eds. Inflammation: Basic Principles and Clinical Correlates, 3rd edn. Philadelphia: Lippincott Williams and Wilkins, 1999.
26. Heinecke JW. Mechanisms of oxidative damage by myeloperoxidase in atherosclerosis and other inflammatory disorders. J Lab Clin Med 1999; 133: 321–5.
27. Knight JA. Free radicals: their history and current status in aging and disease. Ann Clin Lab Sci 1998; 28: 331–46.
28. Wozniak W. Origin and the functional role of microglia. Folia Morphol (Warsz) 1998; 57: 277–85.
29. Naito M, Umeda S, Yamamoto T, et al. Development, differentiation, and phenotypic heterogeneity of murine tissue macrophages. J Leukoc Biol 1996; 59: 133–8.
30. Faust N, Huber MC, Sippel AE, Bonifer C. Different macrophage populations develop from embryonic/fetal and adult hematopoietic tissues. Exp Hematol 1997; 25: 432–44.
31. Jiang Y, Beller DI, Frendl G, Graves DT. Monocyte chemoattractant protein-1 regulates adhesion molecule expression and cytokine production in human monocytes. J Immunol 1992; 148: 2423–8.
32. Schumann RR, Latz E. Lipopolysaccharide-binding protein. Chem Immunol 2000; 74: 42–60.
33. Schlegel RA, Krahling S, Callahan MK, Williamson P. CD14 is a component of multiple recognition systems used by macrophages to phagocytose apoptotic lymphocytes. Cell Death Differ 1999; 6: 583–92.
34. Hammerstrom J. Human macrophage differentiation in vivo and in vitro. A comparison of human peritoneal macrophages and monocytes. Acta Pathol Microbiol Scand [C] 1979; 87C: 113–20.
35. Takahashi K, Naito M, Takeya M. Development and heterogeneity of macrophages and their related cells through their differentiation pathways. Pathol Int 1996; 46: 473–85.
36. Blackwell JM, Searle S. Genetic regulation of macrophage activation: understanding the function of Nramp1 (=Ity/Lsh/Bcg). Immunol Lett 1999; 65: 73–80.
37. Rutherford MS, Witsell A, Schook LB. Mechanisms generating functionally heterogeneous macrophages: chaos revisited. J Leukoc Biol 1993; 53: 602–18.

38. Everson MP, Chandler DB. Changes in distribution, morphology, and tumor necrosis factor-alpha secretion of alveolar macrophage subpopulations during the development of bleomycin-induced pulmonary fibrosis. Am J Pathol 1992; 140: 503–12.

39. Chettibi S, Ferguson MJ. Wound repari: an overview. In: Gallin JI, Synderman R, eds. Inflammation: Basic Principles and Clinical Correlates, 3rd edn. Philadelphia: Lippincott Williams and Wilkins, 1999.

40. Arenberg DA, Strieter RM. Angiogenesis. In: Gallin JI, Synderman R, eds. Inflammation: Basic Principles and Clinical Correlates, 3rd edn. Philadelphia: Lippincott Williams and Wilkins, 1999.

41. Postlewaite AE, Kang AH. Fibroblasts and matrix proteins. In: Gallin JI, Synderman R, eds. Inflammation: Basic Principles and Clinical Correlates, 3rd edn. Philadelphia: Lippincott Williams and Wilkins, 1999.

42. Jackson JR, Seed MP, Kircher CH, Willoughby DA, Winkler JD. The codependence of angiogenesis and chronic inflammation. Faseb J 1997; 11: 457–65.

43. Polverini PJ. How the extracellular matrix and macrophages contribute to angiogenesis-dependent diseases. Eur J Cancer 1996; 32A: 2430–7.

44. Laskin DL, Laskin JD. Macrophages, inflammatory mediators, and lung injury. Methods 1996; 10: 61–70.

45. Hauser CJ. Regional macrophage activation after injury and the compartmentalization of inflammation in trauma. New Horiz 1996; 4: 235–51.

46. Raines EW, Ross R. Is overamplification of the normal macrophage defensive role critical to lesion development? Ann NY Acad Sci 1997; 811: 76–85.

47. Penfold PL, Killingsworth MC, Sarks SH. Senile macular degeneration: the involvement of immunocompetent cells. Graefes Arch Clin Exp Ophthalmol 1985; 223: 69–76.

48. Penfold P, Killingsworth M, Sarks S. An ultrastructural study of the role of leucocytes and fibroblasts in the breakdown of Bruch's membrane. Aust J Ophthalmol 1984; 12: 23–31.

49. Killingsworth MC, Sarks JP, Sarks SH. Macrophages related to Bruch's membrane in age-related macular degeneration. Eye 1990; 4(Pt 4): 613–21.

50. Lopez PF, Grossniklaus HE, Lambert HM, et al. Pathologic features of surgically excised subretinal neovascular membranes in age-related macular degeneration. Am J Ophthalmol 1991; 112: 647–56.

51. Oh H, Takagi H, Takagi C, et al. The potential angiogenic role of macrophages in the formation of choroidal neovascular membranes. Invest Ophthalmol Vis Sci 1999; 40: 1891–8.

52. Cousins SW, Espinosa-Heidmann DG, Csaky KG. Monocyte activation in patients with age-related macular degeneration: a biomarker of risk for choroidal neovascularization? Arch Ophthalmol 2004; 122: 1013–18.

53. Steinman RM. Dendritic Cells. Philadelphia: Lippencott-Raven Publishers, 1999.

54. McMenamin PG. The distribution of immune cells in the uveal tract of the normal eye. Eye 1997; 11(Pt 2): 183–93.

55. Forrester JV, Liversidge J, Dick A, et al. What determines the site of inflammation in uveitis and chorioretinitis? Eye 1997; 11(Pt 2): 162–6.

56. Nilsson G, Costa JJ, Metcalfe DD. Mast cells and basophils. In: Gallin JI, Synderman R, eds. Inflammation: Basic Principles and Clinical Correlates, 3rd edn. Philadelphia: Lippincott Williams and Wilkins, 1999.

57. Dines KC, Powell HC. Mast cell interactions with the nervous system: relationship to mechanisms of disease. J Neuropathol Exp Neurol 1997; 56: 627–40.

58. Meininger CJ. Mast cells and tumor-associated angiogenesis. Chem Immunol 1995; 62: 239–57.

59. Hagiwara K, Khaskhely NM, Uezato H, Nonaka S. Mast cell "densities" in vascular proliferations: a preliminary study of pyogenic granuloma, portwine stain, cavernous hemangioma, cherry angioma, Kaposi's sarcoma, and malignant hemangioendothelioma. J Dermatol 1999; 26: 577–86.

60. Costa JJ, Galli SJ. Mast cells and basophils. In: Rich R, Flesher TA, Schwartz BD, Shearer WT, Strober W, eds. Clinical Immunology: Principles and Practice. Vol. 1. St. Louis: Mosby, 1996.

61. Kovanen PT. Role of mast cells in atherosclerosis. Chem Immunol 1995; 62: 132–70.

62. Ignatescu MC, Gharehbaghi-Schnell E, Hassan A, et al. Expression of the angiogenic protein, platelet-derived endothelial cell growth factor, in coronary atherosclerotic plaques: In vivo correlation of lesional microvessel density and constrictive vascular remodeling. Arterioscler Thromb Vasc Biol 1999; 19: 2340–7.

63. Kaartinen M, van der Wal AC, van der Loos CM, et al. Mast cell infiltration in acute coronary syndromes: implications for plaque rupture. J Am Coll Cardiol 1998; 32: 606–12.

64. Boesiger J, Tsai M, Maurer M, et al. Mast cells can secrete vascular permeability factor/vascular endothelial cell growth factor and exhibit enhanced release after immunoglobulin E-dependent upregulation of fc epsilon receptor I expression. J Exp Med 1998; 188: 1135–45.

65. Kanbe N, Tanaka A, Kanbe M, et al. Human mast cells produce matrix metalloproteinase 9. Eur J Immunol 1999; 29: 2645–9.

66. Johnson JL, Jackson CL, Angelini GD, George SJ. Activation of matrix-degrading metalloproteinases by mast cell proteases in atherosclerotic plaques. Arterioscler Thromb Vasc Biol 1998; 18: 1707–15.

67. May CA. Mast cell heterogeneity in the human uvea. Histochem Cell Biol 1999; 112: 381–6.

68. Tonnesen MG, Feng X, Clark RA. Angiogenesis in wound healing. J Investig Dermatol Symp Proc 2000; 5: 40–6.

69. Azizkhan RG, Azizkhan JC, Zetter BR, Folkman J. Mast cell heparin stimulates migration of capillary endothelial cells in vitro. J Exp Med 1980; 152: 931–44.

70. Tharp MD. The interaction between mast cells and endothelial cells. J Invest Dermatol 1989; 93: 107S–12S.

71. Takehana Y, Kurokawa T, Kitamura T, et al. Suppression of laser-induced choroidal neovascularization by oral tranilast in the rat. Invest Ophthalmol Vis Sci 1999; 40: 459–66.

72. Janeway CA, Tavers P, Walport M. Immunobiology. London: Academic Press, 1999.

73. Roitt IM. Roitt's Essential Immunology. Oxford: Blackwell Science Ltd, 1999.

74. Seder RA, Mosmann TM. Differentiation of Effector Phenotypes of CD4+ and CD8+ cells. Philadelphia: Lippencott-Raven Publishers, 1999.

75. Benoist C, Mathis D. T-lymphocyte Differentiation and Biology. Philadelphia: Lippencott-Raven Publishers, 1999.

76. Robman L, Mahdi O, McCarty C, et al. Exposure to Chlamydia pneumoniae infection and progression of

age-related macular degeneration. Am J Epidemiol 2005; 161: 1013–19.

77. Dunn DE, Jin JP, Lancki DW, Fitch FW. An alternative pathway of induction of lymphokine production by T lymphocyte clones. J Immunol 1989; 142: 3847–56.

78. Lee KP, Harlan DM, June CH. Role of costimulation in the host response to infection. In: Gallin JI, Synderman R, eds. Inflammation: Basic Principles and Clinical Correlates, 3rd edn. Philadelphia: Lippincott Williams and Wilkins, 1999.

79. Augustin AA, Julius MH, Cosenza H. Antigen-specific stimulation and trans-stimulation of T cells in long-term culture. Eur J Immunol 1979; 9: 665–70.

80. Clark MR. IgG effector mechanisms. Chem Immunol 1997; 65: 88–110.

81. Dwyer JM. Immunoglobulins in autoimmunity: history and mechanisms of action. Clin Exp Rheumatol 1996; 14(Suppl 15): S3–7.

82. Reichlin M. Cellular dysfunction induced by penetration of autoantibodies into living cells: cellular damage and dysfunction mediated by antibodies to dsDNA and ribosomal P proteins. J Autoimmun 1998; 11: 557–61.

83. Shoenfeld Y, Alarcon-Segovia D, Buskila D, et al. Frontiers of SLE: review of the 5th International Congress of Systemic Lupus Erythematosus, Cancun, Mexico, April 20–25, 1998. Semin Arthritis Rheum 1999; 29: 112–30.

84. Adamus G, Machnicki M, Elerding H, et al. Antibodies to recoverin induce apoptosis of photoreceptor and bipolar cells in vivo. J Autoimmun 1998; 11: 523–33.

85. Rosenberg HF, Gallin JI. Inflammation. Philadelphia: Lippencott-Raven Publishers, 1999.

86. Descotes J, Choquet-Kastylevsky G, Van Ganse E, Vial T. Responses of the immune system to injury. Toxicol Pathol 2000; 28: 479–81.

87. Cotran RS, Kumar V, Collins T, Robbins SL. Robbins Pathologic Basis of Disease. Philadelphia: WB Saunders Co, 1999.

88. Silverstein RL. The vascular endothelium. In: Gallin JI, Synderman R, editors. Inflammation: Basic Principles and Clinical Correlates, 3rd edn. Philadelphia: Lippincott Williams and Wilkins, 1999.

89. Mims CA, Nash A, Stephen J. Mims Pathogenesis of Infectious Diseases. London: Academic Press, 2001.

90. Blaser MJ, Smith PD. Persistent mucosal colonization by Helicobacter pylori and the induction of inflammation. In: Gallin JI, Synderman R, editors. Inflammation: Basic Principles and Clinical Correlates, 3rd edn. Philadelphia: Lippincott Williams and Wilkins, 1999.

91. Robman L, Mahdi OS, Wang JJ, et al. Exposure to Chlamydia pneumoniae infection and age-related macular degeneration: the Blue Mountains Eye Study. Invest Ophthalmol Vis Sci 2007; 48: 4007–11.

92. Guymer R, Robman L. Chlamydia pneumoniae and age-related macular degeneration: a role in pathogenesis or merely a chance association? Clin Experiment Ophthalmol 2007; 35: 89–93.

93. Miller DM, Espinosa-Heidmann DG, Legra J, et al. The association of prior cytomegalovirus infection with neovascular age-related macular degeneration. Am J Ophthalmol 2004; 138: 323–8.

94. Cousins SW, Espinosa-Heidmann DG, Miller DM, et al. Macrophage activation associated with chronic murine cytomegalovirus infection results in more severe experimental choroidal neovascularization. PLoS Pathog 2012; 8: e1002671.

95. Weiss A. T-lymphocyte activation. Philadelphia: Lippencott-Raven Publishers, 1999.

96. Gregerson DS. Immune privilege in the retina. Ocul Immunol Inflamm 1998; 6: 257–67.

97. Cousins SW, Dix RD. Immunology of the eye. In Immunology of the Nervous System. Keane RW, Hickey WF, eds. New York: Oxford University Press, 1997.

98. Shevach EM. Organ-specific autoimmunity. Philadelphia: Lippencott-Raven Publishers, 1999.

99. Singh VK, Kalra HK, Yamaki K, et al. Molecular mimicry between a uveitopathogenic site of S-antigen and viral peptides. Induction of experimental autoimmune uveitis in Lewis rats. J Immunol 1990; 144: 1282–7.

100. Levine JS, Koh JS. The role of apoptosis in autoimmunity: immunogen, antigen, and accelerant. Semin Nephrol 1999; 19: 34–47.

101. Berden JH, van Bruggen MC. Nucleosomes and the pathogenesis of lupus nephritis. Kidney Blood Press Res 1997; 20: 198–200.

102. Gregerson DS, Torseth JW, McPherson SW, et al. Retinal expression of a neo-self antigen, beta-galactosidase, is not tolerogenic and creates a target for autoimmune uveoretinitis. J Immunol 1999; 163: 1073–80.

103. Ross R. Atherogenesis. In: Gallin JI, Synderman R, editors. Inflammation: Basic Principles and Clinical Correlates, 3rd edn. Philadelphia: Lippincott Williams and Wilkins, 1999.

104. Adler S, Couser W. Immunologic mechanisms of renal disease. Am J Med Sci 1985; 289: 55–60.

105. Dick AD. Immune mechanisms of uveitis: insights into disease pathogenesis and treatment. Int Ophthalmol Clin 2000; 40: 1–18.

106. Smith RE. Commentary on histoplasmosis. Ocul Immunol Inflamm 1997; 5: 69–70.

107. Klein R, Klein BE, Jensen SC. The relation of cardiovascular disease and its risk factors to the 5-year incidence of age-related maculopathy: the Beaver Dam Eye Study. Ophthalmology 1997; 104: 1804–12.

108. Hyman L, Schachat AP, He Q, Leske MC. Hypertension, cardiovascular disease, and age-related macular degeneration. age-related macular degeneration risk factors study group. Arch Ophthalmol 2000; 118: 351–8.

109. Vingerling JR, Dielemans I, Bots ML, et al. Age-related macular degeneration is associated with atherosclerosis. the rotterdam study. Am J Epidemiol 1995; 142: 404–9.

110. Ross R. Atherosclerosis–an inflammatory disease. N Engl J Med 1999; 340: 115–26.

111. Masuda J, Ross R. Atherogenesis during low level hypercholesterolemia in the nonhuman primate. I. Fatty streak formation. Arteriosclerosis 1990; 10: 164–77.

112. Curcio CA, Millican CL, Bailey T, Kruth HS. Accumulation of cholesterol with age in human Bruch's membrane. Invest Ophthalmol Vis Sci 2001; 42: 265–74.

113. Hariri RJ, Alonso DR, Hajjar DP, Coletti D, Weksler ME. Aging and arteriosclerosis. I. Development of myointimal hyperplasia after endothelial injury. J Exp Med 1986; 164: 1171–8.

114. Napoli C. Low density lipoprotein oxidation and atherogenesis: from experimental models to clinical studies. G Ital Cardiol 1997; 27: 1302–14.

115. Nagornev VA, Maltseva SV. The phenotype of macrophages which are not transformed into foam cells in atherogenesis. Atherosclerosis 1996; 121: 245–51.

116. Klaver CC, Kliffen M, van Duijn CM, et al. Genetic association of apolipoprotein E with age-related macular degeneration. Am J Hum Genet 1998; 63: 200–6.

117. Ross R, Masuda J, Raines EW, et al. Localization of PDGF-B protein in macrophages in all phases of atherogenesis. Science 1990; 248: 1009–12.

118. Rajavashisth TB, Xu XP, Jovinge S, et al. Membrane type 1 matrix metalloproteinase expression in human atherosclerotic plaques: evidence for activation by proinflammatory mediators. Circulation 1999; 99: 3103–9.

119. George SJ. Tissue inhibitors of metalloproteinases and metalloproteinases in atherosclerosis. Curr Opin Lipidol 1998; 9: 413–23.

120. Clinton SK, Underwood R, Hayes L, et al. Macrophage colony-stimulating factor gene expression in vascular cells and in experimental and human atherosclerosis. Am J Pathol 1992; 140: 301–16.

121. de Boer OJ, van der Wal AC, Becker AE. Atherosclerosis, inflammation, and infection. J Pathol 2000; 190: 237–43.

122. Saikku P. Epidemiologic association of Chlamydia pneumoniae and atherosclerosis: the initial serologic observation and more. J Infect Dis 2000; 181(Suppl 3): S411–13.

123. Taylor-Robinson D, Thomas BJ. Chlamydia pneumoniae in atherosclerotic tissue. J Infect Dis 2000; 181(Suppl 3): S437–40.

124. Meier CR. Antibiotics in the prevention and treatment of coronary heart disease. J Infect Dis 2000; 181(Suppl 3): S558–62.

125. Leinonen M. Chlamydia pneumoniae and other risk factors for atherosclerosis. J Infect Dis 2000; 181(Suppl 3): S414–16.

126. Kol A, Lichtman AH, Finberg RW, Libby P, Kurt-Jones EA. Cutting edge: heat shock protein (HSP) 60 activates the innate immune response: CD14 is an essential receptor for HSP60 activation of mononuclear cells. J Immunol 2000; 164: 13–17.

127. Kol A, Bourcier T, Lichtman AH, Libby P. Chlamydial and human heat shock protein 60s activate human vascular endothelium, smooth muscle cells, and macrophages. J Clin Invest 1999; 103: 571–7.

128. Tezel G, Wax MB. The mechanisms of hsp27 antibody-mediated apoptosis in retinal neuronal cells. J Neurosci 2000; 20: 3552–62.

129. Leinonen M, Saikku P. Infections and atherosclerosis. Scand Cardiovasc J 2000; 34: 12–20.

130. High KP. Atherosclerosis and infection due to Chlamydia pneumoniae or cytomegalovirus: weighing the evidence. Clin Infect Dis 1999; 28: 746–9.

131. Epstein SE, Zhou YF, Zhu J. Potential role of cytomegalovirus in the pathogenesis of restenosis and atherosclerosis. Am Heart J 1999; 138: S476–8.

132. Silverman GJ, Shaw PX, Luo L, et al. Neo-self antigens and the expansion of B-1 cells: lessons from atherosclerosis-prone mice. Curr Top Microbiol Immunol 2000; 252: 189–200.

133. Wick G, Perschinka H, Xu Q. Autoimmunity and atherosclerosis. Am Heart J 1999; 138: S444–9.

134. Seifert PS, Hugo F, Hansson GK, Bhakdi S. Prelesional complement activation in experimental atherosclerosis. Terminal C5b-9 complement deposition coincides with cholesterol accumulation in the aortic intima of hypercholesterolemic rabbits. Lab Invest 1989; 60: 747–54.

135. Benzaquen LR, Nicholson-Weller A, Halperin JA. Terminal complement proteins C5b-9 release basic fibroblast growth factor and platelet-derived growth factor from endothelial cells. J Exp Med 1994; 179: 985–92.

136. Torzewski M, Torzewski J, Bowyer DE, et al. Immunohistochemical colocalization of the terminal complex of human complement and smooth muscle cell alpha-actin in early atherosclerotic lesions. Arterioscler Thromb Vasc Biol 1997; 17: 2448–52.

137. Hazen SL. Oxidation and atherosclerosis. Free Radic Biol Med 2000; 28: 1683–4.

138. Brenner BM, Rector FC. Brenner and Rector's the Kidney, 6th edn. Philadelphia: Saunders Co, 2000.

139. Makker SP. Mediators of immune glomerular injury. Am J Nephrol 1993; 13: 324–36.

140. Olson JL, Heptinstall RH. Nonimmunologic mechanisms of glomerular injury. Lab Invest 1988; 59: 564–78.

141. Johnson RJ. The glomerular response to injury: progression or resolution? Kidney Int 1994; 45: 1769–82.

142. Neuringer JR, Brenner BM. Glomerular hypertension: cause and consequence of renal injury. J Hypertens Suppl 1992; 10: S91–7.

143. Suzuki D. Metalloproteinases in the pathogenesis of diabetic nephropathy. Nephron 1998; 80: 125–33.

144. Anderson S, Vora JP. Current concepts of renal hemodynamics in diabetes. J Diabetes Complications 1995; 9: 304–7.

145. O'Bryan GT, Hostetter TH. The renal hemodynamic basis of diabetic nephropathy. Semin Nephrol 1997; 17: 93–100.

146. Luft FC, Mervaala E, Muller DN, et al. Hypertension-induced end-organ damage : a new transgenic approach to an old problem. Hypertension 1999; 33: 212–18.

147. Peten EP, Garcia-Perez A, Terada Y, et al. Age-related changes in alpha 1- and alpha 2-chain type IV collagen mRNAs in adult mouse glomeruli: competitive PCR. Am J Physiol 1992; 263: F951–7.

148. Ungar A, Castellani S, Di Serio C, et al. Changes in renal autacoids and hemodynamics associated with aging and isolated systolic hypertension. Prostaglandins Other Lipid Mediat 2000; 62: 117–33.

149. Yang N, Wu LL, Nikolic-Paterson DJ, et al. Local macrophage and myofibroblast proliferation in progressive renal injury in the rat remnant kidney. Nephrol Dial Transplant 1998; 13: 1967–74.

150. Suto TS, Fine LG, Shimizu F, Kitamura M. In vivo transfer of engineered macrophages into the glomerulus: endogenous TGF-beta-mediated defense against macrophage-induced glomerular cell activation. J Immunol 1997; 159: 2476–83.

151. Pawluczyk IZ, Harris KP. Macrophages promote prosclerotic responses in cultured rat mesangial cells: a mechanism for the initiation of glomerulosclerosis. J Am Soc Nephrol 1997; 8: 1525–36.

152. Pawluczyk IZ, Harris KP. Cholesterol feeding activates macrophages to upregulate rat mesangial cell fibronectin production. Nephrol Dial Transplant 2000; 15: 161–6.

153. D'Souza MJ, Oettinger CW, Shah A, et al. Macrophage depletion by albumin microencapsulated clodronate: attenuation of cytokine release in macrophage-dependent glomerulonephritis. Drug Dev Ind Pharm 1999; 25: 591–6.

154. Kamanna VS, Pai R, Ha H, Kirschenbaum MA, Roh DD. Oxidized low-density lipoprotein stimulates monocyte adhesion to glomerular endothelial cells. Kidney Int 1999; 55: 2192–202.

155. Hattori M, Nikolic-Paterson DJ, Miyazaki K, et al. Mechanisms of glomerular macrophage infiltration in lipid-induced renal injury. Kidney Int Suppl 1999; 71: S47–50.

156. Duffield JS, Erwig LP, Wei X, et al. Activated macrophages direct apoptosis and suppress mitosis of mesangial cells. J Immunol 2000; 164: 2110–19.

157. Kitamura M. Adoptive transfer of nuclear factor-kappaB-inactive macrophages to the glomerulus. Kidney Int 2000; 57: 709–16.

158. Lan HY, Yang N, Brown FG, et al. Macrophage migration inhibitory factor expression in human renal allograft rejection. Transplantation 1998; 66: 1465–71.

159. Ponticelli C. Progression of renal damage in chronic rejection. Kidney Int Suppl 2000; 75: S62–70.

160. Bennett WM, Fassett RG, Walker RG, et al. Mesangiocapillary glomerulonephritis type II (dense-deposit disease): clinical features of progressive disease. Am J Kidney Dis 1989; 13: 469–76.

161. Joh K, Aizawa S, Matsuyama N, et al. Morphologic variations of dense deposit disease: light and electron microscopic, immunohistochemical and clinical findings in 10 patients. Acta Pathol Jpn 1993; 43: 552–65.

162. Nangaku M, Couser WG. Mechanisms of immune-deposit formation and the mediation of immune renal injury. Clin Exp Nephrol 2005; 9: 183–91.

163. Nordstrand A, Norgren M, Holm SE. Pathogenic mechanism of acute post-streptococcal glomerulonephritis. Scand J Infect Dis 1999; 31: 523–37.

164. Roos A, Sato T, Maier H, van Kooten C, Daha MR. Induction of renal cell apoptosis by antibodies and complement. Exp Nephrol 2001; 9: 65–70.

165. al-Nawab MD, Jones NF, Davies DR. Glomerular epithelial cell endocytosis of immune deposits in human lupus nephritis. Nephrol Dial Transplant 1991; 6: 316–23.

166. Jansen JH, Hogasen K, Mollnes TE. Extensive complement activation in hereditary porcine membranoproliferative glomerulonephritis type II (porcine dense deposit disease). Am J Pathol 1993; 143: 1356–65.

167. Leys A, Vanrenterghem Y, Van Damme B, et al. Fundus changes in membranoproliferative glomerulonephritis type II. A fluorescein angiographic study of 23 patients. Graefes Arch Clin Exp Ophthalmol 1991; 229: 406–10.

168. Leys A, Michielsen B, Leys M, Vanrenterghem Y, Missotten L, Van Damme B. Subretinal neovascular membranes associated with chronic membranoproliferative glomerulonephritis type II. Graefes Arch Clin Exp Ophthalmol 1990; 228: 499–504.

169. Michielsen B, Leys A, Van Damme B, Missotten L. Fundus changes in chronic membranoproliferative glomerulonephritis type II. Doc Ophthalmol 1990; 76: 219–29.

170. Baud L, Fouqueray B, Philippe C, Ardaillou R. Reactive oxygen species as glomerular autacoids. J Am Soc Nephrol 1992; 2: S132–8.

171. Johnson LV, Ozaki S, Staples MK, Erickson PA, Anderson DH. A potential role for immune complex pathogenesis in drusen formation. Exp Eye Res 2000; 70: 441–9.

172. Mullins RF, Russell SR, Anderson DH, Hageman GS. Drusen associated with aging and age-related macular degeneration contain proteins common to extracellular deposits associated with atherosclerosis, elastosis, amyloidosis, and dense deposit disease. Faseb J 2000; 14: 835–46.

173. Anderson DH, Mullins RF, Hageman GS, Johnson LV. A role for local inflammation in the formation of drusen in the aging eye. Am J Ophthalmol 2002; 134: 411–31.

174. Hageman GS, Luthert PJ, Victor Chong NH, et al. An integrated hypothesis that considers drusen as biomarkers of immune-mediated processes at the RPE-Bruch's membrane interface in aging and age-related macular degeneration. Prog Retin Eye Res 2001; 20: 705–32.

175. Cherepanoff S, McMenamin P, Gillies MC, Kettle E, Sarks SH. Bruch's membrane and choroidal macrophages in early and advanced age-related macular degeneration. Br J Ophthalmol 2010; 94: 918–25.

176. Penfold PL, Madigan MC, Gillies MC, Provis JM. Immunological and aetiological aspects of macular degeneration. Prog Retin Eye Res 2001; 20: 385–414.

177. Grossniklaus HE, Cingle KA, Yoon YD, et al. Correlation of histologic 2-dimensional reconstruction and confocal scanning laser microscopic imaging of choroidal neovascularization in eyes with age-related maculopathy. Arch Ophthalmol 2000; 118: 625–9.

178. Espinosa-Heidmann DG, Suner IJ, Hernandez EP, et al. Macrophage depletion diminishes lesion size and severity in experimental choroidal neovascularization. Invest Ophthalmol Vis Sci 2003; 44: 3586–92.

179. Caicedo A, Espinosa-Heidmann DG, Pina Y, Hernandez EP, Cousins SW. Blood-derived macrophages infiltrate the retina and activate Muller glial cells under experimental choroidal neovascularization. Exp Eye Res 2005; 81: 38–47.

180. Caicedo A, Espinosa-Heidmann DG, Hamasaki D, Pina Y, Cousins SW. Photoreceptor synapses degenerate early in experimental choroidal neovascularization. J Comp Neurol 2005; 483: 263–77.

181. Tsutsumi C, Sonoda KH, Egashira K, et al. The critical role of ocular-infiltrating macrophages in the development of choroidal neovascularization. J Leukoc Biol 2003; 74: 25–32.

182. Apte RS, Richter J, Herndon J, Ferguson TA. Macrophages inhibit neovascularization in a murine model of age-related macular degeneration. PLoS Med 2006; 3: e310.

183. Skeie JM, Mullins RF. Macrophages in neovascular age-related macular degeneration: friends or foes? Eye (Lond) 2009; 23: 747–55.

184. Osusky R, Malik P, Aurora Y, Ryan SJ. Monocyte-macrophage differentiation induced by coculture of retinal pigment epithelium cells with monocytes. Ophthalmic Res 1997; 29: 124–9.

185. Kurtz RM, Elner VM, Bian ZM, et al. Dexamethasone and cyclosporin A modulation of human retinal pigment epithelial cell monocyte chemotactic protein-1 and interleukin-8. Invest Ophthalmol Vis Sci 1997; 38: 436–45.

186. Platts KE, Benson MT, Rennie IG, Sharrard RM, Rees RC. Cytokine modulation of adhesion molecule expression on human retinal pigment epithelial cells. Invest Ophthalmol Vis Sci 1995; 36: 2262–9.

187. Nagineni CN, Kutty RK, Detrick B, Hooks JJ. Inflammatory cytokines induce intercellular adhesion molecule-1 (ICAM-1) mRNA synthesis and protein secretion by human retinal pigment epithelial cell cultures. Cytokine 1996; 8: 622–30.

188. Osusky R, Soriano D, Ye J, Ryan SJ. Cytokine effect on fibronectin release by retinal pigment epithelial cells. Curr Eye Res 1994; 13: 569–74.

189. Cousins SW, Espinosa-Heidmann DG, Csaky KG. Monocyte activation in patients with age-related macular degeneration: a biomarker of risk for choroidal neovascularization? Arch Ophthalmol 2004; 122: 1013–18.

190. Danis RP, Ciulla TA, Pratt LM, Anliker W. Intravitreal triamcinolone acetonide in exudative age-related macular degeneration. Retina 2000; 20: 244–50.

191. Challa JK, Gillies MC, Penfold PL, et al. Exudative macular degeneration and intravitreal triamcinolone: 18 month follow up. Aust NZ J Ophthalmol 1998; 26: 277–81.

192. Shi X, Semkova I, Muther PS, et al. Inhibition of TNF-alpha reduces laser-induced choroidal neovascularization. Exp Eye Res 2006; 83: 1325–34.

193. Nussenblatt RB, Byrnes G, Sen HN, et al. A randomized pilot study of systemic immunosuppression in the treatment of age-related macular degeneration with choroidal neovascularization. Retina 2010; 30: 1579–87.

194. Theodossiadis PG, Liarakos VS, Sfikakis PP, Vergados IA, Theodossiadis GP. Intravitreal administration of the anti-tumor necrosis factor agent infliximab for neovascular age-related macular degeneration. Am J Ophthalmol 2009; 147: 825–30, 830 e821.

195. Arias L, Caminal JM, Badia MB, et al. Intravitreal infliximab in patients with macular degeneration who are nonresponders to antivascular endothelial growth factor therapy. Retina 2010; 30: 1601–8.

196. Pulido JS, Pulido JE, Michet CJ, Vile RG. More questions than answers: a call for a moratorium on the use of intravitreal infliximab outside of a well-designed trial. Retina 2010; 30: 1–5.

197. Simon LS, Yocum D. New and future drug therapies for rheumatoid arthritis. Rheumatology (Oxford) 2000; 39(Suppl 1): 36–42.

198. Lee JE, Liang KJ, Fariss RN, Wong WT. Ex vivo dynamic imaging of retinal microglia using time-lapse confocal microscopy. Invest Ophthalmol Vis Sci 2008; 49: 4169–76.

199. Gupta N, Brown KE, Milam AH. Activated microglia in human retinitis pigmentosa, late-onset retinal degeneration, and age-related macular degeneration. Exp Eye Res 2003; 76: 463–71.

200. Ma W, Zhao L, Fontainhas AM, Fariss RN, Wong WT. Microglia in the mouse retina alter the structure and function of retinal pigmented epithelial cells: a potential cellular interaction relevant to AMD. PLoS One 2009; 4: e7945.

201. Wang M, Ma W, Zhao L, Fariss RN, Wong WT. Adaptive Muller cell responses to microglial activation mediate neuroprotection and coordinate inflammation in the retina. J Neuroinflammation 2011; 8: 173.

202. Damani MR, Zhao L, Fontainhas AM, et al. Age-related alterations in the dynamic behavior of microglia. Aging Cell 2011; 10: 263–76.

203. Malchiodi-Albedi F, Matteucci A, Bernardo A, Minghetti L. PPAR-gamma, microglial cells, and ocular inflammation: new venues for potential therapeutic approaches. PPAR Res 2008; 295784.

204. Edwards AO, Ritter R 3rd, Abel KJ, et al. Complement factor H polymorphism and age-related macular degeneration. Science 2005; 308: 421–4.

205. Hageman GS, Anderson DH, Johnson LV, et al. A common haplotype in the complement regulatory gene factor H (HF1/CFH) predisposes individuals to age-related macular degeneration. Proc Natl Acad Sci USA 2005; 102: 7227–32.

206. Haines JL, Hauser MA, Schmidt S, et al. Complement factor H variant increases the risk of age-related macular degeneration. Science 2005; 308: 419–21.

207. Klein RJ, Zeiss C, Chew EY, et al. Complement factor H polymorphism in age-related macular degeneration. Science 2005; 308: 385–9.

208. Perkins SJ, Nan R, Li K, Khan S, Miller A. Complement factor H-ligand interactions: self-association, multivalency and dissociation constants. Immunobiology 2012; 217: 281–97.

209. Clark SJ, Bishop PN, Day AJ. Complement factor H and age-related macular degeneration: the role of glycosaminoglycan recognition in disease pathology. Biochem Soc Trans 2010; 38: 1342–8.

210. Chen Y, Zeng J, Zhao C, et al. Assessing susceptibility to age-related macular degeneration with genetic markers and environmental factors. Arch Ophthalmol 2011; 129: 344–51.

211. Fritsche LG, Lauer N, Hartmann A, et al. An imbalance of human complement regulatory proteins CFHR1, CFHR3 and factor H influences risk for age-related macular degeneration (AMD). Hum Mol Genet 2010; 19: 4694–704.

212. Sawitzke J, Im KM, Kostiha B, Dean M, Gold B. Association assessment of copy number polymorphism and risk of age-related macular degeneration. Ophthalmology 2011; 118: 2442–6.

213. Sivakumaran TA, Igo RP Jr, Kidd JM, et al. A 32 kb critical region excluding Y402H in CFH mediates risk for age-related macular degeneration. PLoS One 2011; 6: e25598.

214. Anderson DH, Mullins RF, Hageman GS, Johnson LV. A role for local inflammation in the formation of drusen in the aging eye. Am J Ophthalmol 2002; 134: 411–31.

215. Fett AL, Hermann MM, Muether PS, Kirchhof B, Fauser S. Immunohistochemical localization of complement regulatory proteins in the human retina. Histol Histopathol 2012; 27: 357–64.

216. Fett AL, Hermann MM, Muether PS, Kirchhof B, Fauser S. Immunohistochemical localization of complement regulatory proteins in the human retina. Histol Histopathol 2012; 27: 357–64.

217. Isas JM, Luibl V, Johnson LV, et al. Soluble and mature amyloid fibrils in drusen deposits. Invest Ophthalmol Vis Sci 2010; 51: 1304–10.

218. Wang J, Ohno-Matsui K, Morita I. Elevated amyloid beta production in senescent retinal pigment epithelium, a possible mechanism of subretinal deposition of amyloid beta in age-related macular degeneration. Biochem Biophys Res Comm 2012; 423: 73–8.

219. Ding JD, Johnson LV, Herrmann R, et al. Anti-amyloid therapy protects against retinal pigmented epithelium damage and vision loss in a model of age-related macular degeneration. Proc Natl Acad Sci USA 2011; 108: E279–87.

220. Aiyaz M, Lupton MK, Proitsi P, Powell JF, Lovestone S. Complement activation as a biomarker for Alzheimer's disease. Immunobiology 2012; 217: 204–15.

221. Brantley MA Jr, Osborn MP, Sanders BJ, et al. Plasma biomarkers of oxidative stress and genetic variants in age-related macular degeneration. Am J Ophthalmol 2011; 153: 460–61.

222. Chi ZL, Yoshida T, Lambris JD, Iwata T. Suppression of drusen formation by compstatin, a peptide inhibitor of complement C3 activation, on cynomolgus monkey with early-onset macular degeneration. Adv Exp Med Biol 2010; 703: 127–35.

223. Hollyfield JG. Age-related macular degeneration: the molecular link between oxidative damage, tissue-specific inflammation and outer retinal disease: the Proctor lecture. Invest Ophthalmol Vis Sci 2010; 51: 1275–81.

224. Hollyfield JG, Bonilha VL, Rayborn ME, et al. Oxidative damage-induced inflammation initiates age-related macular degeneration. Nat Med 2008; 14: 194–8.

225. Weismann D, Hartvigsen K, Lauer N, et al. Complement factor H binds malondialdehyde epitopes and protects from oxidative stress. Nature 2011; 478: 76–81.

226. Coffey PJ, Gias C, McDermott CJ, et al. Complement factor H deficiency in aged mice causes retinal abnormalities and visual dysfunction. Proc Natl Acad Sci USA 2007; 104: 16651–6.

227. Christenbury JG, Ding JD, Kelly U, Groelle M, Bowes Rickman C. Effect of excess complement activation on AMD-like pathology in the APOE4/cfh knockout transgenic murine model: does loss-of-function exacerbate retinal disease? Invest Ophthalmol Vis Sci 2012; 53: 1641 (ARVO E-Abstract).

228. Ufret-Vincenty RL, Aredo B, Liu X, et al. Transgenic mice expressing variants of complement factor H develop AMD-like retinal findings. Invest Ophthalmol Vis Sci 2010; 51: 5878–87.

229. Hageman GS, Mullins RF, Russell SR, Johnson LV, Anderson DH. Vitronectin is a constituent of ocular drusen and the vitronectin gene is expressed in human retinal pigmented epithelial cells. Faseb J 1999; 13: 477–84.

230. Reynolds R, Hartnett ME, Atkinson JP, et al. Plasma complement components and activation fragments: associations with age-related macular degeneration genotypes and phenotypes. Invest Ophthalmol Vis Sci 2009; 50: 5818–27.

231. Troutbeck R, Al-Qureshi S, Guymer RH. Therapeutic targeting of the complement system in age-related macular degeneration: a review. Clin Experiment Ophthalmol 2012; 40: 18–26.

232. Garcia Filho CAA, Yehoshua Z, Gregori G, et al. Efficacy of the systemic complement inhibitor eculizumab in AMD patients with drusen: the COMPLETE study. Invest Ophthalmol Vis Sci 2012; 53: 2045 (ARVO E-Abstract).

233. Yehoshua Z, Garcia Filho CAA, Gregori G, et al. Systemic complement inhibition with eculizumab for the treatment of geographic atrophy in AMD patients: the COMPLETE study. Invest Ophthalmol Vis Sci 2012; 53: 2046 (ARVO E-Abstract).

234. Winkler BS, Boulton ME, Gottsch JD, Sternberg P. Oxidative damage and age-related macular degeneration. Mol Vis 1999; 5: 32.

235. Rozanowska M, Jarvis-Evans J, Korytowski W, et al. Blue light-induced reactivity of retinal age pigment. In vitro generation of oxygen-reactive species. J Biol Chem 1995; 270: 18825–30.

236. Gottsch JD, Bynoe LA, Harlan JB, Rencs EV, Green WR. Light-induced deposits in Bruch's membrane of protoporphyric mice. Arch Ophthalmol 1993; 111: 126–9.

237. Boulton M, Dontsov A, Jarvis-Evans J, Ostrovsky M, Svistunenko D. Lipofuscin is a photoinducible free radical generator. J Photochem Photobiol B 1993; 19: 201–4.

238. Mettu PS, Wielgus AR, Ong SS, Cousins SW. Retinal pigment epithelium response to oxidant injury in the pathogenesis of early age-related macular degeneration. Mol Aspects Med 2012; 33: 376–98.

239. Florence TM. The role of free radicals in disease. Aust NZ J Ophthalmol 1995; 23: 3–7.

240. Machlin LJ, Bendich A. Free radical tissue damage: protective role of antioxidant nutrients. FASEB J 1987; 1: 441–5.

241. Stohs SJ. The role of free radicals in toxicity and disease. J Basic Clin Physiol Pharmacol 1995; 6: 205–28.

242. Chisolm GM 3rd, Hazen SL, Fox PL, Cathcart MK. The oxidation of lipoproteins by monocytes-macrophages. Biochemical and biological mechanisms. J Biol Chem 1999; 274: 25959–62.

243. St-Pierre Y, Van Themsche C, Esteve PO. Emerging features in the regulation of MMP-9 gene expression for the development of novel molecular targets and therapeutic strategies. current drug targets. Inflamm aller 2003; 2: 206–15.

244. Cribier S, Morrot G, Zachowski A. Dynamics of the membrane lipid phase. Prostaglandins Leukot Essent Fatty Acids 1993; 48: 27–32.

245. Beatty S, Koh H, Phil M, Henson D, Boulton M. The role of oxidative stress in the pathogenesis of age-related macular degeneration. Surv Ophthalmol 2000; 45: 115–34.

246. Wilhelm J. Metabolic aspects of membrane lipid peroxidation. Acta Universitatis Carolinae. Med Monogr 1990; 137: 1–53.

247. Blokhina O, Virolainen E, Fagerstedt KV. Antioxidants, oxidative damage and oxygen deprivation stress: a review. Ann Bot (Lond) 2003; 91: 179–94.

248. Marin-Castano ME, Csaky KG, Cousins SW. Nonlethal oxidant injury to human retinal pigment epithelium cells causes cell membrane blebbing but decreased MMP-2 activity. Invest Ophthalmol Vis Sci 2005; 46: 3331–40.

249. Marin-Castano ME, Striker GE, Alcazar O, et al. Repetitive nonlethal oxidant injury to retinal pigment epithelium decreased extracellular matrix turnover in vitro and induced sub-RPE deposits in vivo. Invest Ophthalmol Vis Sci 2006; 47: 4098–112.

250. Pons M, Cousins SW, Csaky KG, Striker G, Marin-Castano ME. Cigarette smoke-related hydroquinone induces filamentous actin reorganization and heat shock protein 27 phosphorylation through p38 and extracellular signal-regulated kinase 1/2 in retinal pigment epithelium: implications for age-related macular degeneration. Am J Pathol 2010; 177: 1198–213.

251. Bertram KM, Baglole CJ, Phipps RP, Libby RT. Molecular regulation of cigarette smoke induced-oxidative stress in human retinal pigment epithelial cells: implications for age-related macular degeneration. Am J Physiol Cell Physiol 2009; 297: C1200–10.

252. Iwahashi M, Katsuragi T, Tani Y, Tsutsumi K, Kakiuchi K. Mechanism for degradation of poly(sodium acrylate) by bacterial consortium no. L7–98. J Biosci Bioeng 2003; 95: 483–7.

253. Decanini A, Nordgaard CL, Feng X, Ferrington DA, Olsen TW. Changes in select redox proteins of the retinal pigment epithelium in age-related macular degeneration. Am J Ophthalmol 2007; 143: 607–15.

254. Zhao Z, Chen Y, Wang J, et al. Age-related retinopathy in NRF2-deficient mice. PLoS One 2011; 6: e19456.

255. Justilien V, Pang JJ, Renganathan K, et al. SOD2 knock-down mouse model of early AMD. Invest Ophthalmol Vis Sci 2007; 48: 4407–20.

256. Kain HL, Reuter U. Release of lysosomal protease from retinal pigment epithelium and fibroblasts during mechanical stresses. Graefes Arch Clin Exp Ophthalmol 1995; 233: 236–43.

257. Brunk UT, Wihlmark U, Wrigstad A, Roberg K, Nilsson SE. Accumulation of lipofuscin within retinal pigment epithelial cells results in enhanced sensitivity to photo-oxidation. Gerontology 1995; 41(Suppl 2): 201–12.

258. Strunnikova N, Baffi J, Gonzalez A, et al. Regulated heat shock protein 27 expression in human retinal pigment epithelium. Invest Ophthalmol Vis Sci 2001; 42: 2130–8.

259. Zhang C, Baffi J, Cousins SW, Csaky KG. Oxidant-induced cell death in retinal pigment epithelium cells mediated through the release of apoptosis-inducing factor. J Cell Sci 2003; 116: 1915–23.

260. Malorni W, Iosi F, Mirabelli F, Bellomo G. Cytoskeleton as a target in menadione-induced oxidative stress in cultured mammalian cells: alterations underlying surface bleb formation. Chem Biol Interact 1991; 80: 217–36.

261. Campochiaro PA, Soloway P, Ryan SJ, Miller JW. The pathogenesis of choroidal neovascularization in patients with age-related macular degeneration. Mol Vis 1999; 5: 34.

262. Bilato C, Crow MT. Atherosclerosis and the vascular biology of aging. Aging (Milano) 1996; 8: 221–34.

263. Spagnoli LG, Sambuy Y, Palmieri G, Mauriello A. Age-related modulation of vascular smooth muscle cells proliferation following arterial wall damage. Artery 1985; 13: 187–98.

264. Espinosa-Heidmann DG, Suner I, Hernandez EP, et al. Age as an independent risk factor for severity of experimental choroidal neovascularization. Invest Ophthalmol Vis Sci 2002; 43: 1567–73.

265. Suner IJ, Espinosa-Heidmann DG, Marin-Castano ME, et al. Nicotine increases size and severity of experimental choroidal neovascularization. Invest Ophthalmol Vis Sci 2004; 45: 311–17.

266. Jeziorska M, Woolley DE. Local neovascularization and cellular composition within vulnerable regions of atherosclerotic plaques of human carotid arteries. J Pathol 1999; 188: 189–96.

267. Green W. R, Enger C. Age-related macular degeneration histopathologic studies. The 1992 Lorenz E. Zimmerman Lecture. Ophthalmol 1993; 100: 1519–153.

268. Tisher CC, Hostetter TH, Diabetic nephropathy. In: Tisher CC, Brenner BM, eds. Renal Pathology with Clinical and Functional Correlations. Philadelphia: J.B. Lippincott, 1994.

269. Sarks JP, Sarks SH, Killingsworth MC. Evolution of geographic atrophy of the retinal pigment epithelium. Eye 1988; 2: 552–77.

270. Duvall-Young J, MacDonald MK, McKechnie NM. Fundus changes in (type II) mesangiocapillary glomerulonephritis simulating drusen: a histopathological report. Br J Ophthalmol 1989; 73: 297–302.

3

Genetics of age-related macular degeneration

Divakar Gupta and Jennifer R. Chao

INTRODUCTION

Age-related macular degeneration (AMD), like Alzheimer's disease and atherosclerosis, is a late-onset degenerative disease. Environmental factors, such as cigarette smoking and nutrition, are associated with AMD (1,2). Heritability also explains much of the risk of developing AMD (3,4). The multifactorial nature of AMD has made the search for absolute genetic contributions challenging. However, advances in understanding the pathology of AMD has helped advance the study of genetic associations, providing evidence that there are strong genetic contributions to this disease.

Three methods of identifying genes contributing to AMD are candidate gene screening, linkage mapping, and case association studies (5). Candidate gene screening involves evaluating genes believed to contribute to the pathophysiology of AMD and those responsible for phenotypically similar diseases. Linkage analysis searches for chromosomal regions that co-segregate with the AMD disease trait by evaluating the segregation of chromosomal regions in families with AMD. Finally, case–control association studies find genetic variants of genes that are associated with AMD by evaluating differences in frequency between those variants in persons with AMD and their matched controls. All of the above methods have yielded our current understanding of the genetics of AMD.

EARLY SUSPICIONS: TWIN AND FAMILIAL AGGREGATION STUDIES

Twin studies were the earliest to implicate a heritability risk for AMD. A report of genetically tested monozygotic twins affected by AMD showed high concordance in both degree of disease severity and onset of vision loss (6). Klein reported that eight of nine twin pairs (seven confirmed monozygotic) examined between 1984 and 1993 demonstrated similar fundus appearances and incidence of visual impairment (7). In 1995, Meyers reported a statistically different concordance of AMD between monozygotic twin pairs (100%, 25 of 25) and dizygotic twin pairs (42%, five of 12), further emphasizing the importance of a genetic etiology (8). Two additional studies confirmed this finding, demonstrating a significantly higher concordance of AMD in monozygotic versus dizygotic twin pairs or twin/spouse pairs (9–11).

Seddon and colleagues evaluated 840 elderly male twins (210 monozygotic and 181 dizygotic), of which 509 were diagnosed with maculopathy and 106 had evidence of severe disease (12). They reported heritability estimates of 46% for the overall five-step grade assignment (based on the Clinical Age-Related Eye Disease study), 67% for intermediate and advanced disease (grades 3, 4, and 5), and 71% for advanced disease only (grades 4 and 5). It has been suggested from this data that advanced disease may have higher heritability. The heritability estimates of the Seddon report are similar to that described in an earlier twin study by Hammond and colleagues of 45% (9). The latter study found that the most heritable phenotypes were soft drusen $\geq 125\,\mu m$ (57%) and ≥ 20 hard drusen (81%), although it should be noted that none of the study participants demonstrated lesions consistent with advanced AMD.

Other groups have studied the concordance rates among persons with AMD and their non-twin siblings, offsprings, and spouses (13–18). Klaver et al. studied the first-degree relatives (siblings and offspring) of 87 persons with late AMD and 135 control subjects (13). They report that the lifetime risk estimate of late AMD for first-degree relatives of patients was 50% (95% CI = 26–73%), while the risk estimate of nonaffected controls was 12% (95% CI = 2.6–6.8). The risk for first-degree relatives was significantly higher among relatives of affected individuals ($P < 0.001$). These data confirmed the findings reported by Seddon et al., who also found that the prevalence of AMD was significantly higher among first-degree relatives (mostly siblings) of patients with neovacular AMD as compared with those of unaffected controls (26.9% and 11.6%, respectively). Together, these early studies provided important clues that there exists a strong role for genetics and heritability in the etiology of AMD.

PATHOGENESIS OF AMD: CANDIDATE GENES

Histological studies of drusen observed in AMD patients reveal that they are most likely products of an inflammatory response. Drusen are composed of proteins and lipids similar to deposit profiles seen in diseases where inflammatory and oxidative damages play a significant role (19–24). Multiple complement factors, apolipoproteins B and E, immunoglobulins, MHC class II antigens, human leukocyte antigen (HLA) DR, cholesterol esters, phospholipids, and carboxyethyl pyrrole protein adducts are found in drusen (23–26). Systemic inflammatory markers such as C-reactive protein (CRP) and interleukin-6 have been shown to be independent risk factors for AMD and progression of the disease (27,28). Drusen seen in membranoproliferative glomerulonephritis type II (MPGNII) are believed to result from a complement-mediated immune system dysfunction and they are immunohistochemically similar to drusen found in AMD (29). There is also a distinct similarity between proteins contained in drusen in AMD and extracellular deposits seen in atherosclerosis (19). As a result, multiple genes involved in inflammatory pathways, Retinal pigmented epithelium (RPE) basement membrane proteins, and extracellular deposits of atherosclerotic disease, amyloidosis, and Alzheimer's disease have been considered as candidates for the pathogenesis of AMD.

Complement-Related Genes and Other Inflammatory Genes with Association to AMD

Complement Factor H

Complement factor H (CFH) regulates the alternative pathway of complement activation (30). Three research groups, each working with distinct cohorts of persons with AMD, reported that a common allelic variant of the *CFH* gene was found at a significantly higher frequency in affected individuals as compared with controls (31–33). The AMD participants, all Americans of European origin, exhibited a range of clinical findings, including extensive drusen, geographic atrophy, and neovascular complications (31,33). The studies utilized single-nucleotide polymorphisms (SNPs) and haplotype blocks to test for associations among AMD cases and they independently found a strong signal at a *CFH* SNP (rs1061170). In doing so, they were able to map a specific chromosomal location to the disease manifested in their study populations (34). The *CFH* polymorphism is located in exon 9, and the allelic variant results in the replacement of the amino acid tyrosine with histidine at amino acid 402 (Tyr402His). The tyrosine to histidine substitution is located within a region of the CFH protein (SCR7) that contains overlapping binding sites for CRP, heparin, and streptococcal M protein (35). The Tyr402His variant of CFH binds CRP more weakly than wild type (30). This substitution is thought to alter the level of inflammation in the outer retina.

Persons heterozygous (carrying a single copy) for the histidine allele in the Tyr402His polymorphism were noted to have a 2.45- to 4.6-fold increased risk of AMD, while individuals homozygous for the histidine allele have a 5.57- to 7.4-fold increased likelihood compared with those who do not carry the allele. The attributable risk of AMD due to the histidine allele is estimated to be approximately 50% in their study populations (31–33). A later study has shown the attributable risk of the Tyr402His polymorphism to be >50% in a Finnish population (36). Subsequent studies of individuals of European descent (American, Icelandic, and French) manifesting a wide clinical range of AMD, including drusen only, geographic atrophy, and/or neovascular, confirmed the finding that the Tyr402His variant was significantly associated with AMD in their populations as well (37–42). More recently, the ALIENOR study, a population-based study in France, showed this CFH polymorphism to be associated with late neovascular

AMD and central soft drusen (43). One prospective study confirmed the association between the Tyr402His variant and an increased risk of AMD, reporting an estimated population attributable risk for CFH Tyr402His of 25% (44).

Environmental factors may have a synergistic effect on the risk of developing AMD in patients with the CFH allele. An incidence study of the Rotterdam population in the Netherlands, reported that the presence of two histidine alleles (homozygous) increased the risk of developing AMD by 12.5 times. However, smoking, in combination with being homozygous for the allele, increased the risk 34-fold (smoking alone increased the risk by 3.3 times) (45). The particularly high risk for AMD in smokers who are homozygous for the Tyr402His allele was confirmed by another study involving participants from England (46).

In contrast to studies involving persons of European descent, reports of AMD in persons of other ethnicities describe a more tenuous association between the disease and the Tyr402His polymorphism. A case–control study of Japanese individuals with neovascular AMD reported that affected patients were at no greater frequency of having the histidine allele in the Tyr402His polymorphism than unaffected individuals (47). A meta-analysis of case–control population studies of Asian individuals revealed that the Tyr402His variant accounted only for 8.8% of the population attributable risk for AMD (48). Another study reported wide ethnic variations in the frequencies of the Tyr402His allele in control populations: African-Americans 0.35 ± 0.04, Caucasians 0.34 ± 0.03, Somalis 0.34 ± 0.03, Hispanics 0.17 ± 0.03, and Japanese 0.07 ± 0.02 (49). Because the frequencies of the Tyr402His polymorphism are not proportionate to the frequencies of AMD in their respective populations, there is a suggestion that the Tyr402His polymorphism may not play as integral a role in AMD of some ethnic groups as in those of European descent (49). Finally, a study evaluating the Tyr402His polymorphism in Latinos suggests that the allele is not a major risk factor for AMD in this population (50). It is important to note, however, that in contrast to the original *CFH* studies, the large majority of affected individuals in the latter study demonstrated only early AMD. This argues that there may be some association between the Tyr402His allele and the severity of AMD. Postel et al. reported that the polymorphism is associated with an increased risk of developing grades 3, 4, and 5 AMD, but not grades 1 and 2 (51). Together, these studies indicate that the relative importance of the *CFH* polymorphism in AMD is in part dictated by both the particular ethnic population in question and also by the severity of AMD exhibited in the population.

Interestingly, one *CFH* polymorphism, rs800292, Ile62Val has been shown to be protective against AMD (38). The Ile62 variant is thought to bind complement factor C3b more strongly, resulting in greater C3b decay and a decreased complement response (52).

Complement Factor H Related Genes: CFHR1 and CFHR3

Near the location of the *CFH* gene on chromosome 1 are the complement factor H-related genes (*CFHR1-5*). Hageman and colleagues characterize a deletion that encompasses the *CFHR1* and *CFHR3* genes and found that nearly 63% of deletions lie on CFH haplotypes that are thought to be protective against AMD (53). Interestingly, the population frequency of deletion alleles varied by ethnicity, with the CFHR1 deletion being most common in African-Americans (16%) and least common in European Americans (4.7%). In another study of 173 individuals with neovascular AMD and 170 controls, the *CFHR1/CFHR3* deletion haplotype was found in 20% of controls and 8% of patients with AMD (54). Characterization of CFHR3 in 2006 has shown that it inhibits complement activation and competes with CFH for binding of complement C3 (55). Deficiency of *CFHR3* is speculated to be protective as it allows for greater CFH regulation of complement activation.

Factor B and Complement Component 2

Given the significant association of the *CFH* polymorphism to AMD, Gold et al. screened for polymorphisms in two other regulatory genes in the same pathway, factor B and complement component 2 (56). They report a statistically significant common risk haplotype (H1) and two protective haplotypes, the L9H variant of *BF* and the E318D variant of *C2*, as well as a variant in intron 10 of *C2* and the R32Q variant of *BF*. The latter two combinations of haplotypes confer a significantly reduced risk of AMD, with an odds ratio (OR) of 0.45 and 0.36, respectively (56).

Complement C3

A study by Yates and colleagues in English and Scottish individuals reported that a single polymorphism on exon 3 of the *C3* gene (rs2230199), causing an Arg80Gly substitution, is a risk factor for AMD (57). They estimated a population attributable risk of 22% for this variant with ORs of 1.7 and 2.6 for heterozygotes and homozygotes of the allele, respectively. After adjusting for age, smoking, CFH Y402H, LOC387715 A69S, and CFB R32Q, Spencer found this risk variant to have a population attributable risk of 17% (58). Hemolysis assays show that the rs2230199 Arg80Gly polymorphism activates the complement alternative pathway more efficiently than wild type (59).

Chromosome 10q26: PLEKHA1, LOC387715, PRSS11, HTRA1

Jakobsdottir and colleagues had previously identified a strong association of chromosome 10q26 and AMD, and they conducted a follow-up study in order to identify candidate genes in that region (42). Three overlying genes, *PLEKHA1*, *LOC387715*, and *PRSS11*, and their respective nonsynonymous SNPs were identified. Genotyping yielded a highly significant association between *PLEKHA1/LOC387715* and AMD, with the SNPs in *PLEKHA1* being more highly associated to AMD than those of *LOC387715*. *PLEKHA1* encodes the protein TAPP1, which is an activator of lymphocytes, and *PLEKHA1* transcripts are expressed in the central macula. They report that the association of either a single or double copy of the high-risk allele in the *PLEKHA1/LOC387715* locus accounts for an OR of 5.0 and an attributable risk of 57% in their study population (42). Additionally, the study notes a weaker association of the *GRK5/RGS10* locus with AMD. All of these associations were independent of the association of AMD with the Tyr402His allele of *CFH*.

Another study reported a significant association of a polymorphism Ala69Ser at *LOC387715* in two case–control cohorts of German descent (60). This polymorphism was associated with AMD, independent of the Tyr402His *CFH* polymorphism. In fact, the contribution of the two genetic alleles was additive. A third study confirmed the role of the Ala69Ser polymorphism at the *LOC287715* gene as another major AMD-susceptibility allele (61). The adjusted population attributable risk percentage estimates reported in their study were 36% for *LOC387715* and 43% for *CFH*, with a significantly higher risk of AMD when coupled with cigarette smoking.

Yang and associates found that an SNP in the promoter region of the *HTRA1* gene, rs11200638, conferred a population attributable risk of 49.3% in a Caucasian cohort of persons with AMD in Utah (62). They demonstrated *HRTA1* expression in drusen from eyes of patients with AMD by labeling with HTRA1 antibody. Additionally, they report elevated expression of *HRTA1* mRNA and protein in the RPE and lymphocytes of AMD patients. HRTA1 is a serine peptidase that appears to regulate the degradation of extracellular matrix proteoglycans and facilitates the access of other degrading matrix enzymes, such as matrix metalloproteinases and collagenases. This study noted an allele dosage effect, where persons homozygous for the allele have an increased risk (OR 7.29 [3.18, 16.74]) over those who are heterozygous [OR 1.83 {1.25, 2.68}]. An estimated population attributable risk from a joint model with the *CFH* Tyr402His allele (i.e., a risk allele at either locus) is 71.4%. DeWan and colleagues concurrently reported an association of the identical SNP from the *HTRA1* promoter in a Chinese population with wet AMD, confirming the significant role of this allelic variation in AMD populations of various ethnicities (63).

OTHER INFLAMMATORY GENES: CXCR1, TLR4, and HLA

Genes encoding other inflammatory factors have been studied, including *CX3CR1*, *TLR4*, and the *HLA* genes (64–69). Two SNPs, V249I and T280M, in the *CX3CR1* gene, which encodes a chemokine receptor expressed in the eye, were screened and found to have a significantly higher prevalence among persons with AMD as compared with controls (68). Additional analysis of ocular tissue with evidence of advanced AMD revealed an even higher prevalence of the T280M allele compared with those with a clinical AMD diagnosis.

Toll-like receptor 4 (*TLR4*) was examined as a possible candidate gene for AMD since the gene is located in a chromosomal region with strong linkage to AMD, chromosome 9q32-33 (64,66,67). The gene product is thought to function as a key mediator of proinflammatory signaling pathways, regulation of cholesterol efflux, and the phagocytosis of photoreceptor outer segments by the RPE (69). Two allelic variants were screened, D299G and T399I, in 667 unrelated AMD patients and 439 controls. The study demonstrated an increased risk of AMD in carriers of the D299G allele. Interestingly, the authors examined the effects of this *TLR4* allelic variant in combination with the *ABCA1* R219K and the APOE-ε4 alleles, and they reported a fourfold increased risk of AMD in carriers who exhibit the D299G *TLR4* and R219K *ABCA1* alleles but not the APOE-ε4 allele (69). This latter finding supports the general idea of a polygenic etiology of AMD.

Principal allele groups of HLA genes, including HLA class I-A, -B, -Cw and class II DRB1 and DQB1, were examined in their relationship to AMD (65). HLA antigens are expressed in eyes, and HLA-DR has been located by immunohistochemistry in both hard and soft drusen (19). The principal allele groups were first screened in a cohort of 100 AMD cases and 92 controls. Alleles with P < 0.1 on initial typing were then screened in an additional 100 AMD cases and 100 controls. Logistic regression for all possible pairwise HLA combinations was performed, along with Bonferroni corrections. The results demonstrate a positive correlation of allele Cw*0701 with AMD, whereas the B*4001 and DRB1*1301 alleles were negatively associated (65).

Extracellular Matrix: *Fibulin*, *CST3*, And *MMP-9*

Fibulins 1–6 were evaluated for their association with AMD because of an association of a *Fibulin 3* mutation to heritable drusen and the significant role played in basement membrane structure by the *Fibulin* family of proteins in general (70–72). While allelic variations in the *Fibulin 1–4* genes could not conclusively be associated with AMD (70), a missense mutation in *Fibulin 5*, was noted to be present in 1.7% of participants with AMD and to be absent in controls (70). Fibulin 5 is thought to connect cellular surface receptors and extracellular elastic fibers, playing a key role in the link between the RPE and Bruch's membrane (71).

An allelic variation in exon 104 of *Fibulin 6* (or *HEMICENTIN-1*) resulted in a nonconserved amino acid substitution, Gln5345Arg in a large AMD family cohort, which segregated exclusively with the presumptive disease haplotype (72). However, multiple subsequent studies were not able to confirm this finding (31,37,64,66,70,73). In a few studies, the allelic variant was not detected in any of the participants with AMD or in controls (64,66,73). The Gln5345Arg variant was found in two of 402 patients and in one of 263 controls in a study by Stone et al., and there was no significant association between the allelic variation and AMD (70). Additionally, in the study population where the Tyr402His variant of *CFH* was found to be significantly

associated with AMD, the Gln5345Arg variant of *HEMICENTIN-1* did not demonstrate allelic association to AMD in the discovery sample (31). Nevertheless, it is possible that the association of this allelic variant of *Fibulin 6* (*HEMICENTIN-1*) with AMD is unique to the family in which it was originally reported, but other allelic variations in *HEMICENTIN-1* should be explored for significant associations in a broader population of affected individuals (72).

Two other genes thought to play a role in the functioning of the RPE and extracellular matrix components are *CST3* and *MMP-9* (74,75). The *CST3* gene encodes for cystatin C, a cysteine protease inhibitor that regulates the activity of cathepsin S, a protease with regulatory functions in the RPE (76). One study of German AMD patients revealed an increased susceptibility to the disease in individuals homozygous for the recessive allele, *CST* B (75). The second gene, *MMP-9*, that encodes the matrix metalloproteinase-9 protein was found to have a polymorphic allele in its promoter region that was significantly associated to neovascular AMD in an Italian study population (74).

Lipid Metabolism: *APOE and PON1*

APOE encodes apolipoprotein E, a protein that plays a central role in lipid transport and distribution in the peripheral and central nervous system (77). It has been found in soft drusen and basal laminar deposits, making it a good candidate gene for AMD (19,78). The gene has three alleles (ε2, ε3, and ε5), each coding for different protein isoforms, with the ε3 allele being the most common. Multiple case–control studies conducted in the Netherlands, Italy, France, United States, Australia, and Iceland have reported that the ε4 allele may confer a protective effect against AMD (79–84). However, there appeared to be no significant association of the ε4 allele to AMD in other case–control studies conducted in Japan, Hong Kong, and the United States (37,85–88). Separately, the *APOE* allele, ε2, has been suggested to confer an increased risk of developing AMD (79,81,83); however, other studies have found no significant association (37,85,87,88). The disparate results of these studies may be a result of the variable baseline distribution of the ε2, ε3, and ε5 alleles in different ethnic populations (89). Additionally, the studies differed greatly in the severity and type of AMD examined, which varied from early stages of the disease to advanced atrophic or neovascular AMD.

One study conducted in the United States examined the combined effect of *APOE* genotypes and smoking history (90). The study was based on the premise of the authors' earlier work that the ε4 allele reduces the risk of AMD and the ε2 allele increases it (83). A later analysis in 2005 suggested that among participants with neovascular AMD (n = 260), smoking conferred the greatest risk in carriers of the ε2 allele, with odds ratios of 1.9 for ε4 carriers (p = 0.11), 2.2 for ε3 homozygotes (p = 0.007), and 4.6 for ε2 carriers (p = 0.001) when compared with nonsmoking ε3 homozygote controls (90). They conclude that smoking likely poses a greater risk in the carriers of the ε2 allele compared with those of other *APOE* alleles.

PON1 encodes paraoxonase, a calcium-dependent glycoprotein that prevents low-density lipoprotein oxidation. It contains two polymorphic sites, Gly192Arg (A/B) and Leu54Met (L/M), which give rise to different protein products of varying enzymatic activities. Ikeda et al. reported a higher frequency of the BB and LL genotypes in participants with neovascular AMD as compared with controls (52.8 *vs.* 35% with P = 0.0127 and 91.7% *vs.* 77.1% with P = 0.009, respectively) in unrelated Japanese participants (72 neovascular AMD and 140 age- and gender-matched controls) (91). Later studies in populations of Anglo-Celtic and Northern Irish descent did not find a significant association of allelic variation to either neovascular or atrophic AMD (92,93). The association of the *PON1* alleles and neovascular AMD may therefore be population-specific.

Other Genes: *LPR6, VEGF, VLDLR, ACE, MnSOD, and EPHX1*
Several candidate genes have been studied in both family-based and case–control cohorts. Low-density lipoprotein receptor-related protein 6 (*LRP6*) and vascular endothelial growth factor (*VEGF*) showed linkage and allelic association in both family-based and case–control data sets (94). In the same study, the gene encoding the very low density lipoprotein receptor (*VLDLR*) did not demonstrate significant linkage, but the family-based result was nominally significant and case–control results were significant (94). The ambiguous *VLDLR* association results echo those previously reported by Conley et al., where *VLDLR* was significant only for the allele-based test but not the linkage analysis (37).

Angiotensin-converting enzyme (ACE) was thought to be a good candidate gene for neovascular AMD because an Alu polymorphism had been associated with proliferative diabetic retinopathy. Hamdi et al. examined the association of the Alu polymorphism in patients with neovascular/wet AMD (n = 86), atrophic AMD (n = 87), and age-matched controls (n = 189). Individuals carrying the Alu element insertion (Alu +/+) in the ACE gene were 4.5 times more frequent in the control population than in the dry/atrophic AMD patients (OR 5, p = 0.004), while the frequency did not differ significantly from the neovascular/wet AMD population (OR 1.4, p = 0.4). The Alu polymorphism in the *ACE* gene was therefore believed to confer protection against dry AMD (95). However, two later multiple candidate gene studies did not find a significant association between the Alu polymorphism in the ACE gene (*DCP1*) and either atrophic or neovascular AMD (37,94).

Some studies have sought to evaluate the role of oxidative damage in AMD (93,96). The genetic polymorphisms of four genes, cytochrome P-450 (*CYP*) 1A1, glutathione S-transferase (*GPX1*), microsomal epoxide hydrolase (*EPHX1*), and manganese superoxide dismutase (*MnSOD*), were evaluated in 102 Japanese participants with neovascular AMD and in 200 controls (96). The results suggested a strong association of a valine/alanine polymorphism of the *MnSOD* gene with neovascular AMD and a weaker association of an exon-3 polymorphism of the *EPHX1* gene. In contrast, multiple candidate gene analysis of patients with neovascular AMD in at least one eye found no significant association with any of the genes evaluated in the earlier study by Kimura et al., including *MnSOD* and multiple *CYP* genes (including *CYP1A1, CYP1A2, CYP2E1, CYP2D6*), *EPHX1*, and *GPX1* (93).

HEREDITARY RETINAL DYSTROPHIES: CANDIDATE GENES
Genes associated with phenotypically similar diseases to AMD were examined as potential candidates for AMD. The genes responsible for monogenic hereditary macular dystrophies such as Stargardt disease, Stargardt-like macular dystrophy (STGD3), autosomal dominant macular dystrophy (adMD), Sorsby fundus dystrophy, Best macular dystrophy, butterfly dystrophy, and Doyne honeycomb retinal dystrophy (malattia leventinese) have been well characterized (97–102). Several of these genes were considered candidate genes for AMD, and their studies are described in this section.

ABCR
ABCR (also *ABCA4* or *STGD1*) is a gene that encodes a photoreceptor-specific ATP-binding cassette transporter of retinaldehyde. *ABCR* is defective in autosomal recessive Stargardt disease, autosomal recessive cone–rod dystrophy, and autosomal recessive retinitis pigmentosa (98). Abnormal function of the transporter, caused by mutations in the *ABCR* gene, is characterized by accumulation of a major lipofuscin fluorophore (A2-E) in the RPE, making this gene attractive as a candidate gene for AMD (103). An early study identified heterozygous mutations of *ABCR* in 16% of AMD patients (104). Subsequently, two specific sequence changes in the *ABCR* gene, G1961E and D2177N, were found to predict a three- and fivefold increased risk of AMD, respectively (105). Further research indicated that in a cohort of families, the AMD-affected relatives of Stargardt disease patients were more likely to be carriers of the pathogenic Stargardt alleles (106). Sixteen specific *ABCR* mutations were found that led to functional abnormalities of the transporter protein, including ATP-binding and ATPase activity (106). Additionally, it is believed that *ABCR* gene variants may be associated with AMD in at least six families (107,108). One study of a group of unrelated multiplex cases of neovascular AMD reported finding six heterozygous missense changes in the *ABCR* gene. Using familial segregation analysis, Souied et al. were able to associate two of the codon changes with familial AMD (107).

In contrast, other studies did not find an association of specific *ABCR* allelic variants to AMD (109–112). The allelic variants, G1961E and D2177N from the initial report by Allikmets et al., were later evaluated in individuals of Somali ancestry, and the allelic frequencies were not significantly different between those with

AMD versus controls (113). Studies evaluating other allelic variations of the *ABCR* gene in participants of Japanese, Chinese, and German origin have also reported no significant difference between allelic variants in participants with AMD and controls (114–116).

The disparate findings encountered in these studies can be difficult to reconcile. A possible consideration is the unique prevalence of *ABCR* polymorphisms in each study population. For example, the most common *ABCR* allele associated with Stargardt disease in patients of European origin was found to be quite common in normal controls of Somali origin (113,117). Moreover, there is a large spectrum in allelic variations of the *ABCR* gene in both populations as a whole, making the differentiation between disease-causing mutations and non-pathogenic polymorphisms difficult.

ELOVL4

A five-base pair deletion in the gene located on chromosome 6q14, *ELOVL4*, has been reported to be closely associated with two forms of autosomal dominant macular dystrophy, STGD3 and adMD, in two families (99). The clinical findings of STGD3 and adMD are similar to the atrophic form of AMD. The normal gene product, ELOVL4, is a retinal photoreceptor-specific protein that functions in the biosynthesis of very long chain fatty acids. A study examining *ELOVL4* polymorphisms in unrelated individuals with predominantly atrophic AMD revealed eight variants in the coding region; however, none of them were significantly associated with susceptibility to AMD (118). Interestingly, a later case–control study of predominantly neovascular AMD in familial cases observed that a variant of the *ELOVL4* gene previously described by Ayyagari, et al., Met299Val, was significantly associated with AMD (37). The discrepancy in these findings may be due to differences in the type of AMD examined (atrophic *vs.* neovascular) or in the sampling of study participants (sporadic *vs.* familial).

Other Genes: VMD2, TIMP3, Peripherin/RDS, Fibulin 3/EFEMP1

A variety of genes responsible for phenotypically similar, monogenic macular dystrophies have had less promising associations with AMD (66,97,101,119–127). Mutations in *VMD2* ((Best macular dystrophy), *TIMP3* (Sorsby fundus dystrophy), *peripherin/RDS* (butterfly dystrophy), and *Fibulin 3/EFEMP1* (Doyne honeycomb retinal dystrophy or malattia leventinese) were studied and have not been found to be significantly associated with AMD.

GENES NOT ASSOCIATED WITH AMD
IMPG2

IMPG2 is a gene encoding the retinal inter-photoreceptor matrix (IPM) proteoglycan IMP200, which is thought to be integral to the interaction of RPE and photoreceptors, specifically regulating the turnover of photoreceptor outer segments. Kuehn et al. screened 92 individuals with AMD and 92 controls and reported three coding and one intronic polymorphism in *IMPG2*. However, none of the allelic variants were present at a significantly different frequency in the AMD versus control participants (128).

GPR75

Rhodopsin is a G-protein coupled receptor, and when it became known that the gene *GPR75* encoded another G-protein coupled receptor expressed in the retina, it was thought to be a possible candidate gene for AMD. However, in a screening of 535 AMD and 252 control cases, only six allelic variants were found once in single AMD patients (129). These rare mutations were deemed unlikely to be significantly associated with AMD pathology in the majority of affected patients.

LAMC1, LAMC2, and LAMB3

The *LAMC1, LAMC2, and LAMB3* genes were selected as positional and functional candidate genes. They are located in a region on chromosome 1q25-31 that has been strongly linked to AMD (64,66,67,87,130–134). The genes code for laminins, which are extracellular matrix proteins located in the basal lamina of the RPE, Bruch's membrane, and choriocapillaris (73). A total of 69 sequence variants, 25 in coding regions, were detected in the three laminin genes. However, none were found to be at a significantly higher frequency in the AMD population as compared with the controls (73). In a separate study, polymorphisms in *LAMC1* and *LAMC2* were also not significantly different between the affected individuals and control cases (37).

Multi-Candidate Gene Screening

Several large candidate genetic screening studies have searched for genes with significant associations to AMD (37,93,94). Esfandiary and colleagues examined genes involved in the detoxification of reactive oxygen species, including *CYP1A1, CYP1A2, CYP2E1, CYP2D6, EPHX1, MnSOD, AhR, NAT2, CAT, GPX1, PON1, and ADPRT1*. Their study population from Northern Ireland was comprised of 94 persons with neovascular AMD and 95 controls (93). They screened a number of SNPs for 12 genes, but none of them revealed a significant association with AMD (93). Conley et al. examined a second category of genes involved in fatty acid biosynthesis and inflammatory pathways (37). They reported a significant association for allelic variants of *CFH* and ELOVL4 as described earlier; however, no association was noted for other genes, including *GLRX2, OCLM, PRELP, RGS16, TGFβ2, ApoH, and ITGB4*. This study also did not find an association with *ACE* and *APOE*, and these genes are described elsewhere in detail. Finally, Haines and colleagues conducted a large screening study of family-based and case–control data sets, and evaluated several genes, of which α-2 macroglobulin (*A2M*), creatine kinase (*CKB*), ACE (*DCP1*), interleukin-1α (*IL1A*), and microsomal glutathione-*S*-transferase 1 (*MGST1*) were found to have no significant association to AMD in both data sets (94).

LINKAGE MAPPING

Linkage mapping has provided a wealth of possible genetic associations to AMD. The multifactorial nature of the disease is reflected in the number and variety of chromosomal associations detected. Genetic markers covering several human chromosomes have been tested for segregation in multiple combined subsets of AMD families. Genetic loci purportedly linked to AMD include 1q25-31, 2q14.3, 2q31.2-2q32.3, 2p21, 3p13, 4q32, 4p16, 5p, 5q34, 6q25.3, 6q14, 8, 9p24, 9q31, 9q33, 10q26, 12q13, 12q23, 14q13, 15q21, 16p12, 17q25, 18p11, 19p, 20q13, 22q, and X (64,66,67,131–136). Once a chromosomal region has been identified, finer mapping narrows the search for possible candidate genes. Two chromosomal loci that are most consistently associated with AMD are discussed here.

One of the first disease loci mapped by linkage analysis to AMD was a 9-cM region of chromosome 1q25-31 (gene symbol, *ARMD1*) (137). The association was demonstrated in a family which demonstrated a predominantly dry phenotype of AMD. While the disease segregated as an autosomal dominant trait in this family, two individuals were identified as having the disease allele but not the phenotype, that is, the allele was nonpenetrant. At this time, the Stargardt disease gene (*ABCR*) was known to be located near this new disease locus at chromosome 1p21, but linkage analysis excluded it as an AMD disease locus in this family. Since then, this region of chromosome 1 has been the most commonly found site to segregate with AMD, both dry and neovascular types, in genome-wide scans involving large numbers (34–530) of families (64,66,67,87,130–134). Interestingly, one study of 70 families did not demonstrate linkage to chromosome 1q (138). Nevertheless, genes located in this region were viewed as possible candidate genes for AMD, including *CFH, HEMICENTIN-1* (or *Fibulin 6*), *LAMC1, LAMC2,* and *LAMB3* (37,72,73). These genes are discussed in detail elsewhere in this chapter.

Another locus consistently associated with AMD was found during an early full genome-wide scan of 225 families with both wet and dry forms of AMD, revealing a strong linkage to chromosome 10 (135). Further evidence from independent studies of different family cohorts narrowed the region to chromosome 10q26 (67,132), and follow-up studies confirmed this finding, including a meta-analysis of genome scans (66,130,134,138). Three genes in this locus have since been implicated in AMD, including *PLEKA1, LOC387715,* and *PRSS11* (42).

EPIGENETICS OF AMD

AMD is a unique complex disease in that relatively few allelic variants explain a large amount (>50%) of the genetic risk (139). Genetics, however, does not explain all of the heritability, nor does it explain variable phenotypes in monozygotic twins. Epigenetics, modifications to the genome that affect structure or function but not sequence, offers a new way to investigate the nonheritable risk of developing disease. Studies in systemic lupus erythematosus have shown that epigenetics may explain some of the discordant phenotypes seen in monozygotic twins with disease. A recent study of monozygotic twins with discordant phenotypes of AMD showed that the twin with more advanced AMD (determined by fundus photos using the Wisconsin Grading System) had a greater smoking history (140). The twin with an earlier-form AMD, smaller drusen and/or less pigmentary change, had a higher intake of vitamin D, betaine, or methionine. The authors conclude that there may be epigenetic mechanisms that link nutritional/environmental factors to AMD pathogenesis. Further studies are needed to better understand the role of epigenetics in AMD.

CONCLUSION

The discovery of specific allelic variants of major disease genes has come after many years of searching for the genetic etiology of AMD. The early twin and familial aggregation studies strongly suggested the disease was heritable, and this was soon followed by linkage analyses implicating large regions of chromosomes and candidate gene screenings describing possible culprit disease genes. Case association studies, in conjunction with the completion of the human genome project, enabled the identification of SNPs in major disease genes, including *CFH* gene, factor B/component 2 locus, *PLEKIIA1, LOC387715,* and *HTRA1.*

Despite the discovery of major disease loci, our understanding of the fundamental nature of AMD etiology has remain unchanged. Current evidence still suggests the disease to be multifactorial, shaped by multiple genes as well as environmental influences. For example, as reviewed above, several studies have demonstrated an additive effect in the population risk of having more than one allelic variant from a major disease locus. Additionally, there appears to be an increased risk of developing AMD when both the disease allele and certain environmental factors, such as cigarette smoking, are present. Moreover, the varying effects of the major disease loci on AMD development across different ethnic groups underscore the multifactorial nature of the disease.

Future progress in studying the etiology of AMD includes the discovery of not only other disease loci throughout the genome, but also the protein products of identified allelic variants. SNPs that result in coding changes need to be studied for their effect on resultant messenger RNA and protein function. An understanding of this next step after genetic coding is fundamental to providing important confirmation of the significance of these genetic variations. In addition, the identification of these genetic allelic variants has opened a window into studying the pathophysiologic mechanisms of disease development, as well as our best hopes for disease intervention.

SUMMARY POINTS

- Twin studies and familial aggregation studies provided the earliest evidence for the heritability of AMD
- Candidate genes were derived from genes involved in pathways thought to contribute to the pathophysiology of AMD and from phenotypically similar diseases
- Case-association studies have identified allelic variations of several genes that are major risk loci for AMD: complement factor H (*CFH*) gene, factor B/component 2 locus, *PLEKHA1*, *LOC387715*, and *HTRA1*
- Linkage mapping, which searches for chromosomal regions that co-segregate with the AMD disease trait, and multi-candidate gene screening have implicated multiple genetic loci in almost every chromosome, including 1q25-31, 2q14.3, 2q31.2-2q32.3, 2p21, 3p13, 4q32, 4p16, 5p, 5q34, 6q25.3, 6q14, 8, 9p24, 9q31, 9q33, 10q26, 12q13, 12q23, 14q13, 15q21, 16p12, 17q25, 18p11, 19p, 20q13, 22q, and X
- Understanding epigenetic influences may explain some of the genetic risk of AMD
- The etiology of AMD is multifactorial, requiring the presence of multiple disease loci as well as environmental factors

REFERENCES

1. Chiu CJ, Klein R, Milton RC, et al. Does eating particular diets alter the risk of age-related macular degeneration in users of the Age-Related Eye Disease Study supplements? Br J Ophthalmol 2009; 93: 1241–6.
2. Chakravarthy U, Wong TY, Fletcher A, et al. Clinical risk factors for age-related macular degeneration: a systematic review and meta-analysis. BMC Ophthalmol 2010; 10: 31.
3. Bok D. Contributions of genetics to our understanding of inherited monogenic retinal diseases and age-related macular degeneration. Arch Ophthalmol 2007; 125: 160–4.
4. Leveziel N, Puche N, Zerbib J, et al. Genetic factors associated with age-related macular degeneration. Med Sci (Paris) 2010; 26: 509–15.
5. Daiger SP. Genetics. Was the human genome project worth the effort? Science 2005; 308: 362–4.
6. Meyers SM, Zachary AA. Monozygotic twins with age-related macular degeneration. Arch Ophthalmol 1988; 106: 651–3.
7. Klein ML, Mauldin WM, Stoumbos VD. Heredity and age-related macular degeneration. Observations in monozygotic twins. Arch Ophthalmol 1994; 112: 932–7.
8. Meyers SM, Greene T, Gutman FA. A twin study of age-related macular degeneration. Am J Ophthalmol 1995; 120: 757–66.
9. Hammond CJ, Webster AR, Snieder H, et al. Genetic influence on early age-related maculopathy: a twin study. Ophthalmology 2002; 109: 730–6.
10. Grizzard SW, Arnett D, Haag SL. Twin study of age-related macular degeneration. Ophthalmic Epidemiol 2003; 10: 315–22.
11. Gottfredsdottir MS, Sverrisson T, Musch DC, et al. Age related macular degeneration in monozygotic twins and their spouses in Iceland. Acta Ophthalmol Scand 1999; 77: 422–5.
12. Seddon JM, Cote J, Page WF, et al. The US twin study of age-related macular degeneration: relative roles of genetic and environmental influences. Arch Ophthalmol 2005; 123: 321–7.
13. Klaver CC, Wolfs RC, Assink JJ, et al. Genetic risk of age-related maculopathy. Population-based familial aggregation study. Arch Ophthalmol 1998; 116: 1646–51.
14. Klein BE, Klein R, Lee KE, et al. Risk of incident age-related eye diseases in people with an affected sibling: The Beaver Dam Eye Study. Am J Epidemiol 2001; 154: 207–11.
15. Seddon JM, Ajani UA, Mitchell BD. Familial aggregation of age-related maculopathy. Am J Ophthalmol 1997; 123: 199–206.
16. Silvestri G, Johnston PB, Hughes AE. Is genetic predisposition an important risk factor in age-related macular degeneration? Eye 1994; 8(Pt 5): 564–8.
17. Heiba IM, Elston RC, Klein BE, et al. Sibling correlations and segregation analysis of age-related maculopathy: the Beaver Dam Eye Study. Genet Epidemiol 1994; 11: 51–67.
18. Piguet B, Wells JA, Palmvang IB, et al. Age-related Bruch's membrane change: a clinical study of the relative role of heredity and environment. Br J Ophthalmol 1993; 77: 400–3.
19. Mullins RF, Russell SR, Anderson DH, Hageman GS. Drusen associated with aging and age-related macular degeneration contain proteins common to extracellular deposits associated with atherosclerosis, elastosis, amyloidosis, and dense deposit disease. FASEB J 2000; 14: 835–46.
20. Donoso LA, Kim D, Frost A, et al. The role of inflammation in the pathogenesis of age-related macular degeneration. Surv Ophthalmol 2006; 51: 137–52.
21. Killingsworth MC, Sarks JP, Sarks SH. Macrophages related to Bruch's membrane in age-related macular degeneration. Eye 1990; 4(Pt 4): 613–21.
22. Gurne DH, Tso MO, Edward DP, et al. Antiretinal antibodies in serum of patients with age-related macular degeneration. Ophthalmology 1991; 98: 602–7.
23. Hageman GS, Luthert PJ, Victor Chong NH, et al. An integrated hypothesis that considers drusen as biomarkers of immune-mediated processes at the RPE-Bruch's membrane interface in aging and age-related macular degeneration. Prog Retin Eye Res 2001; 20: 705–32.
24. Crabb JW, Miyagi M, Gu X, et al. Drusen proteome analysis: an approach to the etiology of age-related macular degeneration. Proc Natl Acad Sci USA 2002; 99: 14682–7.
25. Zarbin MA. Current concepts in the pathogenesis of age-related macular degeneration. Arch Ophthalmol 2004; 122: 598–614.
26. Johnson LV, Ozaki S, Staples MK, et al. A potential role for immune complex pathogenesis in drusen formation. Exp Eye Res 2000; 70: 441–9.
27. Seddon JM, Gensler G, Milton RC, et al. Association between C-reactive protein and age-related macular degeneration. JAMA 2004; 291: 704–10.

28. Seddon JM, George S, Rosner B, et al. Progression of age-related macular degeneration: prospective assessment of C-reactive protein, interleukin 6, and other cardiovascular biomarkers. Arch Ophthalmol 2005; 123: 774–82.

29. Mullins RF, Aptsiauri N, Hageman V. Structure and composition of drusen associated with glomerulonephritis: implications for the role of complement activation in drusen biogenesis. Eye 2001; 15(Pt 3): 390–5.

30. Perkins SJ, Nan R, Li K, et al. Complement Factor H-ligand interactions: Self-association, multivalency and dissociation constants. Immunobiology 2012; 217: 281–97.

31. Edwards AO, Ritter R, Abel KJ, et al. Complement factor H polymorphism and age-related macular degeneration. Science 2005; 308: 421–4.

32. Haines JL, Hauser MA, Schmidt S, et al. Complement factor H variant increases the risk of age-related macular degeneration. Science 2005; 308: 419–21.

33. Klein RJ, Zeiss C, Chew EY, et al. Complement factor H polymorphism in age-related macular degeneration. Science 2005; 308: 385–9.

34. Clark AG. The role of haplotypes in candidate gene studies. Genet Epidemiol 2004; 27: 321–33.

35. Giannakis E, Jokiranta TS, Male DA, et al. A common site within factor H SCR 7 responsible for binding heparin, C-reactive protein and streptococcal M protein. Eur J Immunol 2003; 33: 962–9.

36. Seitsonen SP, Onkamo P, Peng G, et al. Multifactor effects and evidence of potential interaction between complement factor H Y402H and LOC387715 A69S in age-related macular degeneration. PLoS One 2008; 3: e3833.

37. Conley YP, Thalamuthu A, Jakobsdottir J, et al. Candidate gene analysis suggests a role for fatty acid biosynthesis and regulation of the complement system in the etiology of age-related maculopathy. Hum Mol Genet 2005; 14: 1991–2002.

38. Hageman GS, Anderson DH, Johnson LV, et al. A common haplotype in the complement regulatory gene factor H (HF1/CFH) predisposes individuals to age-related macular degeneration. Proc Natl Acad Sci USA 2005; 102: 7227–32.

39. Magnusson KP, Duan S, Sigurdsson H, et al. CFH Y402H confers similar risk of soft drusen and both forms of advanced AMD. PLoS Med 2006; 3: e5.

40. Souied EH, Leveziel N, Richard F, et al. Y402H complement factor H polymorphism associated with exudative age-related macular degeneration in the French population. Mol Vis 2005; 11: 1135–40.

41. Zareparsi S, Branham KE, Li M, et al. Strong association of the Y402H variant in complement factor H at 1q32 with susceptibility to age-related macular degeneration. Am J Hum Genet 2005; 77: 149–53.

42. Jakobsdottir J, Conley YP, Weeks DE, et al. Susceptibility genes for age-related maculopathy on chromosome 10q26. Am J Hum Genet 2005; 77: 389–407.

43. Delcourt C, Delyfer MN, Rougier MB, et al. Associations of complement factor H and smoking with early age-related macular degeneration: the ALIENOR study. Invest Ophthalmol Vis Sci 2011; 52: 5955–62.

44. Schaumberg DA, Christen WG, Kozlowski P, et al. A prospective assessment of the Y402H variant in complement factor H, genetic variants in C-reactive protein, and risk of age-related macular degeneration. Invest Ophthalmol Vis Sci 2006; 47: 2336–40.

45. Despriet DD, Klaver CC, Witteman JC, et al. Complement factor H polymorphism, complement activators, and risk of age-related macular degeneration. JAMA 2006; 296: 301–9.

46. Sepp T, Khan JC, Thurlby DA, et al. Complement factor H variant Y402H is a major risk determinant for geographic atrophy and choroidal neovascularization in smokers and nonsmokers. Invest Ophthalmol Vis Sci 2006; 47: 536–40.

47. Gotoh N, Yamada R, Hiratani H, et al. No association between complement factor H gene polymorphism and exudative age-related macular degeneration in Japanese. Hum Genet 2006; 120: 139–43.

48. Kondo N, Bessho H, Honda S, et al. Complement factor H Y402H variant and risk of age-related macular degeneration in Asians: a systematic review and meta-analysis. Ophthalmology 2011; 118: 339–44.

49. Grassi MA, Fingert JH, Scheetz TE, et al. Ethnic variation in AMD-associated complement factor H polymorphism p.Tyr402His. Hum Mutat 2006; 27: 921–5

50. Tedeschi-Blok N, Buckley J, Varma R, et al. A population-based study of early age-related macular degeneration: role of the complement factor H Y402H polymorphism in bilateral, but not unilateral, disease. Ophthalmology 2007; 114: 99–103

51. Postel EA, et al. Complement Factor H Increases Risk for Atrophic Age-Related Macular Degeneration. Ophthalmology 2006;

52. Tortajada A, et al. The disease-protective complement factor H allotypic variant Ile62 shows increased binding affinity for C3b and enhanced cofactor activity. Hum Mol Genet 2009; 18: 3452–61.

53. Hageman GS, Hancox LS, Taiber AJ, et al. Extended haplotypes in the complement factor H (CFH) and CFH-related (CFHR) family of genes protect against age-related macular degeneration: characterization, ethnic distribution and evolutionary implications. Ann Med 2006; 38: 592–604.

54. Hughes AE, Orr N, Esfandiary H, et al. A common CFH haplotype, with deletion of CFHR1 and CFHR3, is associated with lower risk of age-related macular degeneration. Nat Genet 2006; 38: 1173–7.

55. Fritsche LG, Lauer N, Hartmann A, et al. An imbalance of human complement regulatory proteins CFHR1, CFHR3 and factor H influences risk for age-related macular degeneration (AMD). Hum Mol Genet 2010; 19: 4694–704.

56. Gold B, Merriam JE, Zernant J, et al. Variation in factor B (BF) and complement component 2 (C2) genes is associated with age-related macular degeneration. Nat Genet 2006; 38: 458–62.

57. Yates JR, Sepp T, Matharu BK, et al. Complement C3 variant and the risk of age-related macular degeneration. N Engl J Med 2007; 357: 553–61.

58. Spencer KL, Olson LM, Anderson BM, et al. C3 R102G polymorphism increases risk of age-related macular degeneration. Hum Mol Genet 2008; 17: 1821–4.

59. Heurich M, Martinez-Barricarte R, Francis NJ, et al. Common polymorphisms in C3, factor B, and factor H collaborate to determine systemic complement activity and disease risk. Proc Natl Acad Sci U S A 2011; 108: 8761–6.

60. Rivera A, Fisher SA, Fritsche LG, et al. Hypothetical LOC387715 is a second major susceptibility gene for

age-related macular degeneration, contributing independently of complement factor H to disease risk. Hum Mol Genet 2005; 14: 3227–36.

61. Schmidt S, Hauser MA, Scott WK, et al. Cigarette smoking strongly modifies the association of LOC387715 and age-related macular degeneration. Am J Hum Genet 2006; 78: 852–64.

62. Yang Z, Camp NJ, Sun H, et al. A Variant of the HRTA1 Gene Increases Susceptibility to Age-Related Macular Degeneration. Science 2006; 314: 992–3.

63. DeWan A, Liu M, Hartman S, et al. HTRA1 promoter polymorphism in wet age-related macular degeneration. Science 2006; 314: 989–92.

64. Abecasis GR, Yashar BM, Zhao Y, et al. Age-related macular degeneration: a high-resolution genome scan for susceptibility loci in a population enriched for late-stage disease. Am J Hum Genet 2004; 74: 482–94.

65. Goverdhan SV, Howell MW, Mullins RF, et al. Association of HLA class I and class II polymorphisms with age-related macular degeneration. Invest Ophthalmol Vis Sci 2005; 46: 1726–34.

66. Iyengar SK, Song D, Klein BE, et al. Dissection of genomewide-scan data in extended families reveals a major locus and oligogenic susceptibility for age-related macular degeneration. Am J Hum Genet 2004; 74: 20–39.

67. Majewski J, Schultz DW, Weleber RG, et al. Age-related macular degeneration--a genome scan in extended families. Am J Hum Genet 2003; 73: 540–50.

68. Tuo J, Smith BC, Bojanowski CM, et al. The involvement of sequence variation and expression of CX3CR1 in the pathogenesis of age-related macular degeneration. Faseb J 2004; 18: 1297–9.

69. Zareparsi S, Buraczynska M, Branham KE, et al. Toll-like receptor 4 variant D299G is associated with susceptibility to age-related macular degeneration. Hum Mol Genet 2005; 14: 1449–55.

70. Stone EM, Braun TA, Russell SR, et al. Missense variations in the fibulin 5 gene and age-related macular degeneration. N Engl J Med 2004; 351: 346–53.

71. Johnson LV, Anderson DH. Age-related macular degeneration and the extracellular matrix. N Engl J Med 2004; 351: 320–2.

72. Schultz DW, Klein ML, Humpert AJ, et al. Analysis of the ARMD1 locus: evidence that a mutation in HEMICENTIN-1 is associated with age-related macular degeneration in a large family. Hum Mol Genet 2003; 12: 3315–23.

73. Hayashi M, Merriam JE, Klaver CC, et al. Evaluation of the ARMD1 locus on 1q25-31 in patients with age-related maculopathy: genetic variation in laminin genes and in exon 104 of HEMICENTIN-1. Ophthalmic Genet 2004; 25: 111–19.

74. Fiotti N, Pedio M, Battaglia Parodi M, et al. MMP-9 microsatellite polymorphism and susceptibility to exudative form of age-related macular degeneration. Genet Med 2005; 7: 272–7.

75. Zurdel J, Finckh U, Menzer G, et al. CST3 genotype associated with exudative age related macular degeneration. Br J Ophthalmol 2002; 86: 214–19.

76. Rakoczy PE, Mann K, Cavaney DM, et al. Detection and possible functions of a cysteine protease involved in digestion of rod outer segments by retinal pigment epithelial cells. Invest Ophthalmol Vis Sci 1994; 35: 4100–8.

77. Ignatius MJ, Gebicke-Harter PJ, Skene JH, et al. Expression of apolipoprotein E during nerve degeneration and regeneration. Proc Natl Acad Sci U S A 1986; 83: 1125–9.

78. Anderson DH, Ozaki S, Nealon M, et al. Local cellular sources of apolipoprotein E in the human retina and retinal pigmented epithelium: implications for the process of drusen formation. Am J Ophthalmol 2001; 131: 767–81.

79. Baird PN, Guida E, Chu DT, et al. The epsilon2 and epsilon4 alleles of the apolipoprotein gene are associated with age-related macular degeneration. Invest Ophthalmol Vis Sci 2004; 45: 1311–15.

80. Klaver CC, Kliffen M, van Duijn CM, et al. Genetic association of apolipoprotein E with age-related macular degeneration. Am J Hum Genet 1998; 63: 200–6.

81. Simonelli F, Margaglione M, Testa F, et al. Apolipoprotein E polymorphisms in age-related macular degeneration in an Italian population. Ophthalmic Res 2001; 33: 325–8.

82. Souied EH, Benlian P, Amouyel P, et al. The epsilon4 allele of the apolipoprotein E gene as a potential protective factor for exudative age-related macular degeneration. Am J Ophthalmol 1998; 125: 353–9.

83. Schmidt S, Klaver C, Saunders A, et al. A pooled case-control study of the apolipoprotein E (APOE) gene in age-related maculopathy. Ophthalmic Genet 2002; 23: 209–23.

84. Zareparsi S, Reddick AC, Branham KE, et al. Association of apolipoprotein E alleles with susceptibility to age-related macular degeneration in a large cohort from a single center. Invest Ophthalmol Vis Sci 2004; 45: 1306–10.

85. Gotoh N, Kuroiwa S, Kikuchi T, et al. Apolipoprotein E polymorphisms in Japanese patients with polypoidal choroidal vasculopathy and exudative age-related macular degeneration. Am J Ophthalmol 2004; 138: 567–73.

86. Pang CP, Baum L, Chan WM, et al. The apolipoprotein E epsilon4 allele is unlikely to be a major risk factor of age-related macular degeneration in Chinese. Ophthalmologica 2000; 214: 289–91.

87. Schultz DW, Klein ML, Humpert A, et al. Lack of an association of apolipoprotein E gene polymorphisms with familial age-related macular degeneration. Arch Ophthalmol 2003; 121: 679–83.

88. Wong TY, Shankar A, Klein R, et al. Apolipoprotein E gene and early age-related maculopathy: the Atherosclerosis Risk in Communities Study. Ophthalmology 2006; 113: 255–9.

89. Corbo RM, Scacchi R. Apolipoprotein E (APOE) allele distribution in the world. Is APOE*4 a 'thrifty' allele? Ann Hum Genet 1999; 63(Pt 4): 301–10.

90. Schmidt S, Haines JL, Postel EA, et al. Joint effects of smoking history and APOE genotypes in age-related macular degeneration. Mol Vis 2005; 11: 941–9.

91. Ikeda T, Obayashi H, Hasegawa G, et al., Paraoxonase gene polymorphisms and plasma oxidized low-density lipoprotein level as possible risk factors for exudative age-related macular degeneration. Am J Ophthalmol 2001; 132: 191-5.

92. Baird PN, Chu D, Guida E, et al. Association of the M55L and Q192R paraoxonase gene polymorphisms with age-related macular degeneration. Am J Ophthalmol 2004; 138: 665–6.

93. Esfandiary H, Chakravarthy U, Patterson C, et al. Association study of detoxification genes in age-related macular degeneration. Br J Ophthalmol 2005; 89: 470–4.

94. Haines JL, Schnetz-Boutaud N, Schmidt S, et al. Functional candidate genes in age-related macular degeneration: significant association with VEGF, VLDLR, and LRP6. Invest Ophthalmol Vis Sci 2006; 47: 329–35.

95. Hamdi HK, Reznik J, Castellon R, et al. Alu DNA polymorphism in ACE gene is protective for age-related macular degeneration. Biochem Biophys Res Commun 2002; 295: 668–72.

96. Kimura K, Isashiki Y, Sonoda S, et al. Genetic association of manganese superoxide dismutase with exudative age-related macular degeneration. Am J Ophthalmol 2000; 130: 769–73.

97. Weber BH, Vogt G, Pruett RC, et al. Mutations in the tissue inhibitor of metalloproteinases-3 (TIMP3) in patients with Sorsby's fundus dystrophy. Nat Genet 1994; 8: 352–6.

98. Allikmets R. A photoreceptor cell-specific ATP-binding transporter gene (ABCR) is mutated in recessive Stargardt macular dystrophy. Nat Genet 1997; 17: 122.

99. Zhang K, Kniazeva M, Han M, et al. A 5-bp deletion in ELOVL4 is associated with two related forms of autosomal dominant macular dystrophy. Nat Genet 2001; 27: 89–93.

100. Petrukhin K, Koisti MJ, Bakall B, et al. Identification of the gene responsible for Best macular dystrophy. Nat Genet 1998; 19: 241–7.

101. Stone EM, Lotery AJ, Munier FL, et al. A single EFEMP1 mutation associated with both Malattia Leventinese and Doyne honeycomb retinal dystrophy. Nat Genet 1999; 22: 199–202.

102. Gregory CY, Evans K, Wijesuriya SD, et al. The gene responsible for autosomal dominant Doyne's honeycomb retinal dystrophy (DHRD) maps to chromosome 2p16. Hum Mol Genet 1996; 5: 1055–9.

103. Weng J, Mata NL, Azarian SM, et al. Insights into the function of Rim protein in photoreceptors and etiology of Stargardt's disease from the phenotype in abcr knockout mice. Cell 1999; 98: 13–23.

104. Allikmets R, Shroyer NF, Singh N, et al. Mutation of the Stargardt disease gene (ABCR) in age-related macular degeneration. Science 1997; 277: 1805–7.

105. Allikmets R. Further evidence for an association of ABCR alleles with age-related macular degeneration. The International ABCR Screening Consortium. Am J Hum Genet 2000; 67: 487–91.

106. Shroyer NF, Lewis RA, Yatsenko AN, et al. Cosegregation and functional analysis of mutant ABCR (ABCA4) alleles in families that manifest both Stargardt disease and age-related macular degeneration. Hum Mol Genet 2001; 10: 2671–8.

107. Souied EH, Ducroq D, Rozet JM, et al. ABCR gene analysis in familial exudative age-related macular degeneration. Invest Ophthalmol Vis Sci 2000; 41: 244-7.

108. Bernstein PS, Leppert M, Singh N, et al. Genotype-phenotype analysis of ABCR variants in macular degeneration probands and siblings. Invest Ophthalmol Vis Sci 2002. 43: 466–73.

109. De La Paz MA, Guy VK, Abou-Donia S, et al. Analysis of the Stargardt disease gene (ABCR) in age-related macular degeneration. Ophthalmology 1999; 106: 1531–6.

110. Kuroiwa S, Kojima H, Kikuchi T, et al. ATP binding cassette transporter retina genotypes and age related macular degeneration: an analysis on exudative non-familial Japanese patients. Br J Ophthalmol 1999; 83: 613–15.

111. Stone EM, Webster AR, Vandenburgh K, et al. Allelic variation in ABCR associated with Stargardt disease but not age-related macular degeneration. Nat Genet 1998; 20: 328–9.

112. Schmidt S, Postel EA, Agarwal A, et al. Detailed analysis of allelic variation in the ABCA4 gene in age-related maculopathy. Invest Ophthalmol Vis Sci 2003; 44: 2868–75.

113. Guymer RH, Héon E, Lotery AJ, et al. Variation of codons 1961 and 2177 of the Stargardt disease gene is not associated with age-related macular degeneration. Arch Ophthalmol 2001; 119: 745–51.

114. Baum L, Chan WM, Li WY, et al. ABCA4 sequence variants in Chinese patients with age-related macular degeneration or Stargardt's disease. Ophthalmologica 2003; 217: 111–14.

115. Fuse N, Suzuki T, Wada Y, et al. Molecular genetic analysis of ABCR gene in Japanese dry form age-related macular degeneration. Jpn J Ophthalmol 2000; 44: 245–9.

116. Rivera A, White K, Stohr H, et al. A comprehensive survey of sequence variation in the ABCA4 (ABCR) gene in Stargardt disease and age-related macular degeneration. Am J Hum Genet 2000; 67: 800–13.

117. Lewis RA, Shroyer NF, Singh N, et al. Genotype/Phenotype analysis of a photoreceptor-specific ATP-binding cassette transporter gene, ABCR, in Stargardt disease. Am J Hum Genet 1999; 64: 422–34.

118. Ayyagari R, Zhang K, Hutchinson A, et al. Evaluation of the ELOVL4 gene in patients with age-related macular degeneration. Ophthalmic Genet 2001; 22: 233–9.

119. Akimoto A, Akimoto M, Kuroiwa S, et al. Lack of association of mutations of the bestrophin gene with age-related macular degeneration in non-familial Japanese patients. Graefes Arch Clin Exp Ophthalmol 2001; 239: 66–8.

120. Allikmets R, Seddon JM, Bernstein PS, et al. Evaluation of the Best disease gene in patients with age-related macular degeneration and other maculopathies. Hum Genet 1999; 104: 449–53.

121. Guymer RH, McNeil R, Cain M, et al. Analysis of the Arg345Trp disease-associated allele of the EFEMP1 gene in individuals with early onset drusen or familial age-related macular degeneration. Clin Experiment Ophthalmol 2002; 30: 419–23.

122. Kramer F, White K, Pauleikhoff D, et al. Mutations in the VMD2 gene are associated with juvenile-onset vitelliform macular dystrophy (Best disease) and adult vitelliform macular dystrophy but not age-related macular degeneration. Eur J Hum Genet 2000: 4): 286–92.

123. Lotery AJ, Munier FL, Fishman GA, et al. Allelic variation in the VMD2 gene in best disease and age-related macular degeneration. Invest Ophthalmol Vis Sci 2000; 41: 1291–6.

124. Sauer CG, White K, Kellner U, et al. EFEMP1 is not associated with sporadic early onset drusen. Ophthalmic Genet 2001; 22: 27–34.

125. Seddon JM, Afshari MA, Sharma S, et al. Assessment of mutations in the Best macular dystrophy (VMD2) gene in patients with adult-onset foveomacular vitelliform dystrophy, age-related maculopathy, and bull's-eye maculopathy. Ophthalmology 2001; 108: 2060–7.

126. Shastry BS, Trese V. Evaluation of the peripherin/RDS gene as a candidate gene in families with age-related macular degeneration. Ophthalmologica 1999; 213: 165–70.

127. Li Z, Clarke MP, Barker MD, et al. TIMP3 mutation in Sorsby's fundus dystrophy: molecular insights. Expert Rev Mol Med 2005; 7: 1–15.

128. Kuehn MH, Stone EM, Hageman GS. Organization of the human IMPG2 gene and its evaluation as a candidate gene in age-related macular degeneration and other retinal degenerative disorders. Invest Ophthalmol Vis Sci 2001; 42: 3123–9.

129. Sauer CG, White K, Stohr H, et al. Evaluation of the G protein coupled receptor-75 (GPR75) in age related macular degeneration. Br J Ophthalmol 2001; 85: 969–75.

130. Fisher SA, Abecasis GR, Yashar BM, et al. Meta-analysis of genome scans of age-related macular degeneration. Hum Mol Genet 2005; 14: 2257–64.

131. Santangelo SL, Yen CH, Haddad S, et al. A discordant sib-pair linkage analysis of age-related macular degeneration. Ophthalmic Genet 2005; 26: 61–7.

132. Seddon JM, Santangelo SL, Book K, et al. A genomewide scan for age-related macular degeneration provides evidence for linkage to several chromosomal regions. Am J Hum Genet 2003; 73: 780–90.

133. Weeks DE, Conley YP, Tsai HJ, et al. Age-related maculopathy: an expanded genome-wide scan with evidence of susceptibility loci within the 1q31 and 17q25 regions. Am J Ophthalmol 2001; 132: 682–92.

134. Weeks DE, Conley YP, Tsai HJ, et al. Age-related maculopathy: a genomewide scan with continued evidence of susceptibility loci within the 1q31, 10q26, and 17q25 regions. Am J Hum Genet 2004; 75: 174–89.

135. Weeks DE, Conley YP, Mah TS, et al. A full genome scan for age-related maculopathy. Hum Mol Genet 2000; 9: 1329–49.

136. Schmidt S, Scott WK, Postel EA, et al. Ordered subset linkage analysis supports a susceptibility locus for age-related macular degeneration on chromosome 16p12. BMC Genet 2004; 5: 18.

137. Klein ML, Schultz DW, Edwards A, et al. Age-related macular degeneration. Clinical features in a large family and linkage to chromosome 1q. Arch Ophthalmol 1998; 116: 1082–8.

138. Kenealy SJ, Schmidt S, Agarwal A, et al. Linkage analysis for age-related macular degeneration supports a gene on chromosome 10q26. Mol Vis 2004; 10: 57–61.

139. Manolio TA, Collins FS, Cox NJ, et al. Finding the missing heritability of complex diseases. Nature 2009; 461: 747–53.

140. Seddon JM, Reynolds R, Shah HR, et al. Smoking, dietary betaine, methionine, and vitamin D in monozygotic twins with discordant macular degeneration: epigenetic implications. Ophthalmology 2011; 118: 1386–94.

4

Choroidal neovascularization: VEGF pathways

Anthony B. Daniels, Ivana K. Kim, Demetrios G. Vavvas, and Joan W. Miller

INTRODUCTION

One of the major developments in our understanding of pathologic angiogenic states, such as in cancer and in choroidal neovascularization (CNV), has been the identification of vascular endothelial growth factor (VEGF) as the primary angiogenic signal. It has now become apparent that VEGF plays an indispensable role in the development of CNV in age-related macular degeneration (AMD), and our growing knowledge of VEGF signaling over the past few decades has led to the development and clinical use of anti-VEGF therapies in the treatment of neovascular AMD, which have dramatically altered the course and outcomes of patients with this disease. This chapter reviews the basic pathogenesis of CNV, and specifically focuses on VEGF and VEGF signaling and the role that it plays in the various aspects of angiogenesis and CNV.

BASIC PATHOGENESIS OF ANGIOGENESIS AND CHOROIDAL NEOVASCULARIZATION

New vessels arise via two main routes: by vasculogenesis during development, in which vessels arise *de novo* where previously none existed, and by angiogenesis, in which new vessels sprout from already established vascular channels (1). The latter is important in the process of CNV, and requires a coordinated series of events to take place. Endothelial cells from the parent vessels are activated in response to angiogenic signals and secrete proteolytic enzymes that digest the adjacent basement membrane (2–4). Sprouting occurs in a coordinated fashion, where the leading tip cell migrates in response to graded angiogenic signals, pushed forward by proliferating stalk cells (2,5). Tip-stalk differentiation occurs by competition between adjacent endothelial cells and by paracrine inhibition of tip cell fate specification in adjacent cells (1,2). Tissue plane digestion allows for migration to occur along the extracellular matrix (ECM) scaffold. Once the new endothelial tubes have formed, proliferation activity must be reined in and vessels must mature, by assembling a leak-proof pericyte coating (1,2).

One of the early steps of CNV is thought to be the degradation or mechanical disruption of the endothelial cell basement membrane, with formation of a discontinuity in Bruch's membrane that allows endothelial cells to migrate into the sub-RPE space. With senescence, retinal pigment epithelium (RPE) function becomes compromised, and the composition and properties of Bruch's membrane change. As lysosome function decreases with aging in RPE, lipofuscin (a by-product of photoreceptor outer segment digestion by lysosomes) accumulates, which is thought to result in further disturbance of RPE function (6). Accumulations between the plasma and basement membranes of the RPE (basal laminar deposits) and thickening of the inner collagenous zone of Bruch's membrane (basal linear deposits) also increase with aging, and are associated with CNV (7). Disturbance of the RPE, softening of hard drusen, and cleavage in basal laminar/linear deposits may aid in the formation of soft drusen, which appear to be an important predisposing feature for CNV (7–11). Thickening of Bruch's membrane and deposits between the RPE and Bruch's are speculated to block diffusion of oxygen, thus causing localized hypoxia and expression of angiogenic factors, such as VEGF (12). In addition, complement and other immune components contained within these deposits may initiate inflammation, thus damaging Bruch's membrane further (13–16).

A discontinuity in Bruch's membrane is required for CNV, as transgenic mice that overexpress VEGF in photoreceptors but have an intact Bruch's membrane develop subretinal neovascularization, but the subretinal vessels extend from retinal vessels rather than from the choroidal vasculature (17). In contrast, transgenic mice that overexpress VEGF in RPE cells show intrachoroidal NV that does not penetrate Bruch's membrane and does not extend into the sub-RPE space (18). These findings support the notion that CNV requires both the expression of an angiogenic factor and a break in Bruch's membrane. This break in Bruch's membrane can develop by any of several methods. Traumatic choroidal rupture is a known cause of CNV (19), as is laser disruption (20,21). In the absence of physical trauma, disruption can occur via proteolytic digestion, as occurs when there is an imbalance between proteolytic enzymes such as matrix metalloproteinases (MMPs) and tissue inhibitors of MMPs. Both RPE cells (22,23) and macrophages (24) are known sources of MMPs, and the accumulation of macrophages near thinned segments of Bruch's membrane might contribute to the degradation of Bruch's membrane (25), thus allowing choroidal endothelial cells to gain entry to the sub-RPE space.

AMD has a significant genetic component, as family members of individuals with AMD are more likely to develop the disease, and there is a higher concordance among monozygotic twins than dizygotic twins (26). The composition of Bruch's membrane and of drusen in patients with AMD gives some idea as to the various genetic pathways that have been implicated in predisposition to the development of AMD. Genes involved in lipid regulation, in the complement pathway, and in inflammation are chief among these. The ApoE protein is involved in the regulation of blood lipids, and the e2 allele of the *APOE* gene may increase susceptibility, while the e4 allele may be protective (27). Very strong evidence exists for the complement factor H (*CFH*) gene, where a single nucleotide polymorphism encoding for the Y402H variant can increase the risk of the disease three- to sevenfold (28–30), and several other components of the complement pathway have been implicated in disease progression in several other studies as well (31–35). The chemokine receptor *CX3CR1* gene and the Toll-like receptor 4 (*TLR4*) gene have been implicated in several, but not all, studies as risk factors for progression of the disease (36–39). Convincing genetic association data exist for a locus on chromosome 10q26 which harbors genes that encode pleckstrin homology domain-containing protein 1 (PLEKHA1), the ARMS2 gene product of unknown function, and the trypsin-like protease HTRA1 (40–42). This locus is associated with a seven- to tenfold increased risk of the disease. However, allelic variation of VEGF, the single gene product known to be the most important therapeutic target in neovascular AMD, has not consistently been found to convey increased susceptibility in genomic analyses (35,43–48).

CNV likely occurs when there is an imbalance between proangiogenic and antiangiogenic growth factors. Angiogenic growth factors that promote CNV include VEGF, its homolog placental growth factor (PlGF), fibroblast growth factor, (FGF) (49) and angiopoietins (50,51). Antiangiogenic growth factors, such as pigment epithelial-derived factor (PEDF) (52), inhibit choroidal angiogenesis. This chapter focuses on VEGF, and describes the role that VEGF plays in initiation of angiogenesis, in promoting endothelial cell sprouting and migration, and in vascular leakiness. The roles that the other angiogenic and antiangiogenic growth factors play in CNV, as well as their implications for future treatment, are discussed in detail in chapter 20.

UPSTREAM CONTROL OF VEGF

The most important stimulus for increased *VEGF* expression (and for angiogenesis in general) is hypoxia (53,54), although other conditions such as hypoglycemia (55) and low pH (56) (both of which occur with ischemia) and reactive oxygen species also modulate *VEGF* expression (57). Like many hypoxia-response factors, *VEGF* expression is under the control of hypoxia-inducible factors (HIFs) such as HIF-1α, which is a dimeric transcription factor composed of two subunits, the oxygen-sensitive HIF-1α and its binding partner HIF-1β (58). Under normoxic conditions, the HIF-1α that is synthesized is subsequently ubiquitinated and targeted for degradation in the proteasome. Ubiquitination of HIF-1α occurs via its association with the von Hippel-Lindau (VHL) tumor suppressor protein, which assembles a complex that contains ubiquitin ligase (59). The VHL–HIF–1α–VEGF axis is dependent on the hydroxylation status of the

proteins, and this is, in turn, dependent on the amount of oxygen in the cellular environment (60). Hydroxylation of HIF-1α on proline residues facilitates complex formation with VHL, thereby targeting it for degradation (61). Under hypoxic conditions, HIF is not hydroxylated, does not complex with VHL, and is not targeted for degradation. Therefore, under hypoxic conditions, HIF-1α accumulates in the cytoplasm, complexes with HIF-1β, translocates to the nucleus, and effects its transcriptional control over hypoxia-inducible genes such as *VEGF* (1,2). In addition, under oxygen-rich conditions, HIF-1α is itself hydroxylated, which prevents its interaction with transcriptional co-activators such as p300 and CBP (62). Under hypoxic conditions, this hydroxylation does not occur, the transcription factor complex can form, and therefore HIF-1α can mediate transcription of *VEGF* (Fig. 4.1).

Other growth factors also modulate expression of *VEGF*. For example, TGFβ induces the expression of VEGF transcripts in human RPE cells via a MAPK-mediated pathway. External cellular stimuli, such as epidermal growth factor, insulin-like growth factor-1, FGF, PDGF, and β-estradiol are also involved in the regulation of *VEGF* gene expression, implicating both paracrine and autocrine control in *VEGF* expression (63). In cancer, oncogenes and tumor suppressor genes promote tumorigenesis not only by causing cell division and proliferation but also by inducing *VEGF* expression. For example, cells transfected with mutant *src* or *ras* have increased mRNA and protein levels of VEGF, while tumor suppressor genes such as *p53* suppress *VEGF* transcription (64).

VEGF AND ITS RECEPTORS

There are five different VEGF proteins, termed VEGF-A, VEGF-B, VEGF-C, VEGF-D, and VEGF-E, in addition to the VEGF homolog, PlGF (64,65). The canonical VEGF family protein is VEGF-A, which was the original vasopermeability factor first discovered (usually simply referred to as "VEGF," a convention to which we will adhere in this chapter as well). VEGF-B plays a role in cardiac and coronary artery development (64). VEGF-C plays a role in arteriovenous segregation during vasculogenesis (2), and is primarily involved in lymphangiogenesis, as is VEGF-D (64,65). VEGF-E is a related viral protein, and functions similarly to VEGF-A (64). The effect of PlGF is similar to that of VEGF-A, possibly in part because PlGF binds VEGF receptor 1 (VEGFR1, see below) which itself serves as a receptor decoy, thus freeing VEGF-A to transduce its signal via VEGF receptor 2 (VEGFR2) (63,66). The possible decoy effect of PlGF, as well as the more direct role that PlGF plays in CNV, is discussed in detail in chapter 20.

The most important member of the VEGF family for angiogenesis is VEGF-A. VEGF is a heparin-binding dimeric glycoprotein with disulfide-linked subunits which shares significant sequence homology with the α and β chains of PDGF (67). The human *VEGF-A* gene is located on chromosome 6p, where it encodes five different polypeptides based on variable splicing of the mRNA

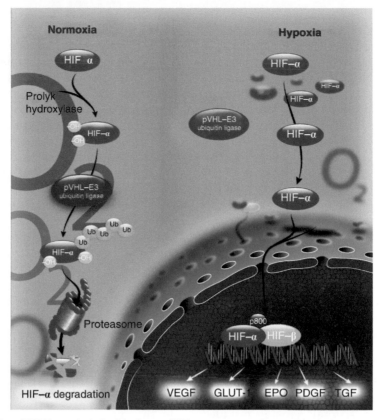

Figure 4.1 The von Hippel-Lindau (**VHL**)/hypoxia-inducible factor (**HIF**) **oxygen-sensing pathway.** In normoxia, HIF-1α that is synthesized is ubiquitinated and targeted for degradation in the proteasome. This process involves hydroxylation of HIF on proline residues, which further facilitates the complex formation with the VHL-E3 ligase and subsequent ubiquitination of HIF-1α. Under hypoxic conditions, HIF-1α is not hydroxylated, does not complex with VHL, and therefore not degraded by the proteasome. Thus, HIF-1α accumulates in the cytoplasm, complexes with HIF-1β, and translocates to the nucleus, where it interacts with transcriptional co-activators such as p300 and affects its transcriptional control over hypoxia-inducible genes such as VEGF, GLUT1, EPO, PDGF, and TGF among others. *Source: Courtesy of Dr Aristomenis Thanos.*

transcript. These transcripts encode proteins that are 121, 145, 165, 189, and 206 amino acids in length in humans (120, 144, 164, and 188 in mice) (64). All presumably have the same functions *in vivo*, but differ in their binding affinities to cell surface proteins and to ECM proteins, and this affects their localization (5,63, 68–72). $VEGF_{165}$, the isoform most important in pathologic angiogenesis, binds heparin and other proteoglycans. $VEGF_{121}$ does not bind heparin or other ECM proteoglycans, and thus diffuses freely over long distances. In contrast, $VEGF_{189}$ binds heparin very strongly, and therefore does not diffuse. The implications of these different binding affinities of VEGF for ECM proteins relate to their ability to cause VEGF-gradient-guided migration of endothelial cells during angiogenesis, which requires both long- and short-range guidance cues (5,72). $VEGF_{121}$, which is soluble and freely diffusible, is effective at long-range guidance, but not short-range guidance (72). On the other hand, $VEGF_{189}$, which is matrix bound, can mediate short-range guidance, but not long-range guidance (72). Only the 165 amino acid isoform, $VEGF_{165}$, exists in both soluble and matrix-bound forms (73), and thus mediates both long-range and short-range migration guidance effectively. Thus, mice engineered to express only $VEGF_{120}$ or $VEGF_{188}$ develop severe anomalies, while mice expressing only $VEGF_{164}$ develop normally (72).

There are three high-affinity VEGF receptors (VEGFRs): VEGFR1 (FMS-like tyrosine kinase or FLT-1 in human) and VEGFR2 (fetal liver kinase 1 or Flk-1 in the mouse; TKR-C in the rat; kinase insert domain receptor or KDR in the human) are expressed on vascular endothelial cells, whereas VEGFR3 (FLT4) is primarily found on lymphatic endothelial cells and primarily binds VEGF-C and VEGF-D (63–65). VEGFR1 has a 10-fold higher affinity than VEGFR2 for VEGF-A, but VEGFR2 is expressed in higher copy numbers than VEGFR1, and it is VEGFR2 that is predominantly responsible for transducing the VEGF angiogenic signal, resulting in mitogenesis, survival, and permeability (65). Corroborating this is the fact that VEGFR2-null mice die *in utero* at approximately day E9 from a failure to initiate vasculogenesis and hematopoiesis, due to defective blood island formation from impaired cell migration (1,74,75). In contrast, VEGFR1-null mice die from vascular defects characterized by angioblasts localized inappropriately to the central regions of the blood islands instead of the periphery, indicative of endothelial cell overgrowth (1,76).

While VEGFR2 transduces the main VEGF signal, VEGFR1 appears to be only weakly stimulated by VEGF binding. This has led to the hypothesis that VEGFR1, either in its membrane-bound or soluble form, may serve as a receptor decoy for VEGF, decreasing VEGF–VEGFR2 signaling by soaking up the available soluble VEGF (63,66,77,78). Several facts support this conclusion: VEGFR1 exists in a soluble form, which appears to have the same effect on angiogenic signaling as the membrane-bound form (79,80); mice expressing only the extracellular domain of VEGFR1, without the kinase domain, develop normally (77); PlGF, which binds specifically to VEGFR1, increases angiogenic signaling, presumably by displacing VEGF from the VEGFR1 decoy receptor, and thus making more VEGF available to stimulate the active VEGFR2 receptor (66).

VEGF also binds to neuropilins (Nrp) 1 and 2, which are transmembrane glycoproteins with short cytoplasmic domains, which function as co-receptors for VEGFRs (1,78). It is not clear if neuropilins are capable of independent VEGF-mediated signaling, but rather enhance VEGFR2 signaling by increasing $VEGF_{165}$-VEGFR2 binding, perhaps by presenting VEGF to VEGFR2 (1). Interestingly, they also form complexes with VEGFR1 (as well as with VEGFR3). Nrp1 mutants display vascular defects (81), since Nrp1 is found on arterial endothelium, while Nrp2 mutants display defective lymphangiogensis (1), consistent with Nrp2's lymphatic and venous restriction.

VEGFR2 undergoes ligand-dependent dimerization and autophosphorylation of several tyrosine residues. Phosphorylated Tyr^{1175} binds and activates phospholipase C-gamma (PLC-γ), which activates mitogen-activated protein kinase (MAPK), promoting cell proliferation (82). Phosphorylation of PLC-γ also leads to release of calcium stores and activates protein kinase C (PKC) pathways (1). PKC activation stimulates the Raf/MEK/ERK pathway important for cell proliferation (65). The vasopermeability effect of VEGF appears to be a result of this calcium mobilization and PKC activation, via activation of endothelial nitric oxide synthase (65). Src homology 2 domain-containing adapter protein B (Shb) binds Tyr^{1175} and serves as an adaptor for phosphatidylinositol 3 kinase (PI3K), resulting in increased levels of phosphatidylinositol-3,4,5-triphosphate, and thereby inducing activation of Akt/PKB (83). Once activated, the Akt/PKB pathway mediates endothelial cell survival by phosphorylating and thus inhibiting proapoptotic proteins BAD and caspase-9 (65). VEGFR2-activation also leads to endothelial cell migration by activation of actin cytoskeleton remodeling mediated by cdc42 and p38 MAPK (84), and also by Tyr^{951}-mediated Src stimulation via the adaptor protein T-cell specific adaptor (TsAd) (85). The net effect of these downstream signaling pathways is to increase endothelial cell survival, migration, proliferation, and vascular permeability.

ROLE OF VEGF IN CHOROIDAL NEOVASCULARIZATION

There are many lines of evidence that confirm the central role of VEGF in pathologic retinal and CNV. In a rabbit model with ischemic hind limb, a single intra-arterial bolus of VEGF was sufficient to stimulate angiogenesis and collateralization (86). This has led to studies of the therapeutic use of VEGF in peripheral vascular and coronary artery disease. VEGF also results in neovascularization in the corneal micropocket and in the chick chorioallantoic membrane bioassays (87,88).

In vivo work has demonstrated VEGF to be spatially and temporally correlated with iris neovascularization in a monkey model of ischemic retinopathy and iris neovascularization (89). Injections of recombinant human VEGF in normal monkey eyes led to iris neovascularization and neovascular glaucoma, as well as many of the changes of diabetic retinopathy, including vessel dilation, tortuosity, microaneurysm formation, hemorrhage, edema, capillary dropout, and intraretinal neovascularization (90,91). *In situ* hybridization identified the inner retina as the source of VEGF, and VEGF protein levels in serial aqueous samples have been shown to correlate with the severity of induced retinal ischemia and iris neovascularization (89,92). To demonstrate the causal role of VEGF in neovascularization secondary to ischemia, VEGF activity was specifically blocked using anti-VEGF antibodies, soluble VEGF receptors, or antisense oligonucleotides to VEGF. Intravitreous injection of anti-VEGF antibodies completely prevented the development of iris neovascularization in the monkey model (93). Work in models of retinopathy of prematurity (ROP) also demonstrates the importance of VEGF in the development of retinal neovascularization (94–96). In the mouse ROP model, dominant-negative VEGF receptors and VEGF antisense oligonucleotides substantially decreased retinal neovascularization (97,98).

VEGF also plays an important role in the development of CNV. Immunostaining of surgical specimens of choroidal neovascular membranes showed increased VEGF expression (99,100). *In situ* hybridization studies have demonstrated a correlation between VEGF expression and the development of CNV in laser injury models in the rat and monkey (101). Oxidative stress may stimulate the overexpression of growth factors from the RPE, a possible inflammatory state, and subsequent damage and thickening of Bruch's membrane from recruited macrophages (102,103). It has been suggested that the abnormally thickened Bruch's membrane may interfere with polarized RPE secretion of VEGF necessary for maintenance of the choriocapillaris. Atrophy of the choriocapillaris, often seen clinically, may result in a state of outer retinal hypoxia, stimulating VEGF-induced angiogenesis (104). Studies have also shown that despite the absence of hypoxia in the laser injury models, specific compounds which bind VEGF and its receptors virtually eliminate CNV (105–108). These data have important clinical implications, as specific pharmacologic inhibitors of VEGF have been approved for the treatment of neovascular AMD and shown to be effective (see chapter 19 for a detailed review of these).

VEGF plays a direct role in many of the crucial steps of CNV. The initial obligatory step in CNV is the ability of the capillary endothelial cells to cross the basement membrane which otherwise envelops them. VEGF is known to increase levels of MMPs, which are responsible for proteolysis of endothelial cell basement membrane and for digestion through tissue planes. When exposed to VEGF, endothelial cells begin to generate and secrete MMP-2 within three hours of stimulation (109). Vascular smooth muscle cells, which normally envelop the endothelial cells in vessel walls, also upregulate MMP-1, 3, and 9 in response to VEGF (110). Lastly, RPE cells, which normally secrete low basal levels of MMP-2 *in vitro* at rest, show increased levels of secreted MMP-2 in response to VEGF stimulation, and also begin to secrete MMP-9 as well (22). Interestingly, exogenous (and presumably endogenous) MMP-9 also feeds back to further increase gene expression and secretion of VEGF from the RPE cells (23).

The next step in angiogenesis is determination of cell fate as the leading tip cell, which will form the leading edge in migration, and the proliferating stalk cells which will form the ensuing vessel channel walls. This cell fate determination relies on expression of Delta-like ligand 4 (DLL4) on tip cells, suppressing tip cell behavior on adjacent stalk cells (which express the DLL4 receptor, Notch), all of which are under the control of VEGF (1,2). In the absence of an intact DLL4-Notch axis, all cells assume the default tip cell phenotype, and therefore blockade of DLL4 or Notch leads to a hypersprouting phenotype with an excessive number of tip cells and no coordinated vessel formation (111). VEGF, signaling via VEGFR2, increases DLL4 expression in tip cells, thus suppressing tip cell phenotype in adjacent endothelial cells (which therefore assume a stalk cell phenotype) (1,2,112,114). VEGFR3, which is usually confined to lymphatics post-developmentally, is re-expressed in tip cells, and its pharmacological inhibition reduces sprouting (113). VEGFR1, on the other hand, suppresses sprouting, and its loss causes increased sprouting and vascularization (2). Interestingly, a soluble or kinase-deficient variant of VEGFR1 rescues this increased sprouting phenotype (2), again corroborating that VEGFR1 serves as a VEGF trap. DLL4-mediated activation of Notch on adjacent endothelial cells inhibits tip cell behavior in these cells by downregulating VEGFR2, VEGFR3, and Nrp1, while upregulating VEGFR1 (112,114).

Once endothelial cells have assumed their respective tip or stalk cell phenotypes, each type responds differently to VEGF. Stalk cells proliferate in response to the concentration of VEGF, while tip cells do not; rather, they form filopodia via VEGF-mediated activation of cdc42, and then migrate in the direction of the VEGF gradient (2,5). As mentioned above, both long-range and short-range guidance cues are important for nascent vessel migration. Soluble VEGF provides long-range guidance, while ECM-bound VEGF provides short-range guidance cues. $VEGF_{165}$, which binds ECM, but not so tightly that it is unable to diffuse, is therefore ideally suited to this dual guidance task. Evidence for the importance of both short-range and long-range guidance comes from mouse embryos engineered to express solely either $VEGF_{120}$ (the mouse equivalent of human $VEGF_{121}$), which does not have a heparin-binding motif and therefore diffuses freely over long distances, or $VEGF_{188}$ (the mouse equivalent of human $VEGF_{189}$) which is entirely bound to ECM and does not diffuse (72). Mice that only expressed $VEGF_{120}$ and therefore could only provide long-range (but not short-range) cues, exhibit a decrease in capillary branch formation due to altered distribution of endothelial cells within the growing vasculature; thus, they are incorporated into existing vessels to increase their lumen calibers rather than forming additional branches (72). Endothelial cells in these mice have dysfunctional directed extension of filopodia, which is normally provided in a spatially restricted fashion by VEGF (72). In contrast, mice that only express $VEGF_{188}$, and therefore only provide short-range guidance cues, produce excess filopodia in multiple directions, including toward already-existing vessels, and therefore may form many microvessels (72). Thus, it appears that appropriate guidance cues via a VEGF gradient are necessary for appropriate endothelial cell migration and a normal vessel branching pattern.

Lastly, while the proangiogenic VEGF does not directly cause vessel maturation (and therefore termination of the angiogenic signal), it does play a role in this aspect of vessel development as well. VEGF upregulates angiopoietin (Ang)-1 mRNA levels by stabilization of Ang-1 mRNA, and also increases Ang-1 protein secretion (115). Ang-1 plays two related roles: in pericyte and mural cell recruitment for vessel wall stabilization and in maintenance of mature vessel quiescence. Once the vessels become mature and stabilized, they are relatively resistant to VEGF-mediated permeability and angiogenic signalling (2). This suggests that within VEGF stimulation lies the seed to its own termination, by creating a negative feedback loop through Ang-1-mediated vessel maturation, which leads to relative resilience of the vessels to further VEGF stimulation.

CONCLUSIONS

CNV arises from an imbalance of proangiogenic and antiangiogenic signals, and requires a coordinated series of steps to occur. As the primary angiogenic signal, VEGF signaling plays a role in all aspects of CNV formation, causing endothelial cell recruitment, proliferation, migration, and survival. Since VEGF is necessary for CNV initiation and progression, drugs that target VEGF or its receptors can inhibit CNV and its associated vascular leakage. Our expanding knowledge of VEGF–VEGFR interactions and the various VEGF signaling pathways has directly led to our ability to inhibit neovascularization in patients with AMD and other disease states. VEGF inhibition for the treatment of ocular diseases has truly been one of the great success stories in ophthalmology, and a model of bench-to-bedside science, which has dramatically improved the quality of vision—and the quality of life—of a large number of patients.

SUMMARY POINTS

- Choroidal neovascularization (CNV) occurs when there is an imbalance between proangiogenic and antiangiogenic growth factors, but also requires a break in Bruch's membrane to allow choroidal endothelial cells to enter the subretinal space. This can arise from exogenous mechanical disruption (i.e., trauma) or by endogenous proteolytic degradation.

- Vascular endothelial growth factor (VEGF), the primary angiogenic signaling molecule, is produced in response to tissue hypoxia, mainly under the transcriptional control of HIF.
- VEGF-A, the most important VEGF family member for angiogenesis, signals via its receptor, VEGFR2, while VEGFR1 serves as a VEGF trap to decrease angiogenic signaling.
- VEGF signaling plays a role in many steps of angiogenesis:
  - VEGF leads to MMP secretion, causing basement membrane proteolysis to allow endothelial cells to exit pre-existing vessels
  - VEGF provides the angiogenic signal to which phenotypically-different tip and stalk endothelial cells respond, by causing proliferation of stalk cells and by providing the chemical gradient guiding tip cell migration
- Inhibition of VEGF signaling therefore prevents pathologic angiogenesis and CNV.

REFERENCES

1. Patel-Hett S, D'Amore PA. Signal transduction in vasculogenesis and developmental angiogenesis. Int J Dev Biol 2011; 55: 353–63.
2. Potente M, Gerhardt H, Carmeliet P. Basic and therapeutic aspects of angiogenesis. Cell 2011; 146: 873–87.
3. Alexander JP, Bradley JM, Gabourel JD, Acott TS. Expression of matrix metalloproteinases and inhibitor by human retinal pigment epithelium. Invest Ophthalmol Vis Sci 1990; 31: 2520–8.
4. Padgett LC, Lui GM, Werb Z, LaVail MM. Matrix metalloproteinase-2 and tissue inhibitor of metalloproteinase-1 in the retinal pigment epithelium and interphotoreceptor matrix: vectorial secretion and regulation. Exp Eye Res 1997; 64: 927–38.
5. Gerhardt H, Golding M, Fruttiger M, et al. VEGF guides angiogenic sprouting utilizing endothelial tip cell filopodia. J Cell Biol 2003; 161: 1163–77.
6. Kennedy CJ, Rakoczy PE, Constable IJ. Lipofuscin of the retinal pigment epithelium: a review. Eye (Lond) 1995; 9(Pt 6): 763–71.
7. Green WR, Enger C. Age-related macular degeneration histopathologic studies. the 1992 Lorenz E. Zimmerman Lecture. Ophthalmology 1993; 100: 1519–35.
8. Hageman GS, Mullins RF. Molecular composition of drusen as related to substructural phenotype. Mol Vis 1999; 5: 28.
9. Mullins RF, Russell SR, Anderson DH, Hageman GS. Drusen associated with aging and age-related macular degeneration contain proteins common to extracellular deposits associated with atherosclerosis, elastosis, amyloidosis, and dense deposit disease. FASEB J 2000; 14: 835–46.
10. Sarks JP, Sarks SH, Killingsworth MC. Evolution of soft drusen in age-related macular degeneration. Eye (Lond) 1994; 8(Pt 3): 269–83.
11. Abdelsalam A, Del Priore L, Zarbin MA. Drusen in age-related macular degeneration: pathogenesis, natural course, and laser photocoagulation-induced regression. Surv Ophthalmol 1999; 44: 1–29.
12. Starita C, Hussain AA, Patmore A, Marshall J. Localization of the site of major resistance to fluid transport in Bruch's membrane. Invest Ophthalmol Vis Sci 1997; 38: 762–7.
13. Russell SR, Mullins RF, Schneider BL, Hageman GS. Location, substructure, and composition of basal laminar drusen compared with drusen associated with aging and age-related macular degeneration. Am J Ophthalmol 2000; 129: 205–14.
14. Mullins RF, Aptsiauri N, Hageman GS. Structure and composition of drusen associated with glomerulonephritis: implications for the role of complement activation in drusen biogenesis. Eye (Lond) 2001; 15(Pt 3): 390–5.
15. Hageman GS, Luthert PJ, Victor Chong NH, et al. An integrated hypothesis that considers drusen as biomarkers of immune-mediated processes at the RPE-Bruch's membrane interface in aging and age-related macular degeneration. Prog Retin Eye Res 2001; 20: 705–32.
16. Anderson DH, Mullins RF, Hageman GS, Johnson LV. A role for local inflammation in the formation of drusen in the aging eye. Am J Ophthalmol 2002; 134: 411–31.
17. Okamoto N, Tobe T, Hackett SF, et al. Transgenic mice with increased expression of vascular endothelial growth factor in the retina: a new model of intraretinal and subretinal neovascularization. Am J Pathol 1997; 151: 281–91.
18. Schwesinger C, Yee C, Rohan RM, et al. Intrachoroidal neovascularization in transgenic mice overexpressing vascular endothelial growth factor in the retinal pigment epithelium. Am J Pathol 2001; 158: 1161–72.
19. Gross JG, King LP, de Juan E Jr, Powers T. Subfoveal neovascular membrane removal in patients with traumatic choroidal rupture. Ophthalmology 1996; 103: 579–85.
20. van der Zypen E, Fankhauser F, Raess K, England C. Morphologic findings in the rabbit retina following irradiation with the free-running neodymium-YAG laser. disruption of Bruch's membrane and its effect on the scarring process in the retina and choroid. Arch Ophthalmol 1986; 104: 1070–7.
21. Pollack A, Korte GE, Weitzner AL, Henkind P. Ultrastructure of bruch's membrane after krypton laser photocoagulation. I. breakdown of Bruch's membrane. Arch Ophthalmol 1986; 104: 1372–6.
22. Hoffmann S, He S, Ehren M, et al. MMP-2 and MMP-9 secretion by RPE is stimulated by angiogenic molecules found in choroidal neovascular membranes. Retina 2006; 26: 454–61.
23. Hollborn M, Stathopoulos C, Steffen A, et al. Positive feedback regulation between MMP-9 and VEGF in human RPE cells. Invest Ophthalmol Vis Sci 2007; 48: 4360–7.
24. Goetzl EJ, Banda MJ, Leppert D. Matrix metalloproteinases in immunity. J Immunol 1996; 156: 1–4.
25. Killingsworth MC, Sarks JP, Sarks SH. Macrophages related to Bruch's membrane in age-related macular degeneration. Eye (Lond) 1990; 4(Pt 4): 613–21.
26. Hammond CJ, Webster AR, Snieder H, et al. Genetic influence on early age-related maculopathy: a twin study. Ophthalmology 2002; 109: 730–6.
27. Baird PN, Guida E, Chu DT, Vu HT, Guymer RH. The epsilon2 and epsilon4 alleles of the apolipoprotein gene are associated with age-related macular degeneration. Invest Ophthalmol Vis Sci 2004; 45: 1311–15.

28. Haines JL, Hauser MA, Schmidt S, et al. Complement factor H variant increases the risk of age-related macular degeneration. Science. 2005; 308: 419–21.

29. Edwards AO, Ritter R 3rd, Abel KJ, et al. Complement factor H polymorphism and age-related macular degeneration. Science 2005; 308: 421–4.

30. Klein RJ, Zeiss C, Chew EY, et al. Complement factor H polymorphism in age-related macular degeneration. Science 2005; 308: 385–9.

31. Gold B, Merriam JE, Zernant J, et al. Variation in factor B (BF) and complement component 2 (C2) genes is associated with age-related macular degeneration. Nat Genet 2006; 38: 458–62.

32. Yates JR, Sepp T, Matharu BK, et al. Complement C3 variant and the risk of age-related macular degeneration. N Engl J Med 2007; 357: 553–61.

33. Maller JB, Fagerness JA, Reynolds RC, et al. Variation in complement factor 3 is associated with risk of age-related macular degeneration. Nat Genet 2007; 39: 1200–201.

34. Spencer KL, Hauser MA, Olson LM, et al. Deletion of CFHR3 and CFHR1 genes in age-related macular degeneration. Hum Mol Genet 2008; 17: 971–7.

35. Francis PJ, Hamon SC, Ott J, Weleber RG, Klein ML. Polymorphisms in C2, CFB and C3 are associated with progression to advanced age related macular degeneration associated with visual loss. J Med Genet 2009; 46: 300–7.

36. Brion M, Sanchez-Salorio M, Corton M, et al. Genetic association study of age-related macular degeneration in the Spanish population. Acta Ophthalmol 2011; 89: e12–22.

37. Yang X, Hu J, Zhang J, Guan H. Polymorphisms in CFH, HTRA1 and CX3CR1 confer risk to exudative age-related macular degeneration in Han Chinese. Br J Ophthalmol 2010; 94: 1211–14.

38. Zerbib J, Puche N, Richard F, et al. No association between the T280M polymorphism of the CX3CR1 gene and exudative AMD. Exp Eye Res 2011; 93: 382–6.

39. Liu MM, Agron E, Chew E, et al. Copy number variations in candidate genes in neovascular age-related macular degeneration. Invest Ophthalmol Vis Sci 2011; 52: 3129–35.

40. Gotoh N, Yamashiro K, Nakanishi H, et al. Haplotype analysis of the ARMS2/HTRA1 region in Japanese patients with typical neovascular age-related macular degeneration or polypoidal choroidal vasculopathy. Jpn J Ophthalmol 2010; 54: 609–14.

41. Hadley D, Orlin A, Brown G, et al. Analysis of six genetic risk factors highly associated with AMD in the region surrounding ARMS2 and HTRA1 on chromosome 10, region q26. Invest Ophthalmol Vis Sci 2010; 51: 2191–6.

42. Friedrich U, Myers CA, Fritsche LG, et al. Risk- and non-risk-associated variants at the 10q26 AMD locus influence ARMS2 mRNA expression but exclude pathogenic effects due to protein deficiency. Hum Mol Genet 2011; 20: 1387–99.

43. Haines JL, Schnetz-Boutaud N, Schmidt S, et al. Functional candidate genes in age-related macular degeneration: significant association with VEGF, VLDLR, and LRP6. Invest Ophthalmol Vis Sci 2006; 47: 329–35.

44. Churchill AJ, Carter JG, Lovell HC, et al. VEGF polymorphisms are associated with neovascular age-related macular degeneration. Hum Mol Genet 2006; 15: 2955–61.

45. Boekhoorn SS, Isaacs A, Uitterlinden AG, et al. Polymorphisms in the vascular endothelial growth factor gene and risk of age-related macular degeneration: the Rotterdam Study. Ophthalmology 2008; 115: 1899–903.

46. Janik-Papis K, Zaras M, Krzyzanowska A, et al. Association between vascular endothelial growth factor gene polymorphisms and age-related macular degeneration in a Polish population. Exp Mol Pathol 2009; 87: 234–8.

47. Fang AM, Lee AY, Kulkarni M, et al. Polymorphisms in the VEGFA and VEGFR-2 genes and neovascular age-related macular degeneration. Mol Vis 2009; 15: 2710–9.

48. Yu Y, Bhangale TR, Fagerness J, et al. Common variants near FRK/COL10A1 and VEGFA are associated with advanced age-related macular degeneration. Hum Mol Genet 2011; 20: 3699–709.

49. Zubilewicz A, Hecquet C, Jeanny JC, et al. Two distinct signalling pathways are involved in FGF2-stimulated proliferation of choriocapillary endothelial cells: a comparative study with VEGF. Oncogene 2001; 20: 1403–13.

50. Hackett SF, Ozaki H, Strauss RW, et al. Angiopoietin 2 expression in the retina: upregulation during physiologic and pathologic neovascularization. J Cell Physiol 2000; 184: 275–84.

51. Otani A, Takagi H, Oh H, et al. Expressions of angiopoietins and Tie2 in human choroidal neovascular membranes. Invest Ophthalmol Vis Sci 1999; 40: 1912–20.

52. Dawson DW, Volpert OV, Gillis P, et al. Pigment epithelium-derived factor: a potent inhibitor of angiogenesis. Science 1999; 285: 245–8.

53. Shima DT, Adamis AP, Ferrara N, et al. Hypoxic induction of endothelial cell growth factors in retinal cells: identification and characterization of vascular endothelial growth factor (VEGF) as the mitogen. Mol Med 1995; 1: 182–93.

54. Shweiki D, Itin A, Soffer D, Keshet E. Vascular endothelial growth factor induced by hypoxia may mediate hypoxia-initiated angiogenesis. Nature 1992; 359: 843–5.

55. Satake S, Kuzuya M, Miura H, et al. Up-regulation of vascular endothelial growth factor in response to glucose deprivation. Biol Cell 1998; 90: 161–8.

56. Fukumura D, Xu L, Chen Y, et al. Hypoxia and acidosis independently up-regulate vascular endothelial growth factor transcription in brain tumors in vivo. Cancer Res 2001; 61: 6020–4.

57. Kuroki M, Voest EE, Amano S, et al. Reactive oxygen intermediates increase vascular endothelial growth factor expression in vitro and in vivo. J Clin Invest 1996; 98: 1667–75.

58. Kelly BD, Hackett SF, Hirota K, et al. Cell type-specific regulation of angiogenic growth factor gene expression and induction of angiogenesis in nonischemic tissue by a constitutively active form of hypoxia-inducible factor 1. Circ Res 2003; 93: 1074–81.

59. Salceda S, Caro J. Hypoxia-inducible factor 1alpha (HIF-1alpha) protein is rapidly degraded by the ubiquitin-proteasome system under normoxic conditions. Its stabilization by hypoxia depends on redox-induced changes. J Biol Chem 1997; 272: 22642–7.

60. Ivan M, Kondo K, Yang H, et al. HIFalpha targeted for VHL-mediated destruction by proline hydroxylation: implications for O2 sensing. Science 2001; 292: 464–8.

61. Jaakkola P, Mole DR, Tian YM, et al. Targeting of HIF-alpha to the von Hippel-Lindau ubiquitylation complex by O2-regulated prolyl hydroxylation. Science 2001; 292: 468–72.

62. Semenza GL. Vasculogenesis, angiogenesis, and arteriogenesis: mechanisms of blood vessel formation and remodeling. J Cell Biochem 2007; 102: 840–7.

63. Ferrara N, Gerber HP, LeCouter J. The biology of VEGF and its receptors. Nat Med 2003; 9: 669–76.

64. Nagy JA, Dvorak AM, Dvorak HF. VEGF-A and the induction of pathological angiogenesis. Annu Rev Pathol 2007; 2: 251–75.

65. Nilsson M, Heymach JV. Vascular endothelial growth factor (VEGF) pathway. J Thorac Oncol 2006; 1: 768–70.

66. Park JE, Chen HH, Winer J, Houck KA, Ferrara N. Placenta growth factor. potentiation of vascular endothelial growth factor bioactivity, in vitro and in vivo, and high affinity binding to Flt-1 but not to Flk-1/KDR. J Biol Chem 1994; 269: 25646–54.

67. Tischer E, Gospodarowicz D, Mitchell R, et al. Vascular endothelial growth factor: a new member of the platelet-derived growth factor gene family. Biochem Biophys Res Commun 1989; 165: 1198–206.

68. Houck KA, Leung DW, Rowland AM, Winer J, Ferrara N. Dual regulation of vascular endothelial growth factor bioavailability by genetic and proteolytic mechanisms. J Biol Chem 1992; 267: 26031–7.

69. Grunstein J, Masbad JJ, Hickey R, Giordano F, Johnson RS. Isoforms of vascular endothelial growth factor act in a coordinate fashion to recruit and expand tumor vasculature. Mol Cell Biol 2000; 20: 7282–91.

70. Maes C, Carmeliet P, Moermans K, et al. Impaired angiogenesis and endochondral bone formation in mice lacking the vascular endothelial growth factor isoforms VEGF164 and VEGF188. Mech Dev 2002; 111: 61–73.

71. Park JE, Keller GA, Ferrara N. The vascular endothelial growth factor (VEGF) isoforms: differential deposition into the subepithelial extracellular matrix and bioactivity of extracellular matrix-bound VEGF. Mol Biol Cell 1993; 4: 1317–26.

72. Ruhrberg C, Gerhardt H, Golding M, et al. Spatially restricted patterning cues provided by heparin-binding VEGF-A control blood vessel branching morphogenesis. Genes Dev 2002; 16: 2684–98.

73. Ferrara N, Houck K, Jakeman L, Leung DW. Molecular and biological properties of the vascular endothelial growth factor family of proteins. Endocr Rev 1992; 13: 18–32.

74. Shalaby F, Rossant J, Yamaguchi TP, et al. Failure of blood-island formation and vasculogenesis in Flk-1-deficient mice. Nature 1995; 376: 62–6.

75. Shalaby F, Ho J, Stanford WL, et al. A requirement for Flk1 in primitive and definitive hematopoiesis and vasculogenesis. Cell 1997; 89: 981–90.

76. Fong GH, Rossant J, Gertsenstein M, Breitman ML. Role of the Flt-1 receptor tyrosine kinase in regulating the assembly of vascular endothelium. Nature 1995; 376: 66–70.

77. Hiratsuka S, Minowa O, Kuno J, Noda T, Shibuya M. Flt-1 lacking the tyrosine kinase domain is sufficient for normal development and angiogenesis in mice. Proc Natl Acad Sci USA 1998; 95: 9349–54.

78. Zachary I, Gliki G. Signaling transduction mechanisms mediating biological actions of the vascular endothelial growth factor family. Cardiovasc Res 2001; 49: 568–81.

79. Kendall RL, Thomas KA. Inhibition of vascular endothelial cell growth factor activity by an endogenously encoded soluble receptor. Proc Natl Acad Sci USA 1993; 90: 10705–709.

80. Roeckl W, Hecht D, Sztajer H, et al. Differential binding characteristics and cellular inhibition by soluble VEGF receptors 1 and 2. Exp Cell Res 1998; 241: 161–70.

81. Kawasaki T, Kitsukawa T, Bekku Y, et al. A requirement for neuropilin-1 in embryonic vessel formation. Development 1999; 126: 4895–902.

82. Takahashi T, Yamaguchi S, Chida K, Shibuya M. A single autophosphorylation site on KDR/Flk-1 is essential for VEGF-A-dependent activation of PLC-gamma and DNA synthesis in vascular endothelial cells. EMBO J 2001; 20: 2768–78.

83. Holmqvist K, Cross MJ, Rolny C, et al. The adaptor protein shb binds to tyrosine 1175 in vascular endothelial growth factor (VEGF) receptor-2 and regulates VEGF-dependent cellular migration. J Biol Chem 2004; 279: 22267–75.

84. Lamalice L, Houle F, Jourdan G, Huot J. Phosphorylation of tyrosine 1214 on VEGFR2 is required for VEGF-induced activation of Cdc42 upstream of SAPK2/p38. Oncogene 2004; 23: 434–45.

85. Matsumoto T, Bohman S, Dixelius J, et al. VEGF receptor-2 Y951 signaling and a role for the adapter molecule TSAd in tumor angiogenesis. EMBO J. 2005; 24: 2342–53.

86. Takeshita S, Zheng LP, Brogi E, et al. Therapeutic angiogenesis. a single intraarterial bolus of vascular endothelial growth factor augments revascularization in a rabbit ischemic hind limb model. J Clin Invest 1994; 93: 662–70.

87. Connolly DT, Heuvelman DM, Nelson R, et al. Tumor vascular permeability factor stimulates endothelial cell growth and angiogenesis. J Clin Invest 1989; 84: 1470–8.

88. Plouet J, Schilling J, Gospodarowicz D. Isolation and characterization of a newly identified endothelial cell mitogen produced by AtT-20 cells. EMBO J 1989; 8: 3801–806.

89. Miller JW, Adamis AP, Shima DT, et al. Vascular endothelial growth factor/vascular permeability factor is temporally and spatially correlated with ocular angiogenesis in a primate model. Am J Pathol 1994; 145: 574–84.

90. Tolentino MJ, Miller JW, Gragoudas ES, et al. Vascular endothelial growth factor is sufficient to produce iris neovascularization and neovascular glaucoma in a nonhuman primate. Arch Ophthalmol 1996; 114: 964–70.

91. Tolentino MJ, Miller JW, Gragoudas ES, et al. Intravitreous injections of vascular endothelial growth factor produce retinal ischemia and microangiopathy in an adult primate. Ophthalmology 1996; 103: 1820–8.

92. Shima DT, Gougos A, Miller JW, et al. Cloning and mRNA expression of vascular endothelial growth factor in ischemic retinas of macaca fascicularis. Invest Ophthalmol Vis Sci 1996; 37: 1334–40.

93. Adamis AP, Shima DT, Tolentino MJ, et al. Inhibition of vascular endothelial growth factor prevents retinal ischemia-associated iris neovascularization in a nonhuman primate. Arch Ophthalmol 1996; 114: 66–71.

94. Dorey CK, Aouididi S, Reynaud X, Dvorak HF, Brown LF. Correlation of vascular permeability factor/vascular endothelial growth factor with extraretinal neovascularization in the rat. Arch Ophthalmol 1996; 114: 1210–17.

95. Pierce EA, Avery RL, Foley ED, Aiello LP, Smith LE. Vascular endothelial growth factor/vascular permeability factor expression in a mouse model of retinal neovascularization. Proc Natl Acad Sci USA 1995; 92: 905–909.

96. Stone J, Chan-Ling T, Pe'er J, et al. Roles of vascular endothelial growth factor and astrocyte degeneration in

the genesis of retinopathy of prematurity. Invest Ophthalmol Vis Sci 1996; 37: 290–9.

97. Aiello LP, Pierce EA, Foley ED, et al. Suppression of retinal neovascularization in vivo by inhibition of vascular endothelial growth factor (VEGF) using soluble VEGF-receptor chimeric proteins. Proc Natl Acad Sci USA 1995; 92: 10457–61.

98. Robinson GS, Pierce EA, Rook SL, et al. Oligodeoxynucleotides inhibit retinal neovascularization in a murine model of proliferative retinopathy. Proc Natl Acad Sci USA 1996; 93: 4851–6.

99. Lopez PF, Sippy BD, Lambert HM, Thach AB, Hinton DR. Transdifferentiated retinal pigment epithelial cells are immunoreactive for vascular endothelial growth factor in surgically excised age-related macular degeneration-related choroidal neovascular membranes. Invest Ophthalmol Vis Sci 1996; 37: 855–68.

100. Kvanta A, Algvere PV, Berglin L, Seregard S. Subfoveal fibrovascular membranes in age-related macular degeneration express vascular endothelial growth factor. Invest Ophthalmol Vis Sci 1996; 37: 1929–34.

101. Ishibashi T, Hata Y, Yoshikawa H, et al. Expression of vascular endothelial growth factor in experimental choroidal neovascularization. Graefes Arch Clin Exp Ophthalmol 1997; 235: 159–67.

102. Beatty S, Koh H, Phil M, Henson D, Boulton M. The role of oxidative stress in the pathogenesis of age-related macular degeneration. Surv Ophthalmol 2000; 45: 115–34.

103. Penfold PL, Madigan MC, Gillies MC, Provis JM. Immunological and aetiological aspects of macular degeneration. Prog Retin Eye Res 2001; 20: 385–414.

104. Schlingemann RO. Role of growth factors and the wound healing response in age-related macular degeneration. Graefes Arch Clin Exp Ophthalmol 2004; 242: 91–101.

105. Ferrara N, Damico L, Shams N, Lowman H, Kim R. Development of ranibizumab, an anti-vascular endothelial growth factor antigen binding fragment, as therapy for neovascular age-related macular degeneration. Retina 2006; 26: 859–70.

106. Campa C, Kasman I, Ye W, et al. Effects of an anti-VEGF-A monoclonal antibody on laser-induced choroidal neovascularization in mice: optimizing methods to quantify vascular changes. Invest Ophthalmol Vis Sci 2008; 49: 1178–83.

107. Kwak N, Okamoto N, Wood JM, Campochiaro PA. VEGF is major stimulator in model of choroidal neovascularization. Invest Ophthalmol Vis Sci 2000; 41: 3158–64.

108. Seo MS, Kwak N, Ozaki H, et al. Dramatic inhibition of retinal and choroidal neovascularization by oral administration of a kinase inhibitor. Am J Pathol 1999; 154: 1743–53.

109. Zucker S, Mirza H, Conner CE, et al. Vascular endothelial growth factor induces tissue factor and matrix metalloproteinase production in endothelial cells: conversion of prothrombin to thrombin results in progelatinase A activation and cell proliferation. Int J Cancer 1998; 75: 780–6.

110. Wang H, Keiser JA. Vascular endothelial growth factor upregulates the expression of matrix metalloproteinases in vascular smooth muscle cells: role of Flt-1. Circ Res 1998; 83: 832–40.

111. Thurston G, Noguera-Troise I, Yancopoulos GD. The Delta paradox: DLL4 blockade leads to more tumour vessels but less tumour growth. Nat Rev Cancer 2007; 7: 327–31.

112. Liu ZJ, Shirakawa T, Li Y, et al. Regulation of notch1 and Dll4 by vascular endothelial growth factor in arterial endothelial cells: implications for modulating arteriogenesis and angiogenesis. Mol Cell Biol 2003; 23: 14–25.

113. Tammela T, Zarkada G, Wallgard E, et al. Blocking VEGFR-3 suppresses angiogenic sprouting and vascular network formation. Nature 2008; 454: 656–60.

114. Jakobsson L, Franco CA, Bentley K, et al. Endothelial cells dynamically compete for the tip cell position during angiogenic sprouting. Nat Cell Biol 2010; 12: 943–53.

115. Hangai M, Murata T, Miyawaki N, et al. Angiopoietin-1 upregulation by vascular endothelial growth factor in human retinal pigment epithelial cells. Invest Ophthalmol Vis Sci 2001; 42: 1617–25.

5

Risk factors for age-related macular degeneration and choroidal neovascularization

Francis Char DeCroos and Julia A. Haller

INTRODUCTION

Age-related macular degeneration (AMD) is a major health problem worldwide and is the most frequent cause of blindness among individuals 55 years or older in developed countries (1). Owing to the progressive increase in the life expectancy and the proportion of elderly persons in the population of the United States, it is estimated that the number of persons having late AMD will increase to 2.95 million in 2020 (1). The increasing prevalence of AMD has led many investigators to search for factors that could be modified to prevent the onset of or delay the natural course of AMD. The modification of risk factors has the potential for widespread public health impact on AMD morbidity and can complement the available therapeutic modalities.

EPIDEMIOLOGIC STUDIES ON RISK FACTORS FOR AMD AND LIMITATIONS OF THESE STUDIES

The exact pathogenesis of AMD remains unknown. Multiple epidemiologic studies have explored risk factors for AMD including case–control, cross-sectional, and prospective cohort studies. The analysis of risk factors for AMD is inherently difficult because many of them are closely interrelated, for example, race, ocular pigmentation, and sunlight exposure, or socioeconomic status, smoking, and nutrition. In addition, the difficulties in establishing a causal link between a disease and a potential risk factor are magnified for a condition such as AMD because this disease manifests late in life. Additional challenges studying this chronic condition include a long lead time, a possible recall bias, and survivor cohort effects.

Another difficulty in the study of AMD is the differences in methodology used in the various studies. In this chapter, we will use the term AMD to include the entire spectrum of the disease. Neovascular AMD and geographic atrophy will be collectively termed *late AMD* and the early lesions of AMD will be termed *early AMD*. Intrinsic to this classification scheme is a handful of limitations. It is possible that the factors associated with early AMD may be different from those associated with progression to neovascular AMD or geographic atrophy. Likewise, although neovascular AMD and geographic atrophy are termed collectively as late AMD (or late ARM), they may have different causes (2). For these reasons, it may be important to pay attention to the different stages of AMD and to separate the two manifestations of late AMD in epidemiologic studies, as has been done in some studies (3–5).

When critically evaluating the AMD risk factor literature one must be mindful that examination of large number variables may find associations by chance alone. For example, the Framingham Eye Study correlated its ophthalmic diagnoses with almost all of 667 variables from the Framingham Heart Study (6). Study of a high number of associations resulting in chance findings are likely contributors partly responsible for inconsistent results between studies. Conversely, repeated finding of the same risk factors in studies conducted in different populations provides compelling evidence of a real association between AMD and a potential risk factor. Finally, while results from epidemiologic studies may identify risk factors for AMD, proof that modifying a particular established risk factor can influence the course of the disease can emerge only from randomized prospective clinical trials.

RISK FACTORS OF AMD

A number of risk factors for AMD have been incriminated from various epidemiologic studies, suggesting that the condition is multifactorial in etiology (Table 5.1). These risk factors may be broadly classified into personal or environmental factors, and the personal factors may be further subdivided into sociodemographic, ocular, and systemic factors.

PERSONAL FACTORS
Sociodemographic Factors
Age

Age is the strongest risk factor associated with AMD. The prevalence, incidence, and progression of all forms of AMD rise steeply with advancing age (7,8). In the Beaver Dam Offspring Study AMD was present in 9.8% of study participants aged 65 years or older compared with 2.4% of study participants aged 21–34 years (8). Although closely linked to the aging process, AMD is not universal and this disease not inevitable with increasing age.

Race/Ethnicity

Several studies have suggested that AMD is more prevalent among whites than blacks. In the Baltimore Eye

Table 5.1 Risk Factors for AMD

Established risk factors

  Age

  Race/ethnicity

  Heredity

  Smoking

Possible risk factors

  Gender

  Socioeconomic status

  Iris color

  Macular pigment optical density

  Cataract and its surgery

  Refractive error

  Cup/disc ratio

  Cardiovascular disease

  Hypertension and blood pressure

  Serum lipid levels and dietary fat intake

  Body mass index

  Hematologic factors including homocysteine

  Chlamydia pneumoniae infection

  Reproductive and related factors

  Antioxidant enzymes

  Sunlight exposure

  Micronutrients

  Dietary fish intake

  Alcohol consumption

Factors probably not associated with AMD

  Diabetes and hyperglycemia

Abbreviation. AMD, age-related macular degeneration.

Survey, drusen (>63 μm) were identified in about 20% of individuals in both blacks and whites, but large drusen (>125 μm) were more common among older whites (15% for whites *vs.* 9% for blacks over 70 years old). Retinal pigmentary abnormalities were also more common among older whites (7.9% for whites *vs.* 0.4% for blacks over 70 years old). The prevalence ratio (white : black) was 10.7 for geographic atrophy, 8.8 for neovascular AMD, and 10.1 for all late AMD (geographic atrophy plus neovascular AMD). In this study, cases of AMD-related blindness were found only in whites (9,10).

Klein et al. reported the prevalence of AMD in four racial/ethnic groups (white, black, Hispanic, and Chinese) that participated in the Multi-Ethnic Study of Atherosclerosis (11). The study found the prevalences of any AMD were 2.4%, 4.2%, 4.6%, and 5.4% for blacks, Hispanics, Chinese, and whites, respectively (*p* < 0.001 for any differences among groups). Estimated prevalences of late AMD were 0.3%, 0.2%, 1.0%, and 0.6% for blacks, Hispanics, Chinese, and whites, respectively. The frequency of neovascular AMD was highest in Chinese (age- and gender-adjusted OR, 4.30; 95% CI, 1.3–14.27) compared with whites. Differences in age, gender, pupil size, body mass index (BMI), smoking, alcohol drinking history, diabetes, and hypertension status did not explain the differences of AMD prevalences among the racial/ethnic groups. For patients of Native American ancestry, the Los Angeles Latino Eye study noted increased association with late AMD (5).

For all such investigations studying racial variation in AMD, it is unclear whether the degree of fundus pigmentation affects the ability to detect lesions such as hyperpigmentation and hypopigmentation of the RPE or drusen. It is plausible that variations in normal fundus pigmentation may lead to errors in detecting subtle early AMD lesions, resulting in some spurious differences among the ethnic groups.

Overall, current evidence suggests that early AMD is common among blacks and Hispanics but less common than among non-Hispanic whites. Also, late AMD is less frequent in these groups compared with non-Hispanic whites. Differences in genetic susceptibility probably explain part of the disparities in the prevalence of AMD in different races.

Heredity

Analysis of heredity in the disease process of AMD is limited by the fact that the disorder is associated with aging, frequently causing its most significant phenotypic manifestations in the later years of life. As a result, usually only one generation in the appropriate age range is available for study. The parents of the proband are often deceased, and the children are often too young to manifest the disease. Because information from several generations of families of multiple affected individuals is often lacking, genetic analysis is limited. An analysis of specific allelic associations with AMD is not detailed in this chapter and can be found in chapter 3 of this book.

Clinical studies indicate that AMD demonstrates familial clustering. For example, in the Blue Mountains Eye Study, subjects with signs of AMD (4.5%) were more likely to report a first-degree family history of AMD than among subjects without AMD (2.3%). The highest rate was reported by subjects with late AMD (6.9%), particularly those with neovascular AMD (8.2%). After adjusting for age, sex, and current smoking, a clear increase in risk associated with family history, from no AMD [OR, 1.0 (index)] to early AMD (OR, 2.17; 95% CI, 1.04–4.55), late AMD (geographic atrophy or neovascular AMD) (OR, 3.92; 95% CI, 1.34–11.46), and neovascular AMD (OR, 4.30; 95% CI, 1.37–13.45) was observed (12). In another study, investigators examined the concordance of AMD in 100 monozygotic twins (50 pairs) and 47 spouses (124). The concordance of AMD was 90% in monozygotic twin pairs which significantly exceeded that of 70% for twin-spouse pairs (*p* = 0.0279). In the nine twin pairs that were concordant, fundus appearance and visual impairment were similar (13).

Gender

Gender has not been consistently found to be a risk factor for AMD. Gender was not associated with AMD in multiple studies worldwide (14–16). In contrast, Smith and associates pooled data from the three large-scale population-based studies using similar diagnostic criteria and techniques, and found significant but modest increase in AMD prevalence among females compared with males, with OR of 1.15 (95% CI, 1.10–1.21) adjusting for 10-year age categories (17). Another study in the Malay population reported both early and late AMD were more common in women after adjusting for age and smoking (4).

Socioeconomic Status and Education

Socioeconomic status and education have not been consistently found to be a risk factor for AMD. The Eye Disease Case–Control study found that persons with higher levels of education had a slightly reduced risk of neovascular AMD, but the association did not remain statistically significant after multiple regression modeling (18). The Beaver Dam Eye Study found no relation of income, educational level, or marital status to AMD (19).

OCULAR FACTORS
Macular Pigment Optical Density

Of late, there is heightened interest in the potential role of macular pigment in protecting against AMD (20). The yellow macular pigment, which characterizes the retinas of primates including man, was shown in 1985 to be composed of two chromatographically separable components, namely lutein and zeaxanthin (21). Of note, lutein and zeaxanthin are entirely of dietary origin.

Although the exact role of the macular pigment remains uncertain, several functions have been hypothesized. These include reducing the damaging photo-oxidative effects of blue light through its pre-receptorial absorption (22), and protecting against the adverse effects of reactive oxygen intermediates through its antioxidant properties (23). Multiple groups have suggested that the absorption characteristics and antioxidant properties of macular pigment confer protection against AMD (23,24). Interestingly, a strong inverse relationship between smoking and macular pigment optical density has been shown by Hammond et al., and this may partly explain how smoking increases the risk of AMD (see below) (25).

Although discussed under the heading of ocular risk factors, macular pigment optical density is inherently related to nutrition since it can be altered by dietary modification or supplementation (26). Consumption of certain vegetables in particular will increase the dietary intake of lutein and zeaxanthin. Examples of such foods include kale, spinach, turnip greens, broccoli, and Brussel sprouts. Because human macular pigment can be augmented with dietary modification and nutritional supplementation, the protective effect of macular pigment, if proven, has potential therapeutic implications. Nevertheless, evidence that dietary modifications or supplementation with lutein and/or zeaxanthin can prevent, delay, or modify the course of AMD is still lacking. The second phase of the National Eye Institute's age-related eye disease study (AREDS 2) is investigating the effect of 10 mg lutein and 2 mg zeaxanthin on AMD (27).

Cataract and Cataract Extraction

Since cataract and AMD are the most frequent causes of visual impairment in older individuals and the prevalence of both conditions is strongly age related, a possible association between the two conditions has long been debated. However, the association between cataract and AMD has not been found consistently. In studies from the United Kingdom and Germany no statistically significant association was found between cataract and AMD (28,29). In the Framingham Eye Study, researchers found a positive association between AMD and cortical changes but a negative association between AMD and nuclear sclerosis (30). The Andhra Pradesh Eye Disease Study also found cortical cataract, but not nuclear sclerotic or posterior subcapsular cataract, to be significantly associated with an increased prevalence of AMD (adjusted OR, 2.87; 95% CI, 1.57–5.27) (16).

A meta-analysis of four prospective studies noted that previous cataract surgery was associated with neovascular AMD (RR, 3.05; 95% CI, 2.05–4.55) (31). Likewise, in the Beaver Dam Eye Study, eyes that had undergone cataract surgery before baseline, compared with eyes that were phakic at baseline, were more likely to have progression of AMD (OR, 2.71; 95% CI, 1.69–4.35) and to develop signs of late AMD (OR, 2.80; 95% CI, 1.03–7.63) after controlling for age (32). These relationships remained after controlling for other risk factors in multivariate analyses. The FRANCE-DMLA study group found an increased risk of AMD in persons with a history of previous cataract surgery compared with those with no lens opacities or cataract surgery (OR, 1.68; 95% CI, 1.45–1.95) (33). Similarly, prior cataract surgery was significantly associated with an increased prevalence of AMD in the Andhra Pradesh Eye Disease Study (adjusted OR, 3.79; 95% CI, 2.1–6.78) (16). Several theories may explain the findings of apparent exacerbation of AMD with cataract surgery including a true association due to factors such as increased light transmittance following cataract surgery or surgical inflammation, or simply an increased detection rate following cataract extraction masquerading as relative disease progression. This latter explanation is supported by a number of studies. For example, the Blue Mountains Eye Study reported the association of increased late AMD in eyes after cataract extraction was not significant after multivariate adjustment (34). The Rotterdam Study also did not find any association between cataract surgery and AMD prevalence (35). Likewise, review of the 8050 eyes monitored in the AREDS trial did not reveal any association between cataract surgery and AMD progression (36). Variations in findings among these reports may have resulted from differences in the study populations and/or from differences in methodology and case definitions.

Iris Color

The mechanism by which iris pigmentation might influence AMD is uncertain, but a plausible explanation is that the lower risk for AMD among subjects with darker iris color may be due to the fact that these individuals have more tissue melanin. This increased pigmentation may provide some protection to the retina from exposure to sunlight, reducing direct photo-oxidative damage and thus reducing the risk of AMD (see below). Despite this theoretic protective effect iris color has not consistently been associated with AMD. Weiter et al. found that 76% of 650 patients with AMD had light irides compared with 40% of 363 controls ($p = 0.0001$) (37). In contrast the Beaver Dam Eye Study did not find any relationship between iris color and the incidence and progression of AMD (32). The reasons for these disparities are not clear.

Refractive Error

Several case–control studies have found an association between AMD and refractive error, with hyperopic eyes at a greater risk of AMD. Hyman et al. found that statistically significant differences in mean refractive error were present between female cases and controls ($p = 0.009$), but not between male cases and controls ($p = 0.16$). Female cases had a more positive refractive error (mean = 1.8 diopters) than female controls (mean = 1.1 diopters) (3). The Eye Disease Case–Control Study found that persons with hyperopia had a slightly higher risk of neovascular AMD, but the association did not remain statistically significant after multivariate modeling (18). One caveat in the interpretation of findings in these case–control studies is that because the controls were recruited from ophthalmologic clinics, the control groups may be enriched in the proportion of myopes compared with the general population.

Cup/Disc Ratio

The Eye Disease Case–Control study found that eyes with large horizontal and vertical cup/disc ratios were at reduced risk for neovascular AMD (18). The horizontal cup/disc ratio persisted as statistically significant after multivariate modeling including adjusting for known and potential confounding factors.

SYSTEMIC FACTORS
Cardiovascular Disease and Its Risk Factors

A number of documented risk factors for cardiovascular disease such as age, hypertension, hypercholesterolemia, diabetes, smoking, and dietary intake of fats, alcohol, and antioxidants have been associated with AMD in some studies (31,38). This raises the possibility that the causal pathways for cardiovascular disease and AMD may share similar risk factors. Not all the results from various investigations, however, have been consistent.

Cardiovascular Disease

Some studies reported an association between AMD and various clinical manifestations of cardiovascular disease. In a case–control study, Hyman et al. found AMD to be positively associated with a history of three cardiovascular conditions. These conditions are arteriosclerosis, circulatory problems, and stroke/transient ischemic attacks, with ORs (95% CI) of 2.3 (1.9–2.7), 2.0 (1.1–3.5), and 2.9 (1.3–6.9), respectively (39). The FRANCE-DMLA study group found an increased risk of AMD in persons with a history of coronary artery disease (OR, 1.31; 95% CI, 1.02–1.68) (33). Other studies, such as the Eye Disease Case–Control Study (18), and the Beaver Dam Study (40), found no statistically significant relationship between a history of stroke or cardiovascular disease and AMD.

Hypertension and Blood Pressure

Some large population-based studies showed a small and consistent significant association between AMD and systemic hypertension. Kahn et al., using the data from Framingham Heart and Eye studies, found a positive association between the presence of AMD and higher levels of diastolic blood pressure measured many years before the eye examination (6). Also using data from the Framingham Heart and Eye studies, Sperduto and Hiller found the age- and sex-adjusted relative risk for any AMD was 1.18 (95% CI, 1.01–1.37) for persons diagnosed with hypertension 25 years before the eye examination and 1.04 (95% CI, 0.96–1.23) for persons with hypertension at the time of the eye examination, when compared with those without hypertension (41). Other population-based cross-sectional studies detected no association between hypertension and AMD including the Blue Mountains Eye Study (42), Atherosclerosis Risk In Communities Study (43), and Andhra Pradesh Eye Disease Study (16).

Serum Lipid Levels and Dietary Fat Intake

Some evidence suggests that dietary fat intake, particularly intake of saturated fat and cholesterol, is associated with an increased risk for atherosclerosis. It is biologically plausible that a higher dietary saturated fat intake increases the risk of AMD by promoting atherosclerosis. For example, The Eye Disease Case–Control Study found that persons with midrange (4.889–6.748 mmol/L) and high (≥6.749 mmol/L) total cholesterol levels compared with those with low levels (≤4.888 mmol/L) had ORs for neovascular AMD of 2.2 (95% CI, 1.3–3.4) and 4.1 (95% CI, 2.3–7.3), respectively, after controlling for other factors. A slight but not statistically significant increased risk in neovascular AMD was seen with increasing levels of serum triglycerides in the same study (18). Conversely, pooled data from three cross-sectional studies (Blue Mountains Eye Study, Beaver Dam Eye Study, and Rotterdam Study) found that total serum cholesterol was associated inversely with incident neovascular AMD (OR, 0.94 per 10 mg/dL; 95% CI, 0.88–0.99) (44). Alternatively, several other studies including the Rotterdam study (45), Blue Mountains Eye Study (42), and Atherosclerosis Risk In Communities study (43) did not find any association between serum cholesterol and HDL cholesterol with AMD.

Several studies have evaluated the relationship of lipid-lowering agents and AMD and found conflicting results. One study suggested that use of 3-hydroxy-3-methylglutaryl-coenzyme A (HMG-CoA) reductase inhibitors (statins) might increase the risk of AMD

(OR, 1.40; 95% CI, 0.99–1.98) after controlling for age, sex, and race (46).The Beaver Dam Eye Study (47) and Blue Mountains Eye Study (48) found no association between the use of a lipid-lowering agent and the risk of developing AMD. Similarly, the Complications of Age-related Macular Degeneration Prevention trial did not observe a strong protective effect of statin usage for advanced AMD (RR, 1.15; 95% CI, 0.87–1.52), choroidal neovascularization (CNV) (RR, 1.35; 95% CI, 0.99–1.83), or for end point GA (RR, 0.80; 95% CI, 0.46–1.39).

Diabetes and Hyperglycemia
Many studies have found no significant association between diabetes and/or hyperglycemia and AMD. For example, the Blue Mountains Eye Study found geographic atrophy to be significantly associated with diabetes (OR, 4.0; 95% CI, 1.6–10.3), but no association was found with either neovascular AMD (OR, 1.2; 95% CI, 0.4–3.5) or early AMD (OR, 1.0; 95% CI, 0.5–1.8). There was also no association found between impaired fasting glucose and AMD in the Blue Mountain Eye Study (49) and the Atherosclerosis Risk In Communities Study (43).

Body Mass Index
Some studies observed that having a BMI [defined as body weight in kilograms divided by height in meter square (kg/m^2)] higher than the accepted normal range was associated with an increased risk of early AMD (42) and late AMD (50). In contrast, no association between BMI and AMD was found in the Atherosclerosis Risk In Communities study (43) or the Andhra Pradesh Eye Disease Study (16).

Hematologic Factors and Other Cardiovascular Biomarkers
The prospective Women's Antioxidant and Folic Acid Cardiovascular Study (WAFACS) noted a lower rate of AMD in women who received the trial combination of B-vitamins (folic acid: 2.5 mg/day, B6: 50 mg/day, and B12: 1 mg/day). This placebo-controlled, double blinded trial that showed after following 5442 women for an average of 7.3 years that 55 cases of AMD were reported in the treatment group compared to 82 cases in the placebo group (RR, 0.66; 95% CI, 0.47–0.93). This intriguing finding is limited by the fact that AMD occurrence was determined by self-reporting and medical record review and not through standardized examination or photography. B-vitamin supplementation has been shown to decrease serum levels of homocysteine and subsequently endothelial dysfunction, which could in turn confer a protective effect to the macula (51).

The Blue Mountains Eye Study found that plasma fibrinogen level was associated with late but not early AMD (42). Another study noted a number of inflammatory biomarkers which are known to be associated with cardiovascular disease were also independently associated with AMD progression including C-reactive protein and interleukin 6 (52). In contrast, a subsequent study did not find an association between AMD and the inflammatory biomarkers intercellular adhesion molecule 1, vascular cellular adhesion molecule, and C-reactive protein (53).

Chlamydia pneumoniae Infection
Chronic inflammatory events have been identified as plausible causes of atherosclerosis and much interest has been focused on infections by Chlamydia pneumoniae. C. pneumoniae can multiply in various host cells including macrophages and endothelial cells. The obligate intracellular prokaryote consumes energy that is needed by the host cells, and in the end, destroys them and then infects nearby cells. Thus, a hallmark of chlamydial disease is persistent infection and chronic inflammation.

The Cardiovascular Health and Age-Related Maculopathy Study in Australia showed that the rate of progression of AMD over a seven-year period was increased in those with higher titers of anti-C. pneumoniae antibodies, after controlling for age, smoking, family history of AMD, and history of cardiovascular diseases (54). Subjects in the two upper tertiles of antibody titer were at a significantly greater risk of AMD progression than those in the lowest tertile. In the upper tertile of antibody titers, the risk of progression was 2.07 (95% CI, 0.92–4.69), 2.58 (95% CI, 1.24–5.41), and 3.05 (95% CI, 1.46–6.37) using different definitions of AMD progression.

Reproductive and Related Factors
No consensus exists as to the association of estrogen-related variables on the risk of AMD in women. The Eye Disease Case–Control Study found that use of post-menopausal exogenous estrogen was negatively associated with neovascular AMD (18). The Pathologies Oculaires Liees a l'Age (POLA) study, however, did not find any association of hormone replacement therapy, hysterectomy, or oophorectomy with soft drusen, pigmentary abnormalities, or late AMD (55).

Antioxidant Enzymes
The POLA study, a large-scale population-based cross-sectional study conducted in Southern France, found that higher levels of plasma glutathione peroxidase were significantly associated with a ninefold increase in late AMD prevalence, but not with prevalence of early AMD. Plasma glutathione peroxidase therefore appears to be strongly associated with late AMD, but the biologic meaning of this finding remains to be elucidated. The authors suggest that oxidative stress may lead to the induction of antioxidant enzymes, and therefore high concentrations of antioxidant enzymes may be indicators of oxidative stress (56). Further discussion of oxidative stress and AMD can be found in chapter 6 (Oxidative Stress) of this book.

ENVIRONMENTAL FACTORS
Cigarette Smoking
Of the environmental influences, smoking has most consistently been associated with increased risk of AMD and is the strongest modifiable environmental risk factor for all forms of AMD (18,57–62). The AMD literature

from Asia particularly supports a linkage between smoking and AMD. In the Funagata Study, smoking was associated with late AMD (adjusted OR, 5.03; 95% CI, 1.0–25.47) (62). In another case–control study, compared with male nonsmokers, the age-adjusted OR of developing neovascular AMD was 2.97 (95% CI, 1.00–8.84) for male current smokers and 2.09 (95% CI, 0.71–6.13) for male former smokers. In addition, smoking habit–related variables such as use of extra filter, smoke inhalation level, age of starting smoking, duration of smoking, and the Brinkman index, defined as the number of cigarettes smoked per day times smoking years, were found to be significantly related to an increased risk of neovascular AMD (61). In the Handan eye study, adjusting for higher smoking rates among men compared to women reduced the increased prevalence of early AMD between men and women by 50% to a nonsignificant level (OR, 1.4; 95% CI, 0.9–2.0).

Likewise, the Beaver Dam Eye Study found that the relative OR for neovascular AMD in men and women who were current smokers compared with those who were former smokers or who never smoked were 3.29 (95% CI, 1.03–10.50) and 2.50 (95% CI, 1.01–6.20), respectively (59). Similarly, the Blue Mountains Eye Study found current cigarette smoking to be significantly associated with both early and late AMD, after adjusting for the effects of age and sex. The odds ratios of early and late AMD when comparing current smokers with those who never smoked were 1.89 (95% CI, 1.25–2.84) and 4.46 (95% CI, 2.20–9.03), respectively. A history of having ever smoked was significant for late AMD (OR, 1.83; 95% CI, 1.07–3.13) but not early AMD. In addition, passive smoking among subjects who never themselves smoked, but lived with a smoking spouse, incurred a moderate but not statistically significant increase in the risk of late AMD (OR, 1.42; 95% CI, 0.62–3.26) (60).

In the POLA study, after adjustment for age and sex, current (OR, 3.6; 95% CI, 1.1–12.4) and former smokers (OR, 3.2; 95% CI, 1.3–7.7) had an increased prevalence of late AMD when compared with nonsmokers. The risk of late AMD increased with increasing number of pack-years, with up to a 5.2–fold increase in risk among participants (current and former smokers combined) who smoked 40 pack-years or more (OR 1.9, 95% CI 0.6–6.4 for 1–19 pack-years; OR 3.0, 95% CI 0.9–9.5 for 20–39 pack-years; and OR 5.2, 95% CI 2.0–13.6 for 40 pack-years and more). In addition, the risk of late AMD remained increased until 20 years after cessation of smoking (63).

Two large prospective cohort studies evaluated the relationship between smoking and AMD (57,58). In the Nurses' Health Study with 12 years of follow-up, women who currently smoked ≥25 cigarettes per day had a risk ratio (RR) of AMD of 2.4 (95% CI, 1.4–4.0) compared with women who never smoked. Risk of AMD also increased with an increasing number of pack-years smoked (p for trend <0.001). Past smokers of this amount also had an RR of 2.0 (95% CI, 1.2–3.4) compared with women who never smoked. Compared with current smokers, little reduction in risk was found even after

quitting smoking for 15 or more years (58). In the Physicians' Health Study, men who were current smokers of ≥20 cigarettes per day had an RR of AMD of 2.5 (95% CI, 1.6–3.8) compared with men who never smoked. Men who were past smokers had a modest elevation in RR of AMD of 1.3 (95% CI, 1.0–1.7) (57).

Despite the strong association between smoking and AMD, the awareness of blindness as another smoking-related condition is low. In a cross-sectional survey of 358 adult patients (both smokers and nonsmokers) attending a district general hospital in the United Kingdom, only 9.5% of patients believed that smoking was definitely or probably a cause of blindness, compared with 92.2% for lung cancer, 87.6% for heart disease, and 70.6% for stroke. Although there was a disparity in the knowledge of these smoking-related conditions, about half of the smokers stated that they would definitely or probably quit smoking if they developed early signs of blindness (64). Increasing the awareness of the link between smoking and blindness may therefore be an effective additional approach to encouraging smoking cessation.

Very little evidence contradicts this link between smoking and AMD. The Framingham Eye Study (65), however, did not find an association, and, one study by West et al. even showed smoking to be protective for AMD (66). However, when this decreased risk of AMD associated with smoking was further investigated, no clear dose–response relationship was demonstrated.

In summary, data from large population-based studies (59,60), case–control studies (18,61), and two large prospective cohort studies (57,58) provide convincing evidence that cigarette smoking is a risk factor for AMD. The strongest risk is for current smokers, suggesting that there may be potential benefits of targeting antismoking patient education, especially for those who are current smokers and have signs of early AMD (60). The benefit of stopping smoking is seen after 10 years with reductions in risk although the risks do not return to that of patients who have never smoked until 20 years after stopping smoking (65).

Sunlight Exposure

It is well established that ultraviolet (UV) and visible radiation has the potential to damage the retina and RPE (67). Fortunately, the human retina is protected from short-wavelength radiation, which is particularly damaging, by the cornea which absorbs below 295 nm and the lens which absorbs strongly below 400 nm (68). The epidemiologic evidence of an association between light exposure and AMD is lacking, with few clinical studies showing a positive association between sun exposure and late AMD (69) with other studies failing to note a positive association (18,70). Margrain and colleagues have suggested that the equivocal findings reported in epidemiologic studies are quite unremarkable because first, the absence of a relationship of AMD with UV exposure simply confirms that the adult lens absorbs almost all radiation below 400 nm. Second, they suggested that the assumption that it is lifetime exposure to sunlight that is the relevant variable is probably incorrect. Instead, they suggested that the phototoxicity of blue light increases with age and is likely to be particularly great for those with lipofuscin "hot spots" (68). In summary, there is currently no convincing data to support strategies to reduce light exposure to the eye for the prevention of AMD. However, since there is little risk to a person wearing sunglasses, and this modifies a potential risk factor, many physicians suggest that individuals wear sunglasses to reduce exposure of UV light to ocular structures.

Nutritional Factors
Antioxidants
Photochemical damage from light can induce the production of activated forms of oxygen, which in turn can cause lipid peroxidation of the photoreceptor outer segment membranes. Antioxidants, such as vitamin C, vitamin E, β-carotene, and glutathione, and antioxidant enzymes, such as selenium-dependent glutathione peroxidase, in theory could act as singlet oxygen and free radical scavengers and thereby prevent cellular damage (71). There is considerable interest in determining whether free radicals contribute to the pathogenesis of AMD and if high levels of these antioxidants may protect against AMD.

The results of the Age-Related Eye Disease Study (AREDS) provide strong evidence to support an association of antioxidant intake with AMD. In the AREDS, 11 centers participated in this double-masked clinical trial that randomized participants to receive oral daily supplementation of (i) antioxidants (vitamin C, 500 mg; vitamin E, 400 IU; and β-carotene, 15 mg); (ii) zinc (zinc, 80 mg as zinc oxide, and copper, 2 mg as cupric oxide to prevent potential anemia); (iii) antioxidants plus zinc; or (iv) placebo (72). The average follow-up of the 3640 enrolled study participants in the AREDS AMD trial was 6.3 years, with 2.4% lost to follow-up.

Compared with patients receiving placebo, patients randomized to supplementation with antioxidants plus zinc had a statistically significant odds reduction for the development of advanced AMD (OR, 0.72; 99% CI, 0.52–0.98). Advanced AMD was defined as photocoagulation or other treatment for CNV, or photographic documentation of any of the following: geographic atrophy involving the center of the macula, nondrusenoid RPE detachment, serous or hemorrhagic retinal detachment, hemorrhage under the retina or RPE, and/or subretinal fibrosis. The ORs for zinc alone and antioxidants alone were 0.75 (99% CI, 0.55–1.03) and 0.80 (99% CI, 0.59–1.09), respectively.

The study found that participants with extensive small drusen (>15 drusen, <63 μm), non-extensive intermediate size drusen (1–20 drusen, 64–124 μm), or pigment abnormalities had only a 1.3% five-year probability of progression to advanced AMD. There was no evidence of any treatment benefit in delaying the progression of these patients to more severe drusen pathology. When these 1063 participants were excluded and analysis performed for the rest of the participants who had more severe age-related macular features and who were at the highest risk for progression to advanced AMD, the odds reduction estimates increased (antioxidants plus zinc: OR 0.66, 99% CI 0.47–0.91; zinc: OR 0.71; 99% CI 0.52–0.99; antioxidants: OR 0.76; 99% CI 0.55–1.05).

Estimates of RRs derived from the ORs suggested risk reductions for those taking antioxidants plus zinc, zinc alone, and antioxidants alone were 25%, 21%, and 17%, respectively. The only statistically significant reduction in rates of at least moderate vision loss [defined as decrease in best-corrected visual acuity score from baseline of ≥15 letters in a study eye (equivalent to a doubling or more of the initial visual angle, e.g., 20/20 to 20/40 or worse, or 20/50 to 20/100 or worse)] occurred in persons randomized to receive antioxidants plus zinc (OR, 0.73; 99% CI, 0.54–0.99). There was no statistically significant serious adverse effect associated with any of the formulations.

The AREDS recommended that persons with extensive intermediate size drusen (more than approximately 20 drusen 64–124 μm in size), at least one large druse (>125 μm), noncentral geographic atrophy in one or both eyes, or advanced AMD or vision loss due to AMD in one eye, and without contraindications such as smoking, should consider taking a supplement of antioxidants plus zinc to reduce their risk of progression to advanced AMD and vision loss. Because results from two other randomized clinical trials suggested increased risk of mortality among smokers supplementing with β-carotene (73,74), persons who smoke cigarettes should avoid taking β-carotene, and they might choose to supplement with only some of the study ingredients.

The role of vitamin E supplementation in AMD remains somewhat controversial. The Vitamin E Cataract and Age-related Maculopathy Trial (VECAT) is a prospective randomized placebo-controlled clinical trial in Australia. One of the major arms of the trial found no protective or deleterious effect of daily dietary vitamin E supplementation on the incidence or progression of AMD. Secondary analyses of visual acuity and visual function also failed to show an intervention effect (75). Similarly in the Finnish Alpha-Tocopherol and Beta-Carotene (ATBC) study, no protective effect was noted between 728 participants receiving antioxidants compared 213 receiving placebo. This finding persisted even when each of the antioxidant groups was analyzed individually (76). Inconsistent with many previously published studies is a population based cohort study that noted increased intake of vitamin E was found to have a 2.83-fold increased risk of late AMD (highest compared to lowest tertile). This study also observed a 2.68-fold increased risk of neovascular AMD in groups supplemented with the β-carotene (highest compared to lowest tertile) (77), an effect which persisted even after stratification of the cohort into smokers and non-smokers. Olson and coworkers advise caution when interpreting these findings due to significant loss of follow-up in the vitamin E group and to borderline statistical significance of associations in the β-carotene (78).

The AREDS 2 trial is currently studying the effects of lutein and zeaxanthin and/or omega-3 fatty acids on AMD progression. Additionally, this study will also evaluate the removal of β-carotene from the AREDS formulation, in order to clarify the effect of various currently available supplements on AMD progression.

Dietary Fish Intake

A high proportion of polyunsaturated omega-3 fatty acids, particularly docosahexaenoic acid, is present in the human retina and macula (79,80). Docosahexaenoic acid appears to play an important role in the normal functioning of the retina and is found predominantly in oily fish and offal (81). Increased consumption of fish and fish oils containing omega-3 fatty acids has been associated with a protective effect against atherosclerosis (82).

The evidence for the protective effect of high levels of omega-3 fatty acids merits consideration. In the AREDS trial, participants with the highest consumption of omega-3 fatty acids were less likely to have neovascular AMD at baseline (OR, 0.61; 95% CI = 0.41–0.90) (83). Another meta-analysis of 9 studies demonstrated that high fish intake was associated with a reduced risk of both early (pooled OR, 0.76; 95% CI, 0.64–0.90) and late (pooled OR, 0.67; 95% CI, 0.53–0.85) AMD (84). The AREDS 2 study is currently prospectively investigating the effect of 1 g of omega-3 fatty acid supplementation and AMD progression (27).

Alcohol Consumption

The association between alcohol consumption and AMD is not consistent. The Andhra Pradesh Eye Disease Study found a lower prevalence of AMD in light alcohol drinkers compared with nondrinkers (adjusted OR, 0.38; 95% CI, 0.19–0.7) (16). In contrast, in the Beaver Dam Eye Study, beer consumption was found to be associated with increased prevalence of retinal pigment and neovascular AMD (85). Prospective data from 111,238 women and men in the Nurses' Health Study and the Health Professionals Follow-Up Study did not detect a substantial association between total alcohol intake and incidence of AMD (86). Prospective data of 21,041 male physicians with an average follow-up of 12.5 years in the Physicians' Health Study also indicate that alcohol intake is not appreciably associated with the risk of AMD (57).

DEVELOPMENT OF CNV IN AMD
Occurrence of CNV in AMD

Several trials help elucidate the risk of CNV in AMD. The Macular Photocoagulation Study (MPS) group examined the data of fellow eyes of study participants in the MPS randomized trial for argon laser photocoagulation for multiple types of CNV secondary to AMD (87,88). In the extrafoveal CNV trial, 33 (26%) fellow eyes of 128 participants developed CNV when no CNV was present at baseline (87). In the other three MPS trials, among patients with no classic or occult CNV in the fellow eye at the time of enrollment, CNV developed in 236 (35%) within five years (88).

The AREDS investigators also evaluated the incidence of neovascular AMD as defined as photocoagulation for CNV, or photographic evidence of any of the following: nondrusenoid RPE detachment, serous or hemorrhagic retinal detachment, hemorrhage under the retina or the RPE, and subretinal fibrosis (89). Of the 2506 participants in the bilateral drusen group, 256 (10%) developed neovascular AMD in at least one eye during the course of the study (median = 6.3 years of follow-up). Of the 788 participants in the unilateral advanced AMD group, 278 (35%) developed neovascular AMD during the study.

Risk Factors for Progression to CNV

The choroidal neovascular lesions of AMD cause the vast majority of severe visual loss from this condition (90). In a meta-analysis of 53 studies of eyes with untreated neovascular AMD, the mean vision loss at one year was three lines with 75.7% of patients demonstrating 20/200 or worse vision at three years (91). Due to this strong link between CNV development and vision morbidity in AMD, risk factors may be particularly helpful in identifying patients at high risk of developing CNV. As the treatment of CNV is most effective when it is new and has not caused irreversible scarring and photoreceptor damage, it is important to identify these high-risk patients early and thoroughly educate them about the importance of daily self-monitoring of the central visual field as well as regular follow-up ocular examinations.

The MPS Group evaluated selected risk factors for development of CNV in the fellow eye of patients enrolled in the MPS (88). Certain drusen and RPE abnormalities within 1500 μm of the foveal center in the fellow eye were identified as risk factors for the development of CNV (88,92). Specific risk factors include the presence of five or more drusen (RR, 2.1; 95% CI, 1.3–3.5), focal hyperpigmentation (RR, 2.0; 95% CI, 1.4–2.9), definite systemic hypertension (systolic pressure ≥140 mmHg, diastolic pressure ≥90 mmHg, or use of antihypertensive medications) (RR, 1.7; 95% CI, 1.2–2.4), and one or more large drusen (greater 63 μm in greatest linear dimension) (RR, 1.5; 95% CI, 1.0–2.2). The risk of CNV developing within five years after presenting with CNV in the first eye ranged from 7% if none of these risk factors was present to 87% if all four risk factors were present. Of note, no strong association was found between female sex, higher frequency of aspirin usage, cigarette smoking, and hyperopia and an increased risk of CNV (88).

Multivariate analysis of the risk factors for progression to CNV in AREDS participants identified two risk factors (89). In persons at risk of advanced AMD in both eyes, white race (OR, white vs. black, 6.77; 95% CI, 1.24–36.9) and smoking >10 pack-years (OR, >10 vs. <10 pack-years, 1.55; 95% CI, 1.15–2.09) were independently associated with incident neovascular AMD after controlling for age, gender, and AREDS treatment group.

CONCLUSION

In summary, many risk factors for AMD have been identified during case–control, cross-sectional, and prospective cohort studies. Risk factors such as advanced age, gender, or family history of the disease cannot be modified. One important modifiable risk factor is cigarette smoking, so encouraging smoking cessation when appropriate is a standard component of clinical care. Dietary habits are also modifiable, so if no contraindications exist, it may be reasonable to encourage a diet that includes green leafy vegetables rich in lutein/zeaxanthin and oily fish rich in omega-3 fatty acids. Similarly, exposure to sunlight can be modified with sunglasses, and evidence-based public health recommendations impacting on cardiovascular and other systemic disease prevention should be adopted. It is important to note, however that definite reduction in AMD risk has not been yet proven for any of these strategies. Findings from AREDS suggest that persons with extensive intermediate size drusen, at least one large druse, noncentral geographic atrophy in one or both eyes, or advanced AMD or vision loss due to AMD in one eye, and without contraindications such as cigarette smoking, should consider taking a supplement of antioxidants plus zinc to reduce their risk of progression to advanced AMD and vision loss. The future goal for researchers is to further elucidate modifiable risk factors and to conduct large-scale prospective intervention trials on these factors so that better preventive measures can be implemented.

SUMMARY POINTS

- *Importance of identifying risk factors for AMD.* The identification and modification of risk factors for AMD has the potential for great public health impact
- *Studies on risk factors for AMD.* Case–control, cross-sectional, and prospective cohort studies can help identify risk factors for AMD. Repeated findings of the same risk factors in well-designed studies conducted in different populations are necessary to provide compelling evidence of a real association between AMD and potential risk factors. However, only randomized prospective clinical trials can prove that modifying a particular established risk factor can influence the course of AMD
- *Classification of risk factors.* Risk factors for AMD may be broadly classified into *personal* or *environmental* factors (e.g., smoking, sunlight exposure, and nutritional factors including micronutrients, dietary fish intake, and alcohol consumption). Personal factors may be further subdivided into *sociodemographic* (e.g., age, gender, race/ethnicity, heredity, and socioeconomic status), *ocular* (e.g., iris color, macular pigment optical density, cataract and its surgery, refractive error, and cup/disc ratio), and *systemic* factors (e.g., cardiovascular disease and its

risk factors, reproductive and related factors, and antioxidant enzymes)
- *Established risk factors.* Age, race/ethnicity, heredity, and smoking
- *Possible risk factors.* Gender, socioeconomic status, iris color, macular pigment optical density, cataract and cataract extraction, refractive error, cup/disc ratio, cardiovascular disease, hypertension, blood pressure, serum lipid levels, dietary fat intake, BMI, hematologic factors including homocysteine, *C. pneumoniae* infection, reproductive and related factors, antioxidant enzymes, sunlight exposure, micronutrients, dietary fish intake, and alcohol consumption
- *Factors probably not associated with AMD.* Diabetes and hyperglycemia
- *Risk factors for progression to choroidal neovascularization.* Presence of five or more drusen, focal hyperpigmentation, systemic hypertension, one or more large drusen (>125 μm in greatest linear dimension), white race, and smoking
- *Current opinion on modifying risk factors.* One modifiable well-established risk factor is cigarette smoking. There may be potential benefits of antismoking patient education for primary and secondary prevention of AMD. The Age-Related Eye Disease Study suggested that persons older than 55 years with extensive intermediate size drusen, at least one large druse, noncentral geographic atrophy in one or both eyes, or advanced AMD or vision loss due to AMD in one eye, and without contraindications such as cigarette smoking, should consider taking a supplement of antioxidants plus zinc to reduce their risk of progression to advanced AMD and vision loss. If no contraindications exist, it may reasonable to encourage a diet that includes green leafy vegetables rich in lutein/zeaxanthin and oily fish rich in omega-3 fatty acids.

REFERENCES

1. Friedman DS, O'Colmain BJ, Munoz B, et al. Prevalence of age-related macular degeneration in the United States. Arch Ophthalmol 2004; 122: 564–72.
2. Bird AC, Bressler NM, Bressler SB, et al. An international classification and grading system for age-related maculopathy and age-related macular degeneration. The International ARM Epidemiological Study Group. Surv Ophthalmol 1995; 39: 367–74.
3. Hyman L, Schachat AP, He Q, et al. Hypertension, cardiovascular disease, and age-related macular degeneration. Age-Related Macular Degeneration Risk Factors Study Group. Arch Ophthalmol 2000; 118: 351–8.
4. Kawasaki R, Wang JJ, Aung T, et al. Prevalence of age-related macular degeneration in a Malay population: the Singapore Malay Eye Study. Ophthalmology 2008; 115: 1735–41.
5. Fraser-Bell S, Donofrio J, Wu J, et al. Sociodemographic factors and age-related macular degeneration in Latinos: the Los Angeles Latino Eye Study. Am J Ophthalmol 2005; 139: 30–8.

6. Kahn HA, Leibowitz HM, Ganley JP, et al. The Framingham Eye Study. II. Association of ophthalmic pathology with single variables previously measured in the Framingham Heart Study. Am J Epidemiol 1977; 106: 33–41.

7. Klein R, Klein BE, Linton KL. Prevalence of age-related maculopathy. The Beaver Dam Eye Study. Ophthalmology 1992; 99: 933–43.

8. Klein R, Cruickshanks KJ, Nash SD, et al. The prevalence of age-related macular degeneration and associated risk factors. Arch Ophthalmol 2010 Jun;128:750–8.

9. Friedman DS, Katz J, Bressler NM, et al. Racial differences in the prevalence of age-related macular degeneration: the Baltimore Eye Survey. Ophthalmology 1999; 106: 1049–55.

10. Sommer A, Tielsch JM, Katz J, et al. Racial differences in the cause-specific prevalence of blindness in east Baltimore. N Engl J Med 1991; 325: 1412–17.

11. Klein R, Klein BE, Knudtson MD, et al. Prevalence of age-related macular degeneration in 4 racial/ethnic groups in the multi-ethnic study of atherosclerosis. Ophthalmology 2006; 113: 373–80.

12. Smith W, Mitchell P. Family history and age-related maculopathy: the Blue Mountains Eye Study. Aust NZ J Ophthalmol 1998; 26: 203–6.

13. Gottfredsdottir MS, Sverrisson T, Musch DC, et al. Age related macular degeneration in monozygotic twins and their spouses in Iceland. Acta Ophthalmol Scand 1999; 77: 422–5.

14. Goldberg J, Flowerdew G, Smith E, et al. Factors associated with age-related macular degeneration. An analysis of data from the first National Health and Nutrition Examination Survey. Am J Epidemiol 1988; 128: 700–10.

15. Schachat AP, Hyman L, Leske MC, et al. Features of age-related macular degeneration in a black population. The Barbados Eye Study Group. Arch Ophthalmol 1995; 113: 728–35.

16. Krishnaiah S, Das T, Nirmalan PK, et al. Risk factors for age-related macular degeneration: findings from the Andhra Pradesh eye disease study in South India. Invest Ophthalmol Vis Sci 2005; 46: 4442–9.

17. Smith W, Mitchell P, Wang JJ. Gender, oestrogen, hormone replacement and age-related macular degeneration: results from the Blue Mountains Eye Study. Aust NZ J Ophthalmol 1997; 25(Suppl 1): S13–15.

18. The_Eye_Disease_Case-Control_Study_Group. Risk factors for neovascular age-related macular degeneration. The Eye Disease Case-Control Study Group. Arch Ophthalmol 1992; 110: 1701–8.

19. Klein R, Klein BE, Jensen SC, et al. The relation of socioeconomic factors to age-related cataract, maculopathy, and impaired vision. The Beaver Dam Eye Study. Ophthalmology 1994; 101: 1969–79.

20. Beatty S, Boulton M, Henson D, et al. Macular pigment and age related macular degeneration. Br J Ophthalmol 1999; 83: 867–77.

21. Bone RA, Landrum JT, Tarsis SL. Preliminary identification of the human macular pigment. Vision Res 1985; 25: 1531–5.

22. Bone RA, Landrum JT. Macular pigment in Henle fiber membranes: a model for Haidinger's brushes. Vision Res 1984; 24: 103–8.

23. Snodderly DM. Evidence for protection against age-related macular degeneration by carotenoids and antioxidant vitamins. Am J Clin Nutr 1995; 62: 1448S–61S.

24. Landrum JT, Bone RA, Kilburn MD. The macular pigment: a possible role in protection from age-related macular degeneration. Adv Pharmacol 1997; 38: 537–56.

25. Hammond BR Jr, Wooten BR, Snodderly DM. Cigarette smoking and retinal carotenoids: implications for age-related macular degeneration. Vision Res 1996; 36: 3003–9.

26. Bone RA, Landrum JT, Guerra LH, et al. Lutein and zeaxanthin dietary supplements raise macular pigment density and serum concentrations of these carotenoids in humans. J Nutr 2003; 133: 992–8.

27. Age-related_Eye_Disease_Study_2. Manual of Procedures. 2009. [Available from: http://www.web.emmes.com/study/areds2/resources/areds2_mop.pdf]

28. Gibson JM, Shaw DE, Rosenthal AR. Senile cataract and senile macular degeneration: an investigation into possible risk factors. Trans Ophthalmol Soc UK 1986; 105(Pt 4): 463–8.

29. Baatz H, Darawsha R, Ackermann H, et al. Phacoemulsification does not induce neovascular age-related macular degeneration. Invest Ophthalmol Vis Sci 2008; 49: 1079–83.

30. Sperduto RD, Hiller R, Seigel D. Lens opacities and senile maculopathy. Arch Ophthalmol 1981; 99: 1004–8.

31. Chakravarthy U, Wong TY, Fletcher A, et al. Clinical risk factors for age-related macular degeneration: a systematic review and meta-analysis. BMC Ophthalmol 2010; 10: 31.

32. Klein R, Klein BE, Jensen SC, et al. The relationship of ocular factors to the incidence and progression of age-related maculopathy. Arch Ophthalmol 1998; 116: 506–13.

33. Chaine G, Hullo A, Sahel J, et al. Case-control study of the risk factors for age related macular degeneration. France-DMLA Study Group. Br J Ophthalmol 1998; 82: 996–1002.

34. Wang JJ, Mitchell PG, Cumming RG, et al. Cataract and age-related maculopathy: the Blue Mountains Eye Study. Ophthalmic Epidemiol 1999; 6: 317–26.

35. Ho L, Boekhoorn SS, Liana, et al. Cataract surgery and the risk of aging macula disorder: the rotterdam study. Invest Ophthalmol Vis Sci 2008; 49: 4795–800.

36. Chew EY, Sperduto RD, Milton RC, et al. Risk of advanced age-related macular degeneration after cataract surgery in the Age-Related Eye Disease Study: AREDS report 25. Ophthalmology 2009; 116: 297–303.

37. Weiter JJ, Delori FC, Wing GL, et al. Relationship of senile macular degeneration to ocular pigmentation. Am J Ophthalmol 1985; 99: 185–7.

38. Snow KK, Seddon JM. Do age-related macular degeneration and cardiovascular disease share common antecedents? Ophthalmic Epidemiol 1999; 6: 125–43.

39. Hyman LG, Lilienfeld AM, Ferris FL 3rd, et al. Senile macular degeneration: a case-control study. Am J Epidemiol 1983; 118: 213–27.

40. Klein R, Klein BE, Franke T. The relationship of cardiovascular disease and its risk factors to age-related maculopathy. The Beaver Dam Eye Study. Ophthalmology 1993; 100: 406–14.

41. Sperduto RD, Hiller R. Systemic hypertension and age-related maculopathy in the Framingham Study. Arch Ophthalmol 1986; 104: 216–19.

42. Smith W, Mitchell P, Leeder SR, et al. Plasma fibrinogen levels, other cardiovascular risk factors, and age-related maculopathy: the Blue Mountains Eye Study. Arch Ophthalmol 1998; 116: 583–7.

43. Klein R, Clegg L, Cooper LS, et al. Prevalence of age-related maculopathy in the Atherosclerosis Risk in Communities Study. Arch Ophthalmol 1999; 117: 1203–10.

44. Klein R, Klein BE, Marino EK, et al. Early age-related maculopathy in the cardiovascular health study. Ophthalmology 2003; 110: 25–33.

45. Vingerling JR, Dielemans I, Bots ML, et al. Age-related macular degeneration is associated with atherosclerosis. The Rotterdam Study. Am J Epidemiol 1995; 142: 404–9.

46. McGwin G Jr, Modjarrad K, Hall TA, et al. 3-hydroxy-3-methylglutaryl coenzyme a reductase inhibitors and the presence of age-related macular degeneration in the Cardiovascular Health Study. Arch Ophthalmol 2006; 124: 33–7.

47. Klein R, Klein BE, Jensen SC, et al. Medication use and the 5-year incidence of early age-related maculopathy: the Beaver Dam Eye Study. Arch Ophthalmol 2001; 119: 1354–9.

48. Mitchell P, Wang JJ, Foran S, et al. Five-year incidence of age-related maculopathy lesions: the Blue Mountains Eye Study. Ophthalmology 2002; 109: 1092–7.

49. Mitchell P, Wang JJ. Diabetes, fasting blood glucose and age-related maculopathy: The Blue Mountains Eye Study. Aust NZ J Ophthalmol 1999; 27: 197–9.

50. Seddon JM, Cote J, Davis N, et al. Progression of age-related macular degeneration: association with body mass index, waist circumference, and waist-hip ratio. Arch Ophthalmol 2003; 121: 785–92.

51. Christen WG, Glynn RJ, Chew EY, et al. Folic acid, pyridoxine, and cyanocobalamin combination treatment and age-related macular degeneration in women: the Women's Antioxidant and Folic Acid Cardiovascular Study. Arch Intern Med 2009; 169: 335–41.

52. Seddon JM, George S, Rosner B, et al. Progression of age-related macular degeneration: prospective assessment of C-reactive protein, interleukin 6, and other cardiovascular biomarkers. Arch Ophthalmol 2005; 123: 774–82.

53. Hogg RE, Woodside JV, Gilchrist SE, et al. Cardiovascular disease and hypertension are strong risk factors for choroidal neovascularization. Ophthalmology 2008; 115: 1046–52, e2.

54. Robman L, Mahdi O, McCarty C, et al. Exposure to Chlamydia pneumoniae infection and progression of age-related macular degeneration. Am J Epidemiol 2005; 161: 1013–19.

55. Defay R, Pinchinat S, Lumbroso S, et al. Sex steroids and age-related macular degeneration in older French women: the POLA study. Ann Epidemiol 2004; 14: 202–8.

56. Delcourt C, Cristol JP, Leger CL, et al. Associations of antioxidant enzymes with cataract and age-related macular degeneration. The POLA Study. Pathologies Oculaires Liees a l'Age. Ophthalmology 1999; 106: 215–22.

57. Christen WG, Glynn RJ, Manson JE, et al. A prospective study of cigarette smoking and risk of age-related macular degeneration in men. JAMA 1996; 276: 1147–51.

58. Seddon JM, Willett WC, Speizer FE, et al. A prospective study of cigarette smoking and age-related macular degeneration in women. JAMA 1996; 276: 1141–6.

59. Klein R, Klein BE, Linton KL, et al. The Beaver Dam Eye Study: the relation of age-related maculopathy to smoking. Am J Epidemiol 1993; 137: 190–200.

60. Smith W, Mitchell P, Leeder SR. Smoking and age-related maculopathy. The Blue Mountains Eye Study. Arch Ophthalmol 1996; 114: 1518–23.

61. Tamakoshi A, Yuzawa M, Matsui M, et al. Smoking and neovascular form of age related macular degeneration in late middle aged males: findings from a case-control study in Japan. Research Committee on Chorioretinal Degenerations. Br J Ophthalmol 1997; 81: 901–4.

62. Kawasaki R, Wang JJ, Ji GJ, et al. Prevalence and risk factors for age-related macular degeneration in an adult Japanese population: the Funagata study. Ophthalmology 2008; 115: 1376–81, 81 e1–2.

63. Delcourt C, Diaz JL, Ponton-Sanchez A, et al. Smoking and age-related macular degeneration. The POLA Study. Pathologies Oculaires Liees a l'Age. Arch Ophthalmol 1998; 116: 1031–5.

64. Bidwell G, Sahu A, Edwards R, et al. Perceptions of blindness related to smoking: a hospital-based cross-sectional study. Eye (Lond) 2005; 19: 945–8.

65. Khan JC, Thurlby DA, Shahid H, et al. Smoking and age related macular degeneration: the number of pack years of cigarette smoking is a major determinant of risk for both geographic atrophy and choroidal neovascularisation. Br J Ophthalmol 2006; 90: 75–80.

66. West SK, Rosenthal FS, Bressler NM, et al. Exposure to sunlight and other risk factors for age-related macular degeneration. Arch Ophthalmol 1989; 107: 875–9.

67. Ham WT Jr, Mueller HA, Ruffolo JJ Jr, et al. Action spectrum for retinal injury from near-ultraviolet radiation in the aphakic monkey. Am J Ophthalmol 1982; 93: 299–306.

68. Margrain TH, Boulton M, Marshall J, et al. Do blue light filters confer protection against age-related macular degeneration? Prog Retin Eye Res 2004; 23: 523–31.

69. Cruickshanks KJ, Klein R, Klein BE. Sunlight and age-related macular degeneration. The Beaver Dam Eye Study. Arch Ophthalmol 1993; 111: 514–18.

70. Fletcher AE, Bentham GC, Agnew M, et al. Sunlight exposure, antioxidants, and age-related macular degeneration. Arch Ophthalmol 2008; 126: 1396–403.

71. Frei B. Reactive oxygen species and antioxidant vitamins: mechanisms of action. Am J Med 1994; 97: 5S–13S; discussion 22S–8S.

72. AREDS_Study_Group. A randomized, placebo-controlled, clinical trial of high-dose supplementation with vitamins C and E, beta carotene, and zinc for age-related macular degeneration and vision loss: AREDS report no. 8. Arch Ophthalmol 2001; 119: 1417–36.

73. Omenn GS, Goodman GE, Thornquist MD, et al. Effects of a combination of beta carotene and vitamin A on lung cancer and cardiovascular disease. N Engl J Med 1996; 334: 1150–5.

74. The_Alpha-Tocopherol_Beta_Carotene_Cancer_Prevention_Study_Group. The effect of vitamin E and beta carotene on the incidence of lung cancer and other cancers in male smokers. The Alpha-Tocopherol, Beta Carotene Cancer Prevention Study Group. N Engl J Med 1994; 330: 1029–35.

75. Taylor HR, Tikellis G, Robman LD, et al. Vitamin E supplementation and macular degeneration: randomised controlled trial. BMJ 2002; 325: 11.

76. Teikari JM, Laatikainen L, Virtamo J, et al. Six-year supplementation with alpha-tocopherol and beta-carotene and age-related maculopathy. Acta Ophthalmol Scand 1998; 76: 224–9.

77. Tan JS, Wang JJ, Flood V, et al. Dietary antioxidants and the long-term incidence of age-related macular degeneration: the Blue Mountains Eye Study. Ophthalmology 2008; 115: 334–41.

78. Olson JH, Erie JC, Bakri SJ. Nutritional supplementation and age-related macular degeneration. Semin Ophthalmol 2011; 26: 131–6.

79. van Kuijk FJ, Buck P. Fatty acid composition of the human macula and peripheral retina. Invest Ophthalmol Vis Sci 1992; 33: 3493–6.

80. Robison WG, Kuwabara T, Bieri JG. The roles of vitamin E and unsaturated fatty acids in the visual process. Retina 1982; 2: 263–81.

81. Sanders TA, Haines AP, Wormald R, et al. Essential fatty acids, plasma cholesterol, and fat-soluble vitamins in subjects with age-related maculopathy and matched control subjects. Am J Clin Nutr 1993; 57: 428–33.

82. Kromhout D, Bosschieter EB, de Lezenne Coulander C. The inverse relation between fish consumption and 20-year mortality from coronary heart disease. N Engl J Med 1985; 312: 1205–9.

83. SanGiovanni JP, Chew EY, Clemons TE, et al. The relationship of dietary lipid intake and age-related macular degeneration in a case-control study: AREDS Report No. 20. Arch Ophthalmol 2007; 125: 671–9.

84. Chong EW, Kreis AJ, Wong TY, et al. Dietary omega-3 fatty acid and fish intake in the primary prevention of age-related macular degeneration: a systematic review and meta-analysis. Arch Ophthalmol 2008; 126: 826–33.

85. Ritter LL, Klein R, Klein BE, et al. Alcohol use and age-related maculopathy in the Beaver Dam Eye Study. Am J Ophthalmol 1995; 120: 190–6.

86. Cho E, Hankinson SE, Willett WC, et al. Prospective study of alcohol consumption and the risk of age-related macular degeneration. Arch Ophthalmol 2000; 118: 681–8.

87. Macular_Photocoagulation Study_Group. Five-year follow-up of fellow eyes of patients with age-related macular degeneration and unilateral extrafoveal choroidal neovascularization. Arch Ophthalmol 1993; 111: 1189–99.

88. Macular_Photocoagulation_Study_Group. Risk factors for choroidal neovascularization in the second eye of patients with juxtafoveal or subfoveal choroidal neovascularization secondary to age-related macular degeneration. Macular Photocoagulation Study Group. Arch Ophthalmol 1997; 115: 741–7.

89. Clemons TE, Milton RC, Klein R, et al. Risk factors for the incidence of Advanced Age-Related Macular Degeneration in the Age-Related Eye Disease Study (AREDS) AREDS report no. 19. Ophthalmology 2005; 112: 533–9.

90. Ferris FL 3rd, Fine SL, Hyman L. Age-related macular degeneration and blindness due to neovascular maculopathy. Arch Ophthalmol 1984; 102: 1640–2.

91. Wong TY, Chakravarthy U, Klein R, et al. The natural history and prognosis of neovascular age-related macular degeneration: a systematic review of the literature and meta-analysis. Ophthalmology 2008; 115: 116–26.

92. Bressler SB, Maguire MG, Bressler NM, et al. Relationship of drusen and abnormalities of the retinal pigment epithelium to the prognosis of neovascular macular degeneration. The Macular Photocoagulation Study Group. Arch Ophthalmol 1990; 108: 1442–7.

6

Oxidative stress

Milam A. Brantley Jr, Melissa P. Osborn, and Paul Sternberg Jr

INTRODUCTION

Oxidative stress is hypothesized to contribute to the pathophysiology of age-related macular degeneration (AMD) as well as numerous other chronic, multifactorial conditions, including heart disease, diabetes, and neurodegenerative disorders (1–3). Although reactive oxygen species (ROS) are by-products of normal metabolic processes (e.g., glycolysis and the Krebs cycle), aging and disease may disturb the balance between ROS generation and clearance, resulting in oxidative damage to macromolecules (4). The retina is particularly susceptible to oxidative stress because of its high oxygen consumption, lipid composition, and focused light exposure (4,5). The retinas of AMD patients undergo increased oxidation, as indicated by the greater prevalence of oxidative modifications to proteins and DNA in the Bruch's membrane, drusen, and retinal pigment epithelium (RPE) of AMD patients versus controls (6).

Environmental and demographic factors correspond to both increased oxidative stress and a greater likelihood of developing AMD. Two primary risk factors for AMD are aging and smoking. Past studies have demonstrated that the aging process involves progressive oxidation throughout the body (7) and that AMD risk increases dramatically with age (8). Similarly, cigarette smoking has been shown to increase systemic oxidation (9), and current smokers are two to three times more likely to develop AMD than never-smokers (10). Additional oxidative stress-related risk factors include higher body mass index and greater light exposure (11,12).

Genetic studies also support a link between AMD and oxidative stress. Polymorphisms in mitochondrial DNA (mtDNA) and the paraoxonase 1 (*PON1*) gene have been associated with AMD (13–15). Given the role of mitochondria in cellular respiration and the antioxidant activity of PON1, it is plausible that these variants modulate oxidative stress in the retina. To date, the majority of reported genetic risk factors for AMD are related to the complement system. These include single nucleotide polymorphisms (SNPs) in genes coding for complement factor H (*CFH*), complement factor B/C2, C3, complement factor I, and CFH-related proteins 1 and 3 (16–25). Recent evidence suggests a relationship between these inflammatory genetic variants and biomarkers for oxidative stress (1,26).

An impaired antioxidant defense system in the retina may create a physiologic environment that promotes AMD development and progression. High dietary intake of carotenoids and antioxidants has been linked with lower AMD risk (27–28), and supplementation with antioxidants and zinc was shown to reduce risk of progression to advanced AMD in the Age-Related Eye Disease Study (AREDS) (29). Two carotenoids, lutein and zeaxanthin, comprise the macular pigment that protects against retinal ROS. Some studies have reported low macular pigment levels in AMD patients (30–32). Interestingly, a high dietary intake of lutein/zeaxanthin and omega-3 fatty acids has corresponded to reduced prevalence and incidence of AMD, although a definitive cause and effect relationship has not been established (33).

To explore the role of oxidative stress in the pathogenesis of AMD, we will first discuss the mechanisms of oxidative stress affecting the retina. We then will review AMD biomarkers and risk genotypes that suggest an imbalance between oxidative stress and antioxidant defenses. We will also consider the interaction between inflammation and oxidative damage to the retina in AMD pathophysiology. Finally, we will review potential AMD therapies related to protection against oxidative stress.

OXIDATIVE INJURY TO THE RETINA

ROS, including free radicals, peroxides, and singlet oxygen, are a major source of retinal oxidative stress. Free radicals, such as the hydroxyl radical (OH·), hydroperoxyl radical (HO$_2$·), superoxide anion (O$_2^-$·), and lipid peroxyl radicals, are strong oxidizing agents with an unpaired electron in the outer shell. Peroxides [e.g., hydrogen peroxide (H$_2$O$_2$), lipid peroxides] and singlet oxygen (^{1}O$_2$) have a full complement of electrons in an unstable state (5). Most of the endogenous ROS are generated by the mitochondrial electron transport chain, which converts 2–3% of all utilized oxygen into highly reactive ROS (34). Stimuli such as aging, inflammation, irradiation, air pollutants, and cigarette smoke increase ROS production, leading to cellular oxidative injury (5,7,35). Antioxidants and antioxidant enzymes quickly eliminate the majority of ROS in the body. For example, superoxide dismutase (SOD) converts the superoxide anion, produced during cellular respiration, to H$_2$O$_2$ (5). Smaller antioxidant molecules, such as vitamin E, act on free radicals directly, reducing ROS such as the hydroxyl radical.

As most free radical chain reactions are prevented by free radical–scavenging molecules, it appears that free radicals are often not the direct cause of oxidative damage, but rather act to initiate further oxidative damage by non-radical oxidants. The redox hypothesis describes a radical-free oxidative stress in which disrupted thiol redox circuits interfere with the regulation of cellular redox status, affecting cell signaling and physiological regulation. Redox-sensitive thiols include the amino acid cysteine (Cys), the Cys-derived disulfide cystine (CySS), the Cys-containing tripeptide glutathione (GSH), and glutathione disulfide (GSSG). Sulfur redox couples serve as "on/off" switches regulating gene expression and protein function. Because the Cys/CySS and GSH/GSSG couples are not in equilibrium, it is plausible that abnormal levels of non-radical oxidants could be sufficient to disrupt normal cellular function (36).

It has been suggested that the increased oxidative stress associated with AMD can severely impair the morphology and function of the RPE, photoreceptors, and retinal vasculature. Growing evidence also suggests that the mitochondria of retinal cells contribute to oxidative stress-related pathology.

Retinal Pigment Epithelium

Under normal conditions, phagocytosis of photoreceptor outer segments (POS) by the RPE generates ROS via the NADPH oxidase system, upregulating intracellular H_2O_2 and catalase (37). The phosphoinositide 3-kinase (PI3K)-Akt pathway may protect RPE cells from such oxidative stress by inactivating proapoptotic factors, as demonstrated in cultured RPE cells (38). In the case of aging and disease, antioxidant defenses may not counteract the increased oxidative state of the retina, leading to the accumulation of debris (i.e., drusen) and RPE cell death. Abnormally high concentrations of oxidized products may also limit RPE regulation of key angiogenic factors, resulting in retinal or choroidal neovascularization.

Cell culture studies have demonstrated AMD-like retinal damage induced by oxidizing agents. When treated with tert-butyl hydroperoxide (t-BHP) (39) or H_2O_2 (40), RPE cells exhibited signs of senescence, suggesting that oxidative stress may contribute to geographic atrophy (GA). Additionally, RPE cells exposed to hypoxia/reoxygenation experienced an accumulation of extracellular matrix comparable to the thickening of Bruch's membrane seen in early AMD (41).

The RPE undergoes photo-oxidative stress in response to light exposure, as indicated by increased production of ROS (2,42,43), and oxidative modifications to proteins or lipids called advanced glycation end products (AGEs) (43). AGEs appear to damage cells by modifying intracellular proteins (e.g., transcription factors) and altering extracellular proteins and extracellular matrix molecules. These modified proteins can then bind and activate receptor of AGEs (RAGE), triggering an NF-κB-mediated immune response (44). In human donor eyes, RAGE were found to co-localize with AGE deposits and macular disease in AMD retinas, while normal retinas displayed little or no immunolabeling for AGE or RAGE (45). RAGE also increased RPE secretion of vascular endothelial growth factor (VEGF), which stimulates angiogenesis and enhances vascular permeability (46). These results suggest that the AGE-induced activation of RAGE may play a key role in RPE apoptosis and contribute to neovascular AMD.

Further evidence indicates the influence of oxidative stress on VEGF expression in the RPE. Treatment of cultured RPE cells with the oxidant DL-buthionine-(S,R)-sulfoximine (BSO) caused a significant decrease in intracellular GSH and GSH/GSSG ratios. This change in thiol redox status was associated with increased VEGF-A secretion as well as significant induction of VEGF receptors VEGFR-1 and VEGFR-2 (47). VEGF secretion in RPE cells is regulated, in part, by the mitogen-activated protein kinases (MAPK), including c-Jun-activated kinase (JNK), p38, and Erk. Studies in cultured RPE cells have demonstrated that constitutive VEGF secretion is regulated by p38, while oxidative stress-induced VEGF secretion is mediated by both p38 and Erk (48).

Insufficient antioxidant responses may contribute directly to AMD. Mice lacking nuclear factor erythroid 2-related factor 2 (NRF2), a transcription factor critical to antioxidant pathways, demonstrated AMD-like changes in the retina, including drusen-like deposits, the accumulation of lipofuscin, and spontaneous choroidal neovascularization. Autophagy-related vacuoles and multivesicular bodies were found to be accumulated in the RPE and Bruch's membrane of these $Nrf2^{-/-}$ mice (49).

Photoreceptors

Degeneration of the macula disrupts the physiologic balance of oxidants and antioxidants in the retinal spaces. As a source of ROS, photoreceptors contribute to the oxidative burden of the retina, particularly in a pathologic oxidative environment. The vitality of rods and cones is directly affected by the redox status of surrounding tissue. Photoreceptor cell loss or a reduction in energy-demanding activities like phototransduction can lead to elevated tissue oxygen concentrations because choroidal blood vessels are not autoregulated by local oxygen levels. Accordingly, increases in outer retinal oxygen concentrations have been confirmed in multiple animal models (50–52).

Alterations in the cellular redox status appear to mediate photoreceptor cell death. An in vitro model of photoreceptor apoptosis demonstrated an early and sustained increase in intracellular ROS accompanied by a rapid depletion of intracellular GSH (53). Programmed cell death of photoreceptors has been shown to occur via multiple oxidative stress-related mechanisms, including the classic caspase-dependent apoptotic pathways (54,55), the subsequently identified caspase-independent apoptotic pathways (56–58), and autophagy (59). Evidence suggests that calpain activity may play a critical role in caspase-independent apoptosis (60,61). Interestingly, calpains may impair DNA repair mechanisms, making retinal cells more susceptible to oxidative DNA damage (62).

Retinal Vasculature

Oxidative stress may have direct and indirect effects on choroidal endothelial cells (CECs). ROS produced by reoxygenation have been shown to upregulate VEGF both in vitro and in vivo, suggesting that oxidative stress

Table 6.1 Evidence of Oxidative Stress in Age-Related Macular Degeneration

	Oxidative stress in the retina	Relevant findings in AMD
RPE	Increased production of ROS and AGEs in response to photo-oxidative stress (43) Oxidative modifications to proteins and DNA in Bruch's membrane, drusen, and RPE cells (6) Accumulation of extracellular matrix in RPE cells exposed to hypoxia and reoxygenation (41)	Drusen-like deposits and spontaneous choroidal neovascularization in NRF2-deficient mice (49) Signs of senescence observed in RPE cells treated with oxidizing agents (39,40) Co-localization of RAGE with AGE deposits and macular disease in AMD retinas (45)
Photoreceptors	Increased outer retinal oxygen concentrations in animal models (50–52) Oxidative stress as a mediator for programmed cell death in photoreceptors (54–59)	Early and sustained increase in ROS and rapid depletion of GSH in an in vitro model of photoreceptor apoptosis (53)
Vasculature	ROS-induced upregulation of VEGF in vitro and in vivo (63) Release of the proangiogenic basic fibroblast growth factor by RPE cells exposed to oxidation (66)	Increased proliferation and VEGF expression in CECs treated with AGEs (67) Decreased viability and increased proliferation observed in CECs in response to oxidative stress (66)
Mitochondria	High concentration of ROS produced by the electron transport chain and limited capacity for mtDNA repair (68) Light-induced conformational changes in mitochondria of RPE cells (43) Damage to RPE mtDNA by oxidized photoreceptor outer segments (69)	Alterations in the number and structure of RPE mitochondria (70), mitochondrial proteins (72), and mtDNA (73) in AMD donor eyes Development of dry AMD-like lesions in mice with decreased levels of MnSOD (75)

Abbreviations: AMD, age-related macular degeneration; AGEs, advanced glycation end products; CECs, choroidal endothelial cells; GSH, glutathione; MnSOD, manganese superoxide dismutase; mtDNA, mitochondrial DNA; RPE, retinal pigment epithelium; ROS, reactive oxygen species; RAGE, receptor of AGEs; VEGF, vascular endothelial growth factor.

may contribute to the increases in VEGF seen in AMD (63). Increased VEGF expression in vascular endothelial cells may result from peroxynitrite, a highly reactive oxidant that mediates the inhibition of metabolic enzymes, lipid peroxidation, and oxidation of thiol pools (64,65). Treatment of cultured RPE cells and CECs with the oxidant t-BHP decreased the viability and increased the proliferation of both cell types (66). RPE cells exposed to t-BHP released basic fibroblast growth factor, a prominent proangiogenic factor (66). This finding suggests that oxidative stress may stimulate choroidal neovascularization via RPE–mediated growth factor release. Additionally, treatment of CECs with AGEs demonstrated increased proliferation and VEGF upregulation, suggesting that the exposure of CECs to AGES may also contribute to neovascular AMD (67).

Mitochondria

Accumulating evidence suggests a role for mitochondrial damage in AMD pathophysiology (13). Mitochondria are especially susceptible to oxidative injury due to the high concentration of ROS produced by the electron transport chain and the limited capacity for mtDNA repair (68). In cultured RPE cells, photo-oxidative stress caused structural changes in mitochondria (43), and exposure to oxidized POS damaged mtDNA (69). Abnormalities in the number and structure of RPE mitochondria have been reported in AMD donor eyes (70). Proteomic analyses have suggested that mitochondrial proteins (71) and mtDNA (72) are altered in AMD, and long-extension polymerase chain reaction confirmed that mtDNA is increasingly damaged with disease progression (73). Oxidative damage to mitochondria can lead to apoptosis in human RPE cells (74), and decreased

levels of the mitochondrial antioxidant manganese SOD have led to the development of dry AMD-like lesions in mice (75).

Ultimately, these studies indicate that AMD or AMD risk factors alter the redox status of the retina. This increased oxidative state causes damage to retinal tissues by an array of mechanisms and may provide an etiology for AMD symptoms such as waste accumulation, cell death, and angiogenesis (Table 6.1).

BIOMARKERS OF OXIDATIVE STRESS AND ANTIOXIDANT DEFENSE

Biomarkers of oxidative stress and antioxidant defense may reflect an individual's exposure to oxidative stress as well as the individual's ability to maintain a healthy oxidative state in the retina. Past studies have suggested that levels of these markers are associated with AMD as well as risk factors for the disease.

Oxidative Stress

Redox status. Cysteine thiols are critical to the proper functioning of many enzymes, receptors, ion channels, transporters, and transcription factors (7). Redox potentials for the thiol couples Cys/CySS and GSH/GSSG reflect the overall redox status of a system (76) and may be useful for AMD risk assessment. Two major AMD risk factors, aging and smoking, have been linked to higher thiol oxidation. An initial study reported lower plasma GSH levels in older adults compared with younger individuals (77). In the plasma of healthy individuals aged 19–85, Cys/CySS redox status was found to increase linearly with age over the entire age span, whereas GSH/GSSG redox began to decrease sharply after age 45 (7). These data suggest a continuous, linear increase in oxidative events throughout life and a subsequent rapid decline in antioxidant defense (7). Later, plasma Cys/CySS and GSH/GSSG redox were reported to be more oxidized in smokers compared with nonsmokers (9), and mean plasma CySS was found to be higher in AMD patients than in controls prior to adjustment for age (78). While a clear association between thiol redox and AMD remains to be found, the significant age-related changes in redox status reported in these studies may contribute to AMD.

DNA damage. Oxidative damage to genomic DNA may influence AMD development. Recently, polymorphisms in the DNA repair gene *XPD* were found to be associated with AMD, suggesting that abnormal DNA repair mechanisms may contribute to AMD pathophysiology (79). Levels of 8-hydroxy-2′-deoxyguanosine (8-OHdG), an indicator of total oxidative DNA damage, were found to be significantly higher in the plasma (80) and aqueous humor (81) of neovascular AMD patients compared with controls. The potential correlation between aqueous humor and plasma levels of 8-OHdG remains to be determined. Additionally, lymphocytes of AMD patients were reported to undergo heightened basal endogenous DNA damage, oxidative modification to DNA bases, and sensitivity to H_2O_2 and UV radiation (82).

Amino acid and protein modifications. Homocysteine, an intermediary amino acid formed during the conversion of methionine to Cys, rapidly auto-oxidizes in plasma to form homocystine and mixed disulfides, along with ROS (e.g., superoxide anion and H_2O_2) (83). High plasma homocysteine levels are considered an independent risk factor for atherosclerosis, cardiovascular disease, and venous thrombosis (84). An association between elevated homocysteine and advanced AMD was reported in the large Australian Blue Mountains Eye Study Second Survey (BMES2) (85) and an AREDS substudy (86). Multiple smaller case–control studies have also reported higher plasma homocysteine levels in AMD patients (83,87–91), and two studies have demonstrated increased plasma homocysteine levels in patients with neovascular AMD compared with those having dry AMD (90,91). In contrast, no association was detected between plasma homocysteine and AMD status either in a subset of BMES2 patients matched for age, gender, and smoking (92) or in participants in the third National Health and Nutrition Examination Survey (NHANES) (93). It is difficult to draw comparisons among all of these studies given the differences in study design, sample collection, and AMD grading. Nonetheless, it appears that homocysteine remains a good candidate for an AMD biomarker related to systemic oxidative stress.

Lipid peroxidation. Approximately 80% of the phospholipids in the POS discs are composed of docosahexanoic acid (DHA) (22:6ω-3), the most highly abundant polyunsaturated fatty acid (PUFA) in nature (94). The conjugated double bonds present in PUFAs make them particularly susceptible to free radical damage. Lipid radicals can combine with oxygen to form lipid peroxyl radicals and lipid peroxides. These products can achieve a steady state only by stealing electrons from other PUFAs, thus setting off a cascade of reactions that damages molecules and may become cytotoxic to retinal cells.

Carboxyethyl pyrrole (CEP), a protein modification derived from DHA oxidation, has been extensively studied in AMD. Initial experiments demonstrated an abundance of CEP adducts in AMD Bruch's membrane/RPE/choroid tissues (6) as well as elevated plasma anti-CEP immunoreactivity and serum titer in AMD patients compared with age-matched controls (95). Quantification of CEP modifications and autoantibodies revealed higher mean CEP adduct and autoantibody levels in AMD plasma, with odds ratios three fold greater in AMD patients for each measurement (96). Interestingly, participants with elevated CEP markers as well as risk genotypes for SNPs in *ARMS2*, *HTRA1*, and *C3* had a predicted AMD risk that was two- to three fold greater than their risk based on genotype alone (96). In mice, subretinal injections of CEP-modified serum albumin exacerbated laser-induced choroidal neovascularization, suggesting that increased lipid peroxidation may contribute to the abnormal angiogenesis of neovascular AMD (97).

Malondialdehyde (MDA) and 4-hydroxynoneal (HNE) may also promote retinal damage in AMD. These lipid peroxidation products are predominantly generated from DHA, arachidonic acid, and linoleic acid (98). Both MDA and HNE have been shown to inhibit lysosomal degradation of POS proteins in cultured RPE cells (99), inducing apical-to-basolateral transcytosis of the undegraded POS proteins (100). This mechanism may contribute to sub-RPE deposit formation and drusen biogenesis in AMD, as proteins containing HNE adducts are identified in the retinas of donor eyes in progressive stages of AMD (101). Additionally, elevated plasma MDA levels have been reported in AMD patients in multiple small case–control studies (80,102–104).

Oxidized phospholipids, generated from the oxidation of cellular phospholipids containing PUFAs or low-density lipoprotein (LDL), may correspond to AMD status. Increased levels of oxidized phosphatidylcholine were found in photoreceptors and RPE of AMD donor eyes (105). Systemic studies demonstrated higher mean plasma levels of oxidized LDL in AMD patients (14) and increased susceptibility of LDL to oxidation in neovascular AMD patients compared with controls (106).

Antioxidant Defense

Vitamins. Vitamin C (ascorbate), the major aqueous-phase antioxidant in human blood (107), has been shown to protect RPE cells against H_2O_2-induced (108) and blue light–induced (109) oxidative stress in vitro. While two small studies reported lower plasma vitamin C levels in late AMD patients (110,111), no difference in vitamin C levels was detected between AMD cases and controls in multiple larger studies (112–115).

Vitamin E (tocopherol) acts as the major chain-breaking antioxidant of cellular membranes (5). The most prominent isoform of vitamin E in human retina and plasma, α-tocopherol, is a highly effective free radical scavenger. Vitamin E was shown to protect against photo-oxidative damage in rats through decreased MDA production (116). Also, lower serum vitamin E levels have been reported in AMD patients compared with controls in several small studies (110,111,114,117). The French POLA study found a negative association between vitamin E levels and late AMD after adjusting for lipid levels (115). In contrast, no association between vitamin E levels and AMD was observed in the Eye Disease Case–Control Study (EDCCS) (112) or in the Beaver Dam Eye Study after adjustment for cholesterol levels (118).

Carotenoids. Carotenes (α-carotene, β-carotene, and lycopene) and xanthophylls (lutein, zeaxanthin, and β-cryptoxanthin) comprise the class of antioxidant molecules termed carotenoids (119). Retinal carotenoid levels have been linked with the incidence and progression of retinal degeneration in animal models (120,121). Decreased macular pigment level (lutein and zeaxanthin) was found in AMD patients by direct measurement at autopsy (30) and Raman spectroscopy measurement of macular pigment optical density (MPOD) (31,32). Conversely, MPOD values measured by heterochromic flicker photometry and reflectometry were not significantly different between AMD patients and controls (122,123), and longitudinal studies have not correlated lower macular pigment with increased risk of AMD progression (124,125). Physiological and nutritional variation among study populations and different measurement techniques may explain these mixed results (126,127). Higher plasma levels of carotenoids (lutein, zeaxanthin, α- and β-carotene, cryptoxanthin, lycopene) were associated with lower risk for neovascular AMD in the large EDCCS (112). Low serum lycopene, a precursor to β-carotene, was also associated with AMD in multiple studies (110,118,128). The Carotenoids in Age-Related Macular degeneration Italian Study (CARMIS) reported that central retinal dysfunction in AMD patients, as determined by multifocal ERG, could be improved over 12 months with supplements containing vitamin C, vitamin E, zinc, copper, and xanthophylls (lutein, zeaxanthin, and astaxanthin) (129). Patients taking these supplements experienced improved visual acuity, contrast sensitivity, and visual function after 24 months of treatment (130).

Antioxidant enzymes. The thiol enzymes glutathione peroxidase (GPx) and glutathione reductase (GRx) as well as the heme enzyme catalase have been investigated as potential biomarkers for AMD. GPx, found in the human retina, reduces organic hydroperoxides using GSH as an electron donor (5). Two small studies reported significantly-lower GPx levels in AMD patients (104,131), while others found no association between AMD and GPx level (132,133). The large POLA study reported that higher levels of GPx were associated with a nine-fold increase in late AMD prevalence (134). The activity of GRx, which catalyzes the regeneration of GSH from GSSG, was found to be lower in AMD patients in one study (132) but not another (133). Catalase, an iron-dependent enzyme that scavenges H_2O_2, has been localized in human retina and RPE (5). While one study reported lower plasma catalase levels in AMD patients

Table 6.2 Associations of Plasma Biomarkers of Oxidative Stress with AMD or Risk Factors for AMD

Biomarker type	Biomarker	Detected associations
Thiol	GSH	Age (77)
	E_h (Cys/CySS)	Age (7)
		Smoking (9)
	E_h (GSH/GSSG)	Age (7,9)
DNA	8-OHdG	Neovascular AMD (80)
Amino acid	Homocysteine	AMD (83,87–91)
		Late AMD (85,86)
		Neovascular AMD (90,91)
Lipid	CEP	AMD (95,96)
	MDA	AMD (80,102–104)
	Oxidized LDL	AMD (14)

Abbreviations: AMD, age-related macular degeneration; CEP, carboxyethyl pyrrole; Cys, cysteine; CySS, cystine; GSH, glutathione; GSSG, glutathione disulfide; 8-OHdG, 8-hydroxy-2'-deoxyguanosine; LDL, low-density lipoprotein; MDA, malondialdehyde; E_h, reduction potential.

than controls (103), this association was not replicated in another small study (133). These mixed results suggest a limited role for GPx, GRx, or catalase as plasma biomarkers for AMD.

The antioxidant enzymes SOD and PON1 may influence AMD risk. Two small case–control studies reported lower plasma SOD levels in AMD patients (104,131). However, most studies, including the larger POLA study, found no association between SOD and AMD (132–134). The enzyme PON1 metabolizes lipid peroxides and prevents LDL oxidation by hydrolyzing oxidized substrates. One small study found reduced PON1 activity in AMD patients and reported a negative correlation between PON1 and the lipid peroxidation product MDA (135). Lower PON1 levels were also demonstrated in neovascular AMD patients compared with controls (87).

The association of multiple biomarkers of oxidative stress (Table 6.2) and antioxidant responses (Table 6.3) with AMD reflects the influence of redox status on disease development. However, no single biomarker is currently being used in clinical practice for AMD detection or treatment. As a result, current investigations are moving away from the single biomarker approach to combinations of markers and genetic variants.

GENETICS
Polymorphisms in Antioxidant Enzymes
Polymorphisms in genes coding for antioxidant enzymes can modulate enzymatic activity, thus influencing retinal antioxidant defense. Manganese SOD, coded for by the *SOD2* gene, is found in human mitochondria. The investigation of a valine-to-alanine polymorphism (V16A, SNP rs4880) in the *SOD2* gene has yielded conflicting results in Japanese cohorts. Two initial studies reported inverse associations with AMD: Kimura et al. found that

Table 6.3 Plasma Biomarkers of Antioxidant Defense System Associated with AMD

Biomarker type	Biomarker	Detected associations
Antioxidants	Vitamin C	Late AMD (110,111)
	Vitamin E	AMD (110,111,114,117)
		Late AMD (115)
		Neovascular AMD (118)
	Total Carotenoids	Neovascular AMD (112)
	Lycopene	AMD (110,118,128)
Enzymes	SOD*	AMD (104,131)
	GPx	AMD (104,131)
		Late AMD (134)
	GRx	AMD (132)
	Catalase	AMD (103)
	PON1*	AMD (135)
		Neovascular AMD (87)

*Genetic studies have suggested that polymorphisms in genes coding for these proteins are linked with AMD. *Abbreviations*: AMD, Age-related macular degeneration; GPx, glutathione peroxidase; GRx, glutathione reductase; PON1, paraoxonase 1; SOD, superoxide dismutase.

the V16A variant corresponded to a 10-fold increased risk of neovascular AMD (136), whereas Gotoh et al. found the same SNP to be protective against AMD (137). Subsequently, Kondo investigated multiple *SOD2* SNPs and haplotypes (groups of SNPs inherited together) and identified no associations with neovascular AMD or polypoidal choroidal vasculopathy (PCV, an AMD-related disorder characterized by a branching vascular network under the RPE with polypoidal lesions at its edge under the RPE) (138). Studies in Northern Irish and Polish populations also failed to detect an association between *SOD2* SNPs and AMD (139,140).

Two SNPs in the *PON1* gene (L55M and G192A) were found to be associated with neovascular AMD in a small Japanese cohort (14), but no significant associations between the same two SNPs and AMD were found in a small number of patients from Northern Ireland and Australia (141). In a large U.S. study, direct sequencing of *PON1* exons revealed a weak association between L55M and increased AMD risk (15). Subanalysis showed the G192A allele to be less prevalent in neovascular AMD but not in GA (15). It thus appears that the G192A polymorphism may have a protective role in neovascular AMD and L55M may exert a modest risk effect.

The free radical nitric oxide (NO), highly-abundant in the human body, is synthesized by nitric oxide synthase (NOS). The neuronal and endothelial isoforms (nNOS and eNOS, respectively) function constitutively, whereas inducible NOS (iNOS) is typically expressed in response to inflammation. As NOS isoforms control the level of NO in the body, NOS polymorphisms have been examined for a relationship with AMD. Two eNOS variants showed no association with AMD in a small Austrian cohort (142). However, SNP rs8072199 in the iNOS

gene (*NOS2A*) was found to be associated with AMD in a U.S. study (143). As the *NOS2A* variant rs2248814 was closely associated with smoking in this cohort (143), it is possible that *NOS2A* SNPs modulate the effect of smoking on AMD.

Mitochondrial DNA and ARMS2

Variants in mtDNA have been shown to influence AMD risk. In the large Blue Mountains Eye Study, mitochondrial haplogroup H was associated with reduced prevalence of any AMD and early AMD, whereas haplogroups J and U were associated with early AMD only (144). The T2 haplogroup has been linked to a greater risk for advanced AMD (145), and the mtDNA 4917G polymorphism (associated with haplogroup T) independently predicted the presence of AMD (146). The SNPs T16126C and A73G (associated with haplogroups J and T) were more frequent in donor retinas and blood DNA of AMD patients compared with controls (147). As the T haplogroup has been associated with multifactorial age-related diseases such as coronary artery disease (148) and AMD (146), it seems plausible that carriers of haplogroup T may experience a greater oxidative stress or have greater susceptibility to oxidative damage than individuals with other haplogroups.

The A69S polymorphism in *ARMS2*, which has been linked to mitochondrial function in some studies, is strongly associated with AMD (149,150). ARMS2 mRNA encoding a 12-kDa protein has been detected in human retina. Cell culture experiments have localized this protein to the mitochondrial outer membrane (151) and specifically to mitochondria in the ellipsoid region of the photoreceptors (152). These findings suggest a functional role for ARMS2 in mitochondrial homeostasis and have led to an attractive hypothesis linking ARMS2 and oxidative stress. Such a connection fits well with previous reports of an interaction between *ARMS2* A69S and cigarette smoking history (153,154). The localization of ARMS2 to the mitochondria has been called into question, however, by an immunohisotologic study conducted in that found no co-localization of ARMS2 antibodies and mitochondrial markers and instead reported localization of the ARMS2 protein to the cytosol in cultured RPE cells (155). Due to potential inconsistencies in antibodies and visualization, further investigation is necessary to confirm or refute the relationship between ARMS2 and the mitochondria.

These genetic studies support the hypothesis that impaired regulation of oxidative stress in the retina, whether originating from decreased antioxidant defense or increased oxidative stress, contributes to AMD.

OXIDATIVE STRESS AND INFLAMMATION IN AMD

Immunologic and inflammatory processes play a key role in AMD pathophysiology (e.g., drusen formation, complement activation, macrophage recruitment, and microglial activation) (26,156). Complement proteins have been identified in drusen (157,158), and elevated levels of complement activation products have been demonstrated in the plasma of AMD patients (159,160).

Table 6.4 Evidence Supporting the Role of Inflammation and Its Relationship with Oxidative Stress in AMD Pathophysiology

Factor	Evidence
Inflammation	Presence of complement proteins in drusen (157,158)
	High blood complement protein levels associated with AMD (159,160)
	Associations of genetic variants in multiple complement genes (*CFH, C2/BF, C3, CFI*) with AMD (16–25)
Link between inflammation and oxidative stress	Decreased *CFH* expression in the response to oxidized POS (163) and H_2O_2 (164)
	Disruption in RPE function in presence of both H_2O_2 and complement-sufficient serum (166)
	Decreased ability of CFH to bind MDA in individuals with the *CFH* Y402H risk genotype for AMD (165)
	Complement fixation and development of AMD-like lesions in mice treated with CEP (168)
	Sub-RPE deposits of inflammatory proteins found in *Nrf2$^{-/-}$* mice with impaired antioxidant defenses (49)
	Association of increased superoxide and decreased SOD2 with mononuclear phagocyte-induced apoptosis of the RPE in *sod2$^{+/-}$* mice (161)

Abbreviations: AMD, Age-related macular degeneration; CEP, carboxyethyl pyrrole; BF, complement factor B; CFH, complement factor H; CFI, complement factor I; COX-2, cyclooxygenase-2; H_2O_2, hydrogen peroxide; MDA, malondialdehyde; Nrf2, nuclear factor erythroid 2-related factor 2; POS, photoreceptor outer segments; RPE, retinal pigment epithelium; SOD2, superoxide dismutase 2.

Numerous associations between complement gene polymorphisms and AMD have also been reported (26). The results of both cell culture and animal studies point to a mechanistic link between inflammation and oxidative stress. Decreased SOD and increased superoxide production led to mononuclear phagocyte-induced apoptosis of the RPE in *sod2$^{+/-}$* mice (161). In mice with oxygen-induced retinopathy, injections of the serine proteinase inhibitor SERPINA3K reduced expression of proinflammatory factors (e.g., VEGF, TNF-α), decreased ROS production, and upregulated the antioxidants SOD and GSH (162). The anti-inflammatory effect of SERPINA3K was also demonstrated in retinal cells exposed to hypoxia (162). Additionally, sub-RPE deposits of inflammatory proteins were identified in *Nrf2$^{-/-}$* mice with dysfunctional antioxidant responses (49).

Oxidative stress has been shown to reduce *CFH* expression in the RPE. Long-term treatment of RPE cells with oxidized POS, but not normal POS, markedly downregulated *CFH* mRNA expression. Further, phagocytosis of both oxidized and normal POS reduced CFH protein expression (163). Additionally, RPE cells exposed to H_2O_2 or blue light decreased IFN-γ-mediated expression of *CFH* (109,164). A recent study demonstrated that CFH specifically binds oxidatively-modified MDA, but that each H402 variant (C allele) reduces this binding by approximately 25% (165). Oxidized MDA upregulated the proinflammatory cytokine interleukin (IL)-8 and the antioxidant enzymes NAD(P)H dehydrogenase and hemoxygenase-1 (HO-1) in ARPE-19 cells. Interestingly, CFH specifically inhibited MDA-induced production of IL-8. In a murine model, MDA triggered an inflammatory response, and CFH protected against MDA-induced inflammation (165).

The dynamic interplay between oxidative stress and inflammation may contribute to the abnormalities in RPE function evident in AMD. A combination of H_2O_2 and complement-sufficient serum was shown to disrupt RPE barrier function in vitro and evoke polarized secretion of VEGF, although neither H_2O_2 nor serum alone caused these changes (166). These results suggest that oxidative stress and complement together reduce RPE function. They also point to a common mechanism that

relates an oxidizing environment and complement activation with VEGF production. Recently, sublytic membrane-attack-complex activation was found to increase VEGF production via the Src and Ras-Erk pathways (167). Such pathways could play a role in the neovascularization seen in late AMD. Mice immunized with mouse serum albumin adducted with CEP developed AMD-like lesions in the retina (168). Specifically, these mice produced antibodies to the hapten, fixed complement component 3 in Bruch's membrane, and accumulated drusen below the RPE (168).

Taken together, these studies demonstrate a molecular link between oxidative stress and complement in RPE cells and suggest that the interaction between oxidative stress and inflammatory mediators plays a key role in the development of AMD. The evidence supporting the role of inflammation and its link with oxidative stress in AMD is summarized in Table 6.4.

AMD THERAPIES TARGETING OXIDATIVE STRESS
Oxidative stress-related therapies for AMD generally aim to increase antioxidant defense, thus lowering the oxidative stress on the retina, or to protect against apoptosis. Treatment strategies include antioxidant therapy and genetic modification. Therapies under investigation are outlined in Table 6.5.

Supplemental Antioxidants
Currently, care of patients with dry AMD is centered on antioxidant and zinc supplementation, as there are no direct interventions for drusen or GA. The AREDS, a multicenter, randomized clinical trial sponsored by the National Eye Institute, demonstrated that daily intake of supplemental antioxidants (β-carotene, vitamin C, vitamin E) and zinc reduced the risk of progression to advanced AMD by 25% over five years (29). Since this pivotal study, carotenoids (particularly lutein and zeaxanthin) and omega-3 fatty acids have also been associated with decreased AMD risk, greater visual acuity, and improved central retinal function (as measured by multifocal ERG) (129,130,169–171). The AREDS2 study is prospectively investigating the effect of oral supplementation of xanthophylls and omega-3 fatty acids [DHA and

Table 6.5 Possible Retinal Therapies Targeting Oxidative Stress

Directions for retinal therapy	Treatments under investigation
Anti-inflammatory agents	**Canolol downregulated proinflammatory cytokines** in a rodent model (180) **Curcumin decreased expression of inflammatory mediators** (176) and inhibited the NF-κB pathway (175) in human cells *in vitro* **Resveratrol decreased oxidation and proliferation** via inhibition of the NF-κB pathway in human RPE cells (179)
Boost in antioxidant defense	**Supplementation with xanthophylls and omega-3 fatty acids under investigation** for treatment of AMD in AREDS2 clinical trial (33) **Curcumin prevented retinal oxidative damage** via activation of the NRF2-thioredoxin system **and increased antioxidant expression** in rats and human RPE cells (177,178) **Sulforaphane protected against retinal oxidative damage** via activation of the NRF2-thioredoxin system in rodent models (182–184) **Canolol upregulated antioxidant molecules,** such as catalase, HO-1, and NRF2, in human RPE cells (181)
Genetic modification	**Modulation of SOD2 and CAT gene expression protected against oxidative damage to retinal cells** in rodents (188,189) **Oct4 and SirT1 gene therapy upregulated antioxidant enzymes and improved retinal function** by promoting cellular longevity in rats and human RPE cells (191) **XIAP gene transfer protected against apoptosis** caused by oxidative stress in human RPE cells (190)
Inhibition of apoptotic pathways	**Canolol inhibited oxidative stress-induced apoptosis** via an ERK antioxidative pathway in human RPE cells (181) **Paeoniflorin prevented apoptosis** through caspase-3 inhibition in human RPE cells (187) **Quercetin protected against oxidative damage and senescence** in the retina through inhibition of caspase-3 activity in human RPE cells (186)

Abbreviations: AREDS2, Age-Related Eye Disease Study 2; AMD, age-related macular degeneration; CAT, catalase; ERK, extracellular signal regulated kinase; HO-1, hemoxygenase-1; IL-1β, interleukin-1β; NRF2, nuclear factor erythroid 2-related factor 2; NF-κB, nuclear factor kappa B; RPE, retinal pigment epithelium; SOD2, superoxide dismutase; XIAP, X-linked inhibitor of apoptosis.

eicosapentaenoic acid (EPA)] on the risk of AMD progression (33). In this ongoing clinical trial, scheduled to end in 2013, AMD patients are randomly assigned to four treatment groups: (i) xanthophylls only (10 mg lutein and 2 mg zeaxanthin), (ii) omega-3 fatty acids only (350 mg DHA and 650 mg EPA), (iii) xanthophylls and omega-3 fatty acids, and (iv) placebo (33). The results of this trial may alter the recommended regimen for AMD patients currently treated with antioxidant and zinc supplements.

Two AREDS ancillary studies directly examined the relationship between AREDS supplements (antioxidants and zinc) and thiol redox status in AMD. After five years, supplemental antioxidants reduced the Cys/CySS redox potential (E_h Cys) and increased plasma levels of the reduced thiol Cys (172). These data suggest that the beneficial effect of antioxidant supplementation may be explained, in part, by its effect on Cys availability or its effect on E_h Cys. Also, five years of supplemental zinc decreased plasma levels of the oxidized thiol CySS (173), suggesting a potential role for zinc in preventing increased CySS. These studies provide a potential mechanism for the effects of these supplements on AMD progression.

The topical application of the antioxidant OT-551 has been studied for GA treatment. In a small clinical trial, patients with bilateral GA experienced less vision loss in the OT-551-treated eye, but no significant differences in GA area, contrast sensitivity, microperimetry measurements, and total drusen area, were found (174). The larger Phase II OMEGA study, evaluating the ability

of OT-551 to stop GA progression and reduce the size of the GA lesions, showed no evidence of efficacy in reaching the stated end-point (Paul Sternberg, personal communication). With the lack of promising results in the Phase II study, no further clinical trials are planned for this agent.

Dietary Antioxidants

Naturally-occurring compounds found in food may protect against AMD. Curcumin, from the spice turmeric, has been shown to inhibit the NF-κB pathway of immune response (175) and to decrease expression of inflammatory mediators (176). Curcumin also upregulates antioxidants, such as HO-1, quinone reductase, and glutathione S-transferase (177). A two-week diet supplemented with curcumin protected rats from light-induced retinal damage (178). Similarly, treatment of cultured retinal cells with curcumin protected against H_2O_2-induced cell death by increasing production of antioxidant enzymes, such as thioredoxin, and activating the NRF2 antioxidant pathway (178). Another member of the plant-derived polyphenol family, resveratrol, a compound in red wine, has been shown to decrease oxidative damage and RPE proliferation in vitro (179). Evidence suggests that resveratrol may also take effect through NF-κB pathway inhibition.

Molecules that decrease inflammation and increase antioxidant activity, particularly through NRF2, may protect against oxidative damage in AMD. Canolol, a phenolic compound found in crude canola oil, can reduce the production of iNOS and proinflammatory cytokines (180). In human RPE cells, canolol inhibited ROS production and apoptosis induced by t-BH and upregulated HO-1, catalase, GST-pi, and NRF2 (181). It appears that canolol acts via an antioxidative pathway regulated by extracellular signal regulated kinase (ERK) (181). Sulforaphane, an isothiocyanate found in broccoli, appears to exert neuroprotective effects through activation of the NRF2-thioredoxin system. The antioxidant transcription factor NRF2 binds to the antioxidant response element (ARE), activating the antioxidant defense system in response to oxidative stress (182). Thioredoxin has been shown to protect against H_2O_2-induced damage in photoreceptors cells and light damage in mice (183). Sulforaphane induces thioredoxin in light-exposed RPE cells via the NRF2-ARE pathway (184), thus protecting against photo-oxidative damage to the retina.

Additional dietary compounds that may be protective against oxidative damage interfere with caspase-dependent apoptotic pathways. The flavonoid quercetin, found in green tea and red onion, is a chelating agent that can reduce iron-driven lipid peroxidation (185). Quercetin was reported to protect against H_2O_2-induced oxidative damage and senescence in cultured RPE cells by inhibiting caspase-3 activity (186). Paeoniflorin, an active ingredient in a traditional Chinese medicine (Paeoniae Radix) for the treatment of eye disorders, has been reported to protect against oxidative stress and inflammation. In cultured RPE cells exposed to H_2O_2, paeoniflorin also prevented apoptosis through caspase-3 inhibition (187).

Genetic Modification

Gene therapy is being explored for the treatment of retinal degenerations. Toward this end, genes involved in the regulation of cellular oxidative stress are being targeted in animal studies to reduce ROS production, bolster antioxidant defenses, and/or increase cellular repair capacity. In mice with ischemia-induced retinal injury, plasmids encoding the human *SOD2* or catalase (*CAT*) genes significantly decreased ROS generation and retinal endothelial cell apoptosis (188). Another study showed that an adenovirus carrying the *CAT* gene protected against H_2O_2-induced damage to RPE cells and light-induced damage to RPE and photoreceptors in mice (189).

Neuroprotective agents that can defend against oxidative damage to the retina have also been evaluated as candidates for gene therapy. Virus-mediated gene transfer of human X-linked inhibitor of apoptosis (XIAP) was shown to protect against H_2O_2-induced apoptosis of cultured RPE cells (190). The transcription factor Oct4

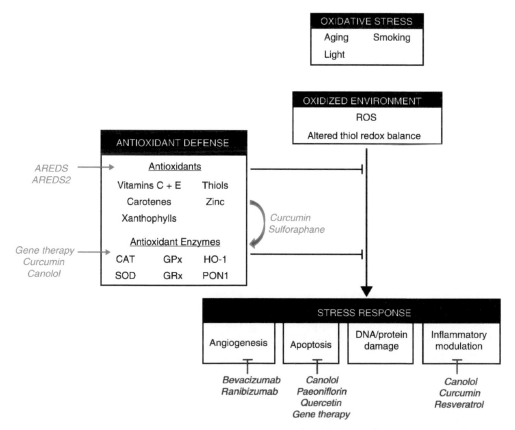

Figure 6.1 Oxidative stress, brought on by factors such as aging and smoking, leads to an oxidized cellular environment that is marked by the accumulation of reactive oxygen species and more oxidized thiol redox status. This oxidized environment triggers stress responses, such as vascular changes, apoptosis, damage to DNA and proteins, and altered inflammatory modulation. Concurrently, the cellular antioxidant defense system, comprised of antioxidants and antioxidant enzymes, is activated, mitigating the damage of oxidative stress. The mechanisms of current and potential treatments for retinal diseases are depicted above, with green representing activation and red representing inhibition. *Abbreviations*: AREDS2, Age-Related Eye Disease Study 2; CAT, catalase; GPx, glutathione peroxidase; GRx, glutathione reductase; HO-1, hemoxygenase-1; PON1, paraoxonase 1; SOD, superoxide dismutase.

(expressed in pluripotent cells) and the mediator of cellular longevity SirT1 have also been investigated. Oct4 and SirT1 were found at lower levels in human aged retina and RPE cells as well as AMD retinas. Introduction of Oct4 and SirT1 increased upregulated GSH, SOD, CAT, and GPx in H_2O_2-exposed RPE cells. This gene transfer also increased antioxidant enzyme levels (e.g., SOD, GSH-Px) and improved retinal function (as measured by ERG) in mice (191). These therapies could help defend against the progression of AMD and perhaps even lead to visual improvement for AMD patients.

CONCLUSIONS

Oxidative stress plays a significant role in the pathogenesis of AMD. ROS, derived primarily from the mitochondria, can threaten the integrity of RPE cells, retinal vascular endothelial cells, and photoreceptors. Increased oxidative stress coupled with depleted antioxidant levels can lead to oxidative damage to DNA, proteins, and lipids in the retina (Figure 6.1). These changes can trigger retinal cell death via modulation of alternative metabolic pathways and stimulation of proapoptotic reactions. Such oxidative injury may contribute to the accumulation of waste deposits, atrophy, and neovascularization seen in AMD. Because oxidative stress appears to be a common mechanism of oxidative damage to the retina, the development of therapy aimed to regulate retinal levels of oxidative stress could significantly reduce vision loss from AMD.

SUMMARY POINTS

- In AMD, the combination of increased oxidative stress and impaired antioxidant defense creates an imbalance between oxidants and antioxidants in the retina, leading to cellular damage.
- Multiple biomarkers of oxidative stress and antioxidant defense as well as genetic variants of oxidative stress and inflammation have been associated with AMD, although no single marker has proven adequate as an independent predictor of AMD risk.
- Therapies that upregulate antioxidant production and exert neuroprotective effects, such as dietary/supplemental antioxidants and genetic modification, have been proposed for AMD.

REFERENCES

1. Khandhadia S, Lotery A. Oxidation and age-related macular degeneration: insights from molecular biology. Expert Rev Mol Med 2010; 12: e34.
2. Winkler BS, Boulton ME, Gottsch JD, et al. Oxidative damage and age-related macular degeneration. Mol Vis 1999; 5: 32.
3. Giacco F, Brownlee M. Oxidative stress and diabetic complications. Circ Res 2010; 107: 1058–70.
4. Cai J, Nelson KC, Wu M, et al. Oxidative damage and protection of the RPE. Prog Retin Eye Res 2000; 19: 205–21.
5. Beatty S, Koh H, Phil M, et al. The role of oxidative stress in the pathogenesis of age-related macular degeneration. Surv Ophthalmol 2000; 45: 115–34.
6. Crabb JW, Miyagi M, Gu X, et al. Drusen proteome analysis: an approach to the etiology of age-related macular degeneration. Proc Natl Acad Sci USA 2002; 99: 14682–7.
7. Jones DP, Mody VC Jr, Carlson JL, et al. Redox analysis of human plasma allows separation of pro-oxidant events of aging from decline in antioxidant defenses. Free Radic Biol Med 2002; 33: 1290–300.
8. Jonasson F, Arnarsson A, Eiriksdottir G, et al. Prevalence of age-related macular degeneration in old persons: Age, Gene/environment Susceptibility Reykjavik study. Ophthalmology 2011; 118: 825–30.
9. Moriarty SE, Shah JH, Lynn M, et al. Oxidation of glutathione and cysteine in human plasma associated with smoking. Free Radic Biol Med 2003; 35: 1582–8.
10. Thornton J, Edwards R, Mitchell P, et al. Smoking and age-related macular degeneration: a review of association. Eye (Lond) 2005; 19: 935–44.
11. Seddon JM, Cote J, Davis N, et al. Progression of age-related macular degeneration: association with body mass index, waist circumference, and waist-hip ratio. Arch Ophthalmol 2003; 121: 785–92.
12. Clemons TE, Milton RC, Klein R, et al. Risk factors for the incidence of advanced age-related macular degeneration in the age-related eye disease study (AREDS) AREDS report no. 19. Ophthalmology 2005; 112: 533–9.
13. Jarrett SG, Lewin AS, Boulton ME. The importance of mitochondria in age-related and inherited eye disorders. Ophthalmic Res 2010; 44: 179–90.
14. Ikeda T, Obayashi H, Hasegawa G, et al. Paraoxonase gene polymorphisms and plasma oxidized low-density lipoprotein level as possible risk factors for exudative age-related macular degeneration. Am J Ophthalmol 2001; 132: 191–5.
15. Pauer GJ, Sturgill GM, Peachey NS, et al. Protective effect of paraoxonase 1 gene variant Gln192Arg in age-related macular degeneration. Am J Ophthalmol 2010; 149: 513–22.
16. Edwards AO, Ritter R 3rd, Abel KJ, et al. Complement factor H polymorphism and age-related macular degeneration. Science 2005; 308: 421–4.
17. Haines JL, Hauser MA, Schmidt S, et al. Complement factor H variant increases the risk of age-related macular degeneration. Science 2005; 308: 419–21.
18. Klein RJ, Zeiss C, Chew EY, et al. Complement factor H polymorphism in age-related macular degeneration. Science 2005; 308: 385–9.
19. Hageman GS, Anderson DH, Johnson LV, et al. A common haplotype in the complement regulatory gene factor H (HF1/CFH) predisposes individuals to age-related macular degeneration. Proc Natl Acad Sci USA 2005; 102: 7227–32.
20. Gold B, Merriam JE, Zernant J, et al. Variation in factor B (BF) and complement component 2 (C2) genes is associated with age-related macular degeneration. Nat Genet 2006; 38: 458–62.
21. Yates JR, Sepp T, Matharu BK, et al. Complement C3 variant and the risk of age-related macular degeneration. N Engl J Med 2007; 357: 553–61.
22. Fagerness JA, Maller JB, Neale BM, et al. Variation near complement factor I is associated with risk of advanced AMD. Eur J Hum Genet 2009; 17: 100–4.
23. Ennis S, Gibson J, Cree AJ, et al. Support for the involvement of complement factor I in age-related macular degeneration. Eur J Hum Genet 2010; 18: 15–16.

24. Hageman GS, Hancox LS, Taiber AJ, et al. Extended haplotypes in the complement factor H (CFH) and CFH-related (CFHR) family of genes protect against age-related macular degeneration: characterization, ethnic distribution and evolutionary implications. Ann Med 2006; 38: 592–604.

25. Hughes AE, Orr N, Esfandiary H, et al. A common CFH haplotype, with deletion of CFHR1 and CFHR3, is associated with lower risk of age-related macular degeneration. Nat Genet 2006; 38: 1173–7.

26. Khandhadia S, Cipriani V, Yates JR, et al. Age-related macular degeneration and the complement system. Immunobiology 2012; 217: 127–46.

27. Seddon JM, Ajani UA, Sperduto RD, et al. Dietary carotenoids, vitamins A, C, and E, and advanced age-related macular degeneration. eye disease case-control study group. JAMA 1994; 272: 1413–20.

28. van Leeuwen R, Boekhoorn S, Vingerling JR, et al. Dietary intake of antioxidants and risk of age-related macular degeneration. JAMA 2005; 294: 3101–7.

29. A randomized, placebo-controlled, clinical trial of high-dose supplementation with vitamins C and E, beta carotene, and zinc for age-related macular degeneration and vision loss: AREDS report no. 8. Arch Ophthalmol. 2001; 119: 1417–36.

30. Bone RA, Landrum JT, Mayne ST, et al. Macular pigment in donor eyes with and without AMD: a case-control study. Invest Ophthalmol Vis Sci 2001; 42: 235–40.

31. Bernstein PS, Zhao DY, Wintch SW, et al. Resonance raman measurement of macular carotenoids in normal subjects and in age-related macular degeneration patients. Ophthalmology 2002; 109: 1780–7.

32. Obana A, Hiramitsu T, Gohto Y, et al. Macular carotenoid levels of normal subjects and age-related maculopathy patients in a Japanese population. Ophthalmology 2008; 115: 147–57.

33. Krishnadev N, Meleth AD, Chew EY. Nutritional supplements for age-related macular degeneration. Curr Opin Ophthalmol 2010; 21: 184–9.

34. Chance B, Sies H, Boveris A. Hydroperoxide metabolism in mammalian organs. Physiol Rev 1979; 59: 527–605.

35. Borish ET, Pryor WA, Venugopal S, et al. DNA synthesis is blocked by cigarette tar-induced DNA single-strand breaks. Carcinogenesis 1987; 8: 1517–20.

36. Jones DP. Radical-free biology of oxidative stress. Am J Physiol Cell Physiol 2008; 295: C849–68.

37. Miceli MV, Liles MR, Newsome DA. Evaluation of oxidative processes in human pigment epithelial cells associated with retinal outer segment phagocytosis. Exp Cell Res 1994; 214: 242–9.

38. Yang P, Peairs JJ, Tano R, et al. Oxidant-mediated Akt activation in human RPE cells. Invest Ophthalmol Vis Sci 2006; 47: 4598–606.

39. Yu AL, Fuchshofer R, Kook D, et al. Subtoxic oxidative stress induces senescence in retinal pigment epithelial cells via TGF-beta release. Invest Ophthalmol Vis Sci 2009; 50: 926–35.

40. Glotin AL, Debacq-Chainiaux F, Brossas JY, et al. Prematurely senescent ARPE-19 cells display features of age-related macular degeneration. Free Radic Biol Med 2008; 44: 1348–61.

41. Fuchshofer R, Yu AL, Teng HH, et al. Hypoxia/reoxygenation induces CTGF and PAI-1 in cultured human retinal pigment epithelium cells. Exp Eye Res 2009; 88: 889–99.

42. Chalam KV, Khetpal V, Rusovici R, et al. A review: role of ultraviolet radiation in age-related macular degeneration. Eye Contact Lens 2011; 37: 225–32.

43. Roehlecke C, Schaller A, Knels L, et al. The influence of sublethal blue light exposure on human RPE cells. Mol Vis 2009; 15: 1929–38.

44. Brownlee M. The pathobiology of diabetic complications: a unifying mechanism. Diabetes 2005; 54: 1615–25.

45. Howes KA, Liu Y, Dunaief JL, et al. Receptor for advanced glycation end products and age-related macular degeneration. Invest Ophthalmol Vis Sci 2004; 45: 3713–20.

46. Ma W, Lee SE, Guo J, et al. RAGE ligand upregulation of VEGF secretion in ARPE-19 cells. Invest Ophthalmol Vis Sci 2007; 48: 1355.61.

47. Sreekumar PG, Kannan R, de Silva AT, et al. Thiol regulation of vascular endothelial growth factor-A and its receptors in human retinal pigment epithelial cells. Biochem Biophys Res Commun 2006; 346: 1200–6.

48. Klettner A, Roider J. Constitutive and oxidative-stress-induced expression of VEGF in the RPE are differently regulated by different mitogen-activated protein kinases. Graefes Arch Clin Exp Ophthalmol 2009; 247: 1487–92.

49. Zhao Z, Chen Y, Wang J, et al. Age-related retinopathy in NRF2-deficient mice. PloS One 2011; 6: e19456.

50. Yu DY, Cringle SJ, Su EN, et al. Intraretinal oxygen levels before and after photoreceptor loss in the RCS rat. Invest Ophthalmol Vis Sci 2000; 41: 3999–4006.

51. Yu DY, Cringle S, Valter K, et al. Photoreceptor death, trophic factor expression, retinal oxygen status, and photoreceptor function in the P23H rat. Invest Ophthalmol Vis Sci 2004; 45: 2013–19.

52. Padnick-Silver L, Kang Derwent JJ, Giuliano E, et al. Retinal oxygenation and oxygen metabolism in abyssinian cats with a hereditary retinal degeneration. Invest Ophthalmol Vis Sci 2006; 47: 3683–9.

53. Carmody RJ, McGowan AJ, Cotter TG. Reactive oxygen species as mediators of photoreceptor apoptosis in vitro. Exp Cell Res 1999; 248: 520–30.

54. Chang GQ, Hao Y, Wong F. Apoptosis: final common pathway of photoreceptor death in rd, rds, and rhodopsin mutant mice. Neuron 1993; 11: 595–605.

55. Tso MO, Zhang C, Abler AS, et al. Apoptosis leads to photoreceptor degeneration in inherited retinal dystrophy of RCS rats. Invest Ophthalmol Vis Sci 1994; 35: 2693–9.

56. Carmody RJ, Cotter TG. Oxidative stress induces caspase-independent retinal apoptosis in vitro. Cell Death Differ 2000; 7: 282–91.

57. Donovan M, Cotter TG. Caspase-independent photoreceptor apoptosis in vivo and differential expression of apoptotic protease activating factor-1 and caspase-3 during retinal development. Cell Death Differ 2002; 9: 1220–31.

58. Doonan F, Donovan M, Cotter TG. Caspase-independent photoreceptor apoptosis in mouse models of retinal degeneration. J Neurosci 2003; 23: 5723–31.

59. Kunchithapautham K, Rohrer B. Autophagy is one of the multiple mechanisms active in photoreceptor degeneration. Autophagy 2007; 3: 65–6.

60. Sanvicens N, Gomez-Vicente V, Masip I, et al. Oxidative stress-induced apoptosis in retinal photoreceptor cells is mediated by calpains and caspases and blocked by the oxygen radical scavenger CR-6. J Biol Chem 2004; 279: 39268–78.

61. Doonan F, Donovan M, Cotter TG. Activation of multiple pathways during photoreceptor apoptosis in the rd mouse. Invest Ophthalmol Vis Sci 2005; 46: 3530–8.

62. Hill JW, Hu JJ, Evans MK. OGG1 is degraded by calpain following oxidative stress and cisplatin exposure. DNA Repair (Amst) 2008; 7: 648–54.

63. Kuroki M, Voest EE, Amano S, et al. Reactive oxygen intermediates increase vascular endothelial growth factor expression in vitro and in vivo. J Clin Invest 1996; 98: 1667–75.

64. Platt DH, Bartoli M, El-Remessy AB, et al. Peroxynitrite increases VEGF expression in vascular endothelial cells via STAT3. Free Radic Biol Med 2005; 39: 1353–61.

65. Abou-Mohamed G, Johnson JA, Jin L, et al. Roles of superoxide, peroxynitrite, and protein kinase C in the development of tolerance to nitroglycerin. J Pharmacol Exp Ther 2004; 308: 289–99.

66. Eichler W, Reiche A, Yafai Y, et al. Growth-related effects of oxidant-induced stress on cultured RPE and choroidal endothelial cells. Exp Eye Res 2008; 87: 342–8.

67. Hoffmann S, Friedrichs U, Eichler W, et al. Advanced glycation end products induce choroidal endothelial cell proliferation, matrix metalloproteinase-2 and VEGF upregulation in vitro. Graefes Arch Clin Exp Ophthalmol 2002; 240: 996–1002.

68. Wallace DC. Mitochondrial diseases in man and mouse. Science 1999; 283: 1482–8.

69. Jin GF, Hurst JS, Godley BF. Rod outer segments mediate mitochondrial DNA damage and apoptosis in human retinal pigment epithelium. Curr Eye Res 2001; 23: 11–19.

70. Feher J, Kovacs I, Artico M, et al. Mitochondrial alterations of retinal pigment epithelium in age-related macular degeneration. Neurobiol Aging 2006; 27: 983–93.

71. Nordgaard CL, Berg KM, Kapphahn RJ, et al. Proteomics of the retinal pigment epithelium reveals altered protein expression at progressive stages of age-related macular degeneration. Invest Ophthalmol Vis Sci 2006; 47: 815–22.

72. Nordgaard CL, Karunadharma PP, Feng X, et al. Mitochondrial proteomics of the retinal pigment epithelium at progressive stages of age-related macular degeneration. Invest Ophthalmol Vis Sci 2008; 49: 2848–55.

73. Karunadharma PP, Nordgaard CL, Olsen TW, et al. Mitochondrial DNA damage as a potential mechanism for age-related macular degeneration. Invest Ophthalmol Vis Sci 2010; 51: 5470–9.

74. Jiang S, Moriarty-Craige SE, Orr M, et al. Oxidant-induced apoptosis in human retinal pigment epithelial cells: dependence on extracellular redox state. Invest Ophthalmol Vis Sci 2005; 46: 1054–61.

75. Justilien V, Pang JJ, Renganathan K, et al. SOD2 knockdown mouse model of early AMD. Invest Ophthalmol Vis Sci 2007; 48: 4407–20.

76. Jones DP, Carlson JL, Samiec PS, et al. Glutathione measurement in human plasma. evaluation of sample collection, storage and derivatization conditions for analysis of dansyl derivatives by HPLC. Clin Chim Acta 1998; 275: 175–84.

77. Samiec PS, Drews-Botsch C, Flagg EW, et al. Glutathione in human plasma: decline in association with aging, age-related macular degeneration, and diabetes. Free Radic Biol Med 1998; 24: 699–704.

78. Brantley MA Jr, Osborn MP, Sanders BJ, et al. Plasma biomarkers of oxidative stress and genetic variants in age-related macular degeneration. Am J Ophthalmol 2012; 153: 460–7.

79. Gorgun E, Guven M, Unal M, et al. Polymorphisms of the DNA repair genes XPD and XRCC1 and the risk of age-related macular degeneration. Invest Ophthalmol Vis Sci 2010; 51: 4732–7.

80. Totan Y, Yagci R, Bardak Y, et al. Oxidative macromolecular damage in age-related macular degeneration. Curr Eye Res 2009; 34: 1089–93.

81. Lau LI, Liu CJ, Wei YH. Increase of 8-hydroxy-2′-deoxyguanosine in aqueous humor of patients with exudative age-related macular degeneration. Invest Ophthalmol Vis Sci 2010; 51: 5486–90.

82. Szaflik JP, Janik-Papis K, Synowiec E, et al. DNA damage and repair in age-related macular degeneration. Mutat Res 2009; 669: 169–76.

83. Coral K, Raman R, Rathi S, et al. Plasma homocysteine and total thiol content in patients with exudative age-related macular degeneration. Eye (Lond) 2006; 20: 203–7.

84. Graham IM, Daly LE, Refsum HM, et al. Plasma homocysteine as a risk factor for vascular disease. The European Concerted Action Project. JAMA 1997; 277: 1775–81.

85. Rochtchina E, Wang JJ, Flood VM, et al. Elevated serum homocysteine, low serum vitamin B12, folate, and age-related macular degeneration: the Blue Mountains Eye Study. Am J Ophthalmol 2007; 143: 344–6.

86. Seddon JM, Gensler G, Klein ML, et al. Evaluation of plasma homocysteine and risk of age-related macular degeneration. Am J Ophthalmol 2006; 141: 201–3.

87. Ates O, Azizi S, Alp HH, et al. Decreased serum paraoxonase 1 activity and increased serum homocysteine and malondialdehyde levels in age-related macular degeneration. Tohoku J Exp Med 2009; 217: 17–22.

88. Nowak M, Swietochowska E, Wielkoszynski T, et al. Changes in blood antioxidants and several lipid peroxidation products in women with age-related macular degeneration. Eur J Ophthalmol 2003; 13: 281–6.

89. Vine AK, Stader J, Branham K, et al. Biomarkers of cardiovascular disease as risk factors for age-related macular degeneration. Ophthalmology 2005; 112: 2076–80.

90. Kamburoglu G, Gumus K, Kadayifcilar S, et al. Plasma homocysteine, vitamin B12 and folate levels in age-related macular degeneration. Graefes Arch Clin Exp Ophthalmol 2006; 244: 565–9.

91. Axer-Siegel R, Bourla D, Ehrlich R, et al. Association of neovascular age-related macular degeneration and hyperhomocysteinemia. Am J Ophthalmol 2004; 137: 84–9.

92. Wu KH, Tan AG, Rochtchina E, et al. Circulating inflammatory markers and hemostatic factors in age-related maculopathy: a population-based case-control study. Invest Ophthalmol Vis Sci 2007; 48: 1983–8.

93. Heuberger RA, Fisher AI, Jacques PF, et al. Relation of blood homocysteine and its nutritional determinants to age-related maculopathy in the third National Health and Nutrition Examination Survey. Am J Clin Nutr 2002; 76: 897–902.

94. Fliesler SJ, Anderson RE. Chemistry and metabolism of lipids in the vertebrate retina. Prog Lipid Res 1983; 22: 79–131.

95. Gu X, Meer SG, Miyagi M, et al. Carboxyethylpyrrole protein adducts and autoantibodies, biomarkers for age-related macular degeneration. J Biol Chem 2003; 278: 42027–35.

96. Gu J, Pauer GJ, Yue X, et al. Assessing susceptibility to age-related macular degeneration with proteomic and genomic biomarkers. Mol Cell Proteomics 2009; 8: 1338–49.

97. Ebrahem Q, Renganathan K, Sears J, et al. Carboxyethyl-pyrrole oxidative protein modifications stimulate neo-vascularization: Implications for age-related macular degeneration. Proc Natl Acad Sci USA 2006 103: 13480–4.

98. Esterbauer H, Schaur RJ, Zollner H. Chemistry and bio-chemistry of 4-hydroxynonenal, malonaldehyde and related aldehydes. Free Radic Biol Med 1991; 11: 81–128.

99. Schutt F, Bergmann M, Holz FG, et al. Proteins modified by malondialdehyde, 4-hydroxynonenal, or advanced glycation end products in lipofuscin of human retinal pigment epithelium. Invest Ophthalmol Vis Sci 2003; 44: 3663–8.

100. Krohne TU, Holz FG, Kopitz J. Apical-to-basolateral transcytosis of photoreceptor outer segments induced by lipid peroxidation products in human retinal pigment epithelial cells. Invest Ophthalmol Vis Sci 2010; 51: 553–60.

101. Ethen CM, Reilly C, Feng X, et al. Age-related macular degeneration and retinal protein modification by 4-hydroxy-2-nonenal. Invest Ophthalmol Vis Sci 2007; 48: 3469–79.

102. Totan Y, Cekic O, Borazan M, et al. Plasma malondialde-hyde and nitric oxide levels in age related macular degeneration. Br J Ophthalmol 2001; 85: 1426–8.

103. Yildirim O, Ates NA, Tamer L, et al. Changes in antioxi-dant enzyme activity and malondialdehyde level in patients with age-related macular degeneration. Oph-thalmologica 2004; 218: 202–6.

104. Evereklioglu C, Er H, Doganay S, et al. Nitric oxide and lipid peroxidation are increased and associated with decreased antioxidant enzyme activities in patients with age-related macular degeneration. Doc Ophthal-mol 2003; 106: 129–36.

105. Suzuki M, Kamei M, Itabe H, et al. Oxidized phospho-lipids in the macula increase with age and in eyes with age-related macular degeneration. Mol Vis 2007; 13: 772–8.

106. Javadzadeh A, Ghorbanihaghjo A, Rashtchizadeh N, et al. Enhanced susceptibility of low-density lipoprotein to oxidation in wet type age-related macular degeneration in male patients. Saudi Med J 2007; 28: 221–4.

107. Frei B, England L, Ames BN. Ascorbate is an outstand-ing antioxidant in human blood plasma. Proc Natl Acad Sci USA 1989; 86: 6377–81.

108. Yin J, Thomas F, Lang JC, et al. Modulation of oxidative stress responses in the human retinal pigment epithe-lium following treatment with vitamin C. J Cell Physiol 2011; 226: 2025–32.

109. Lau LI, Chiou SH, Liu CJ, et al. The effect of photo-oxi-dative stress and inflammatory cytokine on comple-ment factor H expression in retinal pigment epithelial cells. Invest Ophthalmol Vis Sci 2011; 52: 6832–41.

110. Simonelli F, Zarrilli F, Mazzeo S, et al. Serum oxidative and antioxidant parameters in a group of Italian patients with age-related maculopathy. Clin Chim Acta 2002; 320: 111–15.

111. Michikawa T, Ishida S, Nishiwaki Y, et al. Serum anti-oxidants and age-related macular degeneration among older Japanese. Asia Pac J Clin Nutr 2009; 18: 1–7.

112. Eye Disease Case-Control Study Group. Antioxidant status and neovascular age-related macular degenera-tion. Arch Ophthalmol 1993; 111: 104.9.

113. Blumenkranz MS, Russell SR, Robey MG, et al. risk factors in age-related maculopathy complicated by choroidal neovascularization. Ophthalmology 1986; 93: 552–8.

114. Hogg R, Chakravarthy U. AMD and micronutrient anti-oxidants. Curr Eye Res 2004; 29: 387–401.

115. Delcourt C, Cristol JP, Tessier F, et al. POLA Study Group. Age-related macular degeneration and antioxi-dant status in the POLA study. Pathologies Oculaires Liees a l'Age. Arch Ophthalmol 1999; 117: 1384–90.

116. Yilmaz T, Aydemir O, Ozercan IH, et al. Effects of vita-min e, pentoxifylline and aprotinin on light-induced retinal injury. Ophthalmologica 2007; 221: 159–66.

117. Belda JI, Roma J, Vilela C, et al. Serum vitamin E levels negatively correlate with severity of age-related macu-lar degeneration. Mech Ageing Dev 1999; 107: 159–64.

118. Mares-Perlman JA, Brady WE, Klein R, et al. Serum antioxidants and age-related macular degeneration in a population-based case-control study. Arch Ophthalmol 1995; 113: 1518–23.

119. Young AJ, Lowe GM. Antioxidant and prooxidant prop-erties of carotenoids. Arch Biochem Biophys 2001; 385: 20–7.

120. Chucair AJ, Rotstein NP, Sangiovanni JP, et al. Lutein and zeaxanthin protect photoreceptors from apoptosis induced by oxidative stress: relation with docosahexae-noic acid. Invest Ophthalmol Vis Sci 2007; 48: 5168–77.

121. Nakajima Y, Shimazawa M, Otsubo K, et al. Zeaxanthin, a retinal carotenoid, protects retinal cells against oxida-tive stress. Curr Eye Res 2009; 34: 311–18.

122. Berendschot TT, Willemse-Assink JJ, Bastiaanse M, et al. Macular pigment and melanin in age-related maculopa-thy in a general population. Invest Ophthalmol Vis Sci 2002; 43: 1928–32.

123. Ciulla TA, Hammond BR Jr. Macular pigment density and aging, assessed in the normal elderly and those with cataracts and age-related macular degeneration. Am J Ophthalmol 2004; 138: 582–7.

124. Kanis MJ, Berendschot TT, van Norren D. Influence of macular pigment and melanin on incident early AMD in a white population. Graefes Arch Clin Exp Ophthal-mol 2007; 245: 767–73.

125. Robman L, Vu H, Hodge A, et al. Dietary lutein, zeaxan-thin, and fats and the progression of age-related macu-lar degeneration. Can J Ophthalmol 2007; 42: 720–6.

126. Beatty S, van Kuijk FJ, Chakravarthy U. Macular pig-ment and age-related macular degeneration: longitudi-nal data and better techniques of measurement are needed. Invest Ophthalmol Vis Sci 2008; 49: 843–5.

127. Hogg RE, Anderson RS, Stevenson MR, et al. In vivo macular pigment measurements: a comparison of reso-nance Raman spectroscopy and heterochromatic flicker photometry. Br J Ophthalmol 2007; 91: 485–90.

128. Cardinault N, Abalain JH, Sairafi B, et al. Lycopene but not lutein nor zeaxanthin decreases in serum and lipo-proteins in age-related macular degeneration patients. Clin Chim Acta 2005; 357: 34–42.

129. Parisi V, Tedeschi M, Gallinaro G, et al. Carotenoids and antioxidants in age-related maculopathy Italian study: multifocal electroretinogram modifications after 1 year. Ophthalmology 2008; 115: 324–33.

130. Piermarocchi S, Saviano S, Parisi V, et al. Carotenoids in Age-related Maculopathy Italian Study (CARMIS): two-year results of a randomized study. Eur J Ophthalmol 2012; 22: 216–25.

131. Prashar S, Pandav SS, Gupta A, et al. Antioxidant enzymes in RBCs as a biological index of age related macular degeneration. Acta Ophthalmol (Copenh) 1993; 71: 214–18.

132. Cohen SM, Olin KL, Feuer WJ, et al. Low glutathione reductase and peroxidase activity in age-related macular degeneration. Br J Ophthalmol 1994; 78: 791–4.

133. De La Paz MA, Zhang J, Fridovich I. Red blood cell antioxidant enzymes in age-related macular degeneration. Br J Ophthalmol 1996; 80: 445–50.

134. Delcourt C, Cristol JP, Leger CL, et al. The POLA Study. Associations of antioxidant enzymes with cataract and age-related macular degeneration. Pathologies Oculaires Liees a l'Age. Ophthalmology 1999; 106: 215–22.

135. Baskol G, Karakucuk S, Oner AO, et al. Serum paraoxonase 1 activity and lipid peroxidation levels in patients with age-related macular degeneration. Ophthalmologica 2006; 220: 12–16.

136. Kimura K, Isashiki Y, Sonoda S, et al. Genetic association of manganese superoxide dismutase with exudative age-related macular degeneration. Am J Ophthalmol 2000; 130: 769–73.

137. Gotoh N, Yamada R, Matsuda F, et al. Manganese superoxide dismutase gene (SOD2) polymorphism and exudative age-related macular degeneration in the Japanese population. Am J Ophthalmol 2008; 146: 146.

138. Kondo N, Bessho H, Honda S, et al. SOD2 gene polymorphisms in neovascular age-related macular degeneration and polypoidal choroidal vasculopathy. Mol Vis 2009; 15: 1819–26.

139. Esfandiary H, Chakravarthy U, Patterson C, et al. Association study of detoxification genes in age related macular degeneration. Br J Ophthalmol 2005; 89: 470–4.

140. Kowalski M, Bielecka-Kowalska A, Oszajca K, et al. Manganese superoxide dismutase (MnSOD) gene (Ala-9Val, Ile58Thr) polymorphism in patients with age-related macular degeneration (AMD). Med Sci Monit. 2010: 16. CR190.6.

141. Baird PN, Chu D, Guida E, et al. Association of the M55L and Q192R paraoxonase gene polymorphisms with age-related macular degeneration. Am J Ophthalmol 2004; 138: 665–6.

142. Haas P, Aggermann T, Steindl K, et al. Genetic cardiovascular risk factors and age-related macular degeneration. Acta Ophthalmol 2011; 89: 335–8.

143. Ayala-Haedo JA, Gallins PJ, Whitehead PL, et al. Analysis of single nucleotide polymorphisms in the NOS2A gene and interaction with smoking in age-related macular degeneration. Ann Hum Genet 2010; 74: 195–201.

144. Jones MM, Manwaring N, Wang JJ, et al. Mitochondrial DNA haplogroups and age-related maculopathy. Arch Ophthalmol 2007; 125: 1235–40.

145. SanGiovanni JP, Arking DE, Iyengar SK, et al. Mitochondrial DNA variants of respiratory complex I that uniquely characterize haplogroup T2 are associated with increased risk of age-related macular degeneration. PLoS One 2009; 4: e5508.

146. Canter JA, Olson LM, Spencer K, et al. Mitochondrial DNA polymorphism A4917G is independently associated with age-related macular degeneration. PLoS One 2008; 3: e2091.

147. Udar N, Atilano SR, Memarzadeh M, et al. Mitochondrial DNA haplogroups associated with age-related macular degeneration. Invest Ophthalmol Vis Sci 2009; 50: 2966–74.

148. Kofler B, Mueller EE, Eder W, et al. Mitochondrial DNA haplogroup T is associated with coronary artery disease and diabetic retinopathy: a case control study. BMC Med Genet 2009; 10: 35.

149. Rivera A, Fisher SA, Fritsche LG, et al. Hypothetical LOC387715 is a second major susceptibility gene for age-related macular degeneration, contributing independently of complement factor H to disease risk. Hum Mol Genet 2005; 14: 3227–36.

150. Jakobsdottir J, Conley YP, Weeks DE, et al. Susceptibility genes for age-related maculopathy on chromosome 10q26. Am J Hum Genet 2005; 77: 389–407.

151. Kanda A, Chen W, Othman M, et al. A variant of mitochondrial protein LOC387715/ARMS2, not HTRA1, is strongly associated with age-related macular degeneration. Proc Natl Acad Sci USA 2007; 104: 16227–32.

152. Fritsche LG, Loenhardt T, Janssen A, et al. Age-related macular degeneration is associated with an unstable ARMS2 (LOC387715) mRNA. Nat Genet 2008; 40: 892–6.

153. Schmidt S, Hauser MA, Scott WK, et al. Cigarette smoking strongly modifies the association of LOC387715 and age-related macular degeneration. Am J Hum Genet 2006; 78: 852–64.

154. Schaumberg DA, Hankinson SE, Guo Q, et al. A prospective study of 2 major age-related macular degeneration susceptibility alleles and interactions with modifiable risk factors. Arch Ophthalmol 2007; 125: 55–62.

155. Wang G, Spencer KL, Court BL, et al. Localization of age-related macular degeneration-associated ARMS2 in cytosol, not mitochondria. Invest Ophthalmol Vis Sci 2009; 50: 3084–90.

156. Patel M, Chan CC. Immunopathological aspects of age-related macular degeneration. Semin Immunopathol 2008; 30: 97–110.

157. Mullins RF, Russell SR, Anderson DH, et al. Drusen associated with aging and age-related macular degeneration contain proteins common to extracellular deposits associated with atherosclerosis, elastosis, amyloidosis, and dense deposit disease. FASEB J 2000; 14: 835–46.

158. Wang L, Clark ME, Crossman DK, et al. Abundant lipid and protein components of drusen. PLoS One 2010; 5: e10329.

159. Reynolds R, Hartnett ME, Atkinson JP, et al. Plasma complement components and activation fragments: associations with age-related macular degeneration genotypes and phenotypes. Invest Ophthalmol Vis Sci 2009; 50: 5818–27.

160. Scholl HP, Charbel Issa P, Walier M, et al. Systemic complement activation in age-related macular degeneration. PLoS One 2008; 3: e2593.

161. Yang D, Elner SG, Lin LR, et al. Association of superoxide anions with retinal pigment epithelial cell apoptosis induced by mononuclear phagocytes. Invest Ophthalmol Vis Sci 2009; 50: 4998–5005.

162. Zhang B, Hu Y, Ma JX. Anti-inflammatory and antioxidant effects of SERPINA3K in the retina. Invest Ophthalmol Vis Sci 2009; 50: 3943–52.

163. Chen M, Forrester JV, Xu H. Synthesis of complement factor H by retinal pigment epithelial cells is down-regulated by oxidized photoreceptor outer segments. Exp Eye Res 2007; 84: 635–45.

164. Wu Z, Lauer TW, Sick A, et al. Oxidative stress modulates complement factor H expression in retinal pigmented

epithelial cells by acetylation of FOXO3. J Biol Chem 2007; 282: 22414–25.

165. Weismann D, Hartvigsen K, Lauer N, et al. Complement factor H binds malondialdehyde epitopes and protects from oxidative stress. Nature 2011; 478: 76–81.

166. Thurman JM, Renner B, Kunchithapautham K, et al. Oxidative stress renders retinal pigment epithelial cells susceptible to complement-mediated injury. J Biol Chem 2009; 284: 16939–47.

167. Kunchithapautham K, Rohrer B. Sublytic membrane-attack-complex (MAC) activation alters regulated rather than constitutive vascular endothelial growth factor (VEGF) secretion in retinal pigment epithelium mono-layers. J Biol Chem 2011; 286: 23717–24.

168. Hollyfield JG, Bonilha VL, Rayborn ME, et al. Oxidative damage-induced inflammation initiates age-related macular degeneration. Nat Med 2008; 14: 194–8.

169. SanGiovanni JP, Chew EY, Clemons TE, et al. The relationship of dietary carotenoid and vitamin A, E, and C intake with age-related macular degeneration in a case-control study: AREDS Report No. 22. Arch Ophthalmol 2007; 125: 1225–32.

170. Cangemi FE. TOZAL Study: an open case control study of an oral antioxidant and omega-3 supplement for dry AMD. BMC Ophthalmol 2007; 7: 3.

171. Ho L, van Leeuwen R, Witteman JC, et al. Reducing the genetic risk of age-related macular degeneration with dietary antioxidants, zinc, and {omega}-3 fatty acids: the Rotterdam study. Arch Ophthalmol 2011; 129: 758–66.

172. Moriarty-Craige SE, Adkison J, Lynn M, et al. Antioxidant supplements prevent oxidation of cysteine/cystine redox in patients with age-related macular degeneration. Am J Ophthalmol 2005; 140: 1020–6.

173. Moriarty-Craige SE, Ha KN, Sternberg P, Jr., et al. Effects of long-term zinc supplementation on plasma thiol metabolites and redox status in patients with age-related macular degeneration. Am J Ophthalmol 2007; 143: 206–11.

174. Wong WT, Kam W, Cunningham D, et al. Treatment of geographic atrophy by the topical administration of OT-551: results of a phase II clinical trial. Invest Ophthalmol Vis Sci 2010; 51: 6131–9.

175. Singh S, Aggarwal BB. Activation of transcription factor NF-kappa B is suppressed by curcumin (diferuloylmethane). J Biol Chem 1995; 270: 24995–5000.

176. Abe Y, Hashimoto S, Horie T. Curcumin inhibition of inflammatory cytokine production by human peripheral blood monocytes and alveolar macrophages. Pharmacol Res 1999; 39: 41–7.

177. Scapagnini G, Colombrita C, Amadio M, et al. Curcumin activates defensive genes and protects neurons against oxidative stress. Antioxid Redox Signal 2006; 8: 395–403.

178. Mandal MN, Patlolla JM, Zheng L, et al. Curcumin protects retinal cells from light-and oxidant stress-induced cell death. Free Radic Biol Med 2009; 46: 672–9.

179. King RE, Kent KD, Bomser JA. Resveratrol reduces oxidation and proliferation of human retinal pigment epithelial cells via extracellular signal-regulated kinase inhibition. Chem Biol Interact 2005; 151: 143–9.

180. Cao X, Tsukamoto T, Seki T, et al. 4-Vinyl-2,6-dimethoxyphenol (canolol) suppresses oxidative stress and gastric carcinogenesis in Helicobacter pylori-infected carcinogen-treated mongolian gerbils. Int J Cancer 2008; 122: 1445–54.

181. Dong X, Li Z, Wang W, et al. Protective effect of canolol from oxidative stress-induced cell damage in ARPE-19 cells via an ERK mediated antioxidative pathway. Mol Vis 2011; 17: 2040–8.

182. Nguyen T, Sherratt PJ, Pickett CB. Regulatory mechanisms controlling gene expression mediated by the antioxidant response element. Annu Rev Pharmacol Toxicol 2003; 43: 233–60.

183. Tanito M, Agbaga MP, Anderson RE. Upregulation of thioredoxin system via Nrf2-antioxidant responsive element pathway in adaptive-retinal neuroprotection in vivo and in vitro. Free Radic Biol Med 2007; 42: 1838–50.

184. Tanito M, Masutani H, Kim YC, et al. Sulforaphane induces thioredoxin through the antioxidant-responsive element and attenuates retinal light damage in mice. Invest Ophthalmol Vis Sci 2005; 46: 979–87.

185. Murota K, Mitsukuni Y, Ichikawa M, et al. Quercetin-4'-glucoside is more potent than quercetin-3-glucoside in protection of rat intestinal mucosa homogenates against iron ion-induced lipid peroxidation. J Agric Food Chem 2004; 52: 1907–12.

186. Kook D, Wolf AH, Yu AL, et al. The protective effect of quercetin against oxidative stress in the human RPE in vitro. Invest Ophthalmol Vis Sci 2008; 49: 1712–20.

187. Wankun X, Wenzhen Y, Min Z, et al. Protective effect of paeoniflorin against oxidative stress in human retinal pigment epithelium in vitro. Mol Vis 2011; 17: 3512–22.

188. Chen B, Caballero S, Seo S, et al. Delivery of antioxidant enzyme genes to protect against ischemia/reperfusion-induced injury to retinal microvasculature. Invest Ophthalmol Vis Sci 2009; 50: 5587–95.

189. Rex TS, Tsui I, Hahn P, et al. Adenovirus-mediated delivery of catalase to retinal pigment epithelial cells protects neighboring photoreceptors from photo-oxidative stress. Hum Gene Ther 2004; 15: 960–7.

190. Shan H, Ji D, Barnard AR, et al. AAV-mediated gene transfer of human X-linked inhibitor of apoptosis protects against oxidative cell death in human RPE Cells. Invest Ophthalmol Vis Sci 2011; 52: 9591–7.

191. Peng CH, Cherng JY, Chiou GY, et al. Delivery of Oct4 and SirT1 with cationic polyurethanes-short branch PEI to aged retinal pigment epithelium. Biomaterials 2011; 32: 9077–88.

7

Geographic atrophy

Sharon D. Solomon and Janet S. Sunness

INTRODUCTION

Geographic atrophy (GA) of the retinal pigment epithelium (RPE) is the advanced form of non-neovascular age-related macular degeneration (AMD) and is associated with gradual, progressive loss of central vision. Dense scotomas have been shown to correspond to the retinal areas affected by GA (1). These scotomas involve the parafoveal and perifoveal retina early in the course of the disease, often sparing the foveal center until late in the course of the disease (2–5). Consequently, GA is responsible for approximately 20% of the legal blindness secondary to AMD, whereas choroidal neovascularization (CNV), which tends to involve the foveal center much earlier in the course of the disease accounts for nearly 80% of the legal blindness secondary to AMD (6). However, the parafoveal and perifoveal scotomas in the early stages of GA compromise the patient's ability to read and to recognize faces, often despite the retention of good visual acuity, and account for a much larger percentage of moderate visual loss in those affected (7). In addition, GA is present binocularly in most patients. The prevalence of GA in the population 75 years of age or older is approximately 3.5%, half that of neovascular AMD (8,9), and increases to 22% in those 90 years of age or older (10). While there are treatments for choroidal neovascularization, there is presently no definitive treatment available for GA. As our understanding of GA grows, it is hoped that medical and surgical interventions will be developed to completely halt its progression rate and to prevent subsequent moderate and severe visual loss.

CLINICAL FEATURES OF GEOGRAPHIC ATROPHY

GA is easily recognized clinically, as it appears as a well-demarcated area of decreased retinal thickness, compared with the surrounding retina, with a relative change in color that allows for increased visualization of the underlying choroidal vessels. Both the location and pattern of the atrophy may vary in appearance. Drusen, usually a mixture of the soft and calcific types, are present in most eyes until the GA becomes so extensive as to resorb the macular drusen (2). There may be pigmentary alteration, either hypopigmentation or hyperpigmentation preceding and later surrounding the macular atrophy. Forty percent of eyes with macular GA also have peripapillary GA, which may become confluent with the macular atrophy (7). Peripheral reticular degeneration of the pigment epithelium is present in about 41% of eyes (7). The increased choroidal vessel detail in the area of GA is usually the most easily identified fundus change and further reflects the extent of RPE attenuation. On fluorescein angiography, this translates into an area of hyperfluorescence that corresponds to the ophthalmoscopic borders of the GA, secondary to transmission defect and staining. The intensity of hyperfluorescence from the choroidal flush may vary depending on the presence or absence of the underlying choriocapillaris (4). Fluorescein angiography may also aid in distinguishing GA from occult choroidal neovascularization, which may otherwise appear clinically indistinguishable. A recent paper suggests that an area that satisfies one color photographic criterion of GA and also shows hyperfluorescence on FA may be considered GA, allowing for earlier definition of this condition (11).

Fundus autofluorescence imaging is important for the evaluation of GA. Fundus autofluorescence reflects lipofuscin in RPE cells so that where RPE cells are absent there is a loss of autofluorescence. This feature is used to strong advantage in defining and measuring areas of GA in the context of natural history studies and clinical trials because it provides a much more sharp delineation of GA from the surrounding drusen and pigmentary change and lends itself to semiautomated assessment. Many eyes with GA have areas of increased autofluorescence surrounding them, presumably reflecting lipofuscin-laden RPE. Holz's group has shown that eyes with more diffuse increased autofluorescence are likely to progress more rapidly than eyes with little or only focally increased autofluorescence. In addition, the GA tends to grow into the areas of increased autofluorescence. The areas of increased autofluorescence may be associated with a loss of retinal sensitivity, and are considered susceptible areas for the development of GA (12–18). Standard fundus autofluorescence, which uses short wavelengths (blue) cannot provide good definition of the foveal region in many eyes, because the xanthophyll blocks short wavelength light. So, even if the fovea is not atrophic, it may appear dark in the autofluorescence image. In addition, some drusen and pigmentary changes may be associated with a loss of autofluorescence without GA being present, so that clinical correlation with a color fundus image or with infrared reflectance imaging can be helpful (19).

Spectral domain OCT (SD OCT) is very helpful in imaging GA. Investigators are studying how one can best define the edges of GA using SD OCT and en-face images (21). In addition, the changes that occur in the region near the atrophy can be studied.

Hemorrhage may occur in eyes with GA. Though this may be a reflection of the development of CNV and herald a more precipitous decline in visual function secondary to neovascular maculopathy, often the small areas of CNV that develop are transient and may become clinically unapparent a few months later (22). Hemorrhages have also been described in GA in the complete absence of any CNV (22,23). In general, however, the presence of hemorrhage, especially when associated with a sudden change in vision, warrants an angiographic evaluation for the presence of CNV (24).

Although there are frequently small areas of retinal sparing within the GA, especially at the center of the macula, foveal localization may still prove challenging on clinical examination, on the color fundus photograph, and on the angiogram. Clinically, the location of xanthophyll, if visible, is helpful in determining the location of the foveal center. On fluorescein angiography, the intense hyperfluorescence associated with the GA may obscure the view of the entire foveal avascular zone, making foveal localization a less certain task. Under such circumstances, the red-free photographs can often be of significant help. The presence of xanthophyll may suggest that the fovea has visual function, even if the retina appears atrophic and non-functional (25). Testing with devices such as the scanning laser ophthalmoscope (SLO) may help ascertain the remaining central visual potential (1,5,26,27).

HISTOPATHOLOGY AND PATHOGENESIS

Histopathologic examination of eyes with GA demonstrates a loss of RPE cells in the area of atrophy with a secondary loss of overlying photoreceptor cells (28). The choriocapillaris may also be absent, and there is indeed some experimental evidence to suggest that when the RPE is removed or has atrophied, the choriocapillaris involutes secondarily (29–31). GA is associated with thickening of Bruch's membrane secondary to the deposition of basal laminar and basal linear deposits in the surrounding retina (32). Therefore, histologically, GA has been thought of as the end stage of the AMD process if CNV does not develop (33). GA may also occur following the flattening of a retinal pigment epithelial detachment (34,35).

There is controversy as to whether the loss of RPE cells, perhaps related to the deposits in and near Bruch's membrane, is the primary event in the evolution of GA, or whether this RPE atrophy develops secondary to choroidal vascular insufficiency. Green and others have argued that the presence of choroidal vascular insufficiency should result in the subsequent degeneration of all the outer retinal layers (28). This is not seen in eyes with GA. Friedman suggests that choroidal vascular resistance may predispose to the development of AMD, specifically to the development of high-risk drusen and CNV (36). However, a causal association between choroidal vascular resistance and GA has not been established to date. Grunwald has found that foveal choroidal blood flow is reduced in eyes with early atrophic AMD and good visual acuity (37), and this work is continuing

to better characterize the relationship between choroidal blood flow and the development of advanced AMD.

PREVALENCE AND EPIDEMIOLOGY OF GEOGRAPHIC ATROPHY

Population-based studies, such as the Beaver Dam Eye Study and the Rotterdam Study, have examined the prevalence of GA in the elderly and compared it with the prevalence of CNV in the same groups. The prevalence of GA is approximately 3.5% for people age 75 and above in the United States and other developed nations, half that of CNV (8,9). The prevalence of GA increases with age and is actually more common than CNV in older age groups. In the population over age 90, the prevalence of GA can reach levels of 20–35% (10,38). The studies indicate that there is a lower prevalence of GA in African-Americans (39). There does not appear to be a consistent gender difference in prevalence across the populations studied.

In the Beaver Dam Eye Study, 8% of eyes with drusen larger than 250 µm went on to develop GA over a five-year period. Eyes that developed GA all had pigmentary abnormalities and at least 0.2 MPS (Macular Photocoagulation Study) disc areas of drusen at baseline (40). Of the eyes with GA, 42% had a visual acuity of 20/200 or worse. This was similar to the 48% of eyes with neovascular AMD that had a comparable level of severe visual loss (40).

GA is bilateral in 48% to 65% of cases (7,41). The statistics available from the era before anti-VEGF treatments showed that GA is still responsible for a full 20% of the binocular legal blindness secondary to AMD (6). These statistics for severe visual loss measure only the incidence of legal blindness and significantly underestimate the disability associated with GA. A patient with GA and only moderately impaired visual acuity may not be able to read or to recognize faces because the object being visualized does not "fit" into the spared central island of vision (5).

Systemic Risk Factors

A number of population-based studies have attempted to identify possible risk factors for the development of GA and neovascular AMD. The Beaver Dam Eye Study did not demonstrate a relationship between GA and cholesterol level or alcohol intake (8,42). While current or past smoking was a significant risk factor for the presence of GA for women in the Blue Mountains Eye Study, the same association did not reach statistical significance for men (43). In Sunness' study, there was a trend for current smokers to have a more rapid progression of GA than nonsmokers (7). The same study suggested that patients who are pseudophakic or aphakic do not have more rapid progression of GA than their phakic counterparts (7).

The Age-Related Eye Disease Study (AREDS), a multicenter study of the natural history of AMD and cataract, reported its findings on possible risk factors for the development of GA and neovascular AMD. The presence of GA was found to be associated with increasing age and smoking, confirming the findings of previous population-based studies (44). In addition, there appeared to be a positive association between the use of antacids, thyroid hormones, and anti-inflammatory medications and the presence of GA (44,45). These associations have not been previously reported and will certainly prompt further investigation. Level of education was found to be inversely proportional to the presence of GA in that persons with more years of formal schooling seemed to be at lower risk for GA (44,45).

Genetics

The finding, by four groups in 2005, of a correlation between complement factor H polymorphisms and AMD has dramatically transformed thinking about the pathogenetic basis of, and the potential treatment for, GA (46–49). Additional genetic polymorphisms, have been found, including ARMS2/HTRA1, C3, C2, and CFB. Currently, these genetic factors have been felt to account for more than 50% of the risk for developing AMD (50). Additional genetic factors, such as Toll-like receptor 3 (51), have been found to be a risk factor for GA by some groups, but this has not been confirmed by others. Data from another study also suggest that the ApoE epsilon 4 allele may be associated with a reduced risk for the development of AMD (52). There are several new papers published each month regarding genetic factors in AMD.

What is striking, however, is that to date there is no evidence that the genetic polymorphisms present have any effect on the rate of progression of GA (53). This suggests that the role of complement and inflammation may occur earlier in the course of AMD. Drusen contain most of the complement factors (54), additional evidence that inflammation may play a role in AMD prior to the development of GA. It may well be that there is a later role as well, and a number of pharmaceutical companies are testing various anticomplement and anti-inflammatory agents as potential treatments for GA (55).

Interest has also focused on genes responsible for hereditary retinal and macular dystrophies that share some features with GA, including the RDS/peripherin gene associated with Zermatt macular dystrophy (56), the ABCA4 gene associated with Stargardt disease (57–59), but these have not consistently been found to be more common in eyes with GA than in the general population. Twin studies have been used to try to differentiate hereditary from environmental factors in the development of GA.

NATURAL HISTORY OF GEOGRAPHIC ATROPHY

GA typically develops in eyes that, at baseline, have drusen or pigmentary alteration. As drusen fade, focal areas of atrophy may develop in their place, enlarge, and evolve into GA (2,60,61). Alternatively, areas of mottled hypopigmentation may also predispose to the development of GA (2,35). The progression goes through a number of stages. Initially, single or multifocal areas of GA may be found in the region around the fovea. As these areas enlarge and coalesce over time, they can form a horseshoe of atrophy that spares the foveal center (Fig. 7.1). This horseshoe of atrophy may close off into a ring of atrophy that still permits foveal preservation. In the late stages of GA, the fovea itself becomes atrophic and nonseeing, from further coalescence of the GA, requiring the patient to use eccentric retinal loci for fixation and seeing (2).

GA may also occur secondary to RPE detachments, which develop GA in about 20% of cases, when the detachments flatten (34,62–64). This may lead to foveal GA if the RPE detachment was foveal. There also are other patients in whom foveal GA may develop early without evidence of parafoveal or perifoveal GA, and the antecedents of this type of progression is not clear.

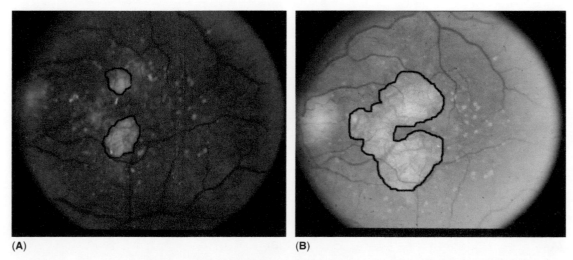

(A) **(B)**

Figure 7.1 Four year progression in geographic atrophy (GA). The GA area is outlined in black. (**A**) There are multifocal areas of GA, along with drusen and pigmentary alteration. (**B**) Four years later, the areas of GA have enlarged and coalesced, forming a horseshoe of atrophy surrounding the fovea.

Because visual loss tends to be gradual and subtle, and takes place over a period of years, patients may not seek medical attention until there is significant encroachment on the fovea, or frank foveal atrophy is present.

While cross-sectionally, the average visual acuity is worse in eyes with larger total atrophic areas, there is a group of patients who have significant foveal resilience in that foveal sparing persists despite marked surrounding GA. In those eyes with foveal-sparing patterns (multifocal GA, horseshoe GA, or ring GA) at baseline, about 75% still had a foveal-sparing pattern at four years of follow-up (65). For eyes with baseline VA 20/50 or better, the rate of enlargement of atrophy was not a risk factor for an increasing rate of visual acuity loss The annual rate of enlargement of GA has been found to be between 1 and 2.5 mm^2 in various studies (16,66,67). Surprisingly, the rate seems to be fairly constant over time, leading to a linear increase in GA area with time (66,67). Neither the phakic status of the study eye nor a history of hypertension in the patient was shown to be a risk factor for the enlargement of total atrophy (7). There was a trend for smokers to have a more rapid enlargement of atrophy (7).

GA is associated with a significant decline in visual acuity over time in many eyes. There was a significantly more rapid rate of moderate and severe vision loss for eyes with a baseline visual acuity of better than 20/50. At two years of follow-up, 40% of these eyes lost three or more lines of visual acuity and 21% lost six or more lines of visual acuity (7). Those numbers grew to 70% at four years of follow-up for three-line loss and 45% at four years for six-line loss (7). Twenty-seven percent of the eyes with visual acuity of 20/50 or better at baseline had visual acuity of 20/200 or worse at four years of follow-up (7). Eyes with baseline visual acuity of 20/60 or worse had a much lower two-year rate of three-line visual loss of about 15%. The presence of CNV in the fellow eye did not appear to affect the rate of visual acuity loss in the GA study eye (7). In Sunness' study, in order to quantify the worsening of visual function in dim illumination, a two log unit neutral density filter was placed over the manifest refraction, and the visual acuity was remeasured with the Early Treatment Diabetic Retinopathy Study (ETDRS) chart. For eyes with visual acuity 20/50 or better at baseline, there was a dramatic worsening of acuity under low luminance, with a median 4.7 lines of worsening. The degree of worsening in dim illumination at baseline was predictive of the subsequent two-year visual acuity loss (68).

The size and rate of progression of atrophy are highly correlated between the two eyes of patients with bilateral GA. This includes the baseline area of total atrophy, the baseline area of central atrophy, the presence of peripapillary atrophy, and the progression of total atrophy (7,69). However, the correlation between eyes for baseline acuity, for acuity at two years, and for two-year change in acuity is significantly smaller, reflecting the importance of the difference in foveal sparing between eyes (Fig. 7.2) (7).

The two parameters used to describe the progression of GA in the Sunness study, namely the enlargement of the atrophic area and visual acuity loss, do not completely gauge the actual impact of GA on visual function and performance. Maximum reading rate can be significantly affected by encroachment of GA on the fovea, even while there may still be little change in visual acuity (5). Some patients may be able to read single letters on acuity charts but are unable to read words because of the size of the preserved foveal island (5). The median maximum reading rate decreased from 110 words per minute (wpm) to 51 wpm over a two-year period in patients with visual acuity better than 20/50, where the normal median rate for the reading test used in elderly people without advanced AMD is 130 wpm. Eighty-three percent of eyes that lost three or more lines of visual acuity had maximum reading rates less than 50 wpm at two-year follow-up. However, even in the group that maintained good acuity at two years,

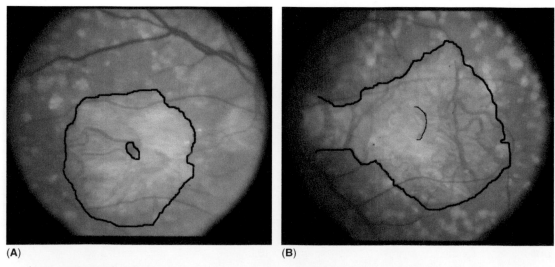

(A)   **(B)**

Figure 7.2 Bilateral geographic atrophy. The geographic atrophy is outlined in black. **(A)** This eye had 20/30 visual acuity; the patient was able to read 80 words per minute, using the small spared central area (inner circle). **(B)** The fellow eye had only a narrow sliver of sparing, whose temporal edge is delineated by the black curve within the atrophy, and had 20/400 visual acuity.

one-third had maximum reading rates below 50 wpm (5). For eyes with visual acuity between 20/80 and 20/200, when the fovea is already involved at baseline, there is evidence to suggest that the maximum reading rate is inversely related to the size of the total atrophic area (70). This may mean that an intervention that could slow the rate of enlargement of atrophy could have a significant impact on preserving visual function, even in the presence of a central scotoma.

DEVELOPMENT OF NEW GEOGRAPHIC ATROPHY

The relatively high prevalence of bilaterality of GA, reported to be anywhere from 48% to 65% (41) in the literature, would suggest that patients with GA in one eye and only drusen or pigmentary changes in the fellow eye are at significant risk for developing GA in the fellow eye. In the Beaver Dam Eye Study, 12 patients had GA in one eye at baseline. After five years of follow-up, three of these patients (25%) had developed GA in the fellow eye (40). Patients with GA in only one eye were found to be 2.8 times more likely to develop advanced AMD in the fellow eye than were patients with only early changes from age-related maculopathy in either eye at baseline. In Sunness' progression study of GA, two of nine patients (22%) with GA in one eye and only drusen or pigmentary changes in the fellow eye developed new GA in the fellow eye during the two-year follow-up period (7).

There is limited information available on the rate of development of GA in the eyes of patients who have only drusen and pigmentary alteration bilaterally at baseline. In the Beaver Dam study population, there was a five-year incidence of new GA of 0.3% (40). Eyes with only drusen less than 125 µm in linear dimension at baseline were not observed to go on to develop GA. Of the eyes with drusen between 125 µm and 250 µm at baseline, 1% were described as developing GA. In comparison, 8% of eyes with drusen 250 µm or larger in linear dimension developed GA over a five-year period. Similarly, only those eyes with greater than 0.2 MPS disc areas of drusen had a tendency toward developing GA. All eyes that developed GA had pigmentary abnormalities at baseline as well (40). In addition to drusen size, there may be some correlation between the type of drusen present in eyes with early age-related maculopathy and the eventual development of GA. Calcific drusen (71), clusters of small, hard drusen, and reticular drusen (72) have all been observed to be present in eyes with GA (35). Finally, other potential risk factors that have been identified in the development of GA include delayed choroidal filling on fluorescein angiography (73,74) and diminished foveal dark-adapted sensitivity (75).

DEVELOPMENT OF CNV IN EYES WITH GEOGRAPHIC ATROPHY

Population-based studies have confirmed that the incidence of CNV in an eye with GA depends, in part, upon the status of the fellow eye. In patients with GA and no CNV in one eye, with GA and CNV in the fellow eye, the eye affected with only GA follows a course that is essentially identical to that of patients with bilateral GA with respect to foveal preservation, rates of acuity loss, and rates of enlargement of atrophy, so long as it does not develop CNV (7). However, when the incidence of developing CNV in these eyes with baseline GA is assessed, it is found to be significantly higher if the fellow eye has CNV at baseline as opposed to GA. Of the patients enrolled in the extrafoveal MPS study with CNV in the study eye, 11 were found to have only GA in the non-study eye at baseline. During the next five years of follow-up, 45% of these eyes went on to develop CNV (76). Findings from the MPS group's juxtafoveal and subfoveal CNV trials support this incidence. Forty-nine percent of patients with CNV in the study eye and only GA in the fellow eye at baseline went on to develop CNV over the five-year follow-up period (77). A prospective study by Sunness et al. in which 31 patients had GA and no CNV in the study eye and CNV in the fellow eye reported a two-year rate of 18% and a four-year rate of 34% for developing CNV in the GA study eye (22). This is in contrast to the results reported by Sunness et al. for patients with bilateral GA at baseline, who had a two-year rate of developing CNV in one eye of 2% and a four-year rate of 11%. Also, none of the patients with GA in one eye and drusen in the fellow eye developed CNV over the two-year period (22). All these data demonstrate that there is a higher incidence of CNV in eyes with GA at baseline that have fellow eyes with CNV.

When CNV does develop in an eye with GA, it seems to have a propensity for areas of preserved retina surrounding the GA or in spared foveal regions. In a study by Schatz and McDonald, 8 of 10 patients who developed CNV in eyes that had only GA previously at baseline, developed CNV at the edge of the atrophy. In the two cases where the CNV developed over the atrophy, fluorescein angiography was able to demonstrate evidence of intact choriocapillaris in those areas (4). Sunness et al. observed the development of CNV over areas of GA only when there were areas of sparing within the atrophy. Otherwise, patients developed CNV in areas that were adjacent to atrophy (22). Some histologic work likewise suggests that CNV does not develop where the choriocapillaris is absent (28).

CNV that is newly developing in eyes with baseline GA may be difficult to detect by clinical examination, OCT, and fluorescein angiography. In the absence of subretinal hemorrhage, it may be difficult to detect subretinal fluid that is shallow and overlying an area of atrophy. On fluorescein angiography, the hyperfluorescence already present from transmission defects and staining due to the GA may obscure any new hyperfluorescence that is secondary to CNV. Because GA does not generally cause an abrupt loss in vision, a patient who presents with subjective and objective evidence of significant changes in baseline visual function should undergo evaluation for the presence of CNV (24). Although GA itself has been associated with subretinal hemorrhages without evidence of CNV (22,23), the presence of hemorrhage should certainly prompt further evaluation to detect newly developing CNV. In some patients, the CNV may spontaneously involute and have an appearance identical to that of GA or may leave small areas of fibrosis as remnants of earlier CNV (22).

IMPAIRMENT OF VISUAL FUNCTION IN EYES WITH GA

Visual acuity alone is an inadequate marker of visual function in patients with GA. In addition to central and paracentral scotoma, eyes with GA have other visual function abnormalities that may be secondary to changes in the function of retina that is not yet atrophic (5). Eyes with GA have marked loss of function in dim environments and benefit greatly from increased lighting (5). Apart from delayed and decreased dark adaptation for both rods and cones (5,78–80), eyes with atrophic AMD may also be compromised by reduced contrast sensitivity (5,81,82). Therefore, despite good visual acuity, the patient's ability to read may be significantly impaired by a combination of factors.

Central and Paracentral Scotomas

Many patients with GA have difficulty reading because of an inability to see a full-enough central field. Even in the presence of good visual acuity, scotomas near the fovea and involving the foveal center compromise visual performance. Patients may complain that they can read small newsprint but not larger news headlines. On clinical examination, it may be apparent that the foveal center remains intact but with only a tiny preserved foveal island, which cannot accommodate the larger headline letters. For this reason, it is important to take into account that such patients may be able to read smaller letters on an eye chart even if they are unable to read the 20/400 letter (5).

The impact that GA has on a patient's lifestyle is not limited solely to the ability to read. Patients with GA may also describe having great difficulty in recognizing faces stemming from their inability to assimilate all the features simultaneously (83). Some find themselves assuming a more reclusive lifestyle after having repeatedly encountered friends and family that they fail to recognize and to greet. Moreover, the same small central islands of preserved retina that impair visual function in the first place also complicate low-vision treatment in these patients. By magnifying the object of interest, these low-vision devices can result in even fewer characters or features being seen by the patient within the spared area.

Conventional visual field measurement is unreliable when an eye lacks steady, central fixation, and can result in plotting scotomas in the wrong location and of the wrong size (1). The SLO provides direct and real-time viewing of stimuli on the retina and permits the precise correlation of visual function with retinal location. SLO macular perimetry has demonstrated that areas of GA are indeed associated with dense scotomas with surrounding retinal sensitivity that may be near normal (1). The fixation behaviors adopted by patients and observed during SLO evaluation may explain the inherent variation in visual acuity in eyes with central scotomas from GA. Approaches combining three-dimensional optical coherence tomography (OCT) images and superimposed SLO microperimetry have also demonstrated correlations between thinning of the neurosensory retina, as seen in GA, and decreases in psychophysical threshold sensitivities (84).

In order for a patient with scotomas that involve the foveal center to realize his visual potential, he has to place the object of regard on functioning retina by adopting an extrafoveal location for fixation, referred to as a preferred retinal locus (PRL). Sunness et al. found that in a study of eyes with central GA and visual acuities ranging from 20/80 to 20/200, all patients who were able to adopt an extrafoveal location for fixation placed their PRL immediately adjacent to the area of atrophy. Most patients fixated with the scotomas to their right or above fixation in visual field space (70). In another study of GA patients by Sunness et al., patients reported improvement in the acuity of their worse-seeing eye when their better-seeing eye worsened somewhat. At baseline, it was noted that these patients had not developed eccentric PRLs in the worse-seeing eye so that they placed the object of regard into their scotoma where it could not be seen. Over three years of follow-up, these patients, with visual acuities ranging from 20/80 to 20/500, did demonstrate a spontaneous mean improvement of 3.2 lines in visual acuity in the worse-seeing eye. This improvement in the worse-seeing eye was concomitant with the deterioration of vision in the previously better-seeing eye. At follow-up with SLO macular perimetry, the patients were observed to have adopted eccentric PRLs, which appeared to account for the improvement in the vision of the previously worse-seeing eye (85).

Awareness of the presence and location of scotomas can aid in the effective utilization of the remaining functional retina, lessening the searching eye movements some patients make when they have no strategy for moving the object of regard away from the scotomas. For example, having the patient fixate superior to the area of atrophy on the retina, that is, placing the scotoma above fixation, is a good strategy because it moves the blind spot out of the most important part of the visual field. Similarly, fixating with the scotoma to the right, that is to the left of the atrophy in a fundus photograph, allows the patient to anchor himself at the beginning of a line while reading (70,86).

With the aid of a macular imaging, a physician can help facilitate the patient's development of a PRL. A fundus photograph has the same left-to-right orientation as visual field space since it has already been reversed by being viewed from the photographer's perspective. Therefore, an area of atrophy to the left of the fovea, or of fixation, corresponds with a scotoma to the left of fixation. The fundus photograph is inverted in superior-inferior orientation relative to visual field space, such that a patient fixating above an area of atrophy in a fundus photograph has the scotoma above fixation in visual field space. If the fundus photograph indicates the likely location of fixation relative to the scotoma, the physician can then instruct the patient to look toward the scotoma in visual field space. This will have the effect of moving the scotoma farther out of the way. For example, if there is a scotoma to the right of fixation, as when a patient neglects the last letters on each line of an eye chart, having the patient look farther to the right should allow the object of regard to come into view.

Difficulties in Dimly Lit Environments

Regardless of their level of visual acuity, most patients with GA have difficulties with reading and with performing other visually related tasks in dimly lit environments. A review of Sunness' questionnaire response found that at least two-thirds of their patients with GA who still had good-enough visual acuity to drive during the day had stopped driving at night (83).

Visual function testing objectively confirms the presence of reduced function in dim illumination in eyes with GA, as demonstrated by Sunness et al. in a study of eyes with GA and visual acuity better than 20/50. When a control group of elderly patients with ocular findings limited to only drusen or pigmentary alteration, without advanced AMD, had a 2-log unit neutral density filter placed over the study eye, the median worsening in acuity was 2.2 lines on the ETDRS acuity chart. No eye worsened more than 5 lines (5). For the study group, there was a median worsening in the acuity of 4.7 lines on the ETDRS acuity chart when a 2-log unit neutral density filter was placed over the study eye (5). The degree of worsening in dim illumination was predictive of the subsequent visual acuity loss (68). When foveal dark-adapted sensitivity was measured by gauging the patient's ability to see a small red target light in the dark after dark adaptation, eyes with GA and good visual acuity had a median sensitivity that was 1.2 log units lower than the sensitivity of the control group of elderly eyes with only early changes from AMD (5).

There is less worsening of visual acuity in dim illumination for eyes that have lost foveal fixation, suggesting that dark-adapted changes may be a sensitive marker for foveal changes even before clinically apparent atrophy of the fovea develops from encroachment of surrounding GA (5). These changes in dark-adapted function may also help predict which patients with high-risk drusen and pigmentary alteration are more likely to eventually develop GA. In a small prospective study of eyes with drusen, Sunness et al. found that the eyes with the most reduced foveal dark-adapted sensitivity were those most likely to develop advanced AMD, including GA (75). Steinmetz et al. observed similar outcomes. Eyes with drusen that had associated delayed choroidal filling and dark-adaptation abnormalities were more likely to develop GA with time (73,74).

In order to maximize the remaining retinal function in these patients, low-vision management of these patients should include an evaluation of lighting needs and appropriate recommendation for the necessary degree of lighting for reading and other tasks. For example, a GA patient may gain an increased sense of independence with the use of a small, handheld penlight to use in a dimly lit restaurant to read a menu. Sloan demonstrated, in a study of visual acuity as a function of chart luminance, that normal eyes reach a plateau and then do not improve further in visual acuity beyond a certain threshold luminance. Though GA was not specifically assessed, she found that eyes with AMD in general continued to improve in acuity with increased luminance for the values tested (87). Eyes with GA and some preservation of central vision likely follow a similar pattern.

Other Visual Function Abnormalities

Several other abnormalities in visual function may occur in eyes affected with GA. Contrast sensitivity has been found to be reduced in eyes with GA and visual acuity better than 20/50 compared with eyes of elderly patients with only drusen and pigmentary alteration. Specifically, contrast sensitivity is reduced at low spatial frequencies, and is even more markedly reduced at higher spatial frequencies (5). Despite the presence of good acuity from preserved foveal islands in eyes affected with GA, the reading rate may be dramatically decreased secondary to paracentral scotomas. In Sunness et al.'s study of visual function in eyes with GA and visual acuity better than 20/50, 50% of eyes had maximum reading rates less than 100 wpm while 17% had maximum reading rates less than 50 wpm. In a comparison group of eyes with only the earliest manifestations of AMD, the median maximum reading rate was found to be 130 wpm, with no eye having a maximum reading rate less than 100 wpm (5). For this reason, visual acuity alone is an inadequate measure of a patient's ability to read.

Patients with small, functional foveal islands may have to find an acceptable compromise between using their central fixation and their eccentric PRL to optimize their visual capacity. While the small foveal region has good acuity, it by definition has a limited visual field extent. Moreover, before the foveal center becomes frankly atrophic, it may still be affected by reduced retinal sensitivity, reduced contrast sensitivity, and a substantial worsening of function in dim illumination. An eccentric, preferred, retinal locus for fixation positioned outside the area of GA will inherently have a lower visual acuity but may be able to offer a larger area of functional retina less affected by dim illumination and reduced contrast sensitivity. Patients may therefore find themselves, often unconsciously, switching back and forth from foveal to eccentric fixation depending upon the visual tasks at hand, illumination conditions, and other factors (5,24,88,89).

The combination of variables that can ultimately affect a GA patient's ability to perform visually related tasks can make it difficult to prescribe low-vision magnification devices that can make the object of regard too large to be accommodated by the intact central region. Evaluation of low-vision requirements should always keep these variables in mind. Good illumination is essential in almost all visually related tasks.

CONDITIONS RESEMBLING GEOGRAPHIC ATROPHY

There are other conditions of the eye that in one stage or other of their progression can resemble GA. Some of these are other manifestations of AMD and simply exist on a different part of the continuum from GA. Other conditions would be classified as retinal or macular degenerations that are not age-related.

CNV that has spontaneously involuted can leave an atrophic scar that resembles GA (91,92). Some scars may have small fibrotic areas that are remnants of previous CNV. Other scars appear identical to GA. In such cases, fluorescein angiography may aid in distinguishing CNV from GA.

Old laser photocoagulation scars may also resemble GA. The history, however, should distinguish the two. Again, fluorescein angiography should demonstrate areas of hypofluorescence that correspond to the laser scars. Areas of GA generally show hyperfluorescence on angiography.

An RPE tear may clinically resemble GA. On fluorescein angiography, however, the straight-line border of hyperfluorescence should be characteristic of a rip. An OCT analysis may also show a disruption in the RPE layer, indicative of an RPE tear. It is unclear whether RPE tears develop atrophy in adjacent areas with time (93).

Eyes with pattern dystrophy and vitelliform changes may develop atrophic changes that progress in a fashion similar to AMD-related GA. These patients may have areas of macular GA, and some may be accompanied by pigmentary alterations characteristic of these conditions and occasionally by reduced electro-oculograms. However, other cases may be difficult to distinguish from age-related GA. The atrophy spreads in a parafoveal pattern with early foveal sparing, often resulting in a similar degree of visual compromise (94).

Central areolar choroidal dystrophy is another degenerative retinal condition that spares the fovea early in the course of disease. This hereditary condition is generally autosomal dominant and causes areas of atrophy in the macular region to develop since early adulthood. Unlike age-related GA, these lesions tend to have early atrophy of the choroidal circulation and choriocapillaris so that involved areas on fluorescein angiography appear as hypofluorescent (95).

Disorders that cause central, atrophic lesions and bull's-eye maculopathies may also mimic age-related GA. Stargardt's disease, cone dystrophy, North Carolina macular dystrophy, benign concentric annular macular dystrophy, and chloroquine and other toxic maculopathies, may all have manifestations similar to GA from AMD. The history, including age of onset of symptoms and prior medication use, may be helpful in differentiating some of these disorders from GA. Associated clinical findings, such as sensitivity to light and significant electroretinographic or color vision abnormalities in cone dystrophy or pisiform flecks and an angiographically dark choroid in Stargardt's disease may also facilitate differentiating the GA that results from these other entities from age-related GA.

POTENTIAL TREATMENTS FOR GEOGRAPHIC ATROPHY

Because GA can be clinically visualized in many patients before the development of moderate or severe vision loss, unlike CNV, there is greater potential for medical intervention to preserve visual function. While there is currently no definitive treatment to reverse the progression of GA, there is currently therapy for retarding disease progression.

The first AREDS trial did not show an effect of the trial medication on the development of GA, and the medication showed no effect on the rate of enlargement of atrophy in GA (96). The AREDS medication may still be recommended to reduce the risk of developing CNV. The second AREDS trial is still ongoing and findings are not available (55).

There are about 10 clinical trials, mainly in the early stages, ongoing for GA. These take a variety of approaches, including antioxidant, anticomplement, and anti-inflammatory agents, visual cycle modulators, neuroprotective agents, and anti-amyloid agents. In one completed phase II study, ciliary neurotrophic factor (CNTF; Neurotech) was delivered via an intraocular encapsulated cell technology implant in patients with GA, who were randomly assigned to receive a high- or low-dose implant or sham surgery (97). CNTF has been found to be protective of cone photoreceptors in animal models of retinal degeneration. CNTF treatment appeared to correlate with a dose-dependent increase in macular thickness (97). Visual acuity stabilization (loss of less than 15 letters) was also more commonly observed in the high-dose group (96.3%) than in the low-dose (83.3%) or sham (75%) groups (97). It was not reported to show an effect on the rate of GA enlargement. Given the fact that for many patients the fovea remains non-atrophic for a number of years, a treatment that improves foveal photoreceptor function may be beneficial in preserving visual function. The phase II trial of oral fenretinide, which competes with vitamin A for retinol binding protein and decreases the amount of vitamin A reaching the retina, found suggestive evidence of an effect on progression (Two-Year Analysis of the Efficacy and Safety of Fenretinide vs. Placebo in the Treatment of Geographic Atrophy. *Presented at the American Academy of Ophthalmology Meeting, 2010, Chicago, IL. Program Number: PA024*), but results have not yet been published.

The first clinical trial of human embryonic stem cell-derived RPE (ACT) for GA is underway. The earliest report of the first patients treated and monitored for four months showed no immediate adverse events (99). Once safety and efficacy of cell incorporation is demonstrated, future trials will provide similar therapy to patients earlier in the course of disease, potentially increasing the chance of photoreceptor rescue.

Currently, patients with GA and visual compromise can be offered rehabilitation in terms of low-vision intervention and new strategies for maximizing their utilization of remaining, healthy retina through the development of PRLs. More cases of GA will continue to be seen in ensuing years as its prevalence grows in an aging population. It is hoped that as more is learned about GA in the future, we can offer more to the patient with respect to the management and eventually prevention of this form of AMD.

SUMMARY POINTS

- The prevalence of geographic atrophy (GA) increases with age, being half as common as CNV at age 75, and more common than chloroidal neovascularization (CNV) in older age groups.
- GA continues to enlarge over time with a median rate of enlargement over a two-year period of 1.8 MPS disc areas.
- Scotomas from GA, the advanced form of nonneovascular AMD, involve the parafoveal and perifoveal retina early in the course of the disease, sparing the foveal center until late in the course of the disease.
- These parafoveal and perifoveal scotomas compromise the ability to read and to recognize faces, often despite the retention of good visual acuity, accounting for a large percentage of moderate visual loss in those affected.
- Hemorrhage may occur in eyes with GA in the absence of CNV. Small areas of CNV that can be associated with hemorrhage may be transient, becoming clinically inapparent, or appearing as increased atrophy, a few months later.
- There is a higher incidence of CNV in eyes with GA at baseline that have fellow eyes with CNV.
- GA is bilateral in more than half of the people with this condition. The size and rate of progression of atrophy are highly correlated between the two eyes of patients with bilateral GA, but the acuities may differ due to central sparing.
- Among eyes with GA with visual acuity better than 20/50, there is a 40% rate of three-line visual loss at two years.
- Maximum reading rate can be significantly affected by encroachment of GA on the fovea, even while there may still be little change in visual acuity.
- Eyes with GA have marked loss of vision in dim environments and benefit greatly from increased lighting.
- Oral supplementation with antioxidants and zinc, per the AREDS protocol, did not show an effect on the rate of enlargement of GA. The indication for supplements is to prevent the development of choroidal neovascularization.
- The development of a preferred retinal locus can aid in the effective utilization of the remaining functional retina.

REFERENCES

1. Sunness JS, Schuchard R, Shen N, et al. Landmark-driven fundus perimetry using the scanning laser ophthalmoscope (SLO). Invest Ophthalmol Vis Sci 1995; 36: 1863–74.
2. Sarks JP, Sarks SH, Killingsworth MC. Evolution of geographic atrophy of the retinal pigment epithelium. Eye 1988; 2: 552–77.
3. Maguire P, Vine AP. Geographic atrophy of the retinal pigment epithelium. Am J Ophthalmol 1986; 102: 621–5.
4. Schatz H, McDonald HR. Atrophic macular degeneration: rate of spread of geographic atrophy and visual loss. Ophthalmology 1989; 96: 1541–51.
5. Sunness JS, Rubin GS, Applegate CA, et al. Visual function abnormalities and prognosis in eyes with age-related geographic atrophy of the macula and good acuity. Ophthalmology 1997; 104: 1677–91.
6. Ferris FL III, Fine SL, Hyman L. Age-related macular degeneration and blindness due to neovascular maculopathy. Arch Ophthalmol 1984; 102: 1640–2.
7. Sunness JS, Gonzalez-Baron J, Applegate CA, et al. Enlargement of atrophy and visual acuity loss in the geographic atrophy form of age-related macular degeneration. Ophthalmology 1999; 106: 1768–79.
8. Klein R, Klein BEK, Franke T. The relationship of cardiovascular disease and its risk factors to age-related maculopathy: the beaver dam eye study. Ophthalmology 1993; 100: 406–14.
9. Vingerling JR, Dielemans I, Hofman A, et al. The prevalence of age-related maculopathy in the rotterdam study. Ophthalmology 1995; 102: 205–10.
10. Quillen D, Blankenship G, Gardner T. Aged eyes: ocular findings in individuals 90 years of age and older. Invest Ophthalmol Vis Sci 1996; 47: S111.
11. Brader HS, Ying GS, Martin ER, Maguire MG. New grading criteria allow for earlier detection of geographic atrophy in clinical trials complications of age-related macular degeneration prevention trial-capt research group. Invest Ophthalmol Vis Sci 2011; 52: 9218 25.
12. Holz FG, Bellmann C, Margaritidis M, et al. Patterns of increased in vivo autofluorescence in the junctional zone of geographic atrophy of the retinal pigment epithelium associated with age-related macular degeneration. Graefe's Arch Clin Exp Ophthalmol 1999; 237: 145–52.
13. Choudhry N, Giani A, Miller JW. Fundus autofluorescence in geographic atrophy: a review. Semin Ophthalmol 2010; 25: 206–13.
14. Delori FC, Dorey CK, Staurenghi G, et al. In vivo fluorescence of the ocular fundus exhibits retinal pigment epithelium lipofuscin characteristics. Invest Ophthalmol Vis Sci 1995; 36: 718–29.
15. Holz FG, Bellman C, Staudt S, Schutt F, Volcker HE. Fundus autofluorescence and development of geographic atrophy in age-related macular degeneration. Invest Ophthalmol Vis Sci 2001; 42: 1051–6.
16. Holz FG, Bindewald-Wittich A, Fleckenstein M, FAM Study Group. Progression of geographic atrophy and impact of fundus autofluorescence patterns in age-related macular degeneration. Am J Ophthalmol 2007; 143: 463–72.
17. Schmitz-Valckenburg S, Bindewald-Wittich A, Dolar-Szczasny J, et al. Fundus autofluorescence in age-related macular degeneration study group. Invest Ophthalmol Vis Sci 2006; 47: 2648–54.
18. Deckert A, Deckert A, Schmitz-Valckenburg S, et al. Automated analysis of digital fundus autofluorescence images of geographic atrophy in age-related macular degeneration using confocal scanning laser ophthalmoscopy (cSLO). BMC Ophthalmol 2005; 5: 8.
19. Sunness JS, Ziegler MD, Applegate CA. Issues in quantifying atrophic macular disease using retinal autofluorescence. Retina 2006; 26: 666–72.
20. Schmitz-Vlackenburg S, Brinkmann CK, Alten F, et al. Semiautomated image processing method for identification and quantification of geographic atrophy in age-related macular degeneration. Invest Ophthalmol Vis Sci 2011; 52: 7640–6.
21. Yehoshua Z, Rosenfeld PJ, Gregori G, et al. Progression of geographic atrophy in age-related macular degeneration

imaged with spectral domain optical coherence tomography. Ophthalmology 2011; 118: 679–86.

22. Sunness JS, Gonzalez-Baron J, Bressler NM, Hawkins B, Applegate CA. The development of choroidal neovascularization in eyes with the geographic atrophy form of age-related macular degeneration. Ophthalmology 1999; 106: 910–19.

23. Nasrallah F, Jalkh AE, Trempe CL, McMeel JW, Schepens CL. Subretinal hemorrhage in atrophic age-related macular degeneration. Am J Ophthalmol 1988; 107: 38–41.

24. Sunness JS, Bressler NM, Maguire MG. Scanning laser ophthalmoscopic analysis of the pattern of visual loss in age-related geographic atrophy of the macula. Am J Ophthalmol 1995; 119: 143–51.

25. Sunness JS, Bressler NM, Tian Y, Alexander J, Applegate CA. Measuring geographic atrophy in advanced age-related macular degeneration. Invest Ophthalmol Vis Sci 1999; 40: 1761–9.

26. Sunness JS, Applegate CA. Long-term follow-up of fixation patterns in eyes with central scotomas from geographic atrophy that is associated with age-related macular degeneration. Am J Ophthalmol 2005; 140: 1085–93.

27. Hartmann KL, Bartsch DU, Cheng L, et al. Scanning laser ophthalmoscope imaging stabilized microperimetry in dry age-related macular degeneration. Retina 2011; 31: 1323–31.

28. Green WR, Key SN III. Senile macular degeneration: a histopathologic study. Trans Am Ophthalmol Soc 1977; 75: 180–254.

29. Korte GE, Reppucci V, Henkind P. Retinal pigment epithelium destruction causes choriocapillary atrophy. Invest Ophthalmol Vis Sci 1984; 25: 1135–45.

30. Leonard DS, Zhang XG, Panozzo G, Sugino IK, Zarbin MA. Clinicopathologic correlation of localized retinal pigment epithelial debridement. Invest Ophthalmol Vis Sci 1997; 38: 1094–09.

31. McLeod DS, Grebe R, Bhutto I, et al. Relationship between RPE and choriocapillaris in age-related macular degeneration. Invest Ophthalmol Vis Sci 2009; 50: 4982–91.

32. Green WR, Enger C. Age-related macular degeneration histopathologic studies: The 1992 Lorenz E. Zimmerman Lecture. Ophthalmology 1993; 100: 1519–35.

33. Sarks SH. Changes in the region of the choriocapillaris in ageing and degeneration. In: XXIII Concilium Ophthalmologicum, Kyoto. Amsterdam-Oxford: Excerpta Medica, 1979.

34. Elman MJ, Fine SL, Murphy RP, Patz A, Auer C. The natural history of serous retinal pigment epithelium detachment in patients with age-related macular degeneration. Ophthalmology 1986; 93: 224–30.

35. Klein ML, Ferris FL 3rd, Armstrong J, AREDS Research Group. Retinal precursors and the development of geographic atrophy in age-related macular degeneration. Ophthalmology 2008; 115: 1026–31.

36. Friedman E, Krupsky S, Lane AM, et al. Ocular blood flow velocity in age-related macular degeneration. Ophthalmology 1995; 102: 640–6.

37. Grunwald JE, Hariprasad SM, Du Pont J, et al. Foveolar choroidal blood flow in age-related macular degeneration. Invest Ophthalmol Vis Sci 1998; 39: 385–90.

38. Hirvela H, Luukinen H, Laara E, Sc L, Laatikainen L. Risk factors of age-related maculopathy in a population 70 years of age or older. Ophthalmology 1996; 103: 871–7.

39. Friedman DS, Katz J, Bressler NM, Rahmani B, Tielsch JM. Racial differences in the prevalence of age-related macular degeneration: the baltimore eye survey. Ophthalmology 1999; 106: 1049–55.

40. Klein R, Klein BE, Jensen SC, Meuer SM. The five-year incidence and progression of age-related maculopathy: the beaver dam eye study. Ophthalmology 1997; 104: 7–21.

41. Porter JW, Thallemer JM. Geographic atrophy of the retinal pigment epithelium: diagnosis and vision rehabilitation. J Am Opt Assoc 1981; 52: 503–8.

42. Ritter LL, Klein R, Klein BE, Mares-Perlman JA, Jensen SC. Alcohol use and age-related maculopathy in the beaver dam eye study. Am J Ophthalmol 1995; 120: 190–6.

43. Smith W, Mitchell P, Leeder SR. Smoking and age-related maculopathy: the blue mountain eye study. Arch Ophthalmol 1996; 114: 1518–23.

44. Age-Related Eye Disease Study Research Group. Risk factors associated with age-related macular degeneration: a case-control study in the age-related eye disease study: age-related eye disease study report number 3. Ophthalmology 2000; 107: 2224–32.

45. Clemons TE, Milton RC, Klein R, Seddon JM, Ferris FL 3rd. Age-related eye disease study research group. risk factors for the incidence of advanced age-related macular degeneration in the age-related eye disease study (AREDS) AREDS report no. 19. Ophthalmology 2005; 112: 533–9.

46. Sepp T, Khan JC, Thurlby DA, et al. Complement factor H variant Y402H is a major risk determinant for geographic atrophy and choroidal neovascularization in smokers and non-smokers. Invest Ophthalmol Vis Sci 2006; 47: 536–40.

47. Yu Y, Reynolds R, Rosner B, Daly MJ, Seddon JM. Prospective assessment of genetic effects on progression to different stages of age-related macular degeneration using multi-state Markov models. Invest Ophthalmol Vis Sci 2012; 53: 1548–56.

48. Raychaudhuri S, Iartchouk O, Chin K, et al. A rare penetrant mutation in CFH confers high risk of age-related macular degeneration. Nat Genet 2011; 43: 1232 6.

49. Stanton CM, Yates JR, den Hollander AI, et al. Complement factor D in age-related macular degeneration. Invest Ophthalmol Vis Sci 2011; 52: 8828–34.

50. Seddon JM, Reynolds R, Yu Y, Daly MJ, Rosner B. Risk models for progression to advanced age-related macular degeneration using demographic, environmental, genetic, and ocular factors. Ophthalmology 2011; 118: 2203–11.

51. Yang Z, Stratton C, Francis PJ, et al. Toll-like receptor 3 and geographic atrophy in age-related macular degeneration. N Engl J Med 2008; 359: 1456–63; Erratum in: N Engl J Med 2009; 361: 431. N Engl J Med 2008; 359: 1859.

52. Yates JR, Moore AT. Genetic susceptibility to age-related macular degeneration. J Med Genet Feb 2000; 37: 83–7.

53. Scholl HP, Fleckenstein M, Fritsche LG, et al. CFH, C3 and ARMS2 are significant risk loci for susceptibility but not for disease progression of geographic atrophy due to AMD. PLoS One 2009; 4: e7418.

54. Gehrs KM, Jackson JR, Brown EN, Allikmets R, Hageman GS. Complement, age-related macular degeneration and a vision of the future. Arch Ophthalmol 2010; 128: 349–58.

55. Yehoshua Z, Rosenfeld PJ, Albini TA. Current clinical trials in dry AMD and the definition of appropriate clinical outcome measures. Semin Ophthalmol 2011; 26: 167–80.

56. Piguet B, Heon E, Munier FL, et al. Full characterization of the maculopathy associated with an Arg-12-Trp

mutation in the RDS/peripherin gene. Ophthalmic Genet 1996; 17: 175–86.

57. Allikmets R, Shroyer NF, Singh N, et al. Mutation of the stargardt disease gene (ABCR) in age-related macular degeneration. Science 1997; 277: 1805–7.

58. Pennisi E. Human genetics: gene found for the fading eyesight of old age. Science 1997; 277: 1765–6.

59. Allikmets and International ABCR screening Consortium. Further evidence for an association of the ABCR alleles with age-related macular degeneration. Am J Human Genetics 2000; 67: 487–91.

60. Gass JDM. Drusen and disciform macular detachment and degeneration. Arch Ophthalmol 1973; 90: 206–17.

61. Peli E, Lahav M. Drusen measurements from fundus photographs using computer image analysis. Ophthalmology 1986; 93: 1575–80.

62. Braunstein RA, Gass JDM. Serous detachments of the retinal pigment epithelium in patients with senile macular disease. Am J Ophthalmol 1979; 88: 652–60.

63. Casswell AG, Kohen D, Bird AC. Retinal pigment epithelial detachments in the elderly: classification and outcome. Br J Ophthalmol 1985; 69: 397–403.

64. Meredith TA, Braley RE, Aaberg TM. Natural history of serous detachments of the retinal pigment epithelium. Am J Ophthalmol 1979; 88: 643–51.

65. Sunness JS, Rubin GS, Zuckerbrod A, Applegate CA. Foveal-sparing scotomas in advanced dry age-related macular degeneration. J Vis Impair Blind 2008; 102: 600–10.

66. Lindblad AS, Lloyd PC, Clemons TE, Age-Related Eye Disease Study Research Group. Change in area of geographic atrophy in the age-related eye disease study: AREDS report number. Arch Ophthalmol 2009; 127: 1168–74.

67. Sunness JS, Margalit E, Srikumaran D, et al. The long-term natural history of geographic atrophy from age-related macular degeneration: enlargement of atrophy and implications for interventional clinical trials. Ophthalmology 2007; 114: 271–7.

68. Sunness JS, Rubin GS, Broman A, et al. Low luminance visual dysfunction as a predictor of subsequent visual acuity loss from geographic atrophy in age-related macular degeneration. Ophthalmology 2008; 115: 1480–8.

69. Fleckenstein M, Schmitz-Valckenberg S, Adrion C, et al. Tracking progression with spectral-domain optical coherence tomography in geographic atrophy caused by age-related macular degeneration. Invest Ophthalmol Vis Sci 2010; 51: 3846–52.

70. Sunness JS, Applegate CA, Haselwood D, Rubin GS. Fixation patterns and reading rates in eyes with central scotomas from advanced atrophic age-related macular degeneration and stargardt disease. Ophthalmology 1996; 103: 1458–66.

71. Sunness JS, Bressler NM, Applegate CA. Ophthalmoscopic features associated with geographic atrophy from age-related macular degeneration (abstract). Invest Ophthalmol Vis Sci 1999; 40: S314.

72. Schmitz-Valckenberg S, Alten F, Steinberg JS, et al. Geographic atrophy progression (GAP) study group. Reticular drusen associated with geographic atrophy in age-related macular degeneration. Invest Ophthalmol Vis Sci 2011; 52: 5009–15.

73. Steinmetz RL, Walter D, Fitzke FW, Bird AC. Prolonged dark adaptation in patients with age-related macular degeneration. Invest Ophthalmol Vis Sci 1991; 32: S711.

74. Steinmetz RL, Haimovici R, Jubb C, Fitzke FW, Bird AC. Symptomatic abnormalities of dark adaptation in patients with age-related bruch's membrane change. Br J Ophthalmol 1993; 77: 549–54.

75. Sunness JS, Massof RW, Johnson MA, et al. Diminished foveal sensitivity may predict the development of advanced age-related macular degeneration. Ophthalmology 1989; 96: 375–81.

76. Macular Photocoagulation Study Group. Five-year follow-up of fellow eyes of patients with age-related macular degeneration and unilateral extrafoveal choroidal neovascularization. Arch Ophthalmol 1993; 111: 1189–99.

77. Macular Photocoagulation Study Group. Risk factors for choroidal neovascularization in the second eye of patients with juxtafoveal or subfoveal choroidal neovascularization secondary to age-related macular degeneration. Arch Ophthalmol 1997; 115: 741–7.

78. Brown B, Kitchin JL. Dark adaptation and the acuity/luminance response in senile macular degeneration (SMD). Am J Optom Physical Opt 1983; 60: 645–50.

79. Brown B, Tobin C, Roche N, Wolanowski A. Cone adaptation in age-related maculopathy. Am J Optom Physical Opt 1986; 63: 450–4.

80. Sunness JS, Massof RW, Johnson MA, Finkelstein D, Fine SL. Peripheral retinal function in age-related macular degeneration. Arch Ophthalmol 1985; 103: 811–16.

81. Brown B, Lovie-Kitchin J. Contrast sensitivity in central and paracentral retina in age-related maculopathy. Clin Exp Optom 1987; 70: 145–8.

82. Midena E, Degli Angeli C, Blarzino MC, Valenti M, Segato T. Macular function impairment in eyes with early age-related macular degeneration. Invest Ophthalmol Vis Sci 1997; 38: 469–77.

83. Applegate CA, Sunness JS, Haselwood DM. Visual symptoms associated with geographic atrophy from age-related macular degeneration. Invest Ophthalmol Vis Sci 1996; 37: S112.

84. Landa G, Rosen RB, Garcia PM, Seiple WH. Combined three-dimensional spectral OCT/SLO topography and microperimetry: steps toward achieving functional spectral OCT/SLO. Ophthalmic Res 2010; 43: 92–8.

85. Sunness JS, Applegate CA, Gonzalez-Baron J. Improvement of visual acuity over time in patients with bilateral geographic atrophy from age-related macular degeneration. Retina 2000; 20: 162–9.

86. Guez JE, Le Gargasson JF, Rigaudiere F, O'Regan JK. Is there a systematic location for the pseudo-fovea in patients with central scotoma? Vision Res 1993; 9: 1271–9.

87. Sloan L. Variation of acuity with luminance in ocular diseases and anomalies. Doc Ophthalmol 1969; 26: 384–93.

88. Schuchard RA, Raasch TW. Retinal locus for fixation: pericentral fixation targets. Clin Vis Sci 1992; 7: 511–20.

89. Lei H, Schuchard RA. Using two preferred retinal loci for different lighting conditions in patients with central scotomas. Invest Ophthalmol Vis Sci 1997; 38: 1812–18.

90. Szlyk JP, Pizzimenti CE, Fishman GA, et al. A comparison of driving in older subjects with and without age-related macular degeneration. Arch Ophthalmol 1995; 113: 1033–40.

91. Bressler NM, Frost LA, Bressler SB, Murphy RP, Fine SL. Natural course of poorly defined choroidal neovascularization in macular degeneration. Arch Ophthalmol 1988; 106: 1537–42.

92. Jalkh AE, Nasrallah FP, Marinelli I, Van de Velde F. Inactive subretinal neovascularization in age-related macular degeneration. Ophthalmology 1990; 97: 1614–19.

93. Yeo JH, Marcus S, Murphy RP. Retinal pigment epithelial tears: patterns and progression. Ophthalmology 1988; 95: 8–13.

94. Marmor MF, McNamara JA. Pattern dystrophy of the retinal pigment epithelium and geographic atrophy. Am J Ophthalmol 1996; 122: 382–92.

95. Krill AE, Archer D. Classification of the choroidal atrophies. Am J Ophthalmol 1971; 72: 562.

96. Age-Related Eye Disease Study Research Group. A randomized, placebo-controlled, clinical trial of high-dose supplementation with vitamins C and E, beta carotene, and zinc for age-related macular degeneration and vision loss: AREDS report No. 8. Arch Ophthalmol 2001; 119: 1417–36.

97. Zhang K, Hopkins JJ, Heier JS, et al. Ciliary neurotrophic factor delivered by encapsulated cell intraocular implants for treatment of geographic atrophy in age-related macular degeneration. Proc Natl Acad Sci USA 2011; 108: 6241–5.

98. Weisz JM, deJuan E, Humayun MS, et al. Allogenic fetal retinal pigment epithelial cell transplant in a patient with geographic atrophy. Retina 1999; 19: 540–5.

99. Schwartz SD, Hubschman JP, Heilwell G, et al. Embryonic stem cells trial for macular degeneration: a preliminary report. Lancet 2012; Epub ahead of print.

8

Non-neovascular age-related macular degeneration

Neelakshi Bhagat and Christina Flaxel

INTRODUCTION

Age-related macular degeneration (AMD), also known as age-related maculopathy (ARM), is the leading cause of severe visual loss in people over 65 years of age in developed countries (1–3). It is also the leading cause of irreversible central vision loss in whites over 50 years of age in the United States (4). The disease affects approximately 8 million people in the United States (5); its advanced form affects more than 1.75 million people (6).

The prevalence and progression of AMD increases with age (Table 8.1), from a prevalence of 1.6% in the age group 52–64 years to 28% in the age group 74–85 years (7). In the Blue Mountain Study, the prevalence of early AMD was reported to increase from 1.3% in the age group 49–54 years to 28.0% for those over 80 years of age; the prevalence of late ARM, on the other hand, increased from 0.1% in the age group 49–54 years to 7.1% in the age group 75–86 years. The population older than 65 years is the fastest growing segment of our society and the prevalence of AMD is predicted to increase dramatically in the next decade (8–10). Recent studies clearly indicate that multiple genetic factors and environment play an important role in developing AMD. Elucidating the pathogenesis will help in developing new therapies to either prevent AMD or treat the neovascular AMD.

CLINICAL FEATURES OF AGE-RELATED MACULAR DEGENERATION

The clinical hallmarks of non-neovascular AMD are soft drusen, localized deposits noted between the basement membrane of the retinal pigment epithelium (RPE) and the Bruch's membrane, associated RPE pigmentary changes, and mild loss in visual acuity (11). The advanced form of non-neovascular AMD, termed geographic atrophy, is characterized by outer retinal and RPE atrophy with loss of choriocapillaris.

The presence of subretinal fluid, subretinal hemorrhage, RPE detachment, a subretinal greenish-greyish membrane, or hard exudates indicates choroidal neovascularization which heralds the onset of neovascular macular degeneration (2). Fluorescein angiography delineates the exact location (subfoveal, juxtafoveal, or extrafoveal), the size, and the pattern of leakage (classic *vs.* occult). Loss of central vision is usually due to RPE atrophy or geographic atrophy in non-neovascular AMD and due to subretinal fluid or subretinal hemorrhage in neovascular AMD.

Early-stage AMD (or early ARM) is defined as the presence of soft drusen (63 μm) alone, RPE depigmentation alone, or a combination of distinct/indistinct drusen with pigment irregularities. Late-stage AMD (or, late ARM) is defined as geographic atrophy (both central and noncentral), signs of neovascular macular degeneration, or a combination of both.

ASSOCIATED FACTORS

Many epidemiologic studies have provided insight on the various factors that may be associated with AMD (12–19). Hereditary influence, photic injury, nutritional deficiency, toxic insult, and systemic factors have been implicated in epidemiologic studies (20–22). These factors can be grouped into the following categories: (i) demographic characteristics, which include age, sex, race, and eye color (23–25); (ii) systemic diseases, such as hypertension, cardiovascular disease, and hypercholesterolemia (1,16,20,26–29); (iii) environmental influences such as smoking, sunlight, and nutrition (16,30–34); (iv) genetic predisposition (34,35).

Demographic Characteristics

The prevalence and progression of all types of AMD increase with age (1,13,24,36–38). A statistically significant increased incidence of ARM lesions is also noted with age (P < 0.05). Individuals 75 years of age or older at baseline have significantly (P < 0.01) higher 10-year incidences of the following characteristics than people who are 43–54 years of age: larger sized drusen (125–249 μm), 26.3% versus 3.3%; ≥250 μm, 16.2% versus 1.0%; soft indistinct drusen 22.2% versus 2.2%; retinal pigment abnormalities, 19.5% versus 0.8%; neovascular macular degeneration, 4.1% versus 0%; and pure geographic atrophy, 3.1% versus 0%. Eyes with soft indistinct drusen or retinal pigmentary abnormalities at baseline, are more likely to develop late ARM at follow-up than eyes without these lesions (15.1% *vs.* 0.4% and 20.0% *vs.* 0.8%, respectively) (39).

AMD is commonly reported to be more prevalent in women (27,40), although conflicting results have been noted. The Beaver Dam Study, after adjusting for age, revealed that the incidence of early AMD was 2.2% higher in women 75 years of age and older than in men in this age group (27). On the other hand, the prevalence of early ARM was higher in men than women in each age category in the Blue Mountains Eye Study (41). However, the pooled data from three different continents (the Beaver Dam Eye Study, the Blue Mountains

Table 8.1   Prevalence of Age-Related Macular Degeneration

Epidemiologic studies	Age (years)	AMD prevalance (%)		
		Early	Late	Early or late
1. Chesapeake Bay (9)	<50	4.0		
	50–59	6.0		
	60–69	13.0		
	70–79	26.0	4.3	
	80+		13.6	
2. Beaver Dam (9)	43–54	8.4	0.1	
	55–64	13.8	0.6	
	65–74	18.0	1.4	
	75+	29.7	7.1	
3. Klein and Klein (27)	45–64			2.3
	65–74			9.0
4. Blue Mountains Study group (36)	49–54	1.3	0.0	
	55–64	2.6	0.2	
	65–74	8.5	0.7	
	75–84	15.5	5.4	
	85+	28.0	18.5	
5. Copenhagen (47)	60–69			4.1
	70–80			20.0
6. Framingham (18)	52–64			1.6
	65–74			11.0
	75–85			27.9

Eye Study, and the Rotterdam Study) did not note such a difference in AMD prevalence between men and women (42).

AMD is noted to be more common in whites than pigmented races (43–45). The prevalence of any ARM in blacks is almost half of noted in whites; 9.1% compared with 18.2% (45). It has been hypothesized that melanin may function as an antioxidant, and protect against lipofuscin accumulation in the RPE cells and development of choroidal neovascularization (46). The association between light-colored irides and AMD has been controversial (47,48). Most of the large case-control and population studies have found no association between iris color and AMD (2,49–52), but a few case-control studies have (53–55).

Systemic Diseases
Hypertension and Cardiovascular Disease
The Framingham Eye Study (1), the Age-Related Eye Disease Study (AREDS) (50), and the Macular Photocoagulation Study (28) reported a positive correlation between AMD and hypertension. This association, however, was not seen in the Beaver Dam Eye Study (29), the Eye Disease Case–Control Study (EDCCS) (51), or in the Cardiovascular Health Study (45). A strong association has been noted between neovascular AMD

and moderate to severe hypertension, particularly in patients on antihypertensive therapy (26,28,40).

In most studies, no justifiable association has been noted between AMD and atherosclerosis (26,27,50) though Hyman and co-workers (53) noted a positive correlation of AMD with stroke, arteriosclerosis, and ischemic attacks.

Hypercholesterolemia
There exist conflicting data regarding the effect of hypercholesterolemia on AMD. A positive correlation has been found between high intake of saturated fat and cholesterol, and AMD (33). A large prospective study of 70,000 individuals (Nurses' Health Study and the Health Professionals Follow-up Study) clearly showed that total fat intake was positively associated with risk of AMD (54). The Eye Disease Case Control Study noted that patients with neovascular ARM were more likely to have higher serum total cholesterol. Some studies, however, have noted a protective effect of serum cholesterol on AMD; the total serum cholesterol has been reported to be inversely related to early AMD (27). A positive relationship has also been noted between high HDL levels and AMD (27).

Environmental Influences
Environmental influences such as photic injury, smoking, and nutrition may have an effect on the development of AMD (31,48,56,57).

Cumulative exposure to light may cause gradual loss of photoreceptor cells in the macula (58). Photo-oxidative damage by reactive oxygen intermediates induced by light may promote the development of AMD (31,32,34). The retina, particularly the macula, is highly susceptible to oxidative stress due to a high polysaturated fatty acid content that is prone to lipid peroxidation (32). There have been, however, conflicting reports regarding the association of ultraviolet or visible light with AMD (56,57). Antioxidants may prevent this damage (32).

Low dietary intake or low plasma concentrations of antioxidants may be associated with AMD (59). High-dose antioxidants, as recommended by AREDS trial, is associated with decreased risk of progression to the neovascular form of AMD (60). In the randomized, placebo-controlled AREDS, supplements containing 5–13 times the recommended daily allowance (RDA) of beta-carotene (15 mg), vitamins C (500 IU) and E (400 IU), and zinc (20 mg) taken by patients with early or monocular late AMD resulted in a 25% reduction in the five-year progression to late AMD and a 19% reduction in severe visual loss in individuals at high risk of developing advanced AMD (60). This benefit did not extend to individuals without AMD or with few drusen.

Much attention has been given to the dietary importance of carotenoids, lutein and zeaxanthin (61), and omega-3 fatty acids. High intake of omega-3 fatty acids and fish is inversely associated with the risk for AMD when intake of linoleic acid is low (62) and high levels of docosahexaenoic acid (DHA) has been associated with a 30% reduced risk of AMD (54). Seddon and co-workers have reported the results of the Eye Disease Case–Control Study trial that revealed that a high dietary intake of carotenoids, particularly dark-green leafy vegetables, is associated with a 43% lower risk of AMD (60). AREDS II, a multicenter, prospective, NIH-sponsored study will evaluate the effects of DHA and omega-3 fatty acids on the progression of AMD. The effects of lutein and zeaxanthin will also be evaluated in AREDS II. Further details about the AREDS study are available in chapter (the AREDS) of this book.

The combined data from the Blue Mountain Eye Study, the Beaver Dam Eye Study, and the Rotterdam Study have clearly shown that current smokers have a significantly higher risk of incident geographic atrophy and late AMD than both past smokers and those who never smoked. The mean age at the time of diagnosis of AMD (geographic atrophy, neovascular AMD, amd late AMD) is lower for current smokers than for past smokers or those who never smoked (63). A statistically significant association has been noted between smoking and any one or more types of AMD, with increased risks for current smokers or past smokers compared with non-smokers; the risk ratio or odds ratio has been described to be between 1.06 and 4.96 (64–66). The mechanism of injury with smoking is not well understood. It is plausible that smoking decreases choroidal flow and potentiates macular hypoxia and ischemia; this may promote AMD by oxidative stress and antioxidant depletion (30,67).

It has also been suggested that a possible small, independent association may exist between high homocysteine levels and AMD (68). Lycopene, a serum carotenoid may be associated with AMD (69).

Genetic Influence

A familial component of AMD has been suggested by twin concordance (70) and first-degree relative studies (71). A population-based study revealed an overall concordance of 37% in monozygotic twins versus 19% for dizygotic twins for early AMD (72). AMD is more likely in first-degree relatives than in age-matched controls (73).

Multiple genes may be associated with AMD. Many studies suggest an association between AMD and the genes that encode for apolipoprotein E (74,75), fibulin (76), Toll-like receptor (77), and hepatic lipase encoding gene (78) and metallopeptidase inhibitor (TIMP3) (79). Major AMD susceptibility alleles have been identified on chromosome 1q32 that encodes complement factor H (CFH) (80–82) and chromosome 10q26 (PLEKHA1, LOC387715, HTRA1). (35,83). The population attributable risk for AMD is estimated to be 71% when disease-associated alleles exist within both the CFH and HTRA1 loci (84). Risk of AMD is increased by two to four fold for hetrozygote carriers and three to seven fold for homozygote carriers for CFH Y402H variant (80,85–88). An in-depth discussion of the genetics of AMD is given in chapter 3 (Genetics of AMD) of this book.

The pathogenesis of AMD is not well understood. However, published literature has demonstrated ties between inflammation and the pathogenesis of AMD (86–88). CFH, expressed in drusen (80), plays an important role in regulating the alternate complement pathway by binding and inactivating C3b. The mutated variant CFH gene may prevent inactivation of the alternate complement pathway, predisposing the eye to persistent inflammation in the retina and choroid. The incidence and progression of AMD may depend on the presence of multiple gene variations and the interplay between genetic and environmental risk factors.

DRUSEN

Drusen were first described in 1854 by Donders (89). They are deposits of membranous debris, extracellular material between the RPE and its basement membrane (basal laminar drusen) or between the RPE basement layer and the inner collagenous layer of Bruch's membrane (basal linear drusen) (18,90–93). Drusen lead to secondary thickening of Bruch's membrane and RPE degeneration. Visual loss in macular degeneration is the result of photoreceptor atrophy that follows RPE atrophy as a result of involution of choriocapillaris (94).

Drusen form as deposition of membranous material between the plasma membrane and the basement membrane of the RPE and can be found as early as the second decade of life. They represent a normal aging change (95,96). Experimental and postmortem human studies have shown that the drusen are RPE–derived (97–99). Ishibashi and coworkers described the formation of drusen under electron microscopy as follows: (i) evagination or budding of the RPE cell in the subepithelial space; (ii) separation of the evaginated portion from the parent RPE cell; (iii) degeneration and disintegration of this evaginated cell components devoid of a nucleus; (iv) accumulation of granular, vesicular, tubular, and linear material in the sub-RPE space (17). The etiology of the evagination is not known.

AMD involves aging changes along with additional pathological changes. In both aging and AMD, the following changes occur: (i) oxidative stress resulting in RPE injury ; (ii) inflammatory response in the Bruch's membrane caused by the RPE injury; (iii) production of abnormal ECM by the injured RPE and choroid; (iv) resultant disturbance in the RPE—Bruch's membrane homeostasis ultimately leading to RPE and choriocapillaris atrophy or growth of choroidal neovascular membrane (100). Environment and genetics may have superimposing effect and most likely alters a given patient's susceptibility to the disease (100).

Types of Drusen

Different types of drusen are noted in the retina: (i) hard, (ii) soft, (iii) crystalline, and (iv) cuticular or basal laminar.

Hard Drusen

Hard drusen are discrete, small, yellow, nodular hyaline deposits in the sub-RPE space, between the basement membrane of RPE and the inner collagenous layer of Bruch's membrane (101). These drusen are smaller than 50 μm in diameter (Fig. 8.1). Focal densifications of Bruch's membrane, termed microdrusen, may precede the formation of hard drusen (102). Preclinical drusen appear ultrastructurally as "entrapment sites" with coated membrane-bound bodies that form adjacent to the inner collagenous layer of Bruch's membrane (102). These are structurally different from basal linear deposit.

Hard drusen are common in young people and do not lead to macular degeneration (90). Small, hard, distinct drusen were found in the macula of 94% of the Beaver Dam Eye Study population (2). These were not noted to increase in number with age. If present in excessive number, however, they may predispose to RPE atrophy (102).

Hard drusen act as window defects on fluorescein angiogram with early hyperfluorecence and fading of fluorescence in late frames (Fig. 8.2).

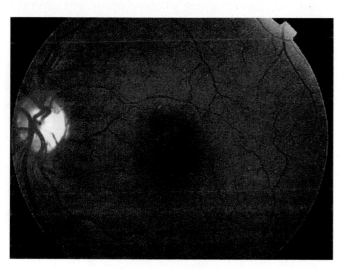

Figure 8.1 Hard drusen.

Soft Drusen

Soft drusen are clinically noted as pale yellow lesions with poorly defined edges (Fig. 8.3). They can also represent focal accentuations of basal linear deposits (91). They also represent localized accumulation of basal laminar deposits in an eye with diffuse basal laminar deposits (103). They gradually enlarge and may coalesce, termed confluent drusen, to form multiple irregular areas of localized RPE detachments. With time, soft drusen can become crystalline in nature. Crystalline drusen are discrete calcific refractile drusen (Fig. 8.4). These are dehydrated soft drusen that predispose to geographic atrophy (Fig. 8.5) (102,104).

Soft drusen are classified by size into small, medium and large. A small soft druse is <63 μm wide, an intermediate druse is between 63–128 μm and a large druse is >128 μm (the width of the retinal vein off the optic nerve is 128 μm). The risk of progression from non-neovascular to neovascular AMD increases with the size and the total area of the drusen (105). Clinical and histological studies have shown that soft drusen precede macular degeneration (106,107). Soft drusen lead to secondary Bruch's membrane thickening and RPE atrophy with subsequent photoreceptor loss, which then promote the development of choroidal neovascularization. (15,93,108).

On fluorescein angiography, soft drusen show early hypofluorescence or hyperfluorescence with no late leakage.

Basal Laminar Drusen

Basal laminar or cuticular drusen are tiny, white deposits found between the plasma membrane of RPE and its basement membrane (Fig. 8.6) (90). Such drusen are mainly composed of collagen, laminin, membrane-bound vesicles, and fibronectin. The deposits tend to accumulate over the thickened Bruch's membrane suggesting that they may be a local response to altered filtration at these sites (101).

Basal laminar drusen are typically very numerous, distributed in a bilaterally symmetrical pattern, and are most prominent in the posterior poles. These unusual

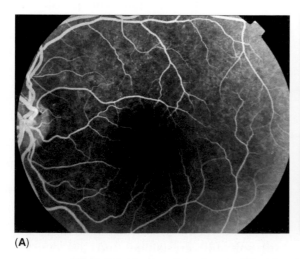

(A)

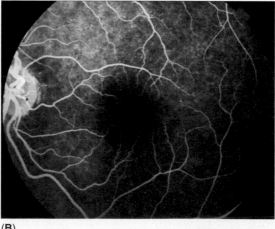

(B)

Figure 8.2 Fluorescein angiogram: (A) early and (B) late frames of hard drusen in the macula.

drusen are often seen in association with other typical hard, soft, or semi-solid drusen. Visual acuity is typically minimally affected despite the large number of these drusen. They tend to occur in younger individuals and in normal eyes and do not predispose to macular degeneration.

On fluorescein angiography, the basal laminar drusen hyperfluoresce early and give an appearance of "starry night" in late frames (Fig. 8.7) (104).

DISAPPEARANCE OF DRUSEN

Various reports have described a spontaneous disappearance of drusen (12,109). Bressler and colleagues noted in their Waterman study that the large drusen disappeared spontaneously in 35% of 47 individuals in five years of follow-up (106). They have also been reported to disappear after laser photocoagulation (Fig. 8.8) (110). RPE atrophy is noted as drusen disappear followed by photoreceptor and choriocapillaris loss (111).

It has been hypothesized that disappearance of drusen may be linked to a lower risk of CNV. This was the basis of undertaking three multicenter trials to evaluate the effect of light laser on drusen, the Choroidal Neovascularization Prevention Trial (CNVPT) (112), the Prophylactic Treatment of AMD study (113,114) and the Drusen Laser Study (115). The CNVPT study, a multicenter, randomized prospective study of laser treatment versus observation evaluated the effect of low-intensity argon laser treatment in eyes with drusen secondary to AMD. The study included two groups: unilateral group, 120 patients with CNVs in one eye and 10 or more drusen larger than 63 mm in diameter in the fellow eye; bilateral drusen group, 156 patients with non-neovascular AMD, 10 or more drusen larger than 63 mm in diameter within 3000 mm of the foveola and good visual acuity (112,116,117). The rate of CNV formation in the bilateral group was found to be not statistically different, 4/152 in the laser-treated group versus 2/156 in the control group, P = 0.42 (112).

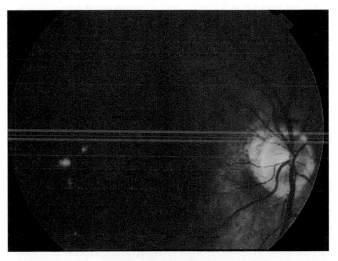

Figure 8.3 Soft drusen.

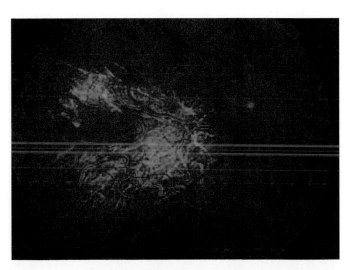

Figure 8.5 Geographic atrophy.

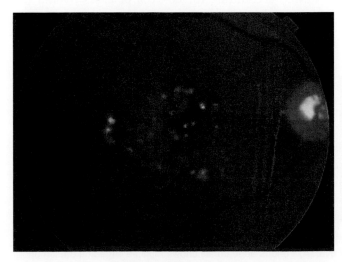

Figure 8.4 Calcific drusen.

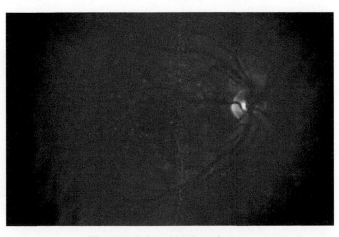

Figure 8.6 Basal laminar drusen.

However, a relatively high rate of CNV development was seen in the unilateral arm and the study was suspended in the treated cohort; 16.9% (10/59) versus 3.2% (2/61 eyes) in the laser treatment and control groups respectively (P = 0.02) (112).

The PTAMD trial, using subthreshold diode laser, has shown similar findings of increased risk of neovascular maculopathy in fellow eyes of patients treated with laser (113). In the phase III PTAMD study, at 1 year, the rate of CNV formation was 15.8% for lasered versus 1.4% for observed eyes (P = 0.05). Most of the intergroup differences in choroidal neovascularization events occurred during the first 2 years of follow-up. Treated eyes showed a higher rate of VA loss (greater than or equal to 3 lines) at 3- and 6-months follow-up relative to observed eyes (8.3% versus 1% and 11.4% versus 4%, respectively; P = 0.02, 0.07). After 6 months, no significant differences were observed in VA loss between groups. Prophylactic subthreshold 810-nm-diode laser treatment to an eye with multiple large drusen in a patient whose fellow eye has already suffered a neovascular event places the treated eye at higher risk of developing choroidal neovascularization (116).

The Drusen Laser Study trial has shown that the incidence of CNV in the unilateral arm was higher in the

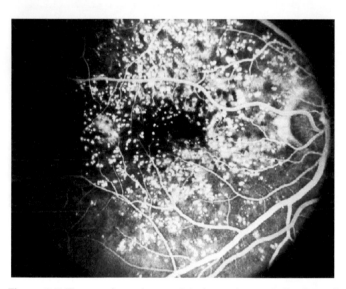

Figure 8.7 Fluorescein angiogram: late frame demonstrating "starry" night" appearance.

laser-treated arm than the control arm, though this was not found to be statistically significant. However, the onset of CNV was approximately six months earlier in the laser-treated group than in the control group, a statistically significant finding (115). The group recommends against prophylactic laser treatment when a neovascular process has already occurred in one eye. However, they were unable to determine the role of prophylactic laser in patients with bilateral drusen and good vision as the event rate is very low in these eyes and a large number of eyes is needed, they were not able to achieve the necessary recruitment goals to answer this question (Fig. 8.9) (115).

Another method of preventing the development of sight-threatening CNV is to deliver a medication to an at-risk eye to slow or stop angiogenesis. The Anecortave Acetate Risk Reduction (AART) trial failed to show any significant reduction in lowering the risk of non-neovascular AMD progressing into neovascular AMD with juxtafoveal injection of anecortave acetate. Other drug trials as with the use of Sirolimus (decreases the production of VEGF-A) are being initiated.

NON-NEOVASCULAR AGE-RELATED MACULAR DEGENERATION

Soft drusen precede macular degeneration (94,106). The mere presence of drusen does not account for significant loss of vision (92). Soft drusen can lead to RPE atrophy with resultant overlying photoreceptor atrophy and vision loss. When the vision falls below or equal to 20/30, the disease process is termed non-neovascular or dry macular degeneration. Subretinal fluid, subretinal hemorrhage, RPE detachment, hard exudates, and subretinal fibrosis, all signs of neovascular maculopathy, are absent in dry macular degeneration. Geographic atrophy (GA) is an advanced form of dry macular degeneration. This involves RPE atrophy with subjacent choriocapillaris and small choroidal vessel atrophy. This condition progresses slowly over years and often spares the center of the foveal avascular zone until late in the course of the disease (118).

Non-neovascular AMD is the most common form of AMD, accounting for 80–90% of cases overall (20). Bressler and co-workers reported a prevalence of 1.8% of AMD in men 50 years of age or older in the Chesapeake

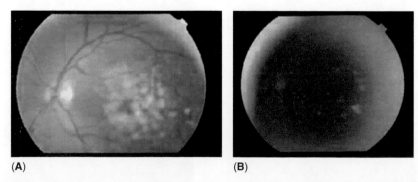

(A)   **(B)**

Figure 8.8 This patient underwent diode laser photocoagulation in his left eye. **(A)** Fundus appearance shows multiple large soft drusen prior to laser. **(B)** Fundus appearance three years later shows a marked reduction in the number of drusen in this eye.

Bay study. Of these, almost 75% had non-neovascular maculopathy (119). It accounts for only 20% of all legal blindness associated with AMD and occurs with geographic atrophy, an advanced form of dry AMD (120).

Soft drusen and retinal pigmentary changes increase with age (12,36). In the five-year period of the Beaver Dam Eye Study, people aged 75 years or more were 3.3–8.4 times as likely to develop drusen between 63 μm and 250 μm in diameter as compared with persons 43–54 years of age. Also persons 75 years of age or over were 16 times more likely to develop confluent drusen when compared with people 43–54 years of age (36). The incidence of early AMD increases with advancing age (Table 8.2). These findings have been noted in all population-based studies: The Beaver Dam Eye Study (36), Blue Mountains-Australian (41), Rotterdam (121), and Colorado-Wisconsin (122) studies of AMD.

Focal hyperpigmentation along with the presence of greater than five soft, large, and confluent drusen is associated with an increased risk of progression of RPE atrophy and choroidal atrophy. These eyes have a higher incidence of developing CNV (92,93). The mere presence of CNV in one eye increases the risk for CNV development in the remaining eye, compared with patients with bilateral drusen. The presence of large drusen in both eyes was a stronger risk factor for progression to advanced AMD than presence in only one eye (123).

The five-year risk of eyes with bilateral soft drusen and good visual acuity to develop CNV is 0.2–18% (12,94,108,124). This risk increases to 7–87% if the fellow eye has CNV (40,93,106,125). Bressler and colleagues, in their age-adjusted analysis, showed that greater than 20 drusen, the presence of soft confluent type, and focal RPE hyperpigmentation were more often noted in the fellow eyes with unilateral neovascular maculopathy than in eyes with bilateral drusen (107). Focal hyperpigmentation and confluence of drusen are associated with an increased risk of progression to neovascular AMD (13). Focal hyperpigmentation may be associated with subclinical subretinal neovascularization that cannot be detected by fluorescein angiogram (124). It may also reflect the changes that have already occurred in the RPE, Bruch's membrane, and choriocapillaris, which facilitate the future development of CNV and may simply suggest the chronicity of the disease process (Fig. 8.10) (124).

The AREDS research study group has described a simplified clinical scale to define risk categories for a five-year risk of developing advanced AMD (105) in eyes without advanced AMD at baseline, or the risk in

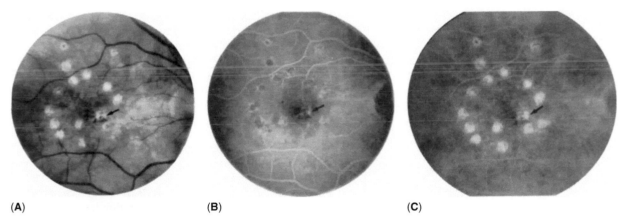

(A)   **(B)**   **(C)**

Figure 8.9 A 76-year-old woman who enrolled and was treated in the unilateral DLS pilot study. Visual acuity in the right eye was 20/30-2; confluent soft drusen were present. By 4 months, drusen had resolved and at 9 months, fleck hemorrhages were evident at the right fovea associated with a laser scar (arrow) **(A)** Fluorescein angiography showed leakage from this laser scar (arrow) **(B,C)**. *Source*: From Ref. 127. Courtesy of Dr Sarah Owens, from the Drusen Laser Study.

Table 8.2 The Beaver Dam Eye Study; 5-Year Incidence of Non-Neovascular AMD Findings

	p-Value	>75 years of age	43–54 years of age
1. Large drusen (125–249 μm)	<0.05	17.6%	2.1%
2. Large drusen (>250 μm)	<0.05	6.5%	0.2%
3. Soft indistinct drusen	<0.05	16.3%	1.8%
4. Retinal pigment abnormalities	<0.05	12.9%	0.9%
5. Pure geographic	<0.05	1.7%	0%

Source: From Ref. 31.

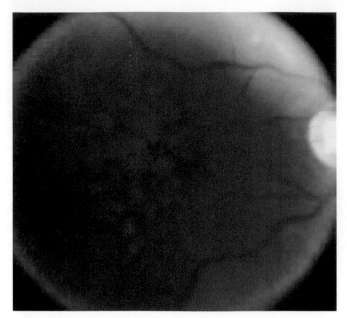

Figure 8.10 High-risk drusen showing large confluent drusen with RPE hyperpigmentation.

the unaffected fellow eye when advanced AMD is present in one eye at baseline. It is a five-step scale (0–4) that predicts an approximately five-year risk of developing advanced AMD in at least one eye as follows: 0 factors, 0.5%; 1 factor, 3%; 2 factors, 12%; 3 factors, 25%; and 4 factors, 50%. The scale sums the retinal risk factors in both eyes. The risk factors are presence of 1 or more large drusen (>125 µm—width of a retinal vein at the disc margin) and pigment stippling; each characteristic gets one point for each eye. Advanced AMD in one eye at baseline is given 2 points. The presence of intermediate drusen (63–128 µm) in both eyes is given 1 point.

The AREDS trial also noted that the drusen area was stronger and a more consistent predictor of progression to advanced AMD than the drusen size. However, for practical clinical purposes, the drusen number and type was used for calculating the severity score.

MONITORING NON-NEOVASCULAR AMD

Patients with intermediate drusen (>63 µm) or those with neovascular AMD in fellow eyes are recommended to take high-dose vitamins as per the AREDS study.

Amsler-grid testing is a sensitive indicator of progression of the disease process. Straight door and window frames may be ways to check for any metamorphopsia. Patients are encouraged to seek medical help if visual distortion, metamorphopsia, loss of central vision, or any new symptoms occur. These herald the growth of choroidal neovascular membranes. The early detection of the choroidal neovascular membranes may facilitate treatment as discussed in other chapters.

SUMMARY

Prevalence of AMD increases with age. Non-neovascular AMD is the most common form of AMD. Factors associated with AMD include advancing age, genetic

component, nutrition, photic injury, smoking, and systemic hypertension. High-risk characteristics of drusen for development of CNV include soft type, large size, greater than five in number, confluent, and presence of RPE stippling. Disappearance of drusen can occur spontaneously or may follow after laser. Geographic atrophy is the advanced form of non-neovascular AMD. Monitoring visual acuity and visual symptoms for the progression to the neovascular AMD is of utmost importance in applying timely treatment (126). Unraveling the multifactorial etiology will be the key to future treatment for AMD (87).

REFERENCES

1. Leibowitz HM, Krueger DE, Maunder LR, et al. The Framingham Eye Study monograph: an ophthalmological and epidemiological study of cataract, glaucoma, diabetic retinopathy, macular degeneration, and visual acuity in a general population of 2631 adults, 1973–1975. Surv Ophthalmol 1980; 24: 335–610.
2. Klein R, Klein BE, Linton KL. Prevalence of age-related maculopathy. The Beaver Dam Eye Study. Ophthalmology 1992; 99: 933–943.
3. Klein R, Klein BE, Tomany SC, et al. Ten-year incidence and progression of age-related maculopathy. The Beaver Dam Eye Study. Ophthalmology 2002; 109: 1767–79.
4. American Academy of Ophthalmology. New therapies for macular degeneration. [Available from: www.aao.org/newsroom/facts/amd.cfm]. 2005.
5. Age-Related Eye Disease Study Research Group. Potential public health impact of age-related eye disease study results: AREDS report no. 11. Arch Ophthalmol 2003; 121: 1621–24.
6. Eye Diseases Prevalence Research Group. Prevalence of age-related macular degeneration in the United States. Arch Ophthalmol 2004; 122: 564–72.
7. Kahn HA, Leibowitz HM, Ganley JP, et al. The Framingham Eye Study. I. Outline and major prevalence findings. Am J Epidemiol 1977; 106: 17–32.
8. Thylefors B. A global initiative for the elimination of avoidable blindness. Am J Ophthalmol 1998; 125: 90–3.
9. Evans J, Wormald R. Is the incidence of registrable age-related macular degeneration increasing? Br J Ophthalmol 1996; 80: 9–14.
10. Friedman DS, O'Colmain BJ, Munoz B, et al. Prevalence of age-related macular degeneration in the United States. Arch Ophthalmol 2004; 122: 564–72.
11. Ambati J, Ambati BK, Yoo SH, Lanchulev S, Adamis AP. Age-related macular degeneration: etiology, pathogenesis, and therapeutic strategies. Surv Ophthalmol 2003; 48: 257–93.
12. Bressler NM, Munoz B, Maguire MG, et al. Five-year incidence and disappearance of drusen and pigment abnormalities. Waterman study. Arch Ophthalmol 1995; 113: 301–8.
13. Sarraf D, Gin T, Yu F, et al. Long-term drusen study. Retina 1999; 19: 513–19.
14. Gragoudas ES, Chandra SR, Friedman E, Klein ML, van Buskirk M. Disciform degeneration of the macula. II. Pathogenesis. Arch Ophthalmol 1976; 94: 755–7.
15. Green WR, McDonnell PJ, Yeo JH. Pathologic features of senile macular degeneration. Ophthalmology 1985; 92: 615–27.

16. Sommerburg O, Kuenen JE, Bird AC, van Kuijk FJ. Fruits and vegetables that are sources for lutein and zeaxanthine: the macular pigment in human eyes. Br J Ophthalmol 1998; 82: 907–10.

17. Ishibashi T, Patterson R, Ohnishi Y, Inomata H, Ryan SJ. Formation of drusen in the human eye. Am J Ophthalmol 1986; 101: 342–53.

18. Abdelsalam A, Del Priore L, Zarbin MA. Drusen in age-related macular degeneration: pathogenesis, natural course, and laser-photociagulation-induced regression. Surv Ophthalmol 1999; 44: 1–29.

19. Gregor Z, Bird AC, Chisolm IH. Senile disciform macular degeneration in the second eye. Br J Ophthalmol 1977; 61: 141–7.

20. Kahn HA, Leibowitz HM, Ganley JP. The Framingham Eye Study. II. Association of ophthalmic pathology with single variables previously measured in the Framingham Heart Study. Am J Epidemmiol 1977; 106: 33–41.

21. Goldberg J, Flowedew G, Smith E, Brody JA, Tso MO. Factors associated with age related macular degeneration. An analysis of data from the first National Health and Nutrition Examination Survey. Am J Epidemiol 1988; 128: 700–10.

22. Vinding T, Appleyard M, Nyboe J, Jensen G. Risk factor analysis for atrophic and neovascular age related macular degeneration. An epidemiologic study of 1000 aged individuals. Acta Ophthalmol (Copenh) 1992; 70: 66–72.

23. Klein ML, Mauldin WM, Stoumbos VD. Hereditary and age related macular degeneration. Observation in monozygotic twins. Arch Ophthalmol 1994; 112: 932–7.

24. Klein ML, Schultz DW, Edwards A, et al. Age-related macular degeneration: clinical features in a large family and linkage to chromosome 1q. Arch Ophthalmol 1998; 116: 1082–8.

25. Maltzman BA, Mulvihill MN, Greenbaum A. Senile maculardegeneration and risk factors; a case-controlled study. Ann Ophthalmol 1979; 11: 1197–201.

26. Hyman L, Schachat AP, He Q, Leske MC. Hypertension, cardiovascular disease, and age-related macular degeneration. Age-related macular degeneration risk factors study group. Arch Ophthalmol 2000; 118: 351–8.

27. Klein R, Klein BE, Jensen SC. The relation of cardiovascular disease and its risk factors to the 5-year incidence of age-related maculopathy: the Beaver Dam Eye Study. Ophthalmology 1997; 104: 1804–12.

28. Macular Photocoagulation Study Group. Laser photocoagulation for juxtafoveal choroidal neovascularization. Five-year results from randomized clinical trials. Arch Ophthalmol 1994; 112: 500–9.

29. Klein BE, Klein R. Cataracts and macular degeneration in older Americans. Arch Ophthalmol 1982; 100: 571–3.

30. Klein R, Klein BE, Moss SE, The Beaver Dam Eye Study. Relation of smoking to the incidence of age-related maculopathy. Am J Epidemiol 1998; 147: 103–10.

31. Gottsch JD, Bynoe LA, Harlan JB, et al. Light-induced deposits in bruch's membrane of protoporphyric mice. Arch Ophthalmol 1993; 111: 126–9.

32. Delcourt C, Cristol JP, Tesseir F, POLA Study Group. Age-related macular degeneration and antioxidant status in the POLA study. Pathologies Oculaires Liees a l'age. Arch Ophthalmol 1999; 117: 1384–90.

33. Mares-Perlman JA, Brady WE, Klein R, et al. Dietary fat and age-related maculopathy. Arch Ophthalmol 1995; 113: 743–8.

34. Tso MO. Pathogenetic factors of aging macular degeneration. Ophthalmology 1985; 92: 628–35.

35. Jakobsdottir J, Conley YP, Weeks DE, et al. Susceptibility genes for age-related maculopathy on chromosome 10q26. Am J Hum Genet 2005; 77: 389–407.

36. Klein R, Klein BEK, Jensen SC, Meuer SM. The five-year incidence and progression of age-related maculopathy: the Beaver Dam Eye Study. Ophthalmology 1997; 104: 7–21.

37. Smith W, Assink J, Klein R, et al. Risk factors for age-related macular degeneration: pooled findings from three continents. Ophthalmology 2001; 108: 697–704.

38. Mitchell P, Wang JJ, Foran S, Smith W. Five-year incidence of age-related maculopathy lesions: the Blue Mountains Eye Study. Ophthalmology 2002; 109: 1092–7.

39. Age-Related Eye Disease Study Research Group. Potential public health impact of age-related eye disease study results: AREDS report no. 11. Arch Ophthalmol 2003; 121: 1621–24.

40. Macular Photocoagulation Study group. Risk factors for choroidal neovascularization in the second eye of patients with juxtafoveal or subfoveal choroidal neovascularization secondary to age-related macular degeneration. Arch Ophthalmol 1997; 115: 741–7.

41. Mitchell P, Smith W, Attebo K, Wang JJ. Prevalence of age-related maculopathy in Australia. The Blue Mountains Study. Ophthalmology 1995; 102: 1450–60.

42. Smith W, Assink J, Klein R, et al. Risk factors for age-related macular degeneration: pooled findings from three continents. Ophthalmology 2001; 108: 697–704.

43. Gregor Z, Joffe L. Senile macular changes in black African. Br J Ophthalmol 1978; 62: 547–50.

44. Friedman DS, Katz J, Bressler NM, et al. Racial differences in the prevalence of age-related macular degeneration: the Baltimore Eye Survey. Ophthalmology 1999; 106: 1049–55.

45. Klein R, Klein BEK, Marino EK, et al. Early age-related maculopathy in the cardiovascular health study. Ophthalmology 2003; 110: 25–33.

46. Sundelin SP, Nilsson SE. Lipofuscin-formation in cultured retinal pigment epithelial cells is related to their melanin content. Free Radic Biol Med 2001; 30: 74–81.

47. Mitchell P, Smith W, Attebo K, Wang JJ. Iris color, skin sun sensitivity and age-related maculopathy. The Blue Mountains Eye Study. Ophthalmology 1998; 105: 1359–63.

48. Smith W, Assink J, Klein R, et al. Risk factors for age-related macular degeneration: pooled findings from three continents. Ophthalmology 2001; 108: 697–704.

49. West SK, Rosenthal FS, Bressler NM, et al. Exposure to sunlight and other risk factors for age-related macular degeneration. Arch Ophthalmol 1989; 107: 875–979.

50. Age-Related Eye Disease Study Research Group. Risk factors associated with age-related macular degeneration. A case-control study in the age-related eye disease study: age-related eye disease study report number 3. Ophthalmology 2000; 107: 2224–32.

51. The Eye Disease Case-Control Study Group. Risk factors for neovascular age related macular degeneration. Arch Ophthalmol 1992; 110: 1701–8.

52. Vinding T. Age-related macular degeneration. Macular changes, prevalence and sex ratio. An epidemiological

study of 1000 aged individuals. Acta Ophthalmol (Copenh) 1989; 67: 609–16.

53. Hyman LG, Lilienfeld AM, Ferris FL III, et al. Senile macular degeneration: a case-control study. Am J Epidemiol 1983; 118: 213–27.

54. Weiter JJ, Delori FC, Wing GL, et al. Relationship of senile macular degeneration to ocular pigmentation. Am J Ophthalmol 1985; 99: 185–7.

55. Frank RN, Puklin JE, Stock C, et al. Race, iris color, and age-related macular degeneration. Trans Am Ophthalmol Soc 2000; 98: 109–15.

56. Cruikshanks KJ, Klein R, Klein BE. The Beaver Dam Eye Study. Sunlight and age-related macular degeneration. Arch Ophthalmol 1993; 111: 514–18.

57. Taylor HR, Munoz B, West S, et al. Visible light and risk of age-related macular degeneration. Trans Am Ophthalmol Soc 1990; 88: 163–73.

58. Gartner S, Henkind P. Aging and degneration of the human macula. 1. outer nuclear layer and photoreceptors. Br J Ophthalmol 1981; 63: 23–8.

59. Evans JR. Risk factors for age-related macular degeneration. Prog Retin Eye Res 2001; 20: 227–53.

60. Age-Related Eye Disease Study Research Group. A randomized, placebo-controlled, clinical trial of high-dose supplementation with vitamins C and E, beta carotene, and zinc for age-related macular degeneration and vision loss: AREDS Report No. 8. Arch Ophthalmol. 2001; 119: 1417–36.

61. Seddon JM, Ajani UA, Sperduto RD, et al. Eye Disease Case-Control Study group. Dietary carotenoids, vitamins A, C and E and advanced age-related macular degeneration. JAMA 1994; 272: 1413–20.

62. Seddon JM, Rosner B, Sperduto RD, et al. Dietary fat and risk for advanced age-related macular degeneration. Arch Ophthalmol 2001; 119: 1191–9.

63. Tomany SC, Mmed JJW, Van Leevuen R, et al. Risk factors for incident age-related macular degeneration: pooled data from 3 continents. Ophthalmology 2004; 111: 1280–7.

64. Thorton J, Edwards R, Mitchell P, et al. Smoking and age-related macular degeneration: a review of assciation. Eye 2005; 19: 935–44.

65. Khan JC, Thurlby DA, Shahid H, Genetic Factors in AMD Study. Smoking and age related macular degeneration: the number of pack years of cigarette smoking is a major determinant of risk for both geographic atrophy and choroidal neovascularisation. Br J Ophthalmol 2006; 90: 75–80.

66. Smith W, Assink J, Klein R, et al. Risk factors for age-related macular degeneration: pooled findings from three continents. Ophthalmology 2001; 108: 697–704.

67. Solberg Y, Rosner M, Belkon M. The association between cigarette smoking and ocular diseases. Surv Ophthalmol 1998; 42: 535–47.

68. Seddon J, Gensler G, Klein ML, Milton RC. Evaluation of plasma homocysteine and age-related macular degeenration. Am J Ophthalmol 2006; 141: 201–3.

69. Mares-Perlman JA, Brady WE, Klein R, et al. Serum antioxidants and age-related macular degeneration in a population-based case-control study. Arch Ophthalmol 1995; 113: 1518–23.

70. Gottfredsdottir MS, Sverrisson T, Musch DC, Stefansson E. Age related macular degeneration in monozygotic twins and their spouces in Iceland. Acta Ophthalmol Scand 1999; 77: 422–5.

71. Klaver CC, Wolfs RC, Assink JJ, et al. Genetic risk of age related maculopathy. population based familial aggregation study. Arch Ophthalmol 1998; 116: 1646–51.

72. Hammond BR Jr, Webster AR, Sneider H, et al. Genetic influence on early age-related maculopathy: a twin study. Ophthalmology 2002; 109: 730–6.

73. Seddon JM, Ajani UA, Mitchell BD. Familial aggregation of age-related maculopathy. Am J Ophthalmol 1997; 123: 199–206.

74. Zareparsi S, Reddick AC, Branham KE, et al. Association of apolipoprotein E alleles with susceptibility to age-related macular degeneration in a large cohort from a single center. Invest Ophthalmol Vis Sc 2004; 45: 1306–10.

75. Souled EH, Benlian P, Amouyel P, et al. The epsilon 4 allele of the apolipoprotein E gene as a potential protective factor for exudatve age-related macular degeneration. Am J Ophthalmol 1998; 125: 353–9.

76. Stone EM, Braun TA, Russell SR, et al. Missense variations in the fibulin 5 gene and age-related macular degeneration. N Engl J Med 2004; 351: 346–3.

77. Zareparsi S, Buraczynska M, Branham KE, et al. Toll-like receptor 4 variant D299G is associated with susceptibility to age-related macular degeneration. Hum Mol Genet 2005; 14: 1449–55.

78. Neale BM, Fagerness J, Reynolds R, et al. Genome-wide association study of advanced age-related macular degeneration identifies a role of the hepatic lipase gene (LIPC). Proc Natl Acad Sci USA 2010; 107: 7395–400.

79. Chen W, Stambolian D, Edwards AO, et al. Genetic variants near TIMP3 and high density lipoprotein associated loci influence susceptibility to age-related macular degeneration. Proc NAtl Acad Sci USA 2010; 107: 7401–6.

80. Hageman GS, Mullins RF. Molecular composition of drusen as related to substructural phenotype. Mol Vis 1999; 5: 28.

81. Zareparsi S, Branham KE, Li M, et al. Strong association of the Y402H variant in complement factor H at 1q32 with susceptibility to age-related macular degeneration. Am J Hum Genet 2005; 77: 149–53.

82. Edwards AO, Ritter R III, Abel KJ, et al. Complement factor H polymorphism and age-related macular degeneration. Science 2005; 308: 421–4.

83. Fisher SA, Abecasis GR, Yashar BM, et al. Meta analussis of genome scans of age-related macular degeneration. Hum Mol Genet 2005; 14: 2257–64.

84. Yang Z, Camp NJ, Sun H, et al. A variant of the HTRA1 gene increases susceptibility to age-related macular degeneration. Science 2006; 314: 992–3.

85. Gold B, Merriam JE, Zernant D, et al. Variation in factorB (BF) and complement component 2 (C2) genes is associated with age-related macular degeneration. Nat Genet 2006; 38: 458–62.

86. Klein RJ, Zeiss C, Chew EY, et al. Complement factor H polymorphism in age-related macular degeneration. Science 2005; 308: 385–9.

87. Swaroop A, Chew EY, Rickman CB, Abecasis GR. Unraveling a multifactorial late-onset disease: from genetic susceptibility to disease mechanisms for age-related macular degeneration. Annu Rev Genomics Hum Genet 2009; 10: 19–43.

88. Haines JL, Hauser MA, Schmidt S, et al. Complement factor H variant increases the risk of age-related macular degeneration. Science 2005; 419–21.

89. Donders FC. Beitrage zur pathologischen anatomie des auges. Arch Ophthalmol 1854; 1: 106–18.

90. Spraul CW, Grossniklaus HE. Characteristics of drusen and bruch's membrane in postmortem eyes with age-related macular degeneration. Arch Ophthalmol 1997; 115: 267–73.

91. Green WR, Enger C. Age-related macular degeneration histopathologic studies. the 1992 lorenz e. zimmerman lecture. Ophthalmology 1993; 100: 12519–1535.

92. Gass JD. Drusen and disciform macular detachment and degeneration. Trans Am Ophthalmol Soc 1972; 70: 409–36.

93. Sarks SH. Council lecture. Drusen and their relationship to snile macular degeneration. Aust J Ophthalmol 1980; 8: 117–30.

94. Gass JD. Drusen and disciform macular detachment and degeneration. Arch Ophthalmol 1973; 90: 206–17.

95. Sarks JP, Sarks SH, Killingsworth MC. Evolution of geographic atrophy of th eretinal pigmnet epithelium. Eye 1988; 2: 552–77.

96. Leu ST, Batni S, Radeke MJ, et al. Drusen are cold spots for proteolysis: expression of matrix metalloproteinases and their tissue inhibitor proteins in age-related macular degeneration. Exp Eye Res 2002; 74: 141–54.

97. Sarks JP, Sarks SH, Killingsworth MC. Evolution of soft drusen in age-related macular degeneration. Eye 1994; 8: 269–83.

98. Green WR, Key SN. Senile macular degeneration: a histopathologic study. Trans Am Ophthalmol Soc 1977; 75: 180–254.

99. Coffey AJ, Brownstein S. The prevalence of macular drusen in postmortem eyes. Am J Ophthalmol 1986; 102: 164–71.

100. Zarbin MA. Current concepts in the pathogenesis of age-related macular degeneration. Arch Ophthalmol 2004; 122: 598–614.

101. Sarks SH, Arnold JJ, Killingsworth MC, Sarks JP. Early drusen formation in the normal and ageing eye and their relation to age-related maculopathy; a clinicopathological study. Br J Ophthalmol 1999; 83: 358–68.

102. Sarks SH. Drusen patterns predisposing to geographic atrophy of the retinal pigment epithelium. Aust J Ophthalmol 1982; 10: 91–7.

103. Bressler NM, Silva JC, Bressler SB, et al. Clinicopathologic correlation of drusen and retinal pigment epithelial abnormalities in age-related macular degeneration. Retina 1994; 14: 130–42.

104. Gass JD. Stereoscopic atlas of macular diseases: Diseases and treatment. Vol.1 St. Louis: CV Mosby, 1987.

105. Age-Related Eye Disease Study Research Group. A simplified severity scale for age-related macular degeneration: AREDS Report No. 18. Arch Ophthalmol 2005; 123: 1570–4.

106. Bressler SB, Maguire MG, Bressler NM, Fine SL, The Macular Photocoagulation Study Group. Relationship of drusen and abnormalities of the retinal pigment epithelium to the prognosis of neovascular macular degeneration. Arch Ophthalmol 1990; 108: 1442–7.

107. Bressler NM, Bressler SB, Seddon JM, Gragoudas ES, Jacobson LP. Drusen characteristics in patients with neovascular vs non-neovascular age-related macular degeneration. Retina 1988; 8: 109–14.

108. Holz FG, Wolfensberger TJ, Piguet B, et al. Bilateral macular drtusen in age-related macular degeneration.

Prognosis and risk factors. Ophthalmology 1994; 101: 1522–8.

109. Javornik NB, Hiner CJ, Marsh MJ, Maguire MG, Bressler NM, For the MPS group. Changes in drusen and RPE abnormalities in age-related macular degeneration. Invest Ophthalmol Vis Sci 1992; 33: 1230.

110. Gass JDM. Drusen and disciform mcular detachment and degeneration. Arch Ophthalmol 1973; 90: 206–17.

111. Smiddy WE, Fine SL. Prognosis of patients with bilateral macular drusen. Ophthalmology 1984; 91: 271–7.

112. Choroidal Neovascularization Prevention Trial Research Group. Laser treatment in fellow eyes with large drusen: updated findings from a pilot randomized clinical trial. Ophthalmology 2003; 110: 971–8.

113. Olk RJ, Friberg TR, Stickney KL, et al. Therapeutic benefits of infrared (810nm) diode laser macular grid photocoagulation in prophylactic treatment of non-neovascular age-related macular degeneration:two-year results of a randomized pilot study. Ophthalmology 1999; 106: 2082–90.

114. Friberg TR, Musch DC, Lim JI, PTAMD Group. Prophylactic treatment of age-related macular degeneration report number 1: 810-nanometer laser to eyes with drusen. unilaterally eligible patients. Ophthalmology 2006; 113: 612–22.

115. Owens SL, Bunce C, Brannon AJ, The Drusen Laser Study Group. Prophylactic laser treatment hastens choroidal neovascularization in the unilateral age-related maculopathy: final results of drusen laser study. Am J Ophthalmol 2006; 141: 276–81.

116. TRIAL Research Group. Laser treatment in eyes with large drusen short-term effects seen in a pilot randomized clinical trial. choroidal neovascularization. Ophthalmology 1998; 105: 11 23.

117. Kaiser RS, Berger JW, Shin DS, Maguire MG, CNVPT Study Group. Laser burn intensity and the risk for choroidal neovascularization in the CNVPT fellow eye study (abstract). Invest Ophthalmol Vis Sci 1999; 40: S377.

118. Sunness JS, Rubin GS, Applegate CA, et al. Visual function abnormalities and prognosis in eyes with age-related geographic atrophy of the macula and good visual acuity. Ophthalmogy 1997; 104: 1677–91.

119. Bressler NM, Bressler SB, West SK, Fine SL, Taylor HR. The grading and prevalence of macular degeneration in chesapeake bay watermen. Arch Ophthalmol 1989; 107: 847–52.

120. Ferris FL, Fine SL, Hyman G. Age-related macular degeneration and blindness due to neovascular maculopathy. Arch Ophthalmol 1984; 102: 1640–2.

121. Vingerling JR, Dielemans I, Hofman A, et al. The prevalence of age-related maculopathy in the rotterdam study. Ophthalmology 1995; 102: 205–10.

122. Cruinshanks KJ, Hamman RE, Klein R, Nondahl DM, Shetterly SM. The prevalence of age-related maculopathy by geographic resion and ethnicity. THE Colorado-wisconsin study of age-related maculopathy. Arch Ophthalmol 1997; 115: 242–50.

123. The Age-Related Eye Disease Study Research Group. A randomized, placebo-controlled, clinical trial of high-dose supplementation with vitamins C and E, beta carotene, and zinc for age-related macular degeneration and vision loss: AREDS report no 8. Arch Ophthalmol 2001; 119: 1417–36.

124. Smiddy WE, Fine SL. Prognosis of patients with bilateral macular drusen. Ophthalmology 1984; 91: 271–7.
125. Strahlman ER, Fine SL, Hillis A. The second eye of patients with senile macular degeneration. Arch Ophthalmol 1983; 101: 1522–8.
126. Mitchell P, Foran S, Age-Related Eye Disease Study. Severity scale and simplified severity scale for age-related macular degeneration. Arch Ophthalmol 2005; 123: 1598–9.
127. Sarah L, Owens MD, Robyn H, et al. Fluorecein angiographic abnormalities after prophylactic macular photocoagulation for high-risk age-related maculopathy. Am J Ophthalmol 1999; 127: 681–7

Neovascular age-related macular degeneration

Jennifer I. Lim

INTRODUCTION

Neovascular (formerly termed exudative) age-related macular degeneration (AMD) was first described and illustrated in the literature in 1875 by Pagenstecher (1), who termed this condition "chorioidioretinitis in regione maculae luteae." In 1905, Oeller first used the term disciform degeneration (degeneratio maculae luteae disciformis) (2). Later, Julius and Kuhnt in 1926 further elaborated on this condition and established it as a disease (3). Further work by clinicians and pathologists over the next several decades led to the revelation that choroidal neovascularization (CNV) was responsible for the manifestations of neovascular AMD. The histopathological association of CNV with disciform scars was discovered in 1928 by Holloway and Verhoeff who described eight eyes with "disc like" degeneration of the retina (4). In 1937, Verhoeff and Grossman similarly demonstrated CNV in their cases of macular degeneration and emphasized that blood vessels erupted through Bruch's membrane (5). It was not until 1951 that clinicopathologic correlations by Ashton and Sorsby demonstrated that CNV with breaks in Bruch's membrane results in subretinal fluid (6). Finally, in 1967 Gass implicated CNV as having a primary role in what was then called "senile disciform macular degeneration" (7,8). In 1971, Blair and Aaberg showed the clinical and fluorescein angiographic characteristics of CNV in these eyes with "senile macular degeneration" (9). In 1976, Small published a clinicopathologic correlation of the evolution of a lesion which was comprised of CNV and a serous pigment epithelial detachment (PED) to a disciform scar (10). In 1977, Green and Key (11) studied the histopathologic features of 176 eyes from 115 patients with AMD. Their work supported the view that drusen predispose to development of CNV. Since then, numerous studies have given us ample histopathologic data on CNV.

Since the earliest description of AMD, there have been numerous refinements in the categorization of the types of AMD. In fact, even the term, AMD, is a relatively recent development. Prior to 1990, the term "senile macular degeneration" was used to refer to what we now know as AMD. More recently, the two main types of AMD, non-neovascular (formerly non-exudative) AMD and neovascular AMD, have been referred to colloquially as dry AMD and wet AMD respectively. Although non-neovascular AMD is typically associated with less severe degrees of visual disturbances than neovascular AMD and may even have no associated visual disturbance, neovascular AMD typically is associated with visual symptoms.

In its untreated state, neovascular AMD may result in devastating loss of vision. Fortunately, both earlier diagnosis of neovascular AMD and more effective therapies for it currently result in less severe visual loss and, in some cases, improvement of visual acuity. This chapter will present an overview of the epidemiology and risk factors associated with the development of neovascular AMD, the clinical features and diagnostic imaging findings in neovascular AMD, and the current and emerging treatment options for neovascular AMD.

EPIDEMIOLOGY

Neovascular AMD, although the less common form of AMD, is the leading cause of new blindness in the older age population in the United States, accounting for 16% of all new cases of blindness over the age of 65 years. Indeed, the majority of patients with severe visual loss have CNV (12). In fact, 79% of eyes legally blind in the Framingham Study and 90% of legally blind eyes in a large case–control study had neovascular AMD (13,14). With the aging of the U.S. population, AMD is reaching epidemic proportions. In the United States alone, there are 50,000 new cases of CNV due to AMD each year. The prevalence of any AMD in the 2005–2008 National Health and Nutrition Examination Survey was 6.5%, which is lower than the 9.4% prevalence reported in the 1988–1994 Third National Health and Nutrition Examination Survey. Nonetheless, this still represents a very large number of affected people. The estimated prevalence of late AMD was 0.8% (95% CI, 0.5–1.3). Non-Hispanic black persons aged 60 years and older had a statistically significantly lower prevalence of any AMD than non-Hispanic white persons aged 60 years and older (odds ratio, 0.37; 95% CI, 0.21–0.67) (15).

The number of persons aged 55 years or older is 38 million in the United States (U.S. census 2000 data) and is projected to increase to 88 million by 2030. The prevalence of AMD, in general, and that of the late forms of AMD increase with advancing age. In a study by Friedman and colleagues, the prevalence of advanced AMD (defined as presence of CNV or foveal geographic atrophy) is estimated to be 1.75 million in the United States. By 2020, the prevalence of advanced AMD is expected to reach 2.95 million. Currently, 1.22 million have neovascular AMD in at least one eye; 973,000 have geographic atrophy in at least one eye; 7.3 million individuals have large drusen in one or both eyes and are at high risk for progression to advanced AMD (16). There is indeed a strong need for the identification of risk factors for neovascular AMD and for preventive therapies. In a recent, multivariate model, age, smoking, body mass index, single nucleotide polymorphisms in the complement factor H (CFH), ARMS2/HTRA1, C3, C2, and CFB genes, as well as presence of advanced AMD in one eye and drusen size in both eyes were all independently associated with progression to advanced AMD (17).

Risk Factors

There are numerous risk factors associated with the development of neovascular AMD. These risk factors include ocular and non-ocular factors; they are discussed in great depth in chapter 5, "Risk Factors for Age-Related Macular Degeneration and Choroidal Neovascularization." Of the non-ocular risk factors, it appears that the epidemiological factors having the strongest association are age, race, smoking, and genetics. Of the ocular risk factors, soft large drusen, retinal pigment epithelium (RPE) pigmentary changes and presence of CNV in the fellow eye have strong associations for development of CNV. It is important to remember that these are only associations and do not imply causation (cause and effect) of AMD.

Non-ocular Risk Factors Associated with Neovascular AMD

Increased age is associated with the increasing risk of neovascular AMD. Patients with neovascular AMD have a mean age of 70.5 years versus 56.8 years for non-neovascular AMD (18). Racial differences in the prevalence of neovascular AMD (and also early AMD) exist. Gregor and Joffe (19) found that the prevalence of disciform AMD was 3.5% of the white South African patients compared with 0.1% of the black South African patients (p < 0.001). The Baltimore Eye Survey revealed a prevalence ratio of 8.8 for white to black neovascular AMD (20). Over a nine-year period, the incidence of AMD in the Barbados Eye Study was 12.6% for early AMD but only 0.7% for late AMD (21). In National Health and Nutritional Examination Survey-III (NHANES-III), the odds ratio for late AMD was 0.34 for non-Hispanic blacks compared with non-Hispanic whites (22). The prevalence of neovascular AMD is higher in Caucasians than African-Americans.

The prevalence rates of neovascular AMD in other racial groups have been investigated. In the Latino Eye Study (6357 Latino patients aged 40 years of age and older), the prevalence of early AMD increased from 6.2% in the 40–49 years old group to 29.7% in the 80 years or older group but that of advanced AMD increased from 0% in the 40–49 years old group to only 8.5% in the 80 years of age or older group (23). Similarly, in the Proyecto group, the prevalence of late AMD increased from 0.1% in 50–59 years old to 4.3% of those 80 years or older (24). These rates of advanced AMD are lower than those in Caucasians. A multivariate analysis from the Latino Eye Study has revealed four-year risk factors for incidence and progression of AMD. Analyses showed older age (OR per decade of age:1.52; 95% CI: 1.29, 1.85) and higher pulse pressure (OR per 10 mm Hg: 2.54; 95%

CI: 1.36, 4.76) were independently associated with the incidence of any AMD. The same factors were associated with early AMD, soft indistinct drusen, and retinal pigmentary abnormalities. Clinically diagnosed diabetes mellitus was independently associated with increased retinal pigment (OR: 1.66;95% CI: 1.01, 2.85), and male gender was associated with retinal pigment epithelial depigmentation (OR 2.50; 95% CI: 1.48, 4.23). Older age (OR per decade of age: 2.20; 95% CI: 1.82, 2.67) and current smoking (OR: 2.85; 95% CI: 1.66,4.90) were independently associated with progression of AMD (25).

In the Multiethnic Study of Atherosclerosis (MESA), the prevalence of AMD was determined in four ethnic cohorts (whites, blacks, Hispanics, and Chinese). The prevalence of any AMD was 5.4% in whites, 2.4% in blacks, 4.2% in Hispanics, and 4.6% in Chinese aged 75–84 years. The prevalence of neovascular AMD was highest for Chinese in which the OR was 4.3 compared with Caucasians (26). Most of the Chinese in MESA were born outside of the United States.

In a subsequent study, 44,103 Asian-Americans who were 40 years of age or older and part of a managed care organization and had at least one eye care visit between 2001 and 2007 were included. There were 2221(5.04%) non-neovascular AMD and 217 (0.49%) neovascular AMD patients. Chinese-Americans [adjusted hazard ratio [HR], 1.63; 95% C, 1.50–1.77) and Pakistani-Americans (HR, 1.97, 95% CI, 1.40–2.77) had a significantly increased risk for non-neovascular AMD compared with non-Hispanic white Americans. By contrast, Japanese-Americans had a 29% decreased risk for non-neovascular AMD compared with non-Hispanic white Americans (HR, 0.71; 95% CI, 0.59–0.85). There were no significant differences in risk for neovascular AMD for any of the Asian ethnicities compared with white Americans (27). This same group also performed a longitudinal study to determine prevalence, incidence, and hazard of non-neovascular and neovascular AMD among difference races in the United States. During the study, of the 2, 259, 061 beneficiaries aged 40 years or more, 113,234 individuals (5.0%) were diagnosed with non-neovascular and 17,181 (0.76%) with neovascular AMD. After adjustment for confounders, blacks had a significantly reduced hazard of non-neovascular (hazard ratio [HR] = 0.75, 95% CI 0.71–0.79) and neovascular AMD (HR = 0.70, 95% CI 0.59–0.83) at age 60 and a reduced hazard of non-neovascular (HR = 0.56, 95% CI 0.52–0.60) and neovascular AMD (HR = 0.45, 95% CI: 0.37–0.54) at age 80 relative to whites. Similar comparisons for Latinos demonstrated an 18% reduced hazard for non-neovascular AMD at age 80 (HR = 0.82, 95% CI: 0.76–0.88) relative to whites. Asian-Americans showed a 28% increased hazard for non-neovascular AMD at age 60 (HR = 1.28, 95% CI: 1.20–1.36) but a 46% decreased hazard for neovascular AMD at age 80 (HR = 0.54, 95% CI: 0.40–0.73) (28). Overall, several studies corroborate the racial differences in the prevalence of AMD in general and the neovascular form.

Family history is a risk factor for the development of AMD, including neovascular AMD. The Blue Mountains

Eye Study showed an odds ratio of 4.30 for neovascular AMD in patients with a family history (29). Klaver and colleagues found the lifetime risk estimate of late AMD to be 50% for relatives of patients versus 12% for relatives of controls (30).

Cigarette smoking has been associated with neovascular AMD in most studies, although it was not linked to AMD in the Framingham Study (13) and the NHANES-III Study (31). The Beaver Dam Eye Study (32) linked smoking to neovascular AMD with a relative risk of 3.29 for current smokers and a relative risk of 2.50 for former smokers compared with those who had never smoked. In the Blue Mountain Eye Study (33), the odds ratio for neovascular AMD was 4.46 for current smokers compared with those who never smoked and 1.83 for former smokers compared with those who never smoked. In the Pathologies Oculaires Liees a l'Age (POLA) study, the odds ratio for neovascular AMD increased with the number of pack-years smoked (34). This higher risk of neovascular AMD persisted until 20 years after cessation of cigarette smoking. In a case–control study by Khan et al. (35) smoking more than 40 pack-years of cigarettes was associated with an odds ratio of 2.49 (95% CI 1.06 to 5.82) for CNV. Stopping smoking was associated with a reduced odds ratio and the risk in those who had not smoked for over 20 years was comparable to non-smokers. Even passive smoking exposure was associated with an increased risk of AMD (OR 1.87; 95% CI 1.03–3.40) in the non-smokers.

In an animal model of rats fed a high-fat diet, exposure to cigarette smoke or the smoke-related redox molecule, hydroquinone, resulted in the formation of sub-RPE deposits, thickening of Bruch's membrane, and accumulation of deposits within Bruch's membrane. This animal model shows that cigarette smoking results in molecules that can cause oxidative injury to the choriocapillaris and RPE, and may explain the association between cigarette smoking and AMD (36). The Carotenoids in Age-Related Eye Disease Study (CAREDS) has shown that women (aged 55–74 years) whose diets scored in the highest quintile compared with the lowest quintile on the modified 2005 Healthy Eating Index had 46% lower odds for early AMD. Women in the highest quintile compared with those in the lowest quintile for physical activity (in metabolic energy task hours per week) had 54% lower odds for early AMD. A combination of three healthy behaviors (healthy diet, physical activity, and not smoking) was associated with 71% lower odds for AMD compared with women who had high-risk scores (P < 0 001) (37).

The association between sunlight exposure and late AMD is not clear. The Chesapeake Bay Watermen Study found an association between late AMD and sunlight (38) as did the Beaver Dam Eye Study (39). Yet, the Eye Disease Case-Control Study (40) and the Australian case-control study on sun exposure and AMD (41) did not show this same association. Since the use of sunglasses (ultraviolet blocking) is relatively inexpensive and also protective against cataract formation, it is reasonable to recommend sunglass protection for older patients.

There have been reports of progression of early to late AMD following cataract surgery. The Beaver Dam Eye Study showed an odds ratio of 2.80 for progression of AMD to late AMD after cataract surgery (and after controlling for age) (42). Pollack and colleagues also noted progression to neovascular AMD occurred in 19.1% of eyes operated on for cataracts versus 4.3% of the fellow eye (43,44). Further investigation is needed in this area.

Ocular Risk Factors Associated with Neovascular AMD

The risk of CNV developing in a patient's eye has been linked to the presence of soft drusen, pigmentary changes, status of the fellow eye, and hypertension. Lanchoney and associates calculated the risk of CNV in patients with bilateral soft drusen to range from 8.6% to 15.9% within 10 years, depending upon the age and sex of the patient (45). These projections were based on natural history studies of Smiddy and Fine (18) and Holz (46).

The Macular Photocoagulation Study (MPS) group has determined the ocular risk factors for development of CNV in the fellow eye (when the opposite eye already has CNV) to include the presence of five or more drusen, focal hyperpigmentation, one or more large drusen (>63 μm), and systemic hypertension (47). The five-year incidence rate for development of CNV ranged from 7% if none of these risk factors was present to 87% if all four risk factors were present. (This was based on the follow-up of patients with juxtafoveal CNV).

The Age-Related Eye Disease Study (AREDS) has also yielded predictive rates of CNV for a patient based upon the ocular findings of both eyes. The AREDS group created a simplified scale for determining the risk of development of neovascular AMD. One risk factor is assigned for the presence of large soft drusen and one risk factor for any pigment abnormality in each eye. Intermediate drusen alone in both eyes is counted as one risk factor. Advanced AMD counts as two points for an affected eye. The values are then summed for both eyes. The five year risk of developing advanced AMD was 0.5% for zero risk factors, 3% for one risk factor, 12% for two risk factors, 25% for three risk factors and 50% for four risk factors (48). The AREDS group has determined the 10-year risk of developing advanced AMD is less than 1% for no risk factor, 10% for one risk factor, 30% for two risk factors, 50% for three risk factors and 70% for four risk factors. (oral communication, Retina Subspecialty Day presentation by Dr Frederick Ferris, AAO Annual Meeting, Las Vegas, Nevada U.S.A., November 10, 2006).

Prevention of CNV and Genetics in AMD

The protective role of antioxidants and vitamins in the prevention of AMD was shown in the AREDS Study (49). The AREDS study enrolled 3640 participants and randomized them to antioxidants alone, antioxidants plus zinc, zinc alone, and placebo. The results showed that beta-carotene (15 mg), vitamin C (500 mg), vitamin E (400 IU), zinc oxide (80 mg), and cupric oxide (2.2 mg) decreased the relative risk of progression of AMD by 28% (OR 0.72, 43–32% absolute risk) and the risk of moderate visual loss by 27% (OR 0.73). Patients with at least one large drusen in either eye, intermediate drusen in both eyes, noncentral geographic atrophy in one or both eyes, and those with visual loss in one eye were considered at high risk for advanced AMD. Patients with these features are recommended to take the supplements. However, those who smoke cigarettes are at increased risk of lung cancer from the beta-carotene component and it is therefore not recommended that they use the AREDS supplements. AREDS2 is a multicenter interventional trial that is investigating the potential protective effects of these supplements without beta-carotene on CNV development in AMD patients who are cigarette smokers as well as the effect of oral supplementation with lutein, zeaxanthin, and omega-3 fatty acids (in addition to the AREDS supplements) on the development of advanced AMD (CNV and geographic atrophy). Further details are available in chapter 26: Prophylactic Treatment: The AREDS Study Results.

The Physicians' Health Study II is also evaluating the role of vitamin E, vitamin C, beta-carotene, and a daily multivitamin. No results are yet available. The Vitamin E, Cataract and Age-related macular degeneration Trial (VECAT) and the Women's Health Study (WHS) are two other randomized trials assessing the risk and benefits of antioxidant vitamins for AMD (50,51). CAREDS was part of the WHS. In the CAREDS, the prevalence of intermediate AMD in 1787 participants was found to not statistically differ with respect to lutein and zeaxanthin intake (51).

Genetic markers for both the risks of AMD and CNV are being determined. (These are discussed in detail in chapter 3, "Genetics of AMD.") One highly associated genetic finding is that of CFH. The inflammatory cascade has been found to play a role in the pathogenesis of AMD. Chapter 2, "Immunology of AMD" discusses the role of inflammation in AMD. Examination of the Submacular Surgery Trial (SST) specimens has revealed that inflammatory cells are found throughout CNV specimens (52,53). The finding of CFH's association with AMD and advanced AMD supports the role of the inflammatory cascade (54–57). (CFH is normally a regulator of the complement cascade and limits the immune reaction to spare host cells. When there is a CFH mutation, the CFH can no longer protect host cells and the host cell undergoes lysis through activation of complement.) In addition to CFH mutations, there are other complement factors being evaluated in the search for the inflammatory component of neovascular AMD.

It is also known that an imbalance between the stimulators and inhibitors of AMD is involved in the development of CNV. For example, pigment epithelial derived factor (PEDF) is a naturally found inhibitor of angiogenesis (58). It is manufactured by RPE cells in the eye. In AMD CNV lesions, levels of PEDF are markedly lower and vascular endothelial growth factor (VEGF) levels markedly higher compared with normal controls. Further details on angiogenesis and rationale of anti-angiogenesis treatments are found in chapter 4, "Choroidal Neovascularization VEGF Pathways."

Pure genetic models are being used to assess risk of progression. The proponents of such a model stress the strengths which include the static nature of the factors (genes do not change) and the objective data (no self-reporting is used unlike that in dietary surveys). One model uses nine SNPs tagging variants in the regulators of complement activation (RCA) locus spanning CFH, complement factor H-related 4(CFHR4), complement factor H-related 5 (CFHR5), and coagulation factor XIII B subunit (F13B) genes; the four remaining SNPs targeted polymorphisms in the complement component 2 (C2), complement factor B (CFB), complement component 3 (C3), and age-related maculopathy susceptibility protein 2 (ARMS2) genes. The pooled sample size was 1132 CNV cases and 822 controls. The test model yielded 82% sensitivity and 63% specificity, comparable with metrics reported with earlier testing models that included environmental risk factors (59).

Until all risk factors and the genetics of AMD are fully determined, prevention of neovascular AMD remains an enigma. Further clinical trials proving the benefit of intervention are necessary before recommendations can be made. However, at this time, modifiable risk factors (such as smoking and hypertension) should be addressed as they are also linked to systemic diseases. Future application of genetic therapy and targeted anti-angiogenesis treatments are now beginning to play a role in the prevention of neovascular AMD and attendant visual acuity loss. It is possible that future treatments of AMD will include targeted genetic therapy to replace defective genes.

SYMPTOMS AND MONITORING FOR NEOVASCULAR AMD

Symptomatic patients with neovascular AMD typically present with complaints of sudden-onset decreased vision, metamorphopsia, and central and/or paracentral scotomas (60,61). Not infrequently, patients are unaware that one of their eyes has already lost vision - until he or she covers the unaffected eye. Other times, patients present with loss of vision in the previously "good eye" and may have been unaware of the visual symptoms in the fellow eye containing a macular scar (62). Yet, other patients may be asymptomatic; routine ophthalmoscopy reveals the CNV in the second eye (prior CNV in the fellow eye) (63). Thus, patients who are at risk for CNV should be periodically screened for CNV and should be encouraged to self-monitor their vision daily. Monitoring options include using an Amsler grid or the preferential hyperacuity perimeter (PHP) (64,65). (See chapter 17, "Microperimetry and Psychophysical Testing to Aid in Determination of Progression of AMD.")

Patients with known cataracts may attribute blurred vision to their cataract and not suspect AMD as the cause. In some patients with dense cataracts, cataract extraction may occur without preoperative detection of the CNV. After the cataract extraction, the ophthalmologist discovers the CNV. A careful preoperative examination for neovascular AMD or advanced non-neovascular AMD is therefore of utmost importance in patients with known AMD. Preoperative fluorescein angiography (FA) and optical coherence tomography (OCT) may help detect CNV. Alternatively, if the cataract density precludes ophthalmoscopy, FA or OCT imaging, an ultrasound examination may be useful in screening for macular fluid or subretinal scar formation to rule out advanced AMD (66).

The Amsler grid is a useful test for detecting the early visual symptoms of neovascular AMD in patients with high-risk AMD eyes (67). Each box on the grid represents one degree of visual field. Thus, the Amsler grid tests the central 10 degrees of visual field beyond fixation. The patient is asked to fixate on the central black dot and to note whether surrounding lines are wavy, missing, or obscured by scotomas (dark areas). If these findings are present, the patient should be instructed to seek attention urgently with his or her ophthalmologist as it is likely that the cause is neovascular AMD. There are limits to Amsler grid testing which includes the cortical completion phenomenon, crowding phenomenon, and lack of forced fixation.

A newly developed computer-automated, three-dimensional (3-D) threshold, Amsler grid visual field test has been shown to be useful in earlier detection of AMD (68). The 3-D Amsler grid utilizes threshold testing. There appear to be different signatures based upon the type of AMD present. The PHP (PreView PHP, Carl Zeiss Meditec, Dublin, California, USA) machine has shown promise in the early detection of neovascular AMD (64,65). The PHP is based upon the concept of vernier (hyperacuity) acuity, the ability to detect a subtle misalignment of an object. The threshold of vernier acuity is three to six seconds of arc in the fovea—10 fold smaller than to resolve an object clearly on the fovea. When photoreceptors are misaligned because of edema, CNV, and or RPE elevation, the brain is able to detect the misalignment. The PHP is useful even in patients with media opacities due to its resistance to retinal image degradation. The central 14 degrees are tested in about five minutes. Patients are shown a series of linear dots with an area of artificial distortion (Fig. 9.1). The artificial distortion is progressively made smaller. If a patient has CNV, the CNV results in a true area of distortion of the dots. When their distortion is larger than the artificial distortion, the patient preferentially chooses that area. A computerized map of these areas is created.

A study comparing retinal specialists' grading of stereoscopic color fundus photos to the PHP has been performed for the detection of CNV. The gold standard for the determination of CNV was FA. In 64 patients with recent-onset CNV and 56 patients with intermediate AMD, retina specialists had a sensitivity of 70%, specificity of 95%, and an overall accuracy of 0.82 in detecting recent-onset CNV. In comparison, PHP had a sensitivity of 83%, specificity of 87%, and an overall accuracy of 0.85 in detecting the same lesions. The PHP may indeed be a useful diagnostic device for patient monitoring. The AREDS2 study is currently studying the usefulness of a home version of the PHP, the ForeseeHome (Notal Vision, Ltd., Tel Aviv, Israel) for detection of progression of non-neovascular AMD.

CLINICAL FEATURES AND IMAGING USED IN THE MANAGEMENT OF NEOVASCULAR AMD

The major clinical features of active neovascular AMD include subretinal fluid, subretinal hemorrhage, sub-RPE fluid, sub-RPE hemorrhage, RPE pigment

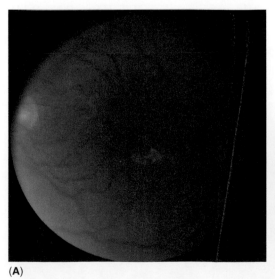
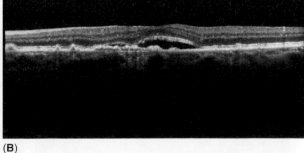

(A)   **(B)**

Figure 9.1 Subretinal fluid. (**A**) There is central blurring of the macular image due to the presence of subretinal fluid (subfoveal and parafoveal), which elevates that portion of the macula from the focal point of the rest of the retina. This is a valuable monocular clue. Clinical examination with stereoscopic viewing showed retinal elevation. (**B**) The corresponding spectral domain optical coherence tomography (SD-OCT) image through the fovea shows the presence of subretinal fluid (dark areas under the retina and above the RPE) elevating the neurosensory retina. Note the adjacent "bumps" of the RPE, which represent some drusen.

alterations, and hard exudates. Chronic neovascular AMD is characterized mainly by the presence of subretinal fibrosis with or without the other features of active exudation. These features may appear clinically as any one or any combination of the following: an area of subretinal fluid (Fig. 9.1), subretinal hemorrhage (Fig. 9.2), hard exudates (Fig. 9.3), serous PED (Fig. 9.4) or a vascularized PED (Fig. 9.5), grayish subretinal membrane (Fig. 9.6), or an area of RPE alteration (Fig. 9.7). The late manifestation of neovascular AMD is a disciform scar (Fig. 9.8) or geographic atrophy (Fig. 9.9), with or without subretinal fluid or subretinal blood. Sometimes, the PED may rip resulting in an RPE rip (Fig. 9.10) which may be associated with active CNV. Spontaneous involution of CNV may manifest as any of the above findings with RPE alterations and or scar formation.

Stereoscopic fundus examination is the best method for examining a patient with suspected CNV. A fundus contact or non-contact lens in conjunction with slit lamp biomicroscopy should be utilized for the examination. For those less comfortable with the non-contact fundus macular lenses, a fundus contact lens is the easiest to use. The fundus contact lens or the 78 diopter lens offers more magnification than the 90 diopter lens. During the examination, it is helpful to have the patient look directly at the thin slit lamp beam and ask the patient whether the beam appears distorted. Elevation of the RPE or retina (due to underlying CNV) causes the patient to perceive distortion of the slit beam.

Using biomicroscopy with a macular lens, the separation of the retina from the underlying RPE, due to underlying subretinal fluid, can be seen. The overlying retina may have cystic changes and may show cystoid macular edema. Sub-RPE fluid appears as a PED and typically has more sharply demarcated borders as compared with subretinal (subneurosensory) fluid (Fig. 9.11). Often, there is a combination of sub-RPE and subretinal fluid associated with the CNV. The CNV itself may be visible as an area of discoloration (Fig. 9.6). Other times, overlying subretinal blood or lipid may be the only clinical clue to the presence of an acute CNV. The definitive test for the presence of CNV has been FA. This is further discussed below and in chapter 12 (Fluorescein Angiography in AMD).

OCT has been an extremely useful tool in the detection and management of CNV in AMD patients. The OCT resolution is noted to range from 3 to 5 μm for spectral domain OCT and was 10 μm for the third-generation OCT machine (69). Microscopic areas of subretinal fluid and areas of elevation can be detected on OCT imaging of the macular area of AMD patients. Areas of CNV appear as RPE thickening with or without intraretinal cysts and subretinal fluid (Fig. 9.12). PEDs are clearly seen on the OCT (Figs. 9.13, 9.14). An OCT,

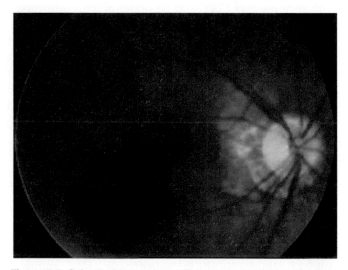

Figure 9.2 Subretinal hemorrhage. Extensive subretinal hemorrhage is present. Note that this myopic patient has large soft drusen as well as an adjacent area of retinal pigment epithelial detachment temporal to the hemorrhage.

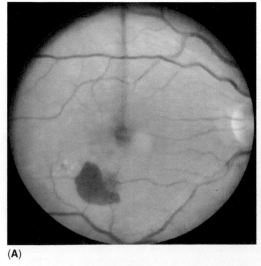

(A)

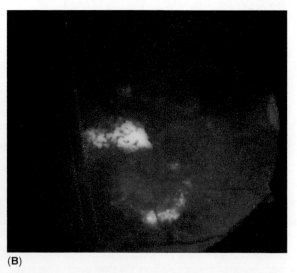

(B)

Figure 9.3 Hard exudates. The presence of hard exudates is sign of neovascular AMD. (**A**) There is a small amount of hard exudates at the inferotemporal periphery of the CNV lesion. Note the presence of subretinal hemorrhage and sub-RPE hemorrhage as well as the subretinal fluid. (**B**) This patient has extensive hard exudates as well as retinal hemorrhages.

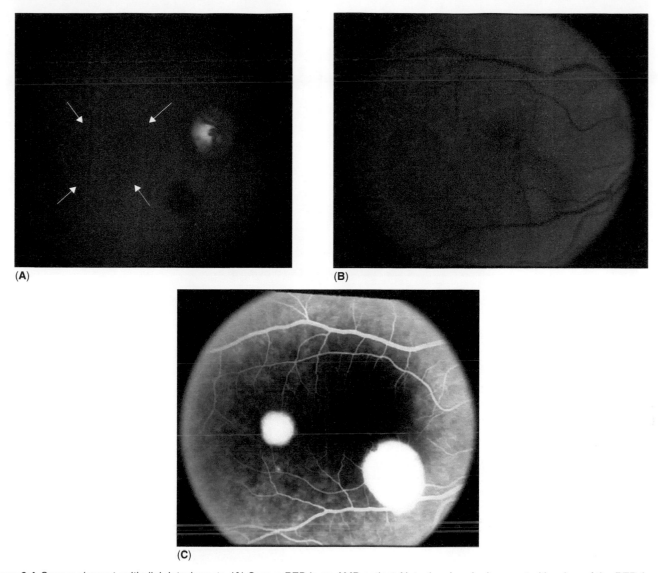

Figure 9.4 Serous pigment epithelial detachments. (**A**) Serous PED in an AMD patient. Note the sharply demarcated borders of the PED (arrows surround PED). There is also an incidental choroidal nevus in this eye. (**B**) Color fundus photo of a patient with AMD and serous PEDs. (**C**) Corresponding fluorescein angiogram shows uniform filling of the PEDs. Note the sharp borders and absence of leakage.

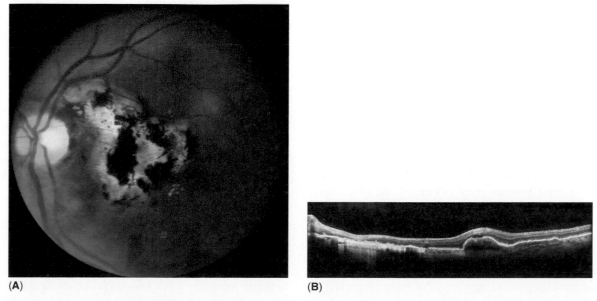

Figure 9.5 Vascularized pigment epithelial detachment (PED) in a patient with polypoidal choroidopathy. (**A**) Color photo. Note the sharply demarcated PED borders and the darkish red coloration of the PED. (B) The SD-OCT shows hyper-reflectivity within the PED. Note the surface of the PED is not smooth and there is overlying subretinal fluid.

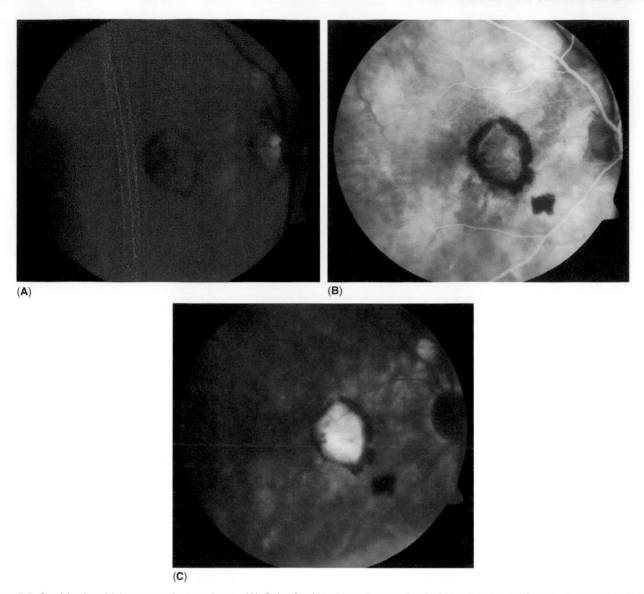

(A)

(B)

(C)

Figure 9.6 Grayish choroidal neovascular membrane. (**A**) Color fundus photo shows subretinal blood and a subfoveal, pigmented lesion surrounded by subretinal hemorrhage. Note the large drusen more temporally. (**B**) Fluorescein angiogram arterial phase shows the lacy, early hyperfluorescence (CNV vessels) in the subfoveal area with surrounding blocked fluorescence (from subretinal blood). (**C**) Fluorescein angiogram from the late venous phase shows leakage of the CNV with less blocked fluorescence around the CNV borders.

however, is not a substitute for fluorescein angiography. At baseline, it is helpful to have a fluorescein angiogram. Investigators have shown that subretinal fluid on SD-OCT is 94% sensitive for but only 27% specific for CNV leakage on FA. Intraretinal hyperreflective flecks and low reflectivity of subretinal deposits were strongly associated with actual leakage on the FA (70). Intraretinal cysts on SD-OCT do not necessarily indicate CNV. Loss of neuronal tissues may occur in old or chronic CNV lesions and result in a cystic space (71). Furthermore, it has been hypothesized that degenerative photoreceptors may form a circular or ovoid conformation advanced pathologies affecting the outer retina and the RPE and result in outer retinal tubulation. The authors suggested that these findings may be misinterpreted as intraretinal or subretinal fluid (72).

When the patient has changes in visual acuity or clinical examination and the OCT is not helpful, a

fluorescein angiogram should be performed to look for areas of CNV. OCT has been used in the recent anti-angiogenesis clinical trials as a secondary outcome measure of treatment outcome. Successful treatment of PEDs and CNVs has been shown to result in normalization of the OCT appearance (Figs. 9.15 and 9.16). Recurrence of the CNV can appear as slight areas of elevation of the RPE, neurosensory retina, or presence of cystic retinal change with intraretinal flecks. OCT is also very helpful in explaining the response or lack of response of treatment to your patient. Further details of the usefulness of OCT imaging in the management of AMD patients is found in chapters 14 and 15.

Further refinements in OCT continue; volumetric evaluation of the CNV lesions is becoming a reality. Other instruments can image the lesions and provide quantitative information. The retinal thickness analyzer can determine lesion dimensions of CNV (73). Quantitative

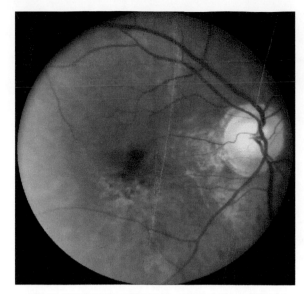

Figure 9.7 RPE alteration. There is increased pigment with some migration into the retina in this eye with neovascular AMD. Note the presence of subretinal blood as well as large soft drusen.

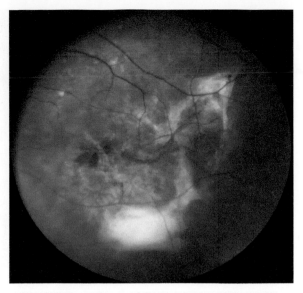

Figure 9.8 Disciform scar. There are both areas of extensive subretinal fibrosis (whitish), which block the view of the choroid, and areas of geographic atrophy in which the deep choroidal vessels are seen. Note there are areas with subretinal hemorrhage, pigment migration into the retina and large drusen. A prominent CNV vessel can be seen within the fibrotic scar superotemporally.

measurements of the retina will undoubtedly prove useful in the management of patients with CNV.

Pigment Epithelial Detachment

The borders of a PED are usually sharply demarcated (Fig. 9.4). Clinically, hemorrhage or hard exudates may or may not be present depending upon the presence or absence of associated CNV. A fluorescein angiogram or indocyanine green (ICG) angiogram is clinically useful to detect the presence of associated CNV. A serous PED shows early hyperfluorescence and uniform fluorescence on the late frames of the angiogram (Fig. 9.4B). The dye pools in the PED on the late phase. The borders remain sharp and the area does not increase in size. On ICG angiography, the PED is hypofluorescent (see chapter 13 on ICG). While a serous PED will show uniform filling of the PED, a vascularized PED shows irregular filling, notching of the PED (Fig. 9.11), or irregular margins on the FA. On the OCT imaging, the RPE elevation is readily seen (Figs. 9.13, 9.14).

If CNV is present within the PED, the occult CNV will frequently show associated subretinal fluid, hard exudate, or subretinal blood. The fluorescein angiogram typically demonstrates irregular filling of the PED and the PED borders may be blurred in the area of the CNV. Leakage on the late frames of the FA is commonly noted (Fig. 9.11). ICG angiography has been shown to be helpful in this regard (74). ICG can identify areas of CNV associated with the PED. Laser photocoagulation of the hot spots may result in the resolution of the PED, subretinal fluid, blood, and lipid (74–76). CNV has been associated with 28–58% of PEDs (75). A study by Elman and colleagues showed that 32% of serous PEDs develop CNV at a mean of 19.6 months (77). Risk factors associated with CNV in these eyes included patient age greater than 65 years, associated sensory retinal detachments and fluorescein

findings of hot spots, notches, late or irregular filling. The association of CNV with PED increases the chance for visual acuity loss (77–79).

In a natural history study by Poliner and associates, the risk of developing CNV was 26% at one year, 42% at two years and 49% at three years in eyes with PEDs followed for 12 or more months (78). The risk of 20/200 or worse visual acuity increased from 17% at one year to 33% at two years and 39% at three years. The majority of eyes (78%) that developed CNV were 20/200 or worse, while only 3% of eyes that did not develop CNV lost vision to that level.

Even with spontaneous flattening of PEDs, the visual acuity outcome is poor (77–80). Unfortunately, most clinical trials have excluded PEDs with CNV and there remains no good treatment for this group of eyes. Currently, off-label treatments are being applied to these CNV lesions with PEDs. Anti-VEGF therapies such as ranibizumab (Lucentis, Genentech Inc., South San Francisco, California, USA), bevacizumab (Avastin, Genentech Inc.), and aflibercept (Eylea, Regeneron Pharmaceuticals, Tarrytown, New York, USA) have been used to treat CNV with PED with some success. The risk of an RPE tear/rip occurring in this setting is a real concern in these eyes (Fig. 9.10). An RPE tear is readily identifiable as a sharply demarcated area of bare choroid with a straight, linear edge. This straight, linear edge corresponds to the location of the associated retracted, scrolled RPE. The fluorescein angiogram shows blocked fluorescence in the area of scrolled RPE and hyperfluorescence in the area without RPE. The natural history of PEDs includes RPE tears, but treatment of CNV with PEDs has also been temporarily associated with RPE tears (81).

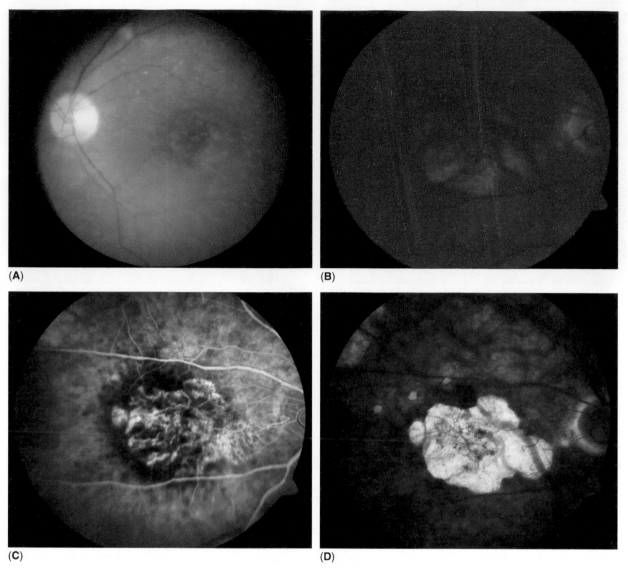

(A)   (B)

(C)   (D)

Figure 9.9 Geographic atrophy. Neovascular AMD sometimes in the late phases can appear as geographic atrophy. (**A**). This patient has geographic atrophy in her left eye after having suffered from neovascular AMD in the distant past (untreated). (**B**) Color fundus photo of a different patient with geographic atrophy. Note the well demarcated area of retinal pigment epithelial and choriocapillaris atrophy. Note the orange color of the atrophic lesion and the visibility of the deep choroidal blood vessels within the area. There are no drusen in the atrophic area but soft drusen in the area adjacent to the lesion. (**C**)The corresponding early fluorescein angiogram frame shows hyperfluorescence corresponding to the atrophic area. (**D**) The corresponding late fluorescein angiogram frame shows well-demarcated borders that match the area of atrophy seen clinically (staining). No fluorescein dye leakage is seen (no blurring of image). The borders remain sharply demarcated. Note that the area stained on the angiogram corresponds with the clinically visible lesion borders.

Choroidal Neovascularization

The MPS group has defined the various forms and components of CNV (82). The entire complex of components termed as "CNV lesion" includes the CNV itself, blood, elevated blocked fluorescence (due to a pigment or scar that obscures the neovascular borders), and any serous detachment of the RPE.

The classic clinical description of a choroidal neovascular membrane is that of a dirty gray-colored membrane (Fig. 9.6). There is associated subretinal fluid and there may or may not be subretinal blood and lipid. Sometimes the outlines of the CNV are clearly visible with the subretinal vessels readily seen. Other times, the CNV is manifest only by a neurosensory detachment or even subretinal blood.

The fluorescein angiogram is a key test in the evaluation of patients with CNV. On FA, a well-demarcated area of choroidal hyperfluorescence is seen early (Figs. 9.6 and 9.17). The MPS group characterized classic CNV as only occasionally showing a lacy pattern of hyperfluorescence in the early fluorescein phases. In the later frames of the angiogram, the boundaries of the CNV were obscured by progressive pooling of dye in the subneurosensory space. With the advent of photodynamic therapy (PDT), the term "predominantly classic" was coined. A predominantly classic lesion is one in which the lesion is more than 50% classic CNV in composition (Fig. 9.17).

Occult CNV has been classified as either fibrovascular PED (FVPED) (Fig. 9.18) or late leakage of

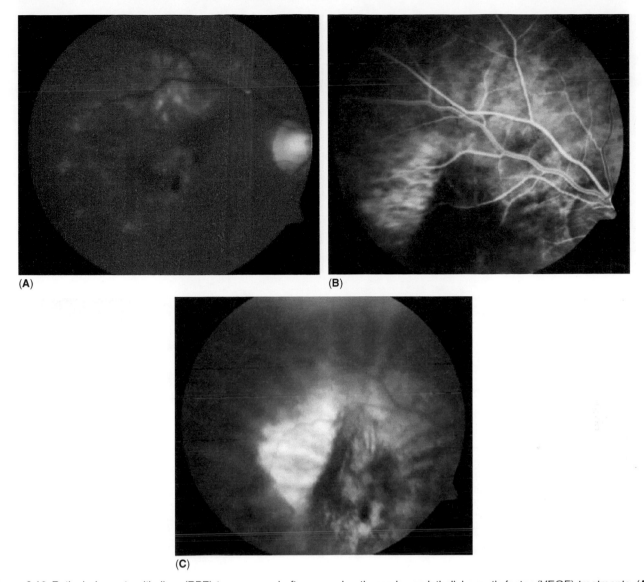

(A)   (B)

(C)

Figure 9.10 Retinal pigment epithelium (RPE) tear occurred after several anti-vascular endothelial growth factor (VEGF) treatments. (**A**) Color fundus photo shows the area of exposed choroid where the RPE tear is located. Note that this area has one linear edge. This linear edge is formed by the scrolled RPE. There are also choroidal folds in the macular area. (**B**) Early fluorescein angiography (FA) phase frame shows hyperfluorescence in the area of denuded RPE and blocked fluorescence in the area of the scrolled RPE tear. (**C**) Late FA phase frame shows hyperfluorescent staining in the area of the RPE rip. There is blocked fluorescence corresponding to the scrolled RPE. The adjacent choroidal neovascularization shows some mild leakage.

undetermined source (LLUS) (Fig. 9.19). These types of occult CNV are differentiated on the basis of the fluorescein angiogram. A stereoscopic FA is very helpful in recognizing occult CNV. FVPEDs show early hyperfluorescence with irregular elevation of the RPE. These areas are not as bright or as discrete as the classic CNV seen on the transit phases. Within one to two minutes, an area of stippled hyperfluorescence is present. By 10 minutes there is persistent fluorescein staining or leakage within the subneurosensory detachment. The borders of the occult CNV may be either well demarcated or poorly demarcated (82). Late leakage is present, although it is not as intense as that seen in classic CNV (82).

Lastly, there is a slow-filling form of classic CNV in which hyperfluorescence is not seen until two minutes. However, in this form of CNV, the late frames of leakage

and pooling of the dye in the sub-neurosensory space correspond to the area seen at two minutes. Further details on FA can be found in chapter 12.

Using ICG angiography, occult CNVs can be further classified into those with hot spots, plaques, combination of these two types, retinal-choroidal anastomosis and polypoidal-type CNV. Using ICG angiography, about one-third of eyes with occult CNV become eligible for treatment (83). ICG angiography is also useful for evaluating eyes with subretinal hemorrhage for the presence of CNV. Further details of the usefulness of ICG angiography and ICG-guided laser photocoagulation of CNV in AMD can be found in chapter 13. With the finding that anti-VEGF drugs work equally well for different types of CNV, the classification of the CNV has become a moot point. The prognostic implication of CNV type on response to treatment remains to be determined.

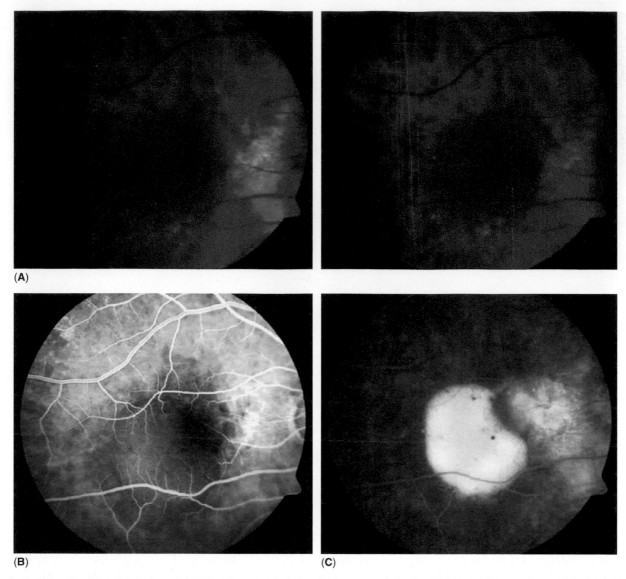

(A)

(B)   (C)

Figure 9.11 Pigment epithelial detachment (PED) with associated choroidal neovascularization (CNV). **(A)** (Stereo photo pair.) The PED is elevated on the stereo images. There is subretinal fluid overlying the entire lesion in addition to the PED fluid. Note the grayish area on the superonasal edge of the PED. This grayish area corresponds to the CNV. **(B)** The corresponding fluorescein angiogram from the late transit phase shows a notch of the PED superonasally. **(C)** The corresponding fluorescein angiogram from the late phase shows fluorescein dye leakage in the area corresponding to the CNV. The adjacent PED shows sharp edges in the areas not involving the CNV.

CNV lesions are further characterized by their location in relation to the foveal center. The location of the CNV is divided into extrafoveal, juxtafoveal, and subfoveal. These definitions were created by the Macular Photocoagulation Study group and are as follows:

Location of Choroidal Neovascularization	Distance from Foveal Avascular Zone Center (µm)
Extrafoveal	200–2500
Juxtafoveal	1–199
Subfoveal	0

A lesion is juxtafoveal if the CNV border closest to the foveal center is within (but not involving the foveal center itself) the foveal avascular zone (FAZ) (Fig. 9.20). A lesion whose closest border to the foveal edge is beyond the FAZ is considered extrafoveal.

Disciform Scar

A disciform scar shows an area of subretinal fibrosis or sub-RPE fibrosis. Dull, white fibrous tissue is seen and may accompany the CNV lesion or replace it over time (Fig. 9.8). Areas of RPE atrophy may or may not be present. FA may show leakage associated with the scar if active CNV is present. The fibrotic scar may otherwise show only staining of the fibrotic tissue.

Patients with CNV typically present with symptoms of metamorphopsia, decreased vision, uniocular diplopia, Amsler grid distortion, scotoma, or macropsia. The severity of the symptoms varies depending upon the location of the CNV. Obviously lesions closer to fixation will cause more noticeable symptoms in the patient's visual field. Patients complaining of such symptoms require prompt clinical evaluation and FA to detect any CNV or PED and to characterize the CNV by type, location, and size. Subfoveal lesions, although

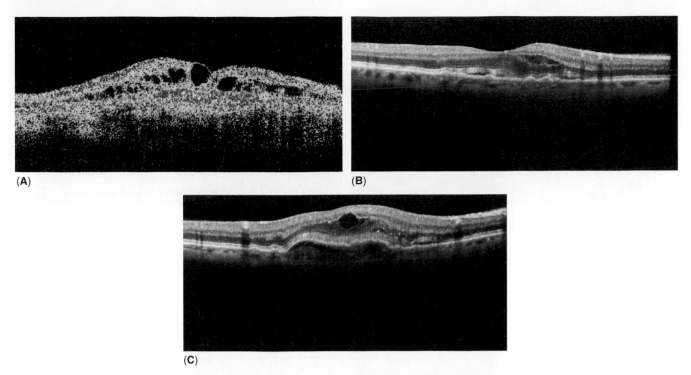

(A)

(B)

(C)

Figure 9.12 (A) Time domain OCT (horizontal cut) from an age-related macular degeneration patient with subfoveal choroidal neovascularization (CNV). The overlying retina shows multiple cysts. The CNV is seen as an area of thickening in the subfoveal zone at the retinal pigment epithelial (RPE) level. (B) Spectral domain (SD-OCT) through the foveal area from an AMD patient with subfoveal CNV. Note the presence of intraretinal cysts and subretinal fluid. (C) SD-OCT through a section just below the fovea of the patient shown in B. Note the presence of intraretinal cysts, subretinal fluid and sub-RPE fluid.

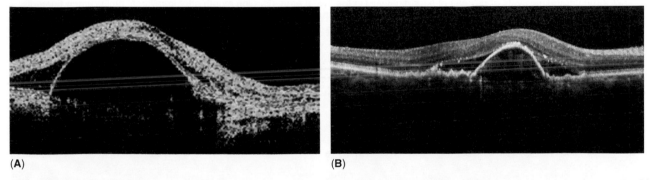

(A)

(B)

Figure 9.13 (A) Time domain OCT from an age-related macular degeneration patient with a subfoveal pigment epithelial detachment (PED) and adjacent choroidal neovascularization. There is a dome-shaped elevation of the retinal pigment epithelium (RPE) reflective border (orange). This represents the PED. The adjacent dark areas under the neurosensory retina and above the RPE represent subretinal fluid. (B). Spectral domain OCT from and age-related macular degeneration patient with choroidal neovascularization and PED. Note the areas of subretinal fluid appear dark under the retina. The PED is dome-shaped with slightly hyper-reflective areas within it. There are hyper-reflective dots within the subretinal space and particularly just beneath the retina. These are often seen in active CNV lesions. The neurosensory retina has tiny cysts present.

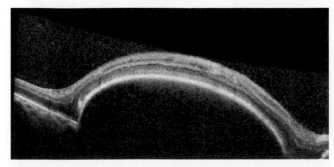

Figure 9.14 Spectral domain OCT shows a pigment epithelial detachment (PED). Note the smooth elevation of the dome of the PED and the hypoechoic characteristics of the sub-RPE fluid.

they may be treated with PDT if the lesion is eligible for PDT, are generally managed by a variety of anti-angiogenic drugs. Anti-angiogenesis treatments should be preceded by fluorescein angiography, for diagnosis and determination of the extent of the CNV, as well as by OCT. OCT prior to treatment and during follow-up is useful to gauge the clinical response. Central retinal thickness and presence of subretinal fluid and retinal cysts are all parameters that can be monitored using the OCT.

Anti-angiogenesis therapies have shown visual improvement is possible even after weeks of untreated disease (84). Thus, because of this potential visual recovery, as long as subfoveal scarring is absent, it seems

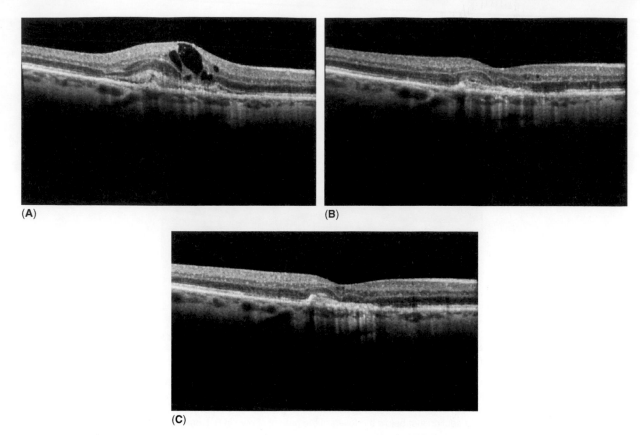

Figure 9.15 Spectral domain OCT (SD-OCT) images of an AMD patient pre-treatment and post-treatment with ranibizumab (Lucentis, Genentech) therapy. New-onset subfoveal choroidal neovascularization (CNV) in the right eye, previously treated with laser in an extrafoveal location. (**A**) SD-OCT shows large intraretinal cysts and areas of subretinal fluid in the foveal area. (**B**) One month after intravitreal ranibizumab (Lucentis, Genentech), there is marked resolution of the cysts and subretinal fluid. The CNV is visible as an area of thickening next to the RPE. The patient underwent another treatment. (**C**) One month later, SD-OCT shows no subretinal fluid and two tiny intraretinal cysts.

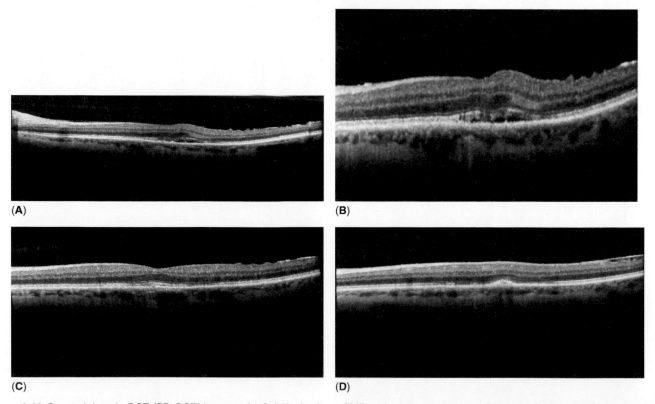

Figure 9.16 Spectral domain OCT (SD-OCT) images of a CNV lesion in an AMD patient pre-treatment and one month post-treatment with aflibercept/VEGF Trap (Eylea, Regeneron). This AMD patient noted sudden visual blurring and metamorphopsia in his previously non-neovascular left eye. (**A**) SD-OCT shows subretinal fluid in the foveal area and outer retinal edema inferior to this area (**B**). One month after an initial treatment with VEGF Trap in that eye, SD-OCT imaging shows resolution of the subretinal fluid (**C**) and resolved retinal edema (**D**).

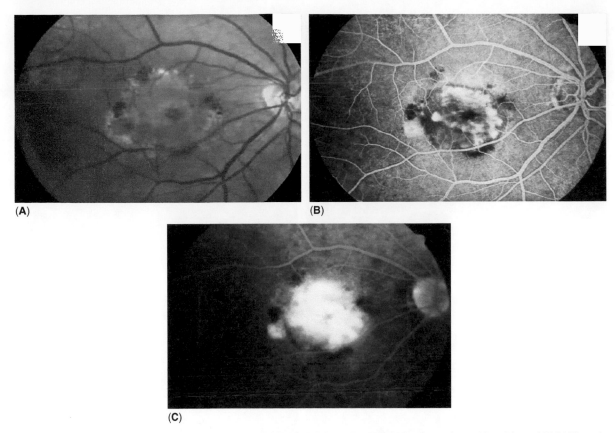

(A) (B)

(C)

Figure 9.17 Predominantly classic choroidal neovascularization (CNV). **(A)** Color fundus photo of a patient with subfoveal CNV. There is subretinal fluid overlying the subfoveal lesion. Areas of hemorrhage and hard exudates are seen in the macular lesion. **(B)** The corresponding early fluorescein angiographic frame shows an area with bright, well-demarcated fluorescence (classic CNV). There is blocked fluorescence corresponding to the areas of hemorrhage. There are also areas of speckled fluorescence (occult CNV) beyond the area of classic CNV. Since the area of classic CNV occupies more than 50% of the entire lesion, the lesion is predominantly classic CNV in composition. **(C)** The corresponding late fluorescein angiographic frame shows intense leakage from the entire CNV component. The areas of blocked fluorescence corresponding to the hemorrhage remain unchanged.

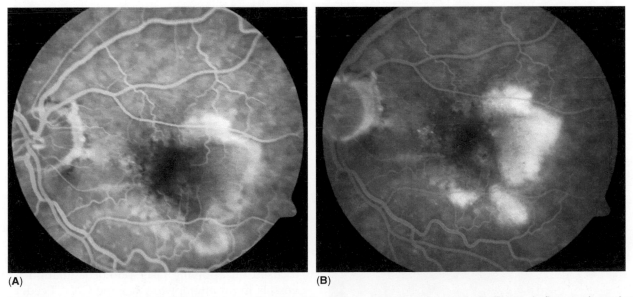

(A) (B)

Figure 9.18 Fibrovascular pigment epithelial detachment. **(A)** The subfoveal area shows hyperfluorescence. The early fluorescein angiographic frame shows hyperfluorescence with some stippled fluorescence. On stereo viewing (not shown) irregular elevation of the retinal pigment epithelium is seen within the area of leakage. The leakage is not as bright as that seen by the same phase of classic choroidal neovascularization. **(B)** On the late fluorescein angiographic frame, at five minutes, more intense fluorescein leakage is seen in this area.

reasonable to treat active CNV even if it is not of recent onset. In the phase I/II ranibizumab trials, nine of the 11 eyes in the untreated group were switched to treatment at day 98. Even at that delayed time interval between onset of CNV and therapy, these eyes experienced a mean visual acuity improvement at six months (7.3 ± 13.1 letters for

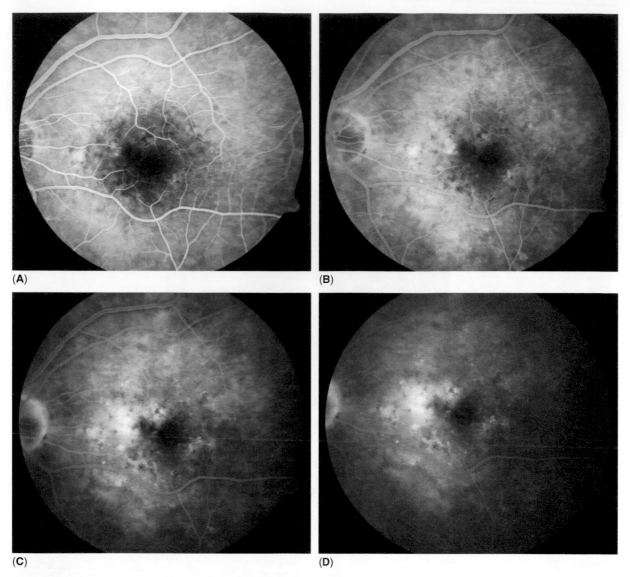

Figure 9.19 Late leakage of undetermined source. **(A, B)** The earlier angiographic frame show no evidence of leakage. **(C, D)** On the late angiographic frames, areas of fluorescein dye leakage appear. This area shows no corresponding area of leakage on the early angiographic frames. The leakage is extrafoveal.

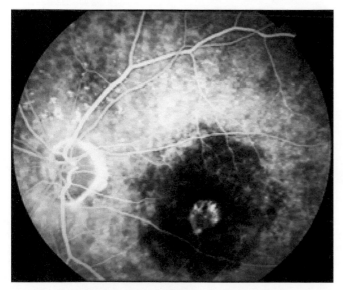

Figure 9.20 Juxtafoveal choroidal neovascularization (CNV). The fluorescein angiography (FA) shows that the closest edge to the foveal center is within the foveal avascular zone. Note however that the edge of the CNV does not involve the foveal center itself.

those switched to 0.3 mg ranibizumab and 3.2 ± 9 letters in the 0.5 mg group).

Feeder Vessels

A feeder vessel is a choroidal vessel that connects the CNV to the underlying choroidal vasculature thus supplying blood to the CNV membrane. Green has suggested that there are two to three feeder vessels crossing Bruch's membrane per CNV (85). Feeder vessels are sometimes ophthalmoscopically visible within the CNV lesion (see chapter 24 for more details). Recent work has focused on applying laser photocoagulation to feeder vessels in an attempt to close the CNV. Feeder vessels have been reported to be present in 15% of cases of CNV. Shiraga and coworkers first reported identification and photocoagulation of feeder vessels using ICG video angiography via a scanning laser ophthalmoscope (86). In 70% of the patients, the neovascular findings resolved; visual acuity improved or stabilized in 68% of patients. Later, Staurenghi and coworkers verified the superiority of dynamic ICG angiography with an scanning laser ophthalmoscope system for identifying feeder vessels in subfoveal CNV (87). Dynamic ICG can detect smaller feeder vessels and enable more targeted treatment of these vessels with a 75% success rate (88).

However, it is possible to detect more feeder vessels in eyes with CNV, using high-speed high-resolution digital angiography. The combined ICG angiography/ dye-enhanced photocoagulation system allows one to synchronize photocoagulation with the arrival of the dye bolus at a targeted vessel site. With the advent of anti-angiogenesis therapies, this method is not often used to treat neovascular AMD.

Pathogenesis of CNV

The pathogenesis of CNV is not fully understood at this time. However it is well accepted that angiogenic factors, such as VEGF, has a primary role in the initiation and maintenance of CNV. There are also non-VEGF pathways that are being elucidated. Chapters 4 and 20 (on VEGF and non-VEGF anti-angiogenesis pathways in the treatment of AMD) explain and discuss these pathways in excellent detail. The primary stimulus resulting in the increase in angiogenic factors remains unknown.

Clues to the pathogenesis of CNV are available from surgically excised membranes (52,53). The most consistent pathological finding is accumulation of abnormal extracellular matrix (ECM) resulting in diffuse thickening of Bruch's membrane (55). Focal areas of thickening form drusen and this diffuse thickening suggests an altered metabolism of the ECM. The available data suggest that altered ECM of RPE cells causes increased secretion of angiogenic growth factors that could contribute to the growth of CNV (52,53). Iatrogenic breaks of Bruch's membrane in animals have led to animal models of CNV (89). Laser-induced CNV in primates has been used to investigate the mechanisms of CNV production and the role of the RPE (90). Chapter 1 (Histopathology of AMD) discusses these changes in detail. It is known that RPE cells produce VEGF and fibroblast growth factor 2. Both are present in fibroblastic cells and in transdifferentiated RPE cells of surgically excised CNV (91–93). Healthy photoreceptors are needed to prevent the choriocapillaris from responding to excess VEGF (94). In addition, inflammatory cells are now felt to be key ingredients to CNV development. In a murine laser-induced model of CNV, CNV volume was significantly suppressed when inflammatory mechanisms were inhibited (95). Angiotensin II type I receptor (AT1-R) signaling blockade with telmisartan inhibited macrophage infiltration and upregulation of VEGF, intercellular adhesion molecule-1 (ICAM-1), monocyte chemoattractant protein-1, and interleukin-6 in the RPE–choroid complex. This research showed that AT1-R-mediated inflammation plays a pivotal role in the development of CNV. Perhaps, AT1-R blockade may serve as another therapeutic strategy to inhibit CNV.

The fact that VEGF is present in CNV has led to the development of drugs that bind VEGF (antibodies or aptamer) or its receptor or drugs that block VEGF signaling. Blockage of VEGF signaling has been shown to inhibit the development of CNV in the laser-induced CNV mouse model (96,97), Initially it was thought that VEGF 165 was the most significant VEGF isoform for CNV. This led to the development of an aptamer to bind VEGF 165 that was used as a treatment for CNV in AMD patients (98). Later, anti-VEGF antibodies were created to treat CNV (99,100). The results of the clinical trials evaluating these treatments will be discussed later in this chapter.

POLYPOIDAL CHOROIDAL VASCULOPATHY

Polypoidal choroidal vasculopathy (PCV) has been classified as a form of CNV that may occur in patients. Yannuzzi and colleagues, in their study, determined the frequency and nature of PCV in patients suspected of harboring neovascular AMD (101). In their prospective study of 167 newly diagnosed patients with neovascular AMD, CNV was diagnosed in 154 (92.2%) and PCV in 13 (7.8%). Non-white race (23.1%), absence of drusen (16.7% had drusen) and peripapillary location were felt to distinguish between PCV and AMD. Since then, it is now recognized that PCV occurs in all races (102). PEDs are commonly seen in PCV (Fig. 9.5). ICG angiography is useful in the diagnosis of this entity. A detailed discussion of PCV is given in chapter 10.

RETINAL ANGIOMATOUS PROLIFERATION

One other distinct type of neovascular AMD is retinal angiomatous proliferation (RAP). This entity is characterized by an anomalous retinal vascular complex which is most commonly associated with retinal and subretinal neovascularization (103,104). It has been described predominantly in elderly Caucasians and is often seen bilaterally. While its natural history is not fully understood, it is thought to progress ultimately to a disciform scar. Prior to the recognition of this entity, it was often misdiagnosed as occult CNV.

A three-stage classification system of RAP has been proposed by Yannuzzi and colleagues to describe the various clinical presentations and to theorize on the disease's natural history (104). In stage I, a nodular mass of intraretinal neovascularization is seen and originates from the deep capillary plexus in the paramacular area. There is usually one or more associated retinal vessels which either perfuse or drain the vascular complex. Intraretinal hemorrhages and intraretinal edema are often present. FA typically shows a focal area of staining corresponding to the intraretinal neovascularization. Surrounding leakage is present and often misinterpreted as occult CNV. ICG angiography can aid in the diagnosis by identifying the neovascularization as a focal "hot spot" and intraretinal cystic spaces as focal hyperfluorescent areas.

Stage II, subretinal neovascularization, involves both retinal and subretinal vascular proliferation. The neovascularization occurs in a tangential direction with minimal horizontal extension. Other common signs include increased intraretinal edema, neurosensory

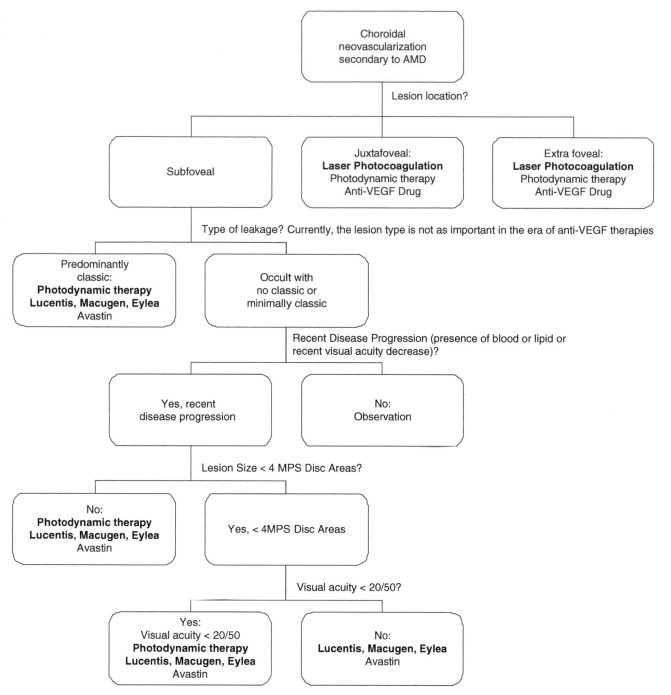

Figure 9.21 Flowchart illustrating treatment options for choroidal neovascular membranes in age-related macular degeneration (AMD) patients. Bold = efficacy proven in phase 3 clinical trials.

retinal detachment, serous PED, and preretinal and subretinal hemorrhages. In many cases, a clear retinal–retinal anastomosis can be seen. FA often shows a diffuse area of leakage which is, again, often misinterpreted as occult CNV.

Stage III of RAP is defined by the stage II findings plus the clear presence of CNV (Fig. 9.21). This is most often documented by the presence of an FVPED or a prior disciform scar. Occasionally, the presence of a retinal–choroidal anastomosis helps confirm the staging. OCT images representative of RAP are found in chapter 14 (Figs. 14.3, 14.4). RAP is discussed in detail in chapter 11.

PROGNOSTIC IMPLICATIONS OF NEOVASCULAR AMD: NATURAL HISTORY OF UNTREATED CNV

The natural history of untreated CNV in the setting of AMD is well established in both retrospective reviews and prospective randomized controlled clinical trials. Untreated, eyes with CNV usually lose visual acuity unless the neovascular complex is not near the foveal area or if it spontaneously scars before reaching the parafoveal regions. The location (extrafoveal, juxtafoveal, and subfoveal) of the CNV is linked with the visual acuity prognosis. Obviously, subfoveal CNV causes more immediate visual symptoms than lesions further away from the foveal center.

Natural History of Extrafoveal CNV

The Macular Photocoagulation Study (MPS) on extrafoveal CNV provides us with robust natural history outcome data for eyes with similar baseline characteristics and extrafoveal CNV. In the MPS untreated group, initial visual acuity was 20/100 or better in these symptomatic eyes.

When untreated, 50% of affected eyes with extrafoveal CNV had, by the time of the first follow-up visit (three months after enrollment for 98 eyes), already lost two or more lines of visual acuity; 10% had suffered a loss of six or more lines of visual acuity (105). Thus, eyes with classic extrafoveal CNV are at high risk for visual acuity loss without prompt treatment. It is important to realize that patients remain in this non-subfoveal phase for only a short time after the onset of symptoms (106).

At the conclusion of the extrafoveal study, in the untreated (natural history) group, 80% of women and 67% of men lost two or more lines of visual acuity from baseline; 43% of women and 47% of men lost six or more lines of visual acuity from baseline (105). Thus, the natural course of extrafoveal CNV may be visually devastating. Although photocoagulation is not a cure for the majority of eyes, the MPS results as summarized below show that there is a statistically significant benefit to photocoagulation versus observation.

Natural History of Juxtafoveal CNV

Thirteen percent of patients with juxtafoveal CNV in the natural history arm (249 eyes) of the MPS lost six or more lines of visual acuity by three months after enrollment and 58% lost six or more lines by 36 months. The juxtafoveal study included eyes with visual acuity 20/400 or better at entry (107). By five years 61% suffered six or more lines of visual acuity loss (108). Only 9.6% of eyes remained unchanged and 5.9% of eyes gained two or more lines of visual acuity by five years.

Natural History of Subfoveal CNV

The MPS Subfoveal Study is the largest study of the natural history of eyes with subfoveal CNV and initial visual acuity of 20/100 or better. This study found that a majority of eyes will lose significant amounts of visual acuity over time if left untreated. In fact, 77% of patients lost four or more lines of visual acuity at 24 months and 64% lost six or more lines. The smaller the lesion at baseline, the better the initial visual acuity (109).

In the MPS subfoveal trials, eyes with subfoveal CNV were enrolled if initial visual acuity was between 20/40 and 20/320. The visual acuity outcomes were dependent upon the baseline visual acuity and the lesion size. For all of the groups (A–D), visual acuity in the natural history group continued to drop during follow-up.

For lesions one disc area or smaller in size with visual acuity 20/125 or worse and for lesions greater than one and up to two disc areas with visual acuity 20/200 or worse (Group A), 14% of untreated eyes lost six or more lines of visual acuity at three months after enrollment. By one year, 25% lost six or more lines of visual acuity. By four years, 35% lost six or more lines of visual acuity. These were eyes with small lesions and poor visual acuity.

For lesions one disc area or smaller in size with visual acuity 20/100 or better and for lesions greater than one and up to two disc areas with visual acuity 20/160 or better (Group B), 11% of the natural history group lost six or more lines of visual acuity at three months, 19% at six months, 38% at one year, 52% at two years and three years and 55% at four years after enrollment. Thus these eyes with better initial acuity and a smaller lesion size had more visual acuity to lose over time.

For lesions two or more disc areas in size and initial visual acuity 20/200 or worse (Group C), 8% lost six or more lines of visual acuity at six months, 15% at one year, 13% at two years, 16% at three years and 25% at four years. Thus eyes with larger lesions and poorer initial acuity had less visual acuity to lose over time.

For lesions more than two disc areas in size and initial visual acuity 20/160 or better (Group D), 13% lost six or more lines of visual acuity by three months, 26% at six months, 31% at one year, 54% at two years, 45% at three years, and 55% at four years. Eyes with larger lesions and better visual acuity had more visual acuity to lose over time.

MACULAR PHOTOCOAGULATION STUDY

The MPS studies represent the first randomized clinical trials for evaluation of treatments of neovascular AMD. The MPS studies gave us robust natural history data for eyes with classic CNV in various locations. Although laser is now rarely used for treatment of CNV, the results will be summarized here for historic purposes. (Further details are found in chapter 18.) The MPS enrolled patients with classic CNV. However, analysis of the data revealed that eyes were enrolled that had classic CNV associated with occult CNV. The MPS treatment recommendations, however, should apply to eyes with classic CNV. Only about 13% of AMD patients with CNV are eligible for treatment by the MPS criteria (110). Patients should be informed that laser treatment results in a permanent scotoma (location, size, and effect on central vision function such as reading) and that there is a high risk of persistent CNV (CNV seen within six weeks of treatment after closure) or recurrent CNV (CNV developing after six weeks of treatment and initial closure). In the current era of anti-vascular endothelial growth factor (VEGF) intravitreal therapy, laser photocoagulation should be considered only for non-subfoveal lesions, particularly extrafoveal lesions.

Extrafoveal CNV

The original MPS report on the efficacy of laser photocoagulation for extrafoveal CNV in the setting of AMD was published in 1982 (105). That study showed an overwhelmingly positive effect of laser treatment for extrafoveal CNV (200–2500 μm from the foveal center). Eligibility criteria included patient age of 50 years or more, best corrected visual acuity at least 20/100, presence of drusen, symptoms due to the CNV, no prior laser treatment, and no other eye diseases that could affect visual acuity. Treatment was applied to the entire CNV and all surrounding blocked fluorescence (based on FA) or subretinal blood. The treatment, performed with 200 μm spots of 0.5 second duration argon blue-green laser, extended 100–125 μm on all sides of the CNV beyond blood, pigment, or blocked fluorescence. The intention was to treat any occult CNV in those regions.

After 18 months' follow-up, 60% of untreated eyes versus 25% of treated eyes suffered severe visual loss (p < 0.001) (severe visual loss was defined as a loss of six or more lines of visual acuity). The study recruitment was halted at 18 months because of this overwhelming treatment benefit and control group patients were offered laser treatment if there were eligible lesions. This report which was the first randomized controlled multicenter clinical trial for the treatment of AMD led to a firm treatment recommendation of laser photocoagulation for extrafoveal CNV due to AMD (105). Three years' and five years data later confirmed the long-term efficacy of laser photocoagulation in treated versus control, despite development of recurrent CNV in the treated eyes (111). Recurrent CNV occurred in 54% of the eyes; these eyes had worse visual acuity outcomes than eyes without recurrences. At the time of the study, no treatment was possible for the eyes that developed subfoveal recurrent CNV. Now, with our current armamentarium of anti-VEGF therapies, better visual results would be expected even in eyes with the subfoveal CNV (98–100,112).

Juxtafoveal CNV

The MPS juxtafoveal AMD studies showed that krypton laser photocoagulation for juxtafoveal CNV was effective for prevention of moderate and severe visual acuity loss. This study incorporated krypton red laser because the red wavelength would not be absorbed by the xanthophyll as much as blue laser light and was thus felt to be safer. CNV lesions lying between 1 and 199 μm off the foveal center or CNV located between 200 and 2500 μm off the center with associated blood or blocked fluorescence within 200 μm of the FAZ center were enrolled. Peripapillary CNV was eligible if the required laser photocoagulation would spare at least 1.5 clock hours along the temporal half of the disc. Treatment of the entire CNV with a 100 μm border was required on the non-foveal border and in areas of blood or blocked fluorescence.

Eighty-six of 174 (49%) treated eyes versus 98 of 169 (58%) observed eyes lost six or more lines of visual acuity at three years (97). At the 36 month visit, 62% of untreated and 49% of treated eyes had visual acuity worse than 20/200 (p = 0.02). The treatment effect depended strongly on the presence or absence of hypertension. Untreated eyes without hypertension were twice as likely to lose six or more lines of visual

acuity compared with treated eyes (64% vs. 31%). This effect was only 1.5 times for the eyes with hypertension (70% vs. 46%). At five years, 71 (52%) of treated eyes versus 83 (61%) of untreated eyes lost six or more lines of visual acuity (95). The effect was greater for normotensive (RR 1.82) than hypertensive (RR 0.93) patients.

The MPS study found 32% of treated eyes showed persistence and an additional 47% of treated eyes developed recurrent CNV within five years after krypton laser to juxtafoveal CNV (113). Eyes without persistent or recurrent CNV maintained 20/80 to 20/100 visual acuity.

Persistent CNV was twice as high when there was 10% or more of the foveal side of the CNV not treated. Central leakage in the MPS studies was not linked to a worse outcome. Forty-one percent of the eyes in the juxtafoveal group did not have adequate coverage of the CNV on the foveal edge in contrast to 14% for the extrafoveal group. The MPS recommended that the visual loss may be reduced by covering the entire CNV lesion with laser treatment. More than 90% of recurrences were on the foveal side following laser treatment of extrafoveal and juxtafoveal CNV.

Subfoveal CNV

Subfoveal CNV was investigated by the MPS group beginning in 1986. Investigators felt that the poor natural history of eyes with subfoveal CNV (109–114) and scattered reports of outcomes of subfoveal laser not resulting in uniformly poor visual acuity warranted trial of photocoagulation of subfoveal CNV lesions (115). In Jalkh et al.'s study of 94 eyes followed up for an average of 15 months, CNV was closed in 88 eyes and visual acuity was stabilized or improved in those eyes (115).

Patients were eligible for inclusion into the MPS subfoveal study if there was some classic CNV, the lesion borders were well defined, the lesion was 3.5 disc areas or less in size, or less than six disc areas (new area of treatment plus old scar) if recurrent CNV was present. Visual acuity had to be at least 20/320 but no better than 20/40. A total of 373 eyes (371 patients) with new-onset CNV and a total of 206 eyes (206 patients) from 13 clinical centers were randomized to laser treatment (argon green or krypton red as assigned during randomization) versus observation. Treatment was performed to all areas of classic and occult CNV within the lesion. Treatment included a border 100 μm beyond the margins for initial treatments or 300 μm into the old treatment scar for recurrent CNV; treatment was based on a fluorescein angiogram not more than 96 hours old. Posttreatment photographs were taken to check adherence to the MPS standards (116).

For treated eyes, visual acuity usually decreased three lines from baseline within three months after treatment and then was stable for 42 months after treatment. In contrast, untreated eyes had less decreased visual acuity initially but continued to decrease throughout the follow-up period. Treated eyes lost 3.3 lines at 12 months versus 3.7 lines for untreated eyes. At 24 months, treated eyes lost 3.0 lines versus 4.4 lines for untreated eyes. At three months, 20% of treated eyes lost six or more lines of visual acuity loss; this remained stable at 42 months. For untreated eyes, 11% at three months had lost six or more lines of vision, but increased to 48% at the 42 months follow-up with p = 0.006. At the 42 months' follow-up, reading speed and contrast sensitivity were better for the treated than untreated eyes (116).

The persistence rate was 24%; recurrence rate was 32% at three years. There was no difference between the argon and the krypton groups. However, persistence and recurrence did not affect visual acuity outcomes, unlike in the extrafoveal and juxtafoveal groups. The three-year rate for subfoveal persistent or recurrent CNV was 56%.

Subgroup analysis showed that treated eyes with smaller CNV lesions (one disc diameter or less) experienced an earlier treatment benefit. Eyes with 20/40 to 20/100 visual acuity lost on average more than four lines of vision post treatment and did not experience any treatment benefit until 18 months later.

For the recurrent CNV subfoveal group, the MPS found a similar treatment benefit. Ninety-seven eyes were treated (49 argon, 48 krypton) and 109 were observed. Treated eyes lost approximately 2.5 lines of visual acuity three months after treatment followed by stable vision for 30 months. Untreated eyes continued to lose visual acuity throughout follow-up such that the average loss was 1.1 lines more than the treated eyes at 24 months. Six or more lines of visual acuity were lost in 14% of treated versus 9% of untreated eyes at three months. This remained about 10% for the treated group but increased to 32% for the untreated group at 18 months of follow-up. Treated eyes retained contrast sensitivity, whereas untreated eyes lost contrast sensitivity.

After thermal laser photocoagulation, patients require close monitoring consisting of visual acuity, Amsler grid, biomicroscopy, and FA to help detect persistent or recurrent CNV. Usually patients are checked three weeks after laser for extrafoveal/subfoveal CNV and two to three weeks after laser for juxtafoveal CNV. The second visit is typically four to six weeks after laser, the third visit is six to twelve weeks after the laser and the fourth visit three to six months after laser. Any symptomatic patient should be examined immediately.

Overall, we no longer recommend thermal laser photocoagulation to patients with subfoveal CNV. PDT and anti-angiogenesis treatments are more efficacious and safe. Instead of an immediate visual loss with laser photocoagulation, these treatments slow down the progression of visual loss in most patients and sometimes even result in improved visual acuity, particularly in the case of anti-VEGF drugs.

OCCULT CHOROIDAL NEOVASCULARIZATION
Natural History
The MPS group reviewed the results of the juxtafoveal study with respect to the presence or absence of occult CNV. In the subgroup, they noted that there were eyes with only occult CNV, occult and classic CNV, and only classic CNV. For eyes with occult CNV that were untreated, 41% within 12 months lost significant visual acuity. Of the 26 symptomatic eyes with occult-only lesions, classic CNV developed in 23% within three months and an additional 23% developed classic CNV by 12 months. For the eyes which developed classic CNV, 58% developed severe visual loss. In the group that did not develop classic CNV, only 18% developed severe visual loss. Overall, 23% of eyes which initially had occult-only CNV lesions remained stable or improved at the 36 months follow-up. Of these, 5% of the occult-only group had a two-line or more increase in visual acuity at 36 months follow-up (117).

Bressler et al. performed a natural history study of 84 eyes in 74 patients with poorly defined fluorescein angiographic CNV (118). The lesions were subfoveal in 89% of the eyes. Initial visual acuity averaged 20/80 and 93% had no classic CNV component. Over a follow-up ranging from 6 to 53 months (mean 28 months), 14% remained stable or improved, 21% lost three to six lines of visual acuity, and 42% lost more than six lines of visual acuity. Additional analysis, which included only those 46 eyes with two or more years of follow-up, similar results were found: 17% remained stable or improved, 22% lost three to six lines of visual acuity and 48% lost more than six lines of visual acuity. Eyes which developed disciform scars had worse visual acuities compared with eyes which had poorly defined CNV and leakage.

Soubrane et al. (119) analyzed visual and angiographic outcomes of 156 patients (82 untreated) with symptomatic occult CNV and initial visual acuity of 20/100 or better. This series excluded eyes with turbid fluid, subretinal blood, PED, or visible CNV. Follow-up ranged from one to eight years. There was no difference between treated and untreated eyes with CNV. Sixty-five percent of eyes with presenting subfoveal CNV had initial visual acuity of 20/50 or better. In this natural history group, visual acuity fell from 20/40 to 20/70. Similar to Bressler et al.'s results (118), when visible new vessels developed, the visual acuity decreased. Treatment, when compared with the natural history group, did not result in better visual acuity outcomes over time (119).

Bressler et al. also evaluated macular scatter (grid) laser treatment of symptomatic eyes with poorly demarcated subfoveal CNV. Visual acuity ranged from 20/25 to 20/320 visual acuity in the 51 treated eyes and the 52 observed eyes (120). For observed eyes, median visual acuity was 20/80 initially and decreased to 20/320 at 24 months. The difference in visual acuity loss was significant between the treated and observed groups only at six months (1.8 lines lost in the observed vs. 3.8 lines lost in the treated group). However, by 24 months, approximately 40% had severe visual acuity loss in both groups; mean change was a loss of 4.3 lines for observed eyes and 4.6 lines for treated eyes. At 12 months, 35% observed and 29% treated had improved or remained stable, with 37% observed and 30% treated losing two to five lines and 28% observed and 41% treated losing six or more lines of visual acuity. At 24 months, 31% observed and 31% treated had improved or remained stable, 31% observed and 28% treated lost two to five lines, and 38% observed and 42% treated lost six or more lines of visual acuity.

Thus, conventional laser photocoagulation (either confluent or scatter) is not beneficial for AMD patients with subfoveal occult CNV. Fortunately, we are now in an era with several effective alternatives to laser photocoagulation. These treatments are not unique to occult CNV and apply to other CNV lesion subtypes.

CURRENT THERAPEUTIC OPTIONS FOR CNV

The last few years have witnessed an explosion in the available non-ablative therapies for subfoveal CNV. The first proven and effective alternative treatment to laser photocoagulation of subfoveal CNV was PDT. Also, data from robust phase III clinical trials demonstrate efficacy and safety of antiangiogenic agents for subfoveal CNV. These agents are capable not only of stabilizing visual acuity but also of improving visual acuity. Experimental therapies are also being developed and are extensively discussed in chapters 19 (Anti-VEGF and Drugs and Clinical Trials) and 20 (Non-VEGF Related Anti-angiogenesis Pathways for Treatment of AMD). An overview of the currently available therapies and experimental therapies follows herein. Currently, FDA-approved therapies for treatment of subfoveal CNV include PDT with verteporfin dye (Visudyne, QLT), pegaptanib sodium (Macugen), ranibizumab (Lucentis), and aflibercept (Eylea, VEGF Trap eye). Retina specialists also use non–FDA approved therapies such as bevacizumab (Avastin) and experimental therapies in clinical trials.

Photodynamic Therapy

PDT utilizes a photosensitizer drug, verteporfin dye (Visudyne, Novartis, East Hanover, New Jersey, USA, QLT, Vancouver, Canada) that is given intravenously and preferentially localizes to CNV. A diode laser is used to deliver the diode wavelength of light (689 nm) to the lesion. PDT was initially demonstrated to be effective for treatment of subfoveal predominantly classic CNV (this comprises more than 50% of the CNV lesion) CNV. PDT treatment of subfoveal CNV offered an obvious advantage over laser photocoagulation, which causes an irreversible scotoma and hence visual acuity loss. The Treatment of AMD with Photodynamic therapy (TAP) study showed PDT with verteporfin for subfoveal CNV resulted in 61% of treated eyes versus 46% of placebo eyes losing less than 15 letters (approximately three lines of visual acuity) at one year. Subgroup analysis showed that eyes with predominantly classic CNV (defined as 50% or more of the lesion as classic CNV) had the best treatment benefit (67% treated vs. 39% placebo lost less than three lines of visual acuity) (121). Two-year results demonstrated continued efficacy with PDT treatment versus placebo (122). For eyes with 50% or less classic CNV, 66% of treated versus 32.5% placebo lost less than

three lines of visual acuity at 24 months. However, with PDT, only a small percentage of patients (16% vs. 7%) gained one or more lines of visual acuity. Thus patients should be told that, although PDT can help prevent severe visual loss, improvement of visual acuity is indeed rare. Despite PDT treatment, a significant proportion of patients will still lose visual acuity. PDT is also useful in situations where the treating ophthalmologist feels that conventional laser (123) could lead to visual loss (e.g., juxtafoveal lesions close to the foveal center) and when there are contraindications for anti-VEGF therapies.

Eyes with occult lesions were studied as part of the Verteporfin in Photodynamic Therapy Study (VIP). The VIP study showed PDT for occult CNV lesions was beneficial at year 2; the one-year data showed no statistically significant difference between Visudyne and placebo, but did show a trend in favor of Visudyne therapy (124). At year 2, 45% of Visudyne eyes versus 31% of placebo eyes (p = 0.03) lost less than three lines of visual acuity and 71% of Visudyne versus 53% of placebo eyes (p = 0.004) lost less than six lines of visual acuity. The treatment effect was best for eyes with 20/50 or less visual acuity and lesion size smaller than four MPS disc areas. Further evaluation of smaller lesion sizes in the Visudyne in Occult CNV (VIO) showed no benefit at year 1 or year 2 (125). PDT treatment is not very beneficial for occult CNV lesions.

The Visudyne in minimally classic (VIM) study evaluated the use of Visudyne PDT using reduced fluence (RF) and standard fluence (SF). RF was investigated as a way to increase selectivity while limiting potential adverse effects to normal tissue. At 12 months, the VIM study showed 14% (5 of 36) of RF eyes and 28% (10 of 36 eyes) of SF eyes, compared with 47% (18 of 38) of placebo eyes (RF, p = 0.002; SF, p = 0.08; RF + SF, p = 0.004) lost three or more lines of visual acuity. At month 24, this loss occurred in 26% (nine of 34) of RF eyes and 53% (17 of 32) of SF eyes, compared with 62% (23 of 37) of placebo eyes (RF, p = 0.003; SF, p = 0.45; RF + SF, p = 0.03) (126). There were more eyes that progressed from minimally to predominantly classic CNV by 24 months in the placebo group than either treatment groups [11 (28%) of 39 patients compared with 2 (5%) of 38 in the RF group (p = 0.007) and 1 (3%) of 37 in the SF group (p = 0.002)]. No unexpected ocular or systemic adverse events were identified. It was concluded that PDT with Visudyne safely reduced the risks of moderate visual loss and progression to predominantly classic CNV for at least two years in individuals with subfoveal, minimally classic lesions due to AMD measuring six MPS disc areas or less.

Combination therapy using PDT with triamcinolone or with antiangiogenic agents has been tried. Although initial case reports show a decreased number of required PDT treatments as well as improved visual acuity results from combined intravitreal steroid injections with PDT, (127–129), some found no visual benefit but a decreased number of required PDT treatments to close the CNV (129). Recently completed multicenter studies investigating the benefit of intravitreal triamcinolone combinations with PDT found no to little benefit. The DENALI study showed that PDT plus ranibizumab was not non-inferior to monthly ranibizumab with regards to visual acuity, although fewer treatments were needed in the combination group than the ranibizumab monotherapy group (130). The MONT Blanc study demonstrated non-inferiority of combination PDT with ranibizumab *pro re nata* (PRN) therapy (131). However, a decreased treatment burden was not found with combination therapy versus ranibizumab monotherapy. With the Reduced Fluence Visudyne-Anti-VEGF-Dexamethasone in Combination for AMD lesions (RADICAL) study, triple therapy (PDT plus dexamethasone plus ranibizumab) using low-fluence PDT showed the best results. Triple therapy with half-fluence group had a mean of 3 and 4.2 re-treatment visits versus 5.4 and 8.9 visits for ranibizumab monotherapy (p < 0.001) at years 1 and 2 respectively. Details of these studies are found in chapter 23 (Photodynamic Therapy) (132).

Anti-angiogenesis Treatments

As mentioned previously, VEGF plays a major role in angiogenesis. Inhibition of VEGF is therefore a rational treatment approach for CNV therapy. The first anti-VEGF treatment study, the VEGF Inhibition Study in Ocular Neovascularization (V.I.S.I.O.N.) trial used a VEGF aptamer (pegaptanib sodium, Macugen) to treat subfoveal CNV. All lesion subtypes and lesions up to 12 disc areas were included. Patients were randomized to receive an intravitreal injection of Macugen (three does) or to a usual care group. The usual care group allowed the use of PDT for predominantly classic lesions (133,134).

In this study of 1186 patients, the 0.3 mg pegaptanib dose was effective in the prevention of visual loss: 70% versus 55% (p < 0.001) lost less than three lines of visual acuity. Overall, 6% of treated eyes gained three or more lines of visual acuity in the 0.3 mg dose versus 2% in the usual care group. Twenty-two percent of eyes gained one or more lines of vision in the 0.3 mg dose group versus 12% in the sham group. Angiographically, there was a slowing in the rate of the CNV lesion growth, CNV size, and leakage by 30 and 54 weeks. No antibodies were detected against pegaptanib. Significant ocular adverse events in the Macugen-treated eyes included endophthalmitis in 1.3% patients, vitreous floaters in 33%, and anterior chamber inflammation. The 0.3 mg dose of Macugen was approved for use for subfoveal CNV due to AMD in 2005. The importance of aseptic technique and avoidance of injection into eyes with anterior segment infections were other lessons learned during the V.I.S.I.O.N. trial. Exploratory subgroup analysis of the V.I.S.I.O.N. trial results showed Macugen was effective for all subgroups and that no single subgroup drove the efficacy results. The use of PDT could have enhanced the usual care group results and lessened the differences between treatment and usual care. This was the first time that a CNV treatment was independent of lesion subtype. The benefit was maintained at year 2

(133). Macugen has been shown to be quite safe, with low rates (about one per thousand injections) of endophthalmitis. The continuous treatment group of eyes did better than the group of eyes in which treatment was halted after one year (and then allowed to resume treatment if losing ten or more letters).

A subgroup analysis of early lesions was subsequently performed (134). Two groups of early lesions were identified: group 1 included small lesions less than two disc areas in size, with >54 letters, without prior therapy and without scarring or atrophy. Group 2 included occult only lesions without lipid and with better visual acuity than the fellow eye. For these early lesions, there was a better response to Macugen therapy. For group 1, 76% of treated eyes versus 50% of usual care eyes lost <15 letters (p = 0.03). Twelve percent of treated and 4% of usual care eyes gained 15 or more letters. For group 2 eyes, 80% of treated versus 57% of usual care eyes lost < 15 letters (p = 0.05). Twenty percent of treated eyes and 0% of usual care eyes gained 15 or more letters.

Another approach to inhibit VEGF uses an antibody directed against VEGF. The first VEGF antibody created for treatment of neovascular AMD was ranibizumab. Ranibizumab (Lucentis) is a humanized monoclonal antibody antigen-binding fragment (Fab) that binds to and neutralizes the biological activities of all known human VEGF-A isoforms including its proteolytic cleavage products. Since ranibizumab blocks all VEGF isoforms, unlike pegabtanib sodium (Macugen), which is an aptamer that specifically binds only VEGF 165, ranibizumab is able to inhibit other stimulators of angiogenesis in neovascular AMD. Ranibizumab was given as an intravitreal injection monthly in the initial clinical trials. In these clinical trials, visual acuity was maintained within three lines of baseline in over 90% of eyes. Visual acuity improved three or more lines in 33–40% of patients (99,100). These one- and two-year studies represented the best visual acuity results than for any prior randomized multicenter clinical trial on neovascular AMD (99,100).

The MARINA (Minimally classic/occult trial of the Anti-VEGF antibody Ranibizumab In the treatment of Neovascular AMD) study was a phase III, multicenter, randomized trial comparing the efficacy of monthly intravitreal injections of ranibizumab compared with sham injections in 716 patients with minimally classic or occult CNV. Eyes were randomized equally to one of three groups: the 0.3 mg ranibizumab, 0.5 mg of ranibizumab, or sham. Approximately 95% (0.3, 0.5 mg) of ranibizumab eyes versus 62% of control eyes maintained or lost less than 15 letters from baseline (p < 0.0001) at one year. Twenty-five percent of 0.3 mg ranibizumab dose eyes and 34% of 0.5 mg dose ranibizumab eyes versus 5% of sham eyes gained three or more letters from baseline at month 12. The results were maintained at two years. Ninety percent of ranibizumab eyes compared with 53% of control eyes lost less than 15 letters (p < 0.0001) at year 2 for the 0.5 mg dose. Thirty-three percent of ranibizumab eyes versus 3.8% of sham eyes gained three of more lines of visual acuity (p < 0.0001) at year 2 for the 0.5 mg dose. Ranibizumab eyes gained an average of 7.2 letters at year 1 and 6.6 letters at year 2 versus control eyes which lost 10.4 letters at year 1 and 14.9 letters at year 2 (99). Anatomic findings (lesion size, area of leakage, OCT thickness) were also in favor of ranibizumab over sham.

The ANCHOR (ANti-VEGF Antibody for the Treatment of Predominantly Classic CHORoidal Neovascularization in AMD) study was a phase III, multicenter, randomized clinical trial comparing efficacy of monthly intravitreal injections of two doses of ranibizumab (0.3 mg, 0.5 mg) with PDT in 423 patients with predominantly classic CNV. Ninety-four percent (0.3 mg) and 96% (0.5 mg) of ranibizumab eyes versus 64% of PDT eyes lost less than 15 letters (p < 0.0001). Forty percent of ranibizumab eyes versus 5.6% of PDT eyes improved at least 15 letters (p < 0.0001) from baseline at one year. The average change was a gain of 11 letters for ranibizumab eyes versus a loss of 9.5 letters for sham eyes at one year (100). This study thus demonstrated the superiority of ranibizumab to PDT for subfoveal CNV lesions.

The PIER (A Phase IIIb, Multi-center, Randomized, Double-Masked, Sham Injection-Controlled Study of the Efficacy and Safety of Ranibizumab in Subjects with Subfoveal Choroidal Neovascularization with or without Classic CNV Secondary to Age-Related Macular Degeneration) study was a phase III study that evaluated the safety and efficacy of intravitreal injections of two different doses (0.3 mg and 0.5 mg) of ranibizumab administered monthly for three doses and then every three months compared with sham for eyes with subfoveal CNV in 184 patients. The one-year results showed no gain in visual acuity gain from baseline in the treated groups versus a loss of 16.3 letters in the sham group (p < 0.0001). Ninety percent of the ranibizumab 0.5 mg dose lost less than 15 letters versus 49% of the sham eyes (p < 0.0001). There was no difference in the percentage of eyes with improvement of 15 or more letters: 15% of ranibizumab eyes versus 10% of sham eyes (p = 0.71) (135). Based on these positive results, the 0.5 mg dose of Lucentis was approved for treatment of subfoveal CNV by the FDA in 2006. The drug was approved for either monthly injection or quarterly injections.

The FOCUS (RhuFab V2 Ocular Treatment Combining the Use of Visudyne® to Evaluate Safety) study was a phase I/II randomized, multicenter, single-masked, controlled study comparing the safety and efficacy of monthly intravitreal injections of ranibizumab (0.5 mg dose) in combination with verteporfin PDT to PDT alone in patients with predominantly classic CNV. PDT was given at baseline and then on an as-needed basis every three months. Eyes receiving ranibizumab and PDT did better than the eyes receiving PDT alone; 90.5% of combination eyes lost less than 15 letters from baseline as compared with 68% of PDT eyes (p = 0.0003) (136). Approximately 24% of ranibizumab and PDT eyes gained 15 letters from baselines as compared with 5% of PDT eyes (p = 0.0033). Subsequent combination PDT plus ranibizumab versus PDT-alone studies

showed no benefit to using combination PDT therapy versus monotherapy with ranibizumab. More detailed information is available in chapters 22 and 23 (Combination Therapy for AMD and PDT chapters).

In all of the ranibizumab studies, the rates of serious adverse events were low. The incidence of hypertension and thromboembolic events did not differ significantly between the ranibizumab-treated patients and the sham or PDT groups. The incidence of endophthalmitis was low, typically between 1% and 2% for the duration of the study. Ocular serious adverse events occurred in 0.1% of intravitreal injections.

Bevacizumab (Avastin®) has been used off-label for treatment of CNV in AMD patients. Avastin is a full-length anti-VEGF antibody, which contrasts with ranibizumab, which is a VEGF antibody fragment specifically developed for intraocular use. Bevacizumab is FDA approved for use in metastatic colorectal cancer and has significant systemic side effects, including hypertension and increased thromboembolic events, when given intravenously in cancer patients (137,138). In the open label Systemic Avastin for Neovascular AMD (SANA) trial, patients with progressive visual loss who were ineligible for PDT were given intravenous bevacizumab (139,140). Based on the risks of bevacizumab therapy, patients were excluded if they had uncontrolled hypertension, a history of thromboembolic events, current anticoagulation therapy, or proteinuria, or if elective surgery was planned within three months. Patients were followed weekly initially and then monthly. Significant improvements in visual acuity and decreased retinal thickness on OCT were seen. Ten of the 18 patients required medication or adjustment of existing medication for systemic hypertension. These systemic side effects led to the exploratory use of intravitreal injection of bevacizumab to treat CNV in AMD patients.

Intravitreal use of bevacizumab involves both an off-label application of the drug and an alternative route of drug delivery. Rapid visual acuity improvement and decreased retinal thickness (139–142) have led to widespread use in the retinal community. The main force driving intravitreal bevacizumab usage is the high percentage of patients who experience symptomatic relief from active subfoveal CNV. The National Eye Institute's (NEI) Comparison of Treatment Trial (CATT) study, directly compared the efficacy and safety of bevacizumab to ranibizumab in monthly and PRN dosing regimens in patients with subfoveal CNV in AMD eyes. This study showed that bevacizumab was non-inferior to ranibizumab in both monthly and PRN dosing regimen comparisons. However, the visual acuity results at year 1 were inconclusive (not non-inferior) for PRN bevacizumab compared with monthly ranibizumab. PRN dosing for ranibizumab was equivalent to monthly ranibizumab. However, PRN bevacizumab was again inconclusive as compared with monthly bevacizumab. In addition, the OCT data showed the greatest reduction from baseline in central subfield thickness occurred in the monthly ranibizumab groups. Interestingly, there were more hospitalizations for the bevacizumab treated patients at year one. No other new adverse events were noted. The year 2 CATT results showed similar findings (visual acuity, OCT, and adverse events) to year 1 (143,144).

The newest drug to be approved for treatment of neovascular AMD is VEGF trap or aflibercept (Eylea). VEGF Trap inhibits all members of the VEGF family: VEGF-A, -B, -C, -D as well as placental growth factors 1 and 2. VEGF Trap is a recombinant, chimeric, VEGF receptor fusion protein. The binding domains of VEGFR-1 and VEGFR-2 are combined with the Fc portion of immunoglobulin G to create a stable, soluble, high-affinity inhibitor. VEGF trap binds VEGF-A with a higher affinity (Kd <1 pmol/L) than currently available anti-VEGF drugs (145). Whether the broader spectrum and higher affinity of VEGF Trap equates to improved efficiency (longer treatment intervals) versus PRN ranibizumab or PRN bevacizumab in the treatment of neovascular AMD is yet to be determined.

The CLEAR-AMD 1 study was a randomized, multicenter, placebo-controlled, dose-escalation study designed to assess the safety, tolerability, and bioactivity of VEGF Trap (146). In this study, 25 AMD patients with subfoveal CNV with lesions less than 12 disc areas in size and more than 50% active leakage were enrolled. Patients were randomized to receive either placebo or one of three doses of VEGF Trap (0.3-, 1.0-, or 3.0 mg/kg) as a single IV dose, followed by a four-week observation period. Three additional doses were given two weeks apart. Dose-limiting toxicity was observed in two of five patients treated with the 3.0 mg/kg dose. One patient developed grade 4 hypertension and the other developed grade 2 proteinuria. The maximum tolerated IV dose of VEGF Trap was 1.0 mg/kg. Reduced leakage on FA and reduced retinal thickening on OCT were observed in the treated patients. No corresponding reduction in CNV lesion size or improvement in visual acuity was observed in these patients over the short 71-day study period. Due to the systemic side effects, the next study done with VEGF Trap utilized intravitreal administration.

The Clinical Evaluation of Anti-angiogenesis in the Retina Intravitreal Trial (CLEAR-IT 1) study assessed the safety, tolerability and bioactivity of VEGF Trap administered as an intravitreal injection in a phase 1 six week, sequential cohort, single-ascending-dose (0.05 to 4 mg) study in patients with neovascular AMD (147). The study enrolled 21 patients using the same inclusion criteria as CLEAR-AMD 1, and randomized them to receive one of six doses of VEGF Trap as single intravitreal injection: 0.05, 0.15, 0.5, 1.0, 2.0, or 4.0 mg. After 43 days of follow-up, no adverse ocular or systemic events were observed. Mean decrease in excess foveal thickness for all patients was 72%. The mean increase in ETDRS visual acuity was 4.75 letters and visual acuity remained stable or improved in 95% of patients. In fact, three out of six patients treated with the higher doses (2.0 or 4.0 mg) gained ≥ 3 lines of visual acuity by day 43.

Monthly dosing was compared with other regimens in the CLEAR-IT 2 study. This study showed that monthly dosing resulted in greater improvements in visual acuity and retinal thickness than quarterly dosing at week 12 and resulted in the recommendation of an intensive monthly loading dose phase, which was used in the phase 3 VEGF Trap-Eye Investigation of Efficacy and safety in Wet age-related macular degeneration 1 and 2 (VIEW 1 and VIEW 2) clinical trials (148). In addition, the PRN phase beginning at week 12 showed that visual acuity results were maintained with less frequent dosing. The 52-week results of the CLEAR-IT 2 study suggest that VEGF Trap-Eye has an extended duration of action. The average time from last mandatory injection to first PRN injection for all groups combined was greater than four months and for the 2 mg every-4-week group, greater than five months.

The VIEW-1 and VIEW-2 studies compared VEGF Trap at doses of 0.5 mg and 2 mg every 4 weeks and 2 mg every 8 weeks after 3 initial monthly doses, with ranibizumab 0.5 mg every 4 weeks during year 1 (149). In the second year, a PRN capped dosing regimen was used (minimum of one injection every 12 weeks). This was a non-inferiority study. At one year, the VIEW 1 (1217 patients) and VIEW 2 (1240 patients) studies showed VEGF-Trap was non-inferior to ranibizumab. In VIEW-1, 96%, 95%, and 95% of the VEGF Trap-Eye 0.5 mg monthly, 2 mg monthly, and 2 mg every 8 weeks groups, respectively, lost less than 15 letters (maintained vision) at one year compared with 94% of ranibizumab eyes. In VIEW-2, 96% of eyes in all VEGF Trap Eye dose groups maintained vision compared with 94% of the ranibizumab group. The visual acuity gain from baseline in the VEGF Trap 2 mg every eight weeks group was 7.6 letters at week 96 compared with 8.4 letters at week 52. Patients received a mean of 11.2 injections over two years; 4.2 injections occurred during the second year. The visual acuity gain from baseline in the monthly ranibizumab group at week 96 was 7.9 letters compared with 8.7 letters at week 52, with an average of 16.5 injections over two years and 4.7 injections during the second year. OCT findings paralleled the visual acuity results. No additional safety signals were found for VEGF Trap. These positive results led to the approval of VEGF Trap in 2011.

The proportion of patients who required frequent injections (six or more) during the second year was lower in the EYLEA 2 mg-every-eight-week group compared with the ranibizumab group (15.9% vs. 26.5%). In the 25% of patients who required the most intense therapy (the greatest number of injections), patients in the EYLEA 2 mg-every-eight-week group required an average of 1.4 fewer injections in the second year compared with the ranibizumab group (6.6 versus 8.0). In the 25% of patients in each group who had the fewest number of injections in the second year, the average number of injections was similar (approximately three for both groups, corresponding to the protocol-mandated minimum number of injections). In the second year of the studies, patients were treated with the same dose per injection as in the first year and were evaluated monthly to determine the need for re-treatment. The current treatment paradigm using these medical treatments is illustrated in Figure 9.21. Treatments with proven efficacy are shown in boldface.

Thermotherapy

Other treatments for subfoveal neovascular AMD include thermotherapy, radiation therapy, other forms of anti-angiogenesis therapy, submacular surgery, submacular surgery with RPE transplantation surgery and translocation surgery. Some of these alternative therapies have shown no benefit whereas others, such as alternative anti-angiogenesis treatments, have shown visual acuity improvement in eyes with CNV.

Thermotherapy (TTT) is the treatment by which a modified diode laser is used to deliver heat to the choroid and RPE through the pupil. Prior success has been demonstrated for treatment of small choroidal melanoma and retinoblastoma with this method (150,151). Reichel and colleagues (152) performed a pilot study in which 16 eyes of 15 patients with occult CNV were treated with TTT. Over a mean follow-up time of 12 months, 19% improved by two or more lines of visual acuity, 56% remained the same, and 25% lost two or more lines of visual acuity. Ninety-four percent showed decreased exudation despite the visual acuity results. Reichel and coworkers have since performed a multicenter, double-masked, placebo-controlled trial, the TTT4CNV trial. The TTT4CNV trial enrolled 303 patients with small (≤ 3 mm) occult subfoveal CNV with visual acuities ranging from 20/50 to 20/400. Patients randomized to treatment received 800 mW TTT over 60 seconds using a 3 mm spot size from the Iris OcuLight SLx 810 nm laser and the large spot size slit lamp adapter. Compared with placebo eyes, treated eyes did not show a beneficial effect on prevention of moderate visual loss at one year. However, for the subgroup of eyes (41% at baseline) with 20/100 or worse visual acuity at baseline, 23% of treated eyes gained one or more lines of visual acuity and 14% gained three of more lines of visual acuity at one year. No further studies are planned using TTT (153) and this treatment is mostly of historical significance in the era of anti-VEGF therapies.

Radiation

Radiation therapy has been advocated as a therapy for neovascular AMD as it is vasculocidal, anti-inflammatory, and also anti-fibrotic. Low-dose radiation inhibits neovascularization (154–156). The key factor in the use of radiation therapy is achieving a balance between destruction of abnormal CNV tissue and preservation of normal retinal and choroidal blood vessels (157). Since proliferating tissues are more radiosensitive, this balance is theoretically achievable. Conflicting data about the efficacy and morbidity of radiation therapy led to the Age-related Macular Degeneration Radiation Trial (AMDRT). AMDRT was an NEI-sponsored pilot study comparing observation to radiation for neovascular AMD. The AMDRT enrolled patients with lesions not amenable to laser treatment (classic, occult, or mixed). No clinically significant difference was found between eyes assigned to radiation and those to observation (158). At 6 months, 9 radiated eyes (26%) and 17 observed eyes (49%) lost ≥ 3 lines of visual acuity [p = 0.04; stratified chi-square test]. At 12 months, 13 radiated eyes (42%) and 9 observed eyes (49%) lost ≥ 3 visual acuity lines (p = 0.60). The radiated group demonstrated smaller lesions and less fibrosis than the nonradiated group (p = 0.05 and 0.004, respectively) at 12 months. Experimental work continues in this area.

The IRay system uses a low-voltage X-ray source that does not require the same degree of radiation shielding as prior external beam treatments. This system divides the x-ray dose into several separate beams that pass into the eye via different locations on the sclera. Because it uses a lower energy X-ray source, it is administered in the clinic. Clinical trials using the IRay in combination with anti-VEGF drugs are ongoing (159). The INTREPID study (IRay plus aNti-VEGF TREatment for Patients wIth wet AMD) uses a stereotactic delivery (I-Ray,) (IRay system; Oraya Therapeutics Inc., Newark, California, USA) and combines up to 24 Gy with anti-VEGF drugs. More information on the use of radiation for treatment of CNV in AMD can be found in chapter 21 (Radiation Therapy for AMD).

A less penetrating form of radiation, beta particle radiation, has been used in patients with neovascular AMD. The epimacular brachytherapy device (VIDION; NeoVista Inc., Fremont, California, USA) delivers 24 Gy from a strontium 90 source to the macular area during a pars plana vitrectomy (160). This device is approved for treatment of neovascular AMD in the European Union. In a phase 2 multicenter, nonrandomized study using the epimacular radiation therapy device, patients received an intravitreal bevacizumab injection at the time of the surgery and again one month later. Thereafter patients received anti-VEGF therapy as needed, based on disease activity. At two years, 90% (22 of 34) lost less than 15 letters (maintained vision) and 15% (5 of 34) gained 15 or more letters of vision. However, 50% (12 of 24 eyes) of phakic eyes developed cataracts. Removal of the cataract resulted in subsequent improvement of vision in most eyes. At three years, 21% (4 of 19) had gained three or more lines of vision. The number of anti-VEGF re-treatments were markedly decreased (160,161). Further work using epimacular radiation therapy continues. Two prospective, randomized, controlled trials in treatment-naive subjects [CNV secondary to AMD Treated with Beta Radiation Epiretinal Therapy (CABERNET)] and in subjects already treated with anti-VEGF therapy [Macular EpiRetinal Brachytherapy versus Lucentis® Only Treatment (MERLOT)] are in progress. Further details on radiation therapy for neovascular AMD are found in chapter 21.

Surgical Treatments

Pilot studies evaluating submacular surgery for CNV in AMD patients showed some promise and led to the definitive Submacular Surgery Trail (SST). The SST was comprised of four studies, which included a pilot trial. One of the arms of the SST, the recurrent CNV arm, showed no difference between surgery or laser treatment and no further study was recommended (162). The other three arms included new subfoveal CNV associated with AMD (Group N), large subfoveal hemorrhage associated with AMD (Group B), and subfoveal histoplasmosis CNV and idiopathic CNV (Group H). Long-term visual outcomes and recurrence rates after submacular surgery compared similarly with the natural history of untreated CNV. Thus, the SST did not show a benefit for removal of CNV and a modest benefit for subretinal hemorrhage evacuation.

Some groups have combined submacular surgery with RPE transplantation. Since the RPE is often removed during submacular surgery or since RPE atrophy often follows submacular surgical procedures, researchers have been evaluating the efficacy of transplanting RPE cells to repopulate the RPE layer. Loss of the RPE leads to choriocapillaris loss. The details of this technique and the rationale for RPE transplantation are given in detail in chapter 28 (Cellular Transplantation for Advanced AMD). Others are using stem cell techniques. These techniques are discussed in detail in chapter 29 (Novel Therapeutic Interventions: Stem Cell).

Retinal translocation and limited macular translocation surgery (163–169) have been described for treatment of subfoveal CNV. The rationale behind these surgical techniques is to move the macular area from the underlying CNV to a healthier RPE environment. The underlying CNV is thus moved relative to the foveal center and can be treated with conventional laser or surgically removed. Limited macular translocation surgery (164) and 360 degree translocation surgery (167–169) are discussed in detail in chapter 25. In the current era of anti-VEGF therapy, translocation surgery is used less often than in the past.

Low Vision
For patients in whom visual acuity is impaired and no treatment is possible or for whom no treatment possibilities remain, visual rehabilitation is of utmost importance. Low-vision rehabilitation may help these patients best utilize their remaining visual acuity and teach them to utilize ancillary tools such as closed circuit television and magnifiers. These patients should also be reminded that AMD affects central and not peripheral vision. Expectations of the magnitude of benefit achievable with low-vision rehabilitation should be realistically explained to the patient. Further details of the devices and the services available for the low-vision patient are detailed in chapter 30 (Clinical Considerations for Visual Rehabilitation).

Emerging Treatments
Newer mechanisms of anti-angiogenesis treatments continue to be developed. Small interfering (short inhibitory) RNA technology (166–169) targeted against VEGF is being evaluated. Non-RNA inhibitors of VEGF receptor tyrosine kinase activity are in development (170,171).

Tubulin-binding agents, such as combretastatin A-4 phosphate, are in clinical trials (172). Some emerging drugs in development have been pulled from the developmental pipeline because the efficacy is much lower than that of anti-VEGF treatments. This has occurred with squalamine lactate. Exciting work with gene therapy is in progress. One can group these experimental therapies into vascular occlusion therapies, anti-angiogenic agents, and combination therapy with anti-VEGF (discussed earlier), immunomodulators (anti-complement), anti-endothelial cell, anti-pericyte, inhibition of non-VEGF mediated angiogenesis and gene therapy.

Small Interfering RNA
In 1998, Fire and Mello (173) discovered that injection of gene-specific double stranded RNA into cells resulted in potent silencing of that gene's expression. This RNA interference is one of the fundamental mechanisms by which a cell regulates gene expression and protects itself against viral infection. (Fire and Mello were awarded the 2006 Nobel Prize for Physiology and Medicine.)

Double-stranded RNA binds to a protein complex called Dicer. The Dicer cleaves the double-stranded RNA into multiple smaller fragments. A second protein complex called RNA-induced silencing complex (RISC) then binds these RNA fragments and eliminates one of the strands. The remaining strand stays bound to RISC, and serves as a probe that recognizes the corresponding messenger RNA transcript in the cell. When the RISC complex finds a complementary messenger RNA transcript, the transcript is cleaved and degraded, thus silencing that gene's expression.

Researchers have used a small interfering RNA (siRNA) inhibitor of VEGF designed for intravitreal injection for treatment of CNV (172,174,175). A phase I, open-label, dose escalation study of 15 patients revealed no serious ocular or systemic adverse effects at a dose up to 3.0 mg. The drug was later named bevasiranib/Cand5 (Acuity Pharmaceuticals, Philadelphia, Pennsylvania, USA) in the phase II trial, known as the CARE study (Cand5 Anti-VEGF RNAi Evaluation). In this multicenter, randomized, double-masked trial of bevasiranib/Cand5 in patients with CNV secondary to AMD (Brucker et al., Retina Society Meeting, Cape Town, October 2006. Thompson et al. AAO Meeting Las Vegas, November 2006), 127 patients with predominantly classic, minimally classic, or RAP lesions (occult no classic lesions excluded) were randomized to receive one of three doses of the drug (0.2, 1.5, and 3.0 mg) at baseline and at six weeks. The primary endpoint was the mean change in Early Treatment Diabetic Retinopathy Study (ETDRS) visual acuity from baseline at 12 weeks. The drug was found to be safe. At 12 weeks, mean change in ETDRS visual acuity was −4 letters (0.2 mg), −7 letters (1.5 mg), and −6 letters (3.0 mg) for the drug doses respectively. The authors theorized that the disappointing visual results resulted from the fact that bevasiranib/Cand5 only blocks the production of new VEGF and not existing VEGF. They postulated that a baseline combination treatment with a VEGF blocker may be required to "mop up" the pre-existing VEGF load. However, the half-life of VEGF is short and it does not explain why the results were not seen by the 12-week time point.

Subsequently, combination therapy using ranibizumab with bevasiranib was tried in a small group of patients. Three arms were included: ranibizumab alone and two with bevasiranib given two weeks after ranibizumab and then at either 8- or 12-week intervals. In the combination group, ranibizumab was given only twice (baseline and one month later) (170). Further information is not available for this study.

However, there are potentially disturbing aspects to siRNA therapy. Ambati and colleagues have shown in their study that siRNA inhibition may not be selective. In fact, this group showed that siRNAs of 21 nucleotides or larger inhibit CNV in a mouse model (171) due to activation of Toll-like receptor 3, a cell-surface receptor for siRNAs and to immunity pathways. This raises the possibility of widespread inhibition of angiogenesis with potential unanticipated vascular and immune effects.

Receptor Tyrosine Kinase Inhibitors

Non-RNA inhibitors of VEGF receptor tyrosine kinase activity have been identified. The anti-angiogenic properties are being investigated for use in the treatment of systemic malignancy, as well as CNV. One advantage of this class of drugs is the possibility of an oral route of administration, thereby avoiding the ocular complications associated with intravitreal injections. One promising compound is PTK787, which is a nonselective inhibitor of all known VEGF receptors. PTK787 has been shown to inhibit retinal neovascularization in a hypoxic mouse model (176,177). Phase I/II clinical trials of PTK787 (Vatalanib, Novartis, Switzerland) have been done in patients with both solid and hematologic malignancies. A multicenter phase I trial, Safety and Efficacy of Oral PTK787 in Patients With Subfoveal Choroidal Neovascularization Secondary to AMD (ADVANCE) treated the CNV lesions with PDT at baseline, and randomized them to receive concurrent treatment with either 500 or 1000 mg of oral PTK787/Vatalanib, or placebo, once daily for three months. Fifty patients were enrolled and some safety issues were found. (http://clinicaltrials.gov/ct2/show/ NCT00138632?term = ADVANCE&rank = 4).

Pazopanib (GlaxoSmithKline, UK) is a second-generation multitargeted tyrosine kinase inhibitor against all VEGF receptors, PDGFRα, PDGFRβ, and c-kit. Topical pazopanib has been studied in rat CNV models. In this study, the use of pazopanib bid significantly ($P < 0.001$) decreased leakage from the laser-induced CNV by 89.5% and the thickness of the developed CNV lesions was significantly inhibited by 71.7% ($P < 0.001$) (178). An early phase trial is evaluating the pharmacodynamics, safety, and pharmacokinetics of pazopanib eye drops in patients with neovascular AMD. A phase 2 study found that doses of up to 10 mg/mL of pazopanib eye drops were well tolerated. No systemic effects were noted. A study is comparing pazopanib with ranibizumab PRN to placebo with

ranibizumab PRN to ranibizumab active comparator. (www.clinicaltrials.gov/ct2/show/NCT01134055).

Anti-VEGF treatment has enabled a sizeable proportion of treated patients to attain significant visual improvement or to maintain vision. Future research will hopefully continue to build on these advances and make restoration of vision a reality for most of these patients. More details on anti-VEGF for treatment of AMD are found in chapter 19 (Anti-VEGF Drugs and Clinical Trials).

Tubulin Binding Agents

Vascular targeting agents are also being investigated as treatments for CNV. These agents have shown efficacy in causing tumor regression. Combretastatin A-4 is a naturally occurring agent that binds tubulin and causes necrosis and shrinkage of tumors by damaging their blood vessels. A CA-4 prodrug, combretastatin A-4-phosphate (CA-4-P, Zybrestat, Oxigene, South San Francisco), has been tested in two models of ocular neovascularization. CA-4-P is a novel agent that binds tubulin and causes endothelial cells which are normally flat to become round, resulting in narrowing of the lumen and cessation of blood flow in the vessels (179). It is only effective on newly formed blood vessels which have no actin and are therefore susceptible to tubulin structure disruption. CA-4-P increases endothelial cell permeability, while inhibiting endothelial cell migration and capillary tube formation predominantly through disruption of vascular endothelial cadherin/beta-catenin/ Akt signaling pathway, thereby leading to rapid vascular collapse and tumor necrosis (180).

Nambu and coworkers quantitatively assessed the effect of CA-4-P to suppress CNV in transgenic mice with overexpression of VEGF in the retina (rho/ VEGF mice) and mice with CNV due to laser-induced rupture of Bruch's membrane. CA-4-P suppressed the development of VEGF-induced neovascularization in the retina. CA-4-P blocked development and promoted regression of CNV. Therefore, CA-4-P shows potential for both prevention and treatment of ocular neovascularization (181).

Immunomodulators

Local inflammation and activation of the complement cascade is involved in CNV (55–57). Immunomodulators and complement inhibitors are being tried in early phase clinical trials. The rationale is discussed further in chapter 2 (Immunology of AMD). ARC1905 is a selective inhibitor of factor C5 of the complement cascade. Inhibition of the complement cascade at the level of C5 prevents the formation of the key terminal fragments, C5a and the membrane attack complex (MAC:C5b-9) that are responsible for tissue pathology. The C5a fragment is pro-inflammatory. The MAC initiates cell lysis and releases proangiogenic molecules (e.g., PDGF and VEGF). Phase 1 studies are combining anti-angiogenesis agents with ARC 1905.

Another complement inhibitor is POT-4 (Potentia Pharmaceuticals, Louisville, Kentucky, USA), which inhibits complement factor 3 (C3). The ASaP1 study was the first human study of complement inhibition therapy.

In this study, evidence of safety was seen. (http://clini-caltrials.gov/ct2/show/NCT00473928?term = POT4+A ND+macular+degeneration&rank = 1) A phase 2 study was planned.

Pericyte Inhibition

The pericyte is required for vessel maturation in angiogenesis. Platelet-derived growth factor beta (PDGF-B) regulates the recruitment of pericytes (182,183). Researchers have shown that anti-PDGF-B blockade (ARC 126 and ARC 127) in transgenic mice (rho/PDGF-B) results in a marked reduction in epiretinal membrane formation and retinal detachment which would otherwise result in an aggressive model of proliferative retinopathy. These study results suggest a potential application for treatment of CNV (180). E10030 (Ophthotech, Princeton, New Jersey, USA) is an anti-PDGF-B aptamer. A phase 1 study of E10030 and ranibizumab showed evidence of safety and efficacy. In the study, 59% of patients treated with E10030 and ranibizumab gained three or more lines of vision at 12 weeks after the start of therapy. More importantly and interestingly, this phase 1 study was the first to use the drug in neovascular AMD which resulted in a mean decrease of 86% in the area of CNV at 12 weeks (184). A phase 2 trial has enrolled 445 patients.

Endothelial Cell Inhibition

Survival of activated endothelial cells downstream of VEGF signaling involves the interaction of the endothelial transmembrane receptor $\alpha5\beta1$ integrin with the extracellular matrix (ECM) ligand fibronectin. This interaction between activated and proliferating endothelial cells and the ECM proteins via this $\alpha5\beta1$ integrin–mediated mechanism regulates multiple key endothelial cellular processes involved in angiogenesis. Use of a monoclonal antibody to bind and inhibit $\alpha5\beta1$ will interfere with angiogenesis. Volociximab is such an antibody (185). Currently, studies are being conducted in animal models of CNV.

Non-VEGF Pathways

Sphingosine-1 phosphate (S1P) is a bioactive lipid molecule that stimulates endothelial cell migration, proliferation, and survival in vitro. Sonepcizumab is a monoclonal antibody that inhibits S1P. In a mouse model of oxygen-induced retinopathy, intraocular injection of sonepcizumab significantly reduced macrophage influx into ischemic retina and strongly suppressed retinal neovascularization. In a laser-induced CNV mouse model, intraocular injection of sonepcizumab significantly reduced the area of CNV and also reduced fluorescein leakage from the remaining CNV. In a non-human primate model of CNV, intraocular injection of up to 1.8 mg of the sonepcizumab resulted in normal electroretinograms and fluorescein angiograms at four weeks without evidence of structural damage. The authors suggested that sonepcizumab could be considered for evaluation in patients with choroidal or retinal neovascularization (186).

Nicotine has been shown to be a potent stimulator of angiogenesis. This effect is mediated by nicotinic acetylcholine receptors (nAChR) (187). Inhibition via the use of subcutaneous mecamylamine (a nonselective nACHR antagonist) suppressed laser induced CNV in a mouse model (188). The authors also used 0.1% or 1% mecamylamine eye drops in these mice 2 hours prior to inducing CNV with the laser and then twice daily. Mice pretreated with drug had smaller areas of CNV than those treated with vehicle alone at 7 and 14 days later. The use of topical mecamylamine is a potential therapy for CNV. ATG003 (CoMentis) is a topical mecamylamine formulation that is being evaluated in a phase 2 study in AMD patients in combination with anti-VEGF.

Gene Therapy

Gene therapy approaches include delivery of adenoviral vectors contained antiangiogenic proteins such as PEDF or RNA that can attenuate VEGF. Use of adenoviral vectors to continuously deliver the protein would eliminate the need for multiple injections. One approach is to use short hairpin RNA (shRNA) that could attenuate VEGF as a potential therapy for AMD (189). Cashman and colleagues developed several shRNAs from recombinant adenovirus. The investigators found potent shRNA sequences that were able to silence VEGF in human RPE cells by 94% at a 1:5 molar ratio (VEGF to shRNA) and 64% at a 1:0.05 molar ratio. Co-injection of VEGF-expressing viruses into mice with shRNA targeting VEGF led to a substantial (84%) reduction in CNV. shRNA may hold promise as a therapy for AMD.

Campochiaro and colleagues have studied the use of human PEDF to treat CNV. PEDF is one of the most potent known anti angiogenic proteins found in humans. Campochiaro and colleagues have used adenovirus-adsorbed PEDF, Ad(GV)PEDF.11D. The natural blood retinal barrier limits the ability of Ad(GV)PEDF.11D to affect tissues other than those in the eye. Intravitreal administration of Ad(GV)PEDF.11D is a convenient means of delivering PEDF "factories" to the relevant cells within the eye, thus resulting in local PEDF production. In three murine disease models (the laser-induced CNV model, the VEGF transgenic model, and the retinopathy of prematurity model) significant inhibition of neovascularization (up to 85%) was shown with doses of Ad(GV)PEDF vectors ranging from 1×10^8 to 1×10^9 particle units (PUs) (190). Toxicology studies in Cynomolgus monkeys showed a dose-related inflammatory response to Ad(GV)PEDF. A dose of 1×10^8 PU caused no adverse effects, while the inflammatory response observed at 1×10^9 PU was minimal and fully reversible. Higher doses produced increasingly severe inflammatory responses (191).

An open-label, dose-escalation, phase I study investigated the safety, tolerability, and potential activity of intravitreal injection of Ad(GV)PEDF.11D in patients with advanced AMD and CNV with visual acuity 20/200 or worse (192). Twenty-eight patients received a single intravitreal injection of Adenovector pigment epithelium-derived factor 11(AdPEDF.11), at doses ranging from 10^6 to $10^{9.5}$ PU. No serious adverse events related to AdPEDF.11 and no dose-limiting toxicities were found. Signs of mild, transient intraocular inflammation occurred in 25% of patients, but there was no severe inflammation. All adenoviral cultures were negative. Six patients had increased intraocular pressures, which were controlled with topical medications. At three and six months after injection, 55% and 50%, respectively, of patients treated with 10^6 to $10^{7.5}$ PU and 94% and 71% of patients treated with 10^8 to $10^{9.5}$ PU had no change or improvement in lesion size from baseline. The median increase in lesion size at 6 and 12 months was 0.5 and 1.0 disc areas in the low-dose group compared with 0 and 0 disc areas in the high-dose group. These data suggest the possibility of anti-angiogenic activity that may last for several months after a single intravitreal injection of doses greater than 10^8 PU of AdPEDF.11. This study provided evidence that adenoviral vector-mediated ocular gene transfer is a viable approach for the treatment of ocular disorders. Further studies investigating the efficacy of AdPEDF in AMD patients with CNV are planned.

Other researchers have developed vectors that secrete an anti-VEGF molecule, sFLT01, which is delivered by intravitreal an injection of an adenoviral vector, AAV2-sFLT01 (193). AAV2-sFLT01 results in persistent expression and is anti-angiogenic in a murine model of retinal neovascularization. AAV2-sFLT01, when injected intravitreally in a non-human primate model, can inhibit laser induced CNV. It may be an effective long-term treatment for CNV (194).

SUMMARY

The era of improvement of visual acuity as a goal in the treatment of AMD patients with CNV has arrived with the advent of the anti-angiogenesis agents. Ultimately, prevention of CNV must be our goal in order to prevent visual loss in patients with AMD. It is an exciting era in the treatment of neovascular AMD. We now possess in our armamentarium several effective treatments for CNV that can actually improve visual acuity in a significant proportion of patients. Now, we face the problem of the need for frequent intravitreal anti-angiogenesis therapy. Better drug delivery and drug stability for depot therapy are needed. Fortunately, we also are in an era in which exciting new forms of adjunctive therapy or novel drugs may be able to improve our treatment results.

The next decade will undoubtedly usher in even more exciting developments in our battle against neovascular AMD. Basic science research into the pathophysiology of AMD and CNV has resulted in, and hopefully will continue to yield translational discoveries for preventive and innovative targeted treatments against CNV in patients with AMD. Clinical trials investigating the efficacy and safety of these new treatments will continue to decipher useful from non-useful therapy. Perhaps, a combination approach using two or more of the following: anti-angiogenesis agents, anti-inflammatory therapy,integrin antagonists, gene therapy, and basement membrane stabilizers may one day be a preferred treatment for CNV. It is even possible that such agents may some day be used as prophylactic treatment in high-risk eyes. Improved drug delivery into the eye may allow for sustained drug release and thus therapeutic effects with fewer injections (195). Although great progress continues to accrue, much remains to be done in the battle against visual acuity loss and in the quest to restore vision in patients with neovascular AMD.

SUMMARY POINTS

- Neovascular AMD is the major cause of visual blindness in patients with AMD.
- Systemic risk factors associated with CNV include increased age, Caucasian race, and smoking.
- Ocular risk factors associated with increased risk of CNV include 5 or more large sized drusen, confluent drusen, and hyperpigmentation.
- The simplified AREDS scale predicts the risk of CNV over the next 5 years and 10 years based upon the presence of drusen and pigment abnormalities in each eye.
- Symptoms may be absent in the presence of CNV. Amsler grid testing and PHP may help detect problems earlier.
- Prompt evaluation of symptomatic patients is essential for preventing visual loss due to CNV.
- Signs of CNV include subretinal fluid, hard exudates, subretinal hemorrhage or intraretinal hemorrhage, and pigmented subretinal lesions.
- OCT imaging is useful for the detection of intraretinal cystic changes, subretinal fluid, sub-RPE fluid and for monitoring the anatomic response to CNV treatment.
- Anti-angiogenesis treatments result in visual acuity improvements in eyes with subfoveal CNV. Ranibizumab (Lucentis) therapy results in visual acuity improvement in about one-third of patients with new-onset subfoveal CNV.
- Bevacizumab (Avastin), an off-label treatment for neovascular AMD, was shown to be non-inferior to ranibizumab (Lucentis) in the CATT study with regards to visual acuity efficacy and safety at one and two years for both monthly and PRN treatment regimens.
- VEGF Trap (Eylea) when dosed monthly for a total of three treatments and then every 8 weeks is non-inferior to ranibizumab dosed monthly.
- Targeted radiation therapy (IRay x-ray or epimacular beta particle radiation) is being investigated as a treatment for neovascular AMD.
- Newer experimental treatments for neovascular AMD include tubulin-binding agents, immunomodulatory agents (complement inhibitors, sphingosine-1 phosphate (S1P) inhibition), VEGF inhibition by tyrosine kinase inhibitors, non-VEGF inhibition, gene therapy and pericyte inhibition.

REFERENCES

1. Pagenstecher H, Genth CP. Atlas Der Patholischen Antomie Des Augapfels. Wiesbaden: CW Kreiden, 1875.
2. Oeller J. Atlas Seltener Ophthalmoscopischer Bufunde. Wiesbaden: Bergmann JF, 1905.

3. Junius P, Kuhnt H. Die Scheibenformige Entartung Der Netzhautmitte (Degeneratio Maculae Luteae Disciformis). Berlin: Karger, 1926.

4. Holloway TB, Verhoeff FH. Disk-like degeneration of the macula. Trans Am Ophthalmol Soc 1928; 26: 206.

5. Verhoeff FH, Grossman HP. Pathogenesis of disciform degeneration of the macula. Arch Ophthalmol 1937; 35: 262–94.

6. Ashton N, Sorsby A. Fundus dystrophy with unusual features: a histological study. Br J Ophthalmol 1951; 35: 751.

7. Gass JDM. Pathogenesis of disciform detachment of the neuroepithelium. III. Senile disciform macular degeneration. Am J Ophthalmol 1967; 63: 617.

8. Gass JDM. Pathogenesis of disciform detachment of the neuroepithelium. IV. fluorescein angiographic study of senile disciform macular degeneration. Am J Ophthalmol 1967; 63: 645.

9. Blair CJ, Aaberg TM. Massive subretinal exudation associated with senile macular degeneration. Am J Ophthalmol 1971; 71: 639–48.

10. Small ML, Green WR, Alpar JJ, Drewry RE. Senile macular degeneration: a clinicopathologic correlation of two cases with neovascularization beneath the retinal pigment epithelium. Arch Ophthalmol 1976; 94: 601–7.

11. Green WR, Key SN III. Senile macular degeneration: a histopathologic study. Trans Am Ophthalmol Soc 1977; 75: 180–254.

12. Ferris FL, Fine SL, Hyman L. Age-related macular degeneration and blindness due to neovascular maculopathy. Arch Ophthalmol 1984; 102: 1640–2.

13. Leibowitz HM, Krueger DE, Maunder LR, et al. The framingham eye study monograph: an ophthalmological and epidemiological study of cataract, glaucoma, diabetic retinopathy, macular degeneration, and visual acuity in a general population of 2631 adults, 1973–1975. Surv Ophthalmol 1980; 24: 335–610.

14. Hyman LG, Lilienfeld AM, Ferris FL III, Fine SL. Senile macular degeneration: a case-control study. Am J Epidemiol 1983; 118: 213–27.

15. Klein R, Chou CF, Klein BE, et al. Prevalence of age-related macular degeneration in the US population. Arch Ophthalmol 2011; 129:75–80.

16. Friedman DS, O'Colmain BJ, Munoz B, et al. Prevelance of age-related macular degeneration in the United States. Arch Ophthalmol 2004; 122: 564–72.

17. Seddon JM, Reynolds R, Yu Y, Daly MJ, Rosner B. Risk models for progression to advanced age-related macular degeneration using demographic, environmental, genetic, and ocular factors. Ophthalmology 2011; 118: 2203–11.

18. Smiddy WE, Fine SL. Prognosis of patients with bilateral macular drusen. Ophthalmology 1984; 91: 271–7.

19. Gregor Z, Joffe L. Senile macular changes in the black African. Br J Ophthalmol 1978; 62: 547–50.

20. Friedman DS, Katz J, Bressler NM, Rahmani B, Tielsch JM. Racial differences in the prevalence of age-related macular degeneration. Ophthalmology 1999; 106: 1049–55.

21. Leske MC, Wu SY, Hennis A, et al. Nine-year incidence of age-related macular degeneration in the barbados eye studies. Ophthalmology 2006; 113: 29–35.

22. Klein R, Rowland ML, Harris MI. Racial/ethnic differences in age-related maculopathy: third national health and nutrition examination survey. Ophthalmology 1995; 102: 371–81.

23. Varma R, Fraser-Bell S, Tan S, Klein R, Azen SP, Los Angeles Latino Eye Study Group. prevalence of age-related macular degeneration in latinos; the los angeles latino eye study. Ophthalmology 2004; 111: 1288–97.

24. Munoz B, Klein R, Rodriguez J, Snyder R, West SK. Prevalence of age-related macular degeneration in a population-based sample of Hispanic people in arizona: Proyecto VER. Arch Ophthalmol 2005; 123: 1575–80.

25. Choudhury F, Varma R, McKean-Cowdin R, Klein R, Azen SP, Los Angeles Latino Eye Study Group. Risk factors for four-year incidence and progression of age-related macular degeneration: the los angeles latino eye study. Am J Ophthalmol 2011; 152: 385–95.

26. Klein R, Klein BEK, Knudson MD, et al. Prevalence of age-related macular degeneration in 4 racial/ethnic groups in the multi-ethnic study of atherosclerosis. Ophthalmology 2006; 113: 373–80.

27. Stein JD, Vanderbeek BL, Talwar N, et al. Rates of non-exudative and exudative age-related macular degeneration among asian american ethnic groups. Invest Ophthalmol Vis Sci 2011; 52: 6842–8.

28. Vanderbeek BL, Zacks DN, Talwar N, et al. Racial differences in age-related macular degeneration rates in the United States: a longitudinal analysis of a managed care network. Am J Ophthalmol 2011; 152: 273–82.

29. Smith W, Mitchell P. Family history and age-related maculopathy: the blue mountain eye study. Aust NZ J Ophthalmol 1998; 26: 203–6.

30. Klaver CCW, Wolfs RCW, Assink JJM, et al. Genetic risk of age-related maculopathy: population-based familial aggregation study. Arch Ophthalmol 1998; 116: 1646–51.

31. Klein R, Klein BEK, Jensen SC, et al. Age-related maculopathy in a multiracial United States population: the national health and nutrition examination survey III. Ophthalmology 1999; 106: 1056–65.

32. Klein R, Klein BEK, Linton KLP, Demets DL. The beaver dam eye study: the relation of age-related maculopathy to smoking. Am J Epidemiol 1993; 137: 190–200.

33. Smith W, Mitchell P, Leeder SR. Smoking and age-related maculopathy: the blue mountain eye study. Arch Ophthalmol 1996; 114: 1518–23.

34. Delacourt C, Diaz JL, Ponton-Sanchez A, Papoz L. Smoking and age-related macular degeneration. the pola study. pathologies oculaires liees a l'age. Arch Ophthalmol 1998; 116: 1031–5.

35. Khan JC, Thurlby DA, Shahid H, et al. Smoking and age related macular degeneration: the number of pack years of cigarette smoking is a major determinant of risk for both geographic atrophy and choroidal neovascularisation. Br J Ophthalmol 2006; 90: 75–80.

36. Espinosa-Heidmann DG, Suner IJ, Catanuto P, et al. Cigarette smoke-related oxidants and the development of sub-RPE deposits in an experimental animal model of dry AMD. Invest Ophthalmol Vis Sci 2006; 47: 729–37.

37. Mares JA, Voland RP, Sondel SA, et al. Healthy lifestyles related to subsequent prevalence of age-related macular degeneration. Arch Ophthalmol 2011; 129: 470–80.

38. Taylor HR, West SK, Munoz B, et al. The long-term effects of visible light on the eye. Arch Ophthalmol 1992; 110: 99–104.

39. Cruickshanks KJ, Klein R, Klein BEK. Sunlight and age-related macular degeneration: the beaver dam eye study. Arch Ophthalmol 1993; 111: 514–18.

40. The Eye Disease Case-Control Study Group (EDCCS). Risk factors for neovascular age-related macular degeneration. Arch Ophthalmol 1992; 110: 1701–8.

41. Darzins P, Mitchell P, Heller RF. Sun exposure and age-related macular degeneration: an australian case-control study. Ophthalmology 1997; 104: 770–6.

42. Klein R, Klein BEK, Jensen SC, Cruickshanks KJ. The relationship of ocular factors to the incidence and progression of age-related maculopathy. Arch Ophthalmol 1998; 116: 506–13.

43. Pollack A, Marcovich A, Bukelman A, Oliver M. Age-related macular degeneration after extracapsular cataract extraction with intraocular lens implantation. Ophthalmology 1996; 103: 1546–54.

44. Pollack A, Marcovich A, Bukelman A, Zalish M, Oliver M. Development of exudative age-related macular degeneration after cataract surgery. Eye 1997; 11: 523–30.

45. Lanchoney DM, Maguire MG, Fine SL. A model of the incidence and consequences of choroidal neovascularization secondary to age-related macular degeneration: comparative effects of current treatment and potential prophylaxis on visual outcomes in high-risk patients. Arch Ophthalmol 1998; 116: 1045–52.

46. Holz FG, Wolfensberger TJ, Piguet B, et al. Bilateral macular drusen in age-related macular degeneration: prognosis and risk factors. Ophthalmology 1994; 101: 1522–8.

47. Macular Photocoagulation Study Group. Risk factors for choroidal neovascularization in the second eye of patients with juxtafoveal or subfoveal choroidal neovascularization secondary to age-related macular degeneration. Arch Ophthalmol 1997; 115: 741–7.

48. Ferris FL, Davis MD, Clemons TE, et al. A simplified severity scale for AMD: AREDS Report No. 18. Arch Ophthalmol 2005; 123: 1570–4.

49. Age-Related Eye Disease Study Research Group. A randomized, placebo-controlled, clinical trial of high-dose supplementation with vitamins C and E, betacarotene, and zinc for age-related macular degeneration and vision loss. AREDS report no. 8. Arch Ophthalmol 2001; 119: 1417–36.

50. Christen WG, Gaziano JM, Hennekens CH. Design of physicians' health study II—a randomized trial of betacarotene, vitamins E and C, and multivitamins, in prevention of cancer, cardiovascular disease, and eye disease, and review of results of completed trials. Ann Epidemiol 2000; 10: 125–34.

51. Moeller SM, Parekh N, Tinker L, et al. Associations between intermediate age-related macular degeneration and lutein and zeaxanthin in the carotenoids in age-related eye disease study (CAREDS). Ancillary study of the women's health initiative. Arch Ophthalmol 2006; 124: 1151–62.

52. Grossniklaus HE, Miskala PH, Green WR, et al. Histopathologic and ultrastructural features of surgically excised subfoveal choroidal neovascular lesions: submacular surgery trials report no. 7. Arch Ophthalmol 2005; 123: 914–21.

53. Grossniklaus HE, Wilson DJ, Bressler SB, et al. Clinicopathologic studies of eyes that were obtained postmortem from four patients who were enrolled in the submacular surgery trials: report no. 16. Am J Ophthalmol 2006; 141: 93–104.

54. Klein RJ, Zeiss C, Chew EY, et al. Complement factor H polymorphism in age-related macular degeneration. Science 2005; 308: 385–9.

55. Edwards AO, Ritter R III, Abel KJ, et al. Complement factor H polymorphism and age-related macular degeneration. Science 2005; 308: 421–4.

56. Haines JL, Hauser MA, Schmidt S, et al. Complement factor H variant increases the risk of age-related macular degeneration. Science 2005; 308: 419–21.

57. Hageman GS, Anderson DH, Johnson LV, et al. A common haplotype in the complement regulatory gene factor H (HF1/CFH) predisposes individuals to age-related macular degeneration. Proc Natl Acad Sci 2005; 102: 7227–32.

58. Mousa SA, Lorelli W, Campochiaro PA. Extracellular matrix-integrin binding modulates secretion of angiogenic growth factors by retinal pigmented epithelial cells. J Cell Biochem 1999; 74: 135–43.

59. Hageman GS, Gehrs K, Lejnine S, et al. Clinical validation of a genetic model to estimate the risk of developing choroidal neovascular age-related macular degeneration. Hum Genomics 2011; 5: 420–40.

60. Bressler NM, Bressler SB, Gragoudas ES. Clinical characteristics of choroidal neovascular membranes. Arch Ophthalmol 1987; 105: 209–13.

61. Bressler NM, Bressler SB, Fine SL. Age-related macular degeneration. Surv Ophthalmol 1988; 32: 375–413.

62. Moisseiev J, Bressler NM. Asymptomatic neovascular membranes in the second eye of patients with visual loss from age-related macular degeneration. Invest Ophthalmol Vis Sci 1990; 31: 462.

63. Alster Y, Bressler NM, Bressler SB, et al. Preferential hyperacuity perimeter (PreView PHP) for detecting choroidal neovascularization study. Ophthalmology 2005; 112: 1758–65.

64. Goldstein M, Loewenstein A, Barak A, et al. Results of a multicenter clinical trial to evaluate the preferential hyperacuity perimeter for detection of age-related macular degeneration. Retina 2005; 25: 296–303.

65. Loewenstein A, Malach R, Goldstein M, et al. Replacing the Amsler grid: a new method for monitoring patients with age-related macular degeneration. Ophthalmology 2003; 110: 966–70.

66. Valencia M, Green RL, Lopez PF. Echographic findings in hemorrhagic disciform lesions. Ophthalmology 1994; 101: 1379–83.

67. Fine AM, Elman MJ, Ebert JE, et al. Earliest symptoms caused by neovascular membranes in the macula. Arch Ophthalmol 1986; 104: 513–14.

68. Nazemi PP, Fink W, Lim JI, Sadun AA. Electronic amsler grid scotomas of age-related macular degeneration detected and characterized by means of a novel three-dimensional computer-automated visual field test. Retina 2005; 25: 446–53.

69. Srinivasan VJ, Wojtkowski M, Witkin AJ, et al. High-definition and 3-dimensional imaging of macular pathologies with high-speed ultrahigh-resolution optical coherence tomography. Ophthalmology 2006; 113: 2054–65.

70. Giani A, Luiselli C, Esmaili DD, et al. Spectral-domain optical coherence tomography as an indicator of fluorescein angiography leakage from choroidal neovascularization. Invest Ophthalmol Vis Sci 2011; 52: 5579–86.

71. Liakopoulos S, Ongchin S, Bansal A, et al. Quantitative optical coherence tomography findings in various subtypes of neovascular age-related macular degeneration. Invest Ophthalmol Vis Sci 2008; 49: 5048–54.

72. Zweifel SA, Engelbert M, Laud K, et al. Outer retinal tubulation: a novel optical coherence tomography finding. Arch Ophthalmol 2009; 127: 1596–602.

73. Shakoor A, Shahidi M, Blair NP, Gieser JL, Zelkha R. Macular thickness mapping in AMD. Retina 2006; 26: 44–8.

74. Lim JI, Aaberg TM Sr, Capone A Jr, Sternberg P Jr. Indocyanine green angiography-guided photocoagulation of choroidal neovascularization associated with retinal pigment epithelial detachment. Am J Ophthalmol 1997; 123: 524–32.

75. Guyer DR, Yannuzzi LA, Slakter JS, et al. Digital indocyanine green videoangiography of occult choroidal neovascularization. Ophthalmology 1994; 101: 1727–37.

76. Slakter JS, Yannuzzi LA, Sorenson JA, et al. A pilot study of indocyanine green videoangiography-guided laser photocoagulation of occult choroidal neovascularization in age-related macular degeneration. Arch Ophthalmol 1994; 112: 465–72.

77. Elman MJ, Fine SL, Murphy RP, Patz A, Auer C. The natural history of serous retinal pigment epithelium detachment in patients with age-related macular degeneration. Ophthalmology 1986; 93: 224–30.

78. Poliner LA, Olk RJ, Burgess D, Gordon ME. Natural history of retinal pigment epithelial detachments in age-related macular degeneration. Ophthalmology 1986; 93: 543–51.

79. Bird AC, Marshall J. Retinal pigment epithelial detachments in the elderly. Trans Ophthalmol Soc UK 1986; 105: 674–82.

80. Casswell AG, Kohen D, Bird AC. Retinal pigment epithelial detachments in the elderly: classification and outcome. Br J Ophthalmol 1985; 69: 397–403.

81. Dhalla MS, Blinder KJ, Tewari A, Hariprasad SM, Apte RS. Retinal pigment epithelial tear following intravitreal pegaptanib sodium. Am J Ophthalmol 2006; 141: 752–4.

82. Macular Photocoagulation Study Group. Subfoveal neovascular lesions in age-related macular degeneration: guidelines for evaluation and treatment in the macular photocoagulation study. Arch Ophthalmol 1991; 109: 1242–57.

83. Lim JI, Sternberg P Jr, Capone A Jr, Aaberg TM Sr, Gilman JP. selective use of indocyanine green angiography for occult choroidal neovascularization. Am J Ophthalmol 1995; 120: 75–82.

84. Heier JS, Antoszyk AN, Pavan PR, et al. Ranibizumab for treatment of neovascular age-related macular degeneration: a phase I/II multicenter, controlled, multidose degeneration: a phase I/II multicenter, controlled, multi-dose study. Ophthalmology 2006; 113: 633–42.

85. Green WR, Enger C. Age-related macular degeneration: histopathologic studies. the 1992 Lorenz E. Zimmerman lecture. Ophthalmology 1993; 100: 1519–35.

86. Shiraga F, Ojima Y, Matsuo T, Takasu I, Matsui N. Feeder vessel photocoagulation of subfoveal choroidal neovascularization secondary to age-related macular degeneration. Ophthalmology 1998; 105: 662–9.

87. Staurenghi G, Orzalesi N, La Capria A, Aschero M. Laser treatment of feeder vessels in subfoveal choroidal neovascular membranes. a revisitation using dynamic indocyanine green angiography. Ophthalmology 1998; 105: 2297–305.

88. Flower RW. Optimizing treatment of choroidal neovascularization feeder vessels associated with age-related macular degeneration. Am J Ophthalmol 2002; 134: 228–39.

89. Ryan SJ. Subretinal neovascularization: natural history of an experimental model. Arch Ophthalmol 1982; 100: 1804–9.

90. Miller H, Miller B, Ryan SJ. The role of the retinal pigmented epithelium in the involution of subretinal neovascularization. Invest Ophthalmol Vis Sci 1986; 27: 1644–52.

91. Amin R, Pulkin JE, Frank RN. Growth factor localization in choroidal neovascular membranes of age-related macular degeneration. Invest Ophthalmol Vis Sci 1994; 35: 3178–88.

92. Frank RN, Amin RH, Eliott D, Puklin JE, Abrams GW. Basic fibroblast growth factor and vascular endothelial growth factor are present in epiretinal and choroidal neovascularization membranes. Am J Ophthalmol 1996; 122: 393–403.

93. Lopez PF, Sippy BD, Lambert HM, Thach AB, Hinton DR. Transdifferentiated retinal pigment epithelial cells are immunoreactive for vascular endothelial growth factor in surgically excised age-related macular degeneration choroidal neovascular membranes. Invest Ophthalmol Vis Sci 1996; 37: 855–68.

94. Yamada H, Yamada E, Kwak N, et al. Cell injury unmasks a latent proangiogenic phenotype in mice with increased expression of FGF2 in the retina. J Cell Physiol 2000; 185: 135–42.

95. Nagai N, Oike Y, Izumi K, et al. Angiotensin II type 1 receptor-mediated inflammation is required for choroidal neovascularization. Arterioscler Thromb Vasc Biol 2006; 26: 2252–9.

96. Seo M-S, Kwak N, Ozaki H, et al. Dramatic inhibition of retinal and choroidal neovascularization by oral administration of a kinase inhibitor. Am J Pathol 1999; 154: 1743–53.

97. Kwak N, Okamoto N, Wood JM, Campochiaro PA. VEGF is an important stimulator in a model of choroidal neovascularization. Invest Ophthalmol Vis Sci 2000; 41: 3158–64.

98. Gragoudas ES, Adamis AP, Cunningham ET, Feinsod M, Guyer DR. VEGF inhibition study in ocular neovascularization clinical trial group. pegaptanib for neovascular age-related macular degeneration. N Engl J Med 2004; 351: 2805–16.

99. Rosenfeld P, Brown DM, Heier J, et al. Ranibizumab for neovascular age-related macular degeneration. N Engl J Med 2006; 355: 1419–31.

100. Brown DM, Kaiser PK, Michels M, et al. Ranibizumab versus verteporfin for neovascular age-related macular degeneration. N Engl J Med 2006; 355: 1432–44.

101. Yannuzzi LA, Wong DWK, Sforzolini BS, et al. Polypoidal choroidal vasculopathy and neovascularized age-related macular degeneration. Arch Ophthalmol 1999; 117: 1503–10.

102. Lafaut BA, Leys AM, Snyders B, Rasquin F, DeLaey JJ. Polypoidal choroidal vasculopathy in caucasians. Graefes Arch Clin Exp Ophthalmol 2000; 238: 752–9.

103. Latfaut BA, Aisenbrey S, Broeck CV, Bartz-Schmidt KU. Clinicopathological correlation of deep retinal vascular anomalous complex in age-related macular degeneration. Br J Ophthalmol 2000; 84: 1269–74.

104. Yannuzzi LA, Negrao S, Iida T, et al. Retinal angiomatous proliferation in age-related macular degeneration. Retina 2001; 21: 416–34.

105. Macular Photocoagulation Study Group. Argon laser photocoagulation for senile macular degeneration. Results of a randomized clinical trial. Arch Ophthalmol 1982; 100: 912–18.

106. Grey RHB, Bird AC, Chisholm IH. Senile disciform macular degeneration: features indicating suitability for photocoagulation. Br J Ophthalmol 1979; 63: 85–9.

107. Macular Photocoagulation Study Group. Krypton laser photocoagulation for neovascular lesion of age-related macular degeneration. results of a randomized clinical trial. Arch Ophthalmol 1990; 108: 816–24.

108. Macular Photocoagulation Study Group. Laser photocoagulation for juxtafoveal choroidal neovascularization. five-year results from randomized clinical trials. Arch Ophthalmol 1994; 112: 500–9.

109. Guyer DR, Fine SL, Maguire MG, et al. Subfoveal choroidal neovascular membranes in age-related macular degeneration. visual prognosis in eyes with relatively good initial visual acuity. Arch Ophthalmol 1986; 104: 702–5.

110. Freund KB, Yannuzzi LA, Sorenson JA. Age-related macular degeneration and choroidal neovascularization. Am J Ophthalmol 1993; 115: 786–91.

111. Macular Photocoagulation Study Group. Argon laser photocoagulation for neovascular maculopathy: five-year results from randomized clinical trials. Arch Ophthalmol 1991; 109: 1109–14.

112. Macular Photocoagulation Study Group. Recurrent choroidal neovascularization after argon laser photocoagulation for neovascular maculopathy. Arch Ophthalmol 1986; 104: 503–12.

113. Macular Photocoagulation Study Group. Persistent and recurrent neovascularization after krypton laser photocoagulation for neovascular lesions of age-related macular degeneration. Arch Ophthalmol 1990; 108: 825–31.

114. Bressler SB, Bressler NM, Fine SL, et al. Natural course of choroidal neovascular membranes within the foveal avascular zone in senile macular degeneration. Am J Ophthalmol 1982; 93: 157–63.

115. Jalkh AE, Avila MP, Trempe CL, Schepens CL. Management of choroidal neovascularization within the foveal avascular zone in senile macular degeneration. Am J Ophthalmol 1983; 95: 818–25.

116. Macular Photocoagulation Study Group. Laser photocoagulation of subfoveal neovascular lesions in age-related macular degeneration. Results of a randomized clinical trial. Arch Ophthalmol 1991; 109: 1220–31.

117. Macular Photocoagulation Study Group. Occult choroidal neovascularization. influence on visual outcome in patients with age-related macular degeneration. Arch Ophthalmol 1996; 114: 400–12.

118. Bressler NM, Frost LA, Bressler SB, Murphy RP, Fine SL. Natural course of poorly defined choroidal neovascularization associated with macular degeneration. Arch Ophthalmol 1988; 106: 1537–42.

119. Soubrane G, Coscas G, Francais C, Koenig F. Occult subretinal new vessels in age-related macular degeneration. Natural history and early laser treatment. Ophthalmology 1990; 97: 649–57.

120. Bressler NM, Maguire MG, Murphy PL, et al. Macular scatter ("grid") laser treatment of poorly demarcated subfoveal choroidal neovascularization in age-related macular degeneration. Arch Ophthalmol 1996; 114: 1456–64.

121. Treatment of Age-related Macular Degeneration with Photodynamic Therapy (TAP) Study Group Principal Investigators. Photodynamic therapy of subfoveal choroidal neovascularization in age-related macular degeneration with verteporfin. One-year results of 2 randomized clinical trials—TAP Report 1. Arch Ophthalmol 1999; 117: 1329–45.

122. Treatment of Age-Related Macular Degeneration with Photodynamic Therapy (TAP) Study Group. Photodynamic therapy of subfoveal choroidal neovascularization in age-related macular degeneration with verteporfin. Two-year results of 2 randomized clinical trials—TAP Report 2. Arch Ophthalmol 2001; 119: 198–207.

123. Verteporfin Roundtable 2000 Participants, Treatment of Age-Related Macular Degeneration with Photodynamic Therapy (TAP) Study Group Principal Investigators, and Verteporfin in Photodynamic Therapy (VIP) study group Principal Investigators. guidelines for using verteporfin (Visudyne™) in photodynamic therapy to treat choroidal neovascularization due to age-related macular degeneration and other causes. Retina 2002; 22: 6–18.

124. Verteporfin In Photodynamic Therapy (VIP) Study Group. Verteporfin therapy of subfoveal choroidal neovascularization in age-related macular degeneration: two-year results of a randomized clinical trial including lesions with occult with no classic choroidal neovascularizationverteporfin in photodynamic therapy report 2. Am J Ophthalmol 2001; 131: 541–60.

125. Kaiser PK; Visudyne In Occult CNV (VIO) study group. (Antoszyk A, Bernstein P, Blinder K, Boyer D, Gottlieb J, Halperin L, Hao Y, Joffe L, Lim JI, Rosa R, Strong HA, Weisberger A, Williams G, Wong K.) Verteporfin PDT for subfoveal occult CNV in AMD: two-year results of a randomized trial. Curr Med Res Opin 2009; 25: 1853–60.

126. Azab M, Boyer DS, Bressler NM, et al. Visudyne in minimally classic choroidal neovascularization study group. verteporfin therapy of subfoveal minimally classic choroidal neovascularization in age-related macular degeneration: 2-year results of a randomized clinical trial. Arch Ophthalmol 2005; 123: 448–57.

127. Spaide RF, Sorenson J, Maranan L. Combined photodynamic therapy with verteporfin and intravitreal triamcinolone acetonide for choroidal neovascularization. Ophthalmology 2003; 110: 1517–25.

128. Rechtman E, Danis RP, Pratt LM, Harris A. Intravitreal triamcinolone with photodynamic therapy for subfoveal choroidal neovascularization in age related macular degeneration. Br J Ophthalmol 2004; 88: 344–7.

129. Ergun E, Maar N, Ansari-Shahrezaei S, et al. Photodynamic therapy with verteporfin and intravitreal triamcinolone acetonide in the treatment of neovascular age-related macular degeneration. Am J Ophthalmol 2006; 142: 10–16.

130. Kaiser PK, Boyer DS, Cruess AF, DENALI Study Group. Verteporfin plus ranibizumab for choroidal neovascularization in age-related macular degeneration: twelve-month results of the denali study. Ophthalmology 2012; 119: 1001–10.

131. Larsen M, Schmidt-Erfurth U, Lanzetta P, MONT BLANC Study Group. Verteporfin plus ranibizumab for choroidal neovascularization in age-related macular degeneration: twelve-month MONT BLANC study results. Ophthalmology 2012; 119: 992–1000.

132. QLT Inc. Reduced Fluence Visudyne-Anti-VEGF-Dexamethasone in Combination for AMD Lesions (RADICAL). [database on the Internet]. 2011 [cited 2012 Jan 9]. Available from: ClinicalTrials.gov, Web site: http://clinicaltrials.gov/ct2/show/study/NCT00492284.

133. VEGF Inhibition Study in Ocular Neovascularization (V.I.S.I.O.N.) Clinical Trial Group. Year 2 efficacy results of 2 randomized controlled clinical trials of pegaptanib for neovascular age-related macular degeneration. Ophthalmology 2006; 113: 1508–21.

134. The VEGF Inhibition Study in Ocular Neovascularization (V.I.S.I.O.N) Clinical Trial Group. Enhanced efficacy associated with early treatment of neovascular age-related macular degeneration with pegaptanib sodium: an exploratory analysis. Retina 2005; 25: 815–27.

135. Regillo CD, Brown DM, Abraham H, Kaiser PK, Mieler WF. Randomized, double-masked, sham-controlled trial of ranibizumab for neovascular age-related macular degeneration: PIER study year 1. Am J Ophthalmol 2008; 145: 239–48.

136. Heier JS, Boyer DS, Ciulla TA, et al. Ranibizumab combined with verteporfin photodynamic therapy in neovascular age-related macular degeneration: year 1 results of the FOCUS study. Arch Ophthalmol 2006; 124: 1532–42.

137. Ferrara N, Hillan KJ, Novotny W. Bevacizumab (Avastin), a humanized anti-VEGF monoclonal antibody for cancer therapy. Biochem Biophys Res Commun 2005; 333: 328–35.

138. Salesi N, Bossone G, Veltri E, et al. Clinical experience with bevacizumab in colorectal cancer. Anticancer Res 2005; 25: 3619–23.

139. Michels S, Rosenfeld PJ, Puliafito CA, Marcus EN, Venkatraman AS. Systemic bevacizumab (Avastin) therapy for neovascular age-related macular degeneration twelve-week results of an uncontrolled open-label clinical study. Ophthalmology 2005; 112: 1035–47.

140. Moshfeghi AA, Rosenfeld PJ, Puliafito CA, et al. Systemic bevacizumab (Avastin) therapy for neovascular age-related macular degeneration: twenty-four-week results of an uncontrolled open-label clinical study. Ophthalmology 2006; 113: 2002–11.

141. Rosenfeld PJ, Moshfeghi AA, Puliafito CA. Optical coherence tomography findings after an intravitreal injection of bevacizumab (Avastin) for neovascular age-related macular degeneration. Ophthalmic Surg Lasers Imaging 2005; 36: 331–5.

142. Rich RM, Rosenfeld PJ, Puliafito CA, et al. Short-term safety and efficacy of intravitreal bevacizumab (Avastin) for neovascular age-related macular degeneration. Retina 2006; 26: 495–511.

143. Comparison of Age-related Macular Degeneration Treatment Trials (CATT) Research Group. Ranibizumab and bevacizumab for neovascular age-related macular degeneration. N Engl J Med 2011; 364: 1897–908.

144. Comparison of Age-related Macular Degeneration Treatment Trials (CATT) Research Group. Ranibizumab and bevacizumab for treatment of neovascular age-related macular degeneration two year results. Ophthalmology 2012; 119: 1388–98.

145. Nguyen QD, Shah SM, Hafiz G, et al. A phase i trial of an IV-administered vascular endothelial growth factor trap for treatment in patients with choroidal neovascularization due to age-related macular degeneration. Ophthalmology 2006; 113: 1522–32, 33.

146. Nguyen QD, Shah SM, Browning DJ, et al. A phase i study of intravitreal vascular endothelial growth factor trap-eye in patients with neovascular age-related macular degeneration. Ophthalmology 2009; 116: 2141–8.

147. Brown DM, Heier JS, Ciulla T, et al. Primary endpoint results of a Phase II study of vascular endothelial growth factor trap-eye in wet age-related macular degeneration. Ophthalmology 2011; 118: 1089–97.

148. Heier JS, Boyer D, Nguyen QD, et al. The 1-year results of CLEAR-IT 2, a phase 2 study of vascular endothelial growth factor trap-eye dosed as-needed after 12-week fixed dosing. Ophthalmology 2011; 6: 1098–106.

149. www.fda.gov/downloads/AdvisoryCommittees/.../UCM259143.pdf

150. Godfrey DG, Waldron RG, Capone A Jr. Transpupillary thermotherapy for small choroidal melanoma. Am J Ophthalmol 1999; 128: 88–93.

151. Shields CL, Santos MC, Diniz W, et al. Thermotherapy for retinoblastoma. Arch of Ophthalmol 1999; 117: 885–93.

152. Reichel E, Berrocal AM, Ip M, et al. Transpupillary thermotherapy of occult subfoveal choroidal neovascularization in patients with age-related macular degeneration. Ophthalmology 1999; 106: 1908–14.

153. Reichel E, Musch DC, Blodi BA, Mainster MA, TTT4CNV Study Group. Results from the TTT4CNV clinical trial. Invest Ophthalmol Vis Sci 2005; 46: E-abstract 2311.

154. Archambeau JO, Mao XW, Yonemoto LT, et al. What is the role of radiation in the treatment of subfoveal membranes: review of radiobiologic, pathologic, and other considerations to initiate a multimodality discussion. Int J Radiat Oncol Biol Phys 1998; 40: 1125–36.

155. Del Gowin RL, Lewis JW, Hoak JC, Mueller AL, Gibson DP. Radiosensitivity of human endothelial cells in culture. J Lab Clin Med 1974; 84: 42–8.

156. Hosoi Y, Yamamoto M, Ono T, Sakamoto K. Prostacyclin production in cultured endothelial cells is highly sensitive to low doses of ionizing radiation. Int J Radiat Biol 1993; 63: 631–8.

157. Sagerman RH, Chung CT, Alterti WE. Radiosensitivity of ocular and orbital structures. In: Alberti WE, Sagerman RH, eds. Radiotherapy of Intraocular and Orbital Tumors. Berlin: Springer, 1993: 375–85.

158. Marcus DM, Peskin E, Maguire M, et al. The age-related macular degeneration radiotherapy trial (AMDRT): one year results from a pilot study. Am J Ophthalmol 2004; 138: 818–28.

159. Moshfeghi DM, Kaiser PK, Gertner M. Stereotactic low-voltage x-ray irradiation for age-related macular degeneration. Br J Ophthalmol 2011; 95: 185–8.

160. Avila MP, Farah ME, Santos A, et al. Twelve-month short-term safety and visual-acuity results from a multicentre prospective study of epiretinal strontium-90 brachytherapy with bevacizumab for the treatment of subfoveal choroidal neovascularisation secondary to age-related macular degeneration. Br J Ophthalmol 2009; 93: 305–309.

161. Avila MP, Farah ME, Santos A, et al. Three-year safety and visual acuity results of epimacular 90 strontium/90 yttrium brachytherapy with bevacizumab for the treatment of subfoveal choroidal neovascularization secondary to age-related macular degeneration. Retina 2012; 32: 10–18.

162. Submacular Surgery Trials Pilot Study Investigators. Submacular surgery trials randomized pilot trial of laser photocoagulation versus surgery for recurrent choroidal neovascularization secondary to age-related macular degeneration: I. ophthalmic outcomes. Am J Ophthalmol 2000; 130: 387–407.

163. de Juan E Jr, Loewenstein A, Bressler NM, Alexander J. Translocation of the retina for management of subfoveal-choroidal neovascularization II: a preliminary report in humans. Am J Ophthalmol 1998; 125: 635–46.

164. Fujii GY, Pieramici D, Humayun MS, et al. Complications associated with limited macular translocation. Am J Ophthalmol 2000; 130: 751–62.

165. Lewis H, Kaiser PK, Lewis S, Estafanous M. Macular translocation for subfoveal choroidal neovascularization in age-related macular degeneration: a prospective study. Am J Ophthalmol 1999; 128: 135–46.

166. Pertile G, Claes C. Macular translocation with 360 degree retinotomy for management of age-related macular degeneration with subfoveal choroidal neovascularization. Am J Ophthalmol 2002; 134: 560–5.

167. Mruthyunjaya P, Stinnett SS, Toth CA. Change in visual function after macular translocation with 360 retinectomy for neovascular age-related macular degeneration. Ophthalmology 2004; 111: 1715–24.

168. Fujikado T, Asonuma S, Ohji M, et al. Reading ability after macular translocation surgery with 360-degree retinotomy. Am J Ophthalmol 2002; 134: 849–56.

169. Toth CA, Lapolice DJ, Banks AD, Stinnett SS. Improvement in near visual function after macular translocation surgery with 360-degree peripheral retinectomy. Graefes Arch Clin Exp Ophthalmol 2004; 242: 541–8.

170. Singerman L. Combination therapy using the small interfering RNA bevasiranib. Retina 2009; 29: S49–50.

171. Kleinman ME, Yamada K, Takeda A, et al. Sequence- and target-independent angiogenesis suppression by siRNA via TLR3. Nature 2008; 452: 591–7.

172. Shen J, Samul R, Silva RL, et al. Suppression of ocular neovascularization with siRNA targeting VEGF receptor 1. Gene Ther 2006; 13: 225–34.

173. Fire A, Xu S, Montgomery MK, et al. Potent and specific genetic interference by double-stranded RNA in caenorhabditis elegans. Nature 1998; 391: 806–11.

174. Reich SJ, Fosnot J, Kuroki A, et al. Small interfering RNA (siRNA) targeting VEGF effectively inhibits ocular neovascularization in a mouse model. Mol Vis 2003; 9: 210–16.

175. Tolentino MJ, Brucker AJ, Fosnot J, et al. Intravitreal injection of vascular endothelial growth factor small interfering RNA inhibits growth and leakage in a nonhuman primate, laser-induced model of choroidal neovascularization. Retina 2004; 24: 132–8.

176. Maier P, Unsoeld AS, Junker B, et al. Intravitreal injection of specific receptor tyrosine kinase inhibitor PTK787/ZK222 584 improves ischemia-induced retinopathy in mice. Graefes Arch Clin Exp Ophthalmol 2005; 243: 593–6.

177. Ozaki H, Seo MS, Ozaki K, et al. Blockade of vascular endothelial cell growth factor receptor signaling is sufficient to completely prevent retinal neovascularization. Am J Pathol 2000; 156: 697–707.

178. Yafai Y, Yang XM, Niemeyer M, et al. Anti-angiogenic effects of the receptor tyrosine kinase inhibitor, pazopanib, on choroidal neovascularization in rats. Eur J Pharmacol 2011; 666: 12–18.

179. West CM, Price P. Combretastatin A4 phosphate. Anticancer Drugs 2004; 15: 179–87.

180. Vincent L, Kermani P, Young LM, et al. Combretastatin A4 phosphate induces rapid regression of tumor neovessels and growth through interference with vascular endothelial-cadherin signaling. J Clin Invest 2005; 115: 2992–3006.

181. Nambu H, Nambu R, Melia M, Campochiaro PA. Combretastatin A-4 phosphate suppresses development and induces regression of choroidal neovascularization. Invest Ophthalmol Vis Sci 2003; 44: 3650–5.

182. Lindahl P, Johansson BR, Levéen P, Betsholtz C. Pericyte loss and microaneurysm formation in PDGF-B-deficient mice. Science 1997; 277: 242–5.

183. Akiyama H, Kachi S, Lima R, et al. Intraocular injection of an aptamer that binds PDGF-B: a potential treatment for proliferative retinopathies. J Cell Physiol 2006; 207: 407–12.

184. Boyer DS. Ophthotech Anti-PDGF in AMD Study Group. Combined Inhibition of Platelet Derived (PDGF) and Vascular Endothelial (VEGF) Growth Factors for the Treatment of Neovascular Age-Related Macular Degeneration (NV-AMD) - results of a phase 1 study. Invest Ophthalmol Vis Sci 2009; ARVO Suppl, ARVO paper May 4, 2009.

185. Integrin Ramakrishnan V, Bhaskar V, Law DA, et al. Preclinical evaluation of an anti-alpha5 beta1 integrin antibody as a novel anti-angiogenic agent. J Exp Ther Oncol 2006; 5: 273–86.

186. Xie B, Dong A, Rashid A, Stoller G, Campochiaro PA. Blockade of sphingosine-1-phosphate reduces macrophage influx and retinal and choroidal neovascularization. J Cell Physiol 2009; 218: 192–8.

187. Heeschen C, Weis M, Aicher A, Dimmeler S, Cooke JP. A novel angiogenic pathway mediated by non-neuronal nicotinic acetylcholine receptors. J Clin Invest 2002; 110: 527–36.

188. Kiuchi K, Matsuoka M, Wu JC, et al. Mecamylamine suppresses basal and nicotine-stimulated choroidal neovascularization. Invest Ophthalmol Vis Sci 2008; 49: 1705–11.

189. Cashman SM, Bowman L, Christofferson J, Kumar-Singh R. Inhibition of choroidal neovascularization by adenovirus-mediated delivery of short hairpin RNAs targeting VEGF as a potential therapy for AMD. Invest Ophthalmol Vis Sci 2006; 47: 3496–504.

190. Mori K, Gelbach P, Ando A, et al. Regression of ocular neovascularization in response to increased expression of pigment epithelium-derived factor. Invest Ophthalmol Vis Sci 2002; 43: 2428–34.

191. Rasmussen H, Chu KW, Campochiaro P, et al. Clinical protocol. an open-label, phase I, single administration, dose-escalation study of ADGVPEDF.11D (ADPEDF) in neovascular age-related macular degeneration (AMD). Hum Gene Ther 2001; 2: 2029–32.

192. Campochiaro PA, Nguyen QD, Shah SM, et al. Adenoviral vector-delivered pigment epithelium-derived factor for neovascular age-related macular degeneration: results of a phase I clinical trial. Hum Gene Ther 2006; 17: 177–9.

193. Maclachlan TK, Lukason M, Collins M, et al. Preclinical safety evaluation of AAV2-sFLT01- a gene therapy for age-related macular degeneration. Mol Ther 2011; 19: 326–34.

194. Lukason M, DuFresne E, Rubin H, et al. Inhibition of choroidal neovascularization in a nonhuman primate model by intravitreal administration of an AAV2 vector expressing a novel anti-VEGF molecule. Mol Ther 2011; 19: 260–5.

195. Lim JI, Niec M, Hung D, Wong V. A pilot study of combination therapy for neovascular AMD using a single injection of liquid sustained release intravitreal triamcinolone acetonide nad intravitreal ranibizumab as needed. Invest Ophthalmol Vis Sci 2012: 2035. ARVO Suppl): D1053; poster May 7, 2012.

10

Polypoidal choroidal vasculopathy

Richard F. Spaide

Polypoidal choroidal vasculopathy (PCV) is a slow growing complex form of neovascularization that has a branching vascular network (BVN) with aneurysmal dilations at the outer border of the network. PCV accounts for a minority of cases of choroidal neovascularization (CNV) seen among Caucasian patients with age-related macular degeneration (AMD), but accounts for a much larger proportion of eyes with neovascular manifestations in Asian and Black populations. The BVN in younger patients or in eyes with long standing disease appears as interconnected, reddish-orange dilated vessels. In older patients, particularly in Caucasians, the BVN can have an appearance indistinguishable from occult CNV. The BVN commonly expands laterally over years. The aneurysmal changes at the outer border of the lesion are more dynamic and can grow, disappear, or be replaced by network vessels over time. The aneurysmal changes are the source of the more dramatic neovascular manifestations such as serous or serosanguineous detachments of the retinal pigment epithelium (RPE) and the retina. There may be impressive amounts of lipid deposition in some cases. PCV may start at a relatively early age, with some patients being in their 40s. The disease can persist for years before threatening the macula or producing enough neovascular manifestations to be symptomatic. The eyes with PCV do not necessarily have the common ophthalmoscopic precursors seen in AMD such as large drusen or focal hyperpigmentation. Although PCV generally appears in fluorescein angiography with occult characteristics, PCV shows a good treatment response to photodynamic therapy in contrast with eyes harboring occult CNV secondary to AMD. Treatment with agents directed against vascular endothelial growth factor (VEGF) may cause improved visual acuity without much change in the underlying anatomic appearance of the neovascularization. Proper recognition of PCV is important because it can threaten visual function and has different demographic features, appearance, and treatment approaches than does typical CNV in AMD.

HISTORY

The first paper published regarding the disease was in 1985 by Stern and colleagues, who called the condition "multiple recurrent serosanguineous retinal pigment epithelial detachments in black women" (1). The name is an accurate description of some things the disease can do, although it is not limited to black women. In their description of three women, they could not find an etiology for the findings, although they suspected CNV (1). In 1990, three papers published simultaneously expanded the understanding of the disease (2–4). Perkovich reported an update on multiple recurrent serosanguineous retinal pigment epithelial detachments in black women by describing nine black women with disease, but did not find a definitive etiology for the hemorrhages. Kleiner and coworkers published a paper concerning "posterior uveal bleeding syndrome" in eight patients, six of whom were female, and all except for one was black. The bleeding was attributed to orange nodular subretinal structures the authors called "posterior uveal bleeding" (PUB) lesions (3). Similar to the Stern paper, these authors named the disease after one nonspecific feature that could come as a result of the disease. Because some of their patients developed findings suggestive of a disciform scar the authors proposed that CNV may happen concurrently in some eyes. An alternate explanation advanced by the authors was that the PUB lesions could have been an atypical form of CNV. The third paper was by Yannuzzi and coworkers who labeled the condition idiopathic polypoidal choroidal vasculopathy (4). This condition was thought to have two main vascular components, a branching network of what may have been vessels and reddish-orange excrescences at the outer border of the lesion. The authors were not sure whether the lesion represented neovascularization, but noted it did grow larger over time. Increasing the pressure in the eye by digital compression did not cause the vessels to collapse. Given this finding and the ophthalmoscopic impression that the vessels were deep in the choroid, the term choroidal vasculopathy was used. It is unclear where the polypoidal came from because polypoid can mean foot or extension, such as what is seen on an amoeba. On the other hand, polypoidal can mean polyp-like. A polyp is either a solid growth of tissue protruding from a mucous membrane or a simple water-dwelling animal with its mouth surrounded by tentacles. Mucous membranes are not found inside the eye and the fundus lesions do not look like marine animals.

Even though the polypoidal part is difficult to parse, and as will be seen later the vascular network is not in the choroid, the term polypoidal choroidal vasculopathy with, or later without, the word idiopathic caught on. It is difficult to know why, but there are probably some important reasons. The paper had a more complete explanation for the disorder and named the condition after the underlying vascular problem instead of a nonspecific consequence of the underlying pathology. Another reason is the same group subsequently produced many of the early papers about the disorder including expanded appreciation for the abnormalities caused by the disease and the locations within the eye in which it could be observed (5–7).

PATIENT DEMOGRAPHICS

In western countries the proportion of eyes with PCV in series of AMD patients with neovascular disease is about 10% or less, while in Asia the proportion is many times higher (8–12). The proportion of PCV is said to be higher in Blacks, as possibly evidenced by the original descriptions being in Blacks, but the actual proportion as seen in various countries in Africa has not been reported. That being said, most people in the United States are neither Asian nor Black so numerically Caucasian patients make up a substantial proportion of the total seen with PCV. Many Asian or Black patients presenting with PCV have no signs of AMD other than the neovascularization. They may have unilateral disease and can develop PCV at a relatively early age. This has led some authorities to consider PCV an entirely different disease from CNV, secondary to AMD or not (13–15). In the United States this differentiation is not commonly made. In Caucasian patients not only is it possible to see stigmata of AMD such as drusen but it can be difficult to distinguish the BVN in older patients with PCV from ordinary occult CNV. This creates diagnostic uncertainty in that some patients appear to have occult CNV but also may have subtle signs of PCV. Smoking and hypertension are risk factors for PCV, much the same as for CNV secondary to AMD (12).

ANGIOGRAPHY

PCV usually has the appearance of occult CNV during fluorescein angiography, although the larger vascular channels may be seen in PCV, which is not common in ordinary occult CNV (4,16). Fluorescein angiography uses excitation and emission wavelengths in the visible light range, which is absorbed by melanin pigment. Indocyanine green angiography has its excitation and emission peak in the near infra-red region, and as a consequence is less hindered by melanin pigment. The vessels in both the choroid and the neovascularization do not have the blood–brain barrier. As a consequence, a dye such as fluorescein can easily leak from vessels to cause obscuration of the underlying vascular detail (Fig. 10.1). Indocyanine green is highly protein bound and as a consequence does not leak very much from either the choroidal vessels or neovascularization. Using these principles, indocyanine green was found to provide dramatic imaging of PCV (17). The interconnecting channels were very easy to visualize and often traced back to the optic disc region. The excrescences in the first PCV paper were found to be aneurysmal enlargements of terminal portions of the BVN (17). These aneurysmal structures filled relatively slowly in that they were often best seen a minute or so after dye injection (Figs. 10.1 and 10.2). During the course

of the angiogram, the area of hyperfluorescence associated with the aneurysms appeared to enlarge somewhat and with time the dye clears from the circulation to leave faint staining shells visible (5,17). With scanning laser ophthalmoscopic systems some polypoidal lesions can be seen to pulsate with the heartbeat (18).

Central serous chorioretinopathy is a condition found predominantly in men and is manifested by serous detachment of the retina caused by leaks from the level of the RPE. These patients were found to have multifocal choroidal vascular hyperpermeability during indocyanine green angiography (19,20). These patients were found to have marked choroidal thickening when examined with optical coherence tomography (OCT) (21). When reviewing larger series of eyes with PCV it became apparent that about one-third had signs of choroidal vascular hyperpermeability (22). Eyes with PCV have thickening of the choroid (22–25), and the thickening is found in eyes with hyperpermeability (22). In these patients there appears to be a simultaneous occurrence of the two conditions in greater frequency than what would be expected from their joint probabilities if they were truly independent. Some patients with PCV have had the diagnosis of central serous chorioretinopathy when they really had PCV, which led to articles about how PCV masqueraded as central serous chorioretinopathy (26). However, there are patients with the diagnosis of central serous chorioretinopathy for decades who later in life show hemorrhage or other neovascular changes and are found to have PCV. It is likely these patients had central serous chorioretinopathy and then later developed PCV.

OPTICAL COHERENCE TOMOGRAPHY AND HISTOPATHOLOGY

The OCT findings of PCV, much like OCT of many other diseases, changed many concepts of the disease. Early OCT reports suggested the lesions were under Bruch's membrane, consistent with the "choroidal vasculopathy" portion of the name (27,28). As time progressed, some of the published histologic reports showed lesions under the RPE (29–32). The resolution of OCT instruments concurrently improved, and subsequently the reported location of the abnormalities shifted to above Bruch's membrane to lie under the RPE (33,34). Eyes with PCV commonly show some variation of the pigment epithelial detachment. There is usually an aneurysmal dilatation located under the RPE, and the dilatation can be the only component in the contents of the RPE or there can be varying admixtures of blood, serous fluid, fibrovascular material, and scar. The BVN can be seen as large vascular elements coursing under the RPE. By histology the BVN is composed of larger vessels, some of which are arterioles that can even have muscular coats.

The published histopathology papers do not agree completely about the nature of the abnormalities present (29–32,35). A large part of the difficulty is that the source of the material analyzed has been excised surgical specimens in almost every report. The origin and the exact

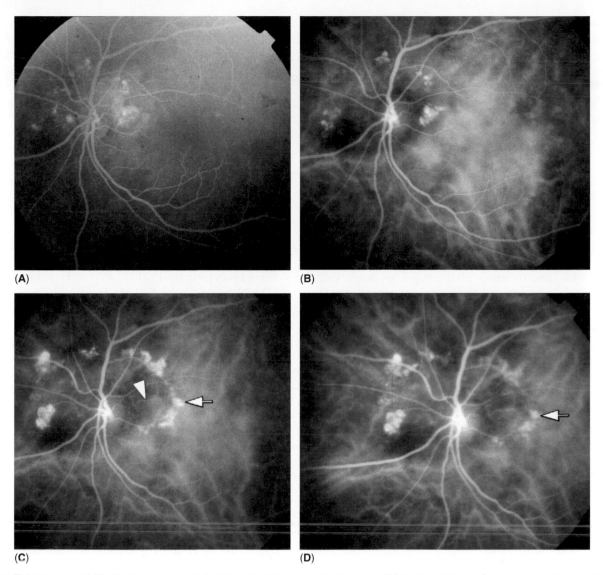

Figure 10.1 This 76-year-old Black woman presented with peripapillary vascular changes. (**A**) In the midphase fluorescein angiogram the patient has what appears to be occult peripapillary choroidal neovascularization. (**B**) The indocyanine green angiogram shows clusters of aneurysmal changes encircling a subtle lesion comprised of branching vessels. (**C**) Two years later the aneurysmal dilations visible in (**B**) are not present, but there are new dilations visible (arrow) at the outer edge of a larger lesion. The branching vascular network was visible (arrowhead). Because the patient had exudation into the macular region the patient was treated with photodynamic therapy to the temporal lesions and given intravitreal bevacizumab. When seen 1 month later the temporal aneurysmal lesions were smaller (arrow).

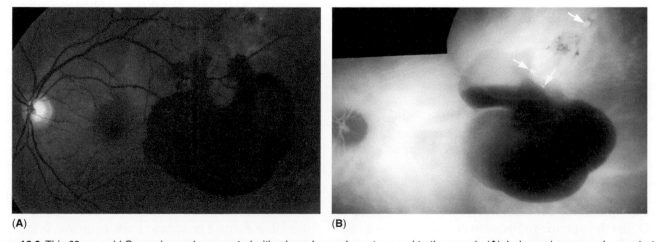

Figure 10.2 This 69-year-old Caucasian male presented with a large hemorrhage temporal to the macula (**A**). Indocyanine green demonstrated a peripheral polypoidal choroidal vasculopathy lesion with aneurysms (arrows) in (**B**).

nature of the vessels have been consequently open to interpretation. For example, some excised specimens consisted of a sample mostly composed of large vessels with some smaller remnants of Bruch's membrane (35). The authors showed angiographic pictures with typical aneurysmal elements with a branching network but the description of the histopathology was of larger choroidal vessels. This implies that the authors thought the blood vessels present in the sample were the choroid, even though the postoperative pictures showed the choroid was still present. An alternate interpretation would be the vessels observed were new vessels proliferating on the inner surface of Burch's membrane as part of the pathologic process involved with PCV. Lafaut and coworkers reported cases of PCV with tissue obtained from surgical specimens that showed large thin-walled vessels and aneurysmal changes. The aneurysmal changes were only one cell-layer thick in some areas (30).

TREATMENT

PCV has been and continues to be treated by a variety of means. Early after recognition of the vascular nature of the disease, laser photocoagulation was used to treat the aneurysmal dilations in some patients to try to control the neovascular and hemorrhagic complications of the disease (4). Because of the chronic nature of PCV the practical consequence was that patients required multiple photocoagulation scars in their macular region. At the end of 2002, two groups reported the results of photodynamic therapy (PDT) using verteporfin in eyes with PCV. One report had two patients (36), one followed for one year, while the other group had 16 patients followed for a mean of one year (37). The patients in both reports showed an improvement in visual acuity. Improvement in acuity is unusual in groups of eyes treated with PDT, particularly since PCV generally has characteristics of occult CNV during fluorescein angiography, a subgroup that ordinarily is thought not to respond well to PDT (38). With PDT there may be slightly less prominence of the BVN, but a much larger change in the appearance of the aneurysmal lesions.

Expansion of the use of PDT after these reports unearthed more potential complications and limitation of the treatment. Some patients treated with PDT had an initial improvement in acuity followed by a slow decline over time. The BVN shows some diminution of vessels diameter after treatment and it is common for many, if not most, of the aneurysmal changes to resolve (38). Isolated treatment of the aneurysmal changes is possible, but this form of therapy does not address potential leakage from the BVN. After treatment with PDT some eyes have experienced serous detachments that generally resolved within a week or so (39). A minority of patients had hemorrhages after PDT, and this seemed to occur more commonly in eyes with clusters of aneurysmal changes. PDT is not possible in eyes with extensive hemorrhages.

The advent of anti-VEGF therapies was a major advance in treating CNV. With typical CNV secondary to AMD, the therapeutic response to bevacizumab is generally similar to ranibizumab. A randomized double masked

trial was not performed to test the response seen in eyes with PCV. However, a nonrandomized comparative trial of 126 eyes with PCV treated with either bevacizumab or ranibizumab found no significant difference between the two drugs, which were administered on an as-needed basis (40). Both groups showed an improvement of between 1 and 2 lines of acuity at 12 months' follow-up. There are relatively few reports about anti-VEGF monotherapy for PCV. Most of the reports involve combination therapy using PDT with ranibizumab or bevacizumab (Fig. 10.1) (40–43). In the EVEREST study, a small randomized trial, 61 Asian patients were randomized to standard-fluence verteporfin PDT, ranibizumab 0.5 mg, or a combination of both (40). The endpoint of the study was regression of the aneurysmal dilations by month 6. By the sixth month a similar proportion of patients had regression of polyps in the PDT (71.4%) and combination groups (77.8%), but a significantly lower proportion in the ranibizumab-only group (28.6%). The study was stated to be not powered to examine visual acuity, and indeed no difference in visual acuity was found. In a non-randomized comparative study, 61 eyes were treated with PDT and ranibizumab and 85 were treated with PDT monotherapy. The mean acuity was better in the combination group (+1.2 lines) at 12 months than in the PDT monotherapy group (+0.4 lines). The use of combination therapy was not seen to reduce the resolution or recurrence of lesions although the authors hypothesized there was a decreased proportion of patients developing hemorrhages (41). In a different study a series of 66 eyes with PCV treated with PDT combined with intravitreal ranibizumab, 5 eyes developed hemorrhage, and the authors suggested post-treatment hemorrhage was still a risk following combination therapy (42). There were no arms in these studies in which the eyes received no treatment, and as such observed hemorrhages in the treated patients could represent the underlying disease, not the treatment.

DIFFERENTIAL DIAGNOSIS

There are two main conditions that produce findings similar to those of PCV. The first condition, radiation-associated choroidal neovasculopathy, was described in eyes that received external beam radiation for CNV secondary to AMD (44). The first series had a relatively low dose of radiation, 20 Gy, and the neovascularization in some appeared to stabilize for a short period of time. Of 193 treated patients, 19 (9.8%) developed an abnormal growth of vessels extending beyond the original neovascular complex. These vessels were best seen with indocyanine green angiography, and at the outer border of the vascular proliferation there were aneurysmal dilations. These eyes showed profuse leakage of fluorescein dye from the aneurysmal lesions and they had a marked propensity for visual acuity loss. This condition was differentiated from typical PCV because of the history of radiation therapy and the explosive progression of the vasculopathy.

The second condition that merges into PCV and may be a variant thereof occurs in patients who have had prolonged treatment with intravitreal anti-VEGF agents. Some of these patients develop persistent fluid after an otherwise-successful treatment and may start to have small hemorrhages. Investigation with indocyanine green angiography in some patients shows a cluster of aneurysmal changes, similar to those seen in PCV. PDT of these lesions results in a decrease in the amount of subretinal exudation (45).

UNRESOLVED ASPECTS OF POLYPOIDAL CHOROIDAL VASCULOPATHY
What is the Relationship Between Polypoidal Choroidal Vasculopathy and Choroidal Neovascularization?

Most eyes, particularly in Asians, do not have typical stigmata of AMD. The affected patients may be younger, are more likely to be male and have with unilateral disease. The eyes show a fortuitously good response to PDT, even though they ostensibly have the fluorescein angiographic characteristics of occult CNV. This has led a number of authors, chiefly from Japan, to conclude PCV is not CNV. In some treatment studies CNV was said to be excluded and in other studies the stated goal was to compare PCV with CNV (38,42). There appears to be a logical dissonance in separating PCV from CNV. PCV is universally viewed as a vascular problem that appears to grow in size. Older ideas attributing the features seen to choroidal vascular abnormalities have given way to the concept that many or most of the findings are due to a peculiar growth of vessels in the sub-RPE space. Since blood vessels aren't ordinarily found there, it is correct to call the process neovascularization. The newly growing vessels are supplied from the choroid, and in an analogous way to conventional CNV it would be proper to call PCV a form of CNV. However, since the accompanying findings in the eye, particularly in Asians or Blacks, do not necessarily or even frequently suggest AMD, it is valid to differentiate PCV as being truly idiopathic.

Several series of patients with PCV have had analysis of candidate genes to evaluate associations that may be present. The reported studies have all been small to medium sized. The observed relationships between single nucleotide polymorphisms in PCV have not varied substantially from those seen in AMD for complement factor H or for ARMS2 in both Japanese and Caucasian populations [reviewed in reference (46)]. One study in Japan found an association between rs2301995 in the elastin locus and PCV (47). A study done in the United States did not find any association between elastin and PCV in Caucasians (48). A subsequent study in Japan found an association between elastin and AMD, but not PCV (49). There have been no consistent differences found in the haplotype associations for CNV in AMD as compared with PCV. These studies suggest there may be genetic risk factors common to both PCV- and CNV-associated AMD that may alter the potential to develop neovascular disease, but not cause a specific phenotypic appearance. It is possible that there are unknown genes or even local factors that modify cause or lead to a specific disease phenotype as there are patients with one phenotype in one eye and the other phenotype in the fellow eye (50).

Why is Hemorrhage Such a Prominent Aspect of Polypoidal Choroidal Vasculopathy?

It is unusual for typical CNV to produce copious hemorrhage unless the patient uses anticoagulants. On the other hand, the early distinguishing characteristic of PCV, particularly considering the precursor name of the condition included hemorrhagic descriptions. One convenient explanation involves use of La Place's law. The wall tension, T, of a sphere is given by the expression $T = (RP)/2$, where R is the radius and P is the pressure. At present the blood pressure in a polypoidal aneurysmal lesion is little more than a guess, but one assumption is the pressure is the same as in the choriocapillaris, which has a luminal diameter of about one-tenth of that of a large polypoid aneurysmal dilatation. The wall tension in a cylinder is shown by the expression $T = PR$. Ordinarily, larger blood vessels have thicker, stronger walls than do smaller vessels. In the case of PCV the aneurysms have nearly the same-wall thickness as the choriocapillaris. The ratio of the wall tensions illustrates one of the unfavorable physiologic aspects of PCV; large thin-walled vessels with high wall tensions may account for at least some of the observed risk PCV patients have for bleeding.

SUMMARY POINTS

- Polypoidal choroidal vasculopathy (PVC) is a slow growing form of neovascularization recognizable by a branching network of reddish-orange interconnecting vessels with aneurysmal dilations at the outer border of the network.
- Indocyanine green angiography is very helpful in visualizing the vascular changes, which originally were thought to be in the choroid, but were later found to be in the sub-retinal pigment epithelial space.
- Fluorescein angiography shows findings consistent with occult choroidal neovascularization (CNV).
- In contrast with typical occult CNV, the neovascular manifestations of PVC typically show favorable treatment response to photodynamic therapy.
- Pharmacologic therapy directed against vascular endothelial growth factor causes decreased exudation and is often used in combination with photodynamic therapy.

REFERENCES

1. Stern RM, Zakov ZN, Zegarra H, Gutman FA. Multiple recurrent serosanguineous retinal pigment epithelial detachments in black women. Am J Ophthalmol 1985; 100: 560–9.
2. Perkovich BT, Zakov ZN, Berlin LA, Weidenthal D, Avins LR. An update on multiple recurrent serosanguineous retinal pigment epithelial detachments in black women. Retina 1990; 10: 18–26.

3. Kleiner RC, Brucker AJ, Johnston RL. The posterior uveal bleeding syndrome. Retina 1990; 10: 9–17.

4. Yannuzzi LA, Sorenson J, Spaide RF, et al. Idiopathic polypoidal choroidal vasculopathy (IPCV). Retina 1990; 10: 1–8.

5. Yannuzzi LA, Ciardella A, Spaide RF, et al. The expanding clinical spectrum of idiopathic polypoidal choroidal vasculopathy. Arch Ophthalmol 1997; 115: 478–85.

6. Moorthy RS, Lyon AT, Rabb MF, et al. Idiopathic polypoidal choroidal vasculopathy of the macula. Ophthalmology 1998; 105: 1380–5.

7. Yannuzzi LA, Nogueira FB, Spaide RF, et al. Idiopathic polypoidal choroidal vasculopathy: a peripheral lesion. Arch Ophthalmol 1998; 116: 382–3.

8. Yannuzzi LA, Wong DW, Sforzolini BS, et al. Polypoidal choroidal vasculopathy and neovascularized age-related macular degeneration. Arch Ophthalmol 1999; 117: 1503–10.

9. Kwok AK, Lai TY, Chan CW, Neoh EL, Lam DS. Polypoidal choroidal vasculopathy in chinese patients. Br J Ophthalmol 2002; 86: 892–7.

10. Uyama M, Matsubara T, Fukushima I, et al. Idiopathic polypoidal choroidal vasculopathy in japanese patients. Arch Ophthalmol 1999; 117: 1035–42.

11. Uyama M, Wada M, Nagai Y, et al. Polypoidal choroidal vasculopathy: natural history. Am J Ophthalmol 2002; 133: 639–48.

12. Sho K, Takahashi K, Yamada H, et al. Polypoidal choroidal vasculopathy: incidence, demographic features, and clinical characteristics. Arch Ophthalmol 2003; 121: 1392–6.

13. Laude A, Cackett PD, Vithana EN, et al. Polypoidal choroidal vasculopathy and neovascular age-related macular degeneration: same or different disease? Prog Retin Eye Res 2010; 29: 19–29.

14. Ozawa S, Ishikawa K, Ito Y, et al. Differences in macular morphology between polypoidal choroidal vasculopathy and exudative age-related macular degeneration detected by optical coherence tomography. Retina 2009; 29: 793–802.

15. Gomi F, Sawa M, Wakabayashi T, et al. Efficacy of intravitreal bevacizumab combined with photodynamic therapy for polypoidal choroidal vasculopathy. Am J Ophthalmol 2010; 150: 48–54.

16. Tamura H, Tsujikawa A, Otani A, et al. Polypoidal choroidal vasculopathy appearing as classic choroidal neovascularisation on fluorescein angiography. Br J Ophthalmol 2007; 91: 1152–9.

17. Spaide RF, Yannuzzi LA, Slakter JS, et al. Indocyanine green video angiography of idiopathic polypoidal choroidal vasculopathy. Retina 1995; 15: 100–10.

18. Okubo A, Ito M, Sameshima M, Uemura A, Sakamoto T. Pulsatile blood flow in the polypoidal choroidal vasculopathy. Ophthalmology 2005; 112: 1436–41.

19. Spaide RF, Campeas L, Haas A, et al. Central serous chorioretinopathy in younger and older adults. Ophthalmology 1996; 103: 2070–80.

20. Spaide RF, Hall L, Haas A, et al. Indocyanine green videoangiography of older adults with central serous chorioretinopathy. Retina 1996; 16: 203–13.

21. Imamura Y, Fujiwara T, Margolis R, Spaide RF. Enhanced depth imaging optical coherence tomography of the choroid in central serous chorioretinopathy. Retina 2009; 29: 1469–73.

22. Koizumi H, Yamagishi T, Yamazaki T, Kawasaki R, Kinoshita S. Subfoveal choroidal thickness in typical age-related macular degeneration and polypoidal choroidal vasculopathy. Graefes Arch Clin Exp Ophthalmol 2011; 249: 1123–8.

23. Chung SE, Kang SW, Lee JH, Kim YT. Choroidal thickness in polypoidal choroidal vasculopathy and exudative age-related macular degeneration. Ophthalmology 2011; 118: 840–5.

24. Kim SW, Oh J, Kwon SS, Yoo J, Huh K. Comparison of choroidal thickness among patients with healthy eyes, early age-related maculopathy, neovascular age-related macular degeneration, central serous chorioretinopathy, and polypoidal choroidal vasculopathy. Retina 2011; 31: 1904–11.

25. Nagase S, Miura M, Makita S, et al. High-penetration optical coherence tomography with enhanced depth imaging of polypoidal choroidal vasculopathy. Ophthalmic Surg Lasers Imaging 2012; 43: e5–9.

26. Yannuzzi LA, Freund KB, Goldbaum M, et al. Polypoidal choroidal vasculopathy masquerading as central serous chorioretinopathy. Ophthalmology 2000; 107: 767–77.

27. Iijima H, Imai M, Gohdo T, Tsukahara S. Optical coherence tomography of idiopathic polypoidal choroidal vasculopathy. Am J Ophthalmol 1999; 127: 301–5.

28. Iijima H, Iida T, Imai M, Gohdo T, Tsukahara S. Optical coherence tomography of orange-red subretinal lesions in eyes with idiopathic polypoidal choroidal vasculopathy. Am J Ophthalmol 2000; 129: 21–6.

29. Spraul CW, Grossniklaus HE, Lang GK. Idiopathic polypoidal choroid vasculopathy. Klin Monatsbl Augenheilkd 1997; 210: 405–6.

30. Lafaut BA, Aisenbrey S, van den Broecke C, et al. Polypoidal choroidal vasculopathy pattern in age-related macular degeneration. a clinicopathologic correlation. Retina 2000; 20: 650–4.

31. Rosa RH Jr, Davis JL, Eifrig CW. Clinicopathologic reports, case reports, and small case series: clinicopathologic correlation of idiopathic polypoidal choroidal vasculopathy. Arch Ophthalmol 2002; 120: 502–8.

32. Nakashizuka H, Mitsumata M, Okisaka S, et al. Clinicopathologic findings in polypoidal choroidal vasculopathy. Invest Ophthalmol Vis Sci 2008; 49: 4729–37.

33. Ojima Y, Hangai M, Sakamoto A, et al. Improved visualization of polypoidal choroidal vasculopathy lesions using spectral-domain optical coherence tomography. Retina 2009; 29: 52–9.

34. Khan S, Engelbert M, Imamura Y, Freund KB. Polypoidal choroidal vasculopathy: simultaneous indocyanine green angiography and eye-tracked spectral domain optical coherence tomography findings. Retina 2012; 32: 1057–68.

35. Kuroiwa S, Tateiwa H, Hisatomi T, Ishibashi T, Yoshimura N. Pathological features of surgically excised polypoidal choroidal vasculopathy membranes. Clin Exp Ophthalmol 2004; 32: 297–302.

36. French

37. Spaide RF, Donsoff I, Lam DL, et al. Treatment of polypoidal choroidal vasculopathy with photodynamic therapy. Retina 2002; 22: 529–35.

38. Honda S, Imai H, Yamashiro K, et al. Comparative assessment of photodynamic therapy for typical age-related macular degeneration and polypoidal choroidal vasculopathy: a multicenter study in hyogo prefecture, japan. Ophthalmologica 2009; 223: 333–8.

39. Wakabayashi T, Gomi F, Sawa M, Tsujikawa M, Tano Y. Marked vascular changes of polypoidal choroidal vasculopathy after photodynamic therapy. Br J Ophthalmol 2008; 92: 936–40.

40. Cho HJ, Kim JW, Lee DW, Cho SW, Kim CG. Intravitreal bevacizumab and ranibizumab injections for patients with polypoidal choroidal vasculopathy. Eye (Lond) 2012; 26: 426–33.

41. Koh A, Lee WK, Chen LJ, et al.; EVEREST STUDY. Efficacy and safety of verteporfin photodynamic therapy in combination with ranibizumab or alone versus ranibizumab monotherapy in patients with symptomatic macular polypoidal choroidal vasculopathy. Retina 2012; 32: 1453–64. [Epub ahead of print].

42. Gomi F, Sawa M, Wakabayashi T, et al. Efficacy of intravitreal bevacizumab combined with photodynamic therapy for polypoidal choroidal vasculopathy. Am J Ophthalmol 2010; 150: 48–54.

43. Kim M, Kim K, Kim do G, Yu SY, Kwak HW. Two-year results of photodynamic therapy combined with intravitreal anti-vascular endothelial growth factor for polypoidal choroidal vasculopathy. Ophthalmologica 2011; 226: 205–13.

44. Spaide RF, Leys A, Herrmann-Delemazure B, et al. Radiation-associated choroidal neovasculopathy. Ophthalmology 1999; 106: 2254–60.

45. Cho M, Barbazetto IA, Freund KB. Refractory neovascular age-related macular degeneration secondary to polypoidal choroidal vasculopathy. Am J Ophthalmol 2009; 148: 70–8.

46. Lima LH, Schubert C, Ferrara DC, et al. Three major loci involved in age-related macular degeneration are also associated with polypoidal choroidal vasculopathy. Ophthalmology 2010; 117: 1567–70.

47. Kondo N, Honda S, Ishibashi K, Tsukahara Y, Negi A. Elastin gene polymorphisms in neovascular age-related macular degeneration and polypoidal choroidal vasculopathy. Invest Ophthalmol Vis Sci 2008; 49: 1101–5.

48. Lima LH, Merriam JE, Freund KB, et al. Elastin rs2301995 polymorphism is not associated with polypoidal choroidal vasculopathy in caucasians. Ophthalmic Genet 2011; 32: 80–2.

49. Yamashiro K, Mori K, Nakata I, et al. Association of elastin gene polymorphism to age-related macular degeneration and polypoidal choroidal vasculopathy. Invest Ophthalmol Vis Sci 2011; 52: 8780–4.

50. Maruko I, Iida T, Saito M, Nagayama D. Combined cases of polypoidal choroidal vasculopathy and typical age-related macular degeneration. Graefes Arch Clin Exp Ophthalmol 2010; 248: 361–8.

11

Variants of neovascular age-related macular degeneration: Type 3 neovascularization (intraretinal neovascularization or retinal angiomatous proliferation)

Adrian T. Fung and K. Bailey Freund

INTRODUCTION

According to the Gass classification of choroidal neovascularization (CNV), neovascular proliferation may occur in two distinct forms (1). In the first, coined "type 1 neovascularization," the neovascular tissue is confined to the sub-retinal pigment epithelial (sub-RPE) space and is usually visible on fluorescein angiography (FA) as "poorly defined" or "occult" leakage. This is the most common form of CNV in age-related macular degeneration (AMD) (2). In contrast, "type 2 neovascularization" refers to neovascular tissue originating in the choroid that gains access to the subretinal space via a breach in the Bruch's membrane/RPE complex. This is usually associated with "well defined" or "classic" leakage on FA. Type 2 neovascularization often occurs in the setting of pathological myopia, choroidal rupture, angioid streaks, and inflammation (3). The existence of intraretinal neovascularization has been described. In a logical progression from the anatomical classification system proposed by Gass, Freund et al. (4) have described this as "type 3 neovascularization." This form of neovascularization has distinct demographic, funduscopic, and prognostic features that set it apart from type 1 and type 2 neovascularization.

ETYMOLOGY

Multiple names have previously been used to describe type 3 neovascularization. It was first described in 1992 by Hartnett et al. (5) as a "retinal vascular abnormality" (RVA). This "outer angiomatous retinal lesion" was described as being located in the deep retina central to a pigment epithelial detachment (PED) and displaying either a feeding retinal arteriole or a draining venule. On FA, the RVA exhibits early hyperfluorescence during dye transit and late leakage. Subsequent to this, the term "deep retinal vascular anomalous complex" (RVAC) (6,7) was used to describe similar lesions. In 2001, Yannuzzi et al. (8) introduced and popularized the term "retinal angiomatous proliferation." "Angiomatous" referred to the compensatory telangiectatic vessels and "proliferation" to the neovascularization. In more advanced cases these lesions were described as becoming associated with the development of a chorioretinal anastomosis (CRA) (9) in the absence of disciform scarring. This distinction is significant since CRA are common in the

presence of disciform scarring but has not otherwise been recognized (8). "Occult chorioretinal anastomosis" (ORCA) (10), "retinal choroidal anastomoses" (RCA), (11) and "retinal anastomosis to the lesion" (12) are synonymous.

Henceforth in this chapter, we will use the term type 3 neovascularization to refer to intraretinal neovascularization. This term has the advantages of conforming to the Gass classification, without suggesting a pathogenic sequence (which has been fervently debated) or the presence of a CRA (which is not always present). It should be remembered that, in many cases, lesion types in AMD may be mixed. Therefore, components of type 1 or type 2 neovascularization may coexist with type 3 neovascularization (4).

RETINAL OR CHOROIDAL ORIGIN (OR BOTH)?

There has been considerable debate regarding whether type 3 neovascularization originates from the retinal or the choroidal circulation (3).

Evidence supporting a retinal origin includes histopathologic studies of transgenic mice that demonstrate development of neovascularization in the outer plexiform layer (13) or deep capillary bed (14) that subsequently migrates into the subretinal space with development of CRA. Of course, the histology of mice retina differs from that of human retina, thus the findings cannot be extrapolated to humans with certainty. More convincing are clinicopathological studies of patients with type 3 neovascularization. Two studies that looked at specimens taken following submacular surgery suggested the presence of intraretinal neovascularization growing into the subretinal space, with some eyes demonstrating CRA (7,15). CNV was not seen, although the absence of intact choroid in these histopathologic specimens means that its presence could not be excluded. In a clinicopathological correlation of a patient with type 3 neovascularization who subsequently died, histology demonstrated intraretinal without sub-RPE neovascularization (16). In a further patient with a clinical diagnosis of type 3 neovascularization, post-mortem histology revealed a plexus of blood vessels in the outer retina abutting the elastic portion of Bruch's membrane (17). The vessels were surrounded by eosinophilic extracellular matrix (17). Although a PED with loss of RPE cells was present underneath the vessels, there was no

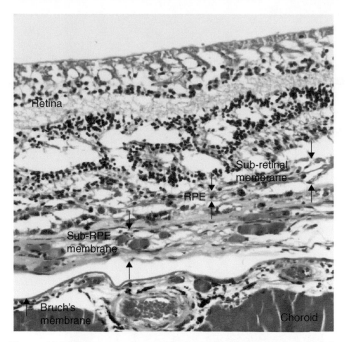

Figure 11.1 High-powered magnification (20x, Hematoxylin and Eosin stain) of a type 3 neovascular membrane. Subretinal pigment and sub-retinal epithelial membrane components are visible, but there is no penetration of Bruch's membrane to the choroid. The intraretinal component of the membrane was present on other sections from the same eye. *Source*: Histopathology slide, courtesy of Dr Sander Dubovy.

communication with the choroid. An example of type 3 neovascularization with subretinal and sub-RPE components (but no penetration of Bruch's membrane) is shown in Figure 11.1. Both Zachs et al. (18) and Brancato et al. (19) described type 3 neovascularization in which optical coherence tomography (OCT) clearly demonstrated intraretinal localization of the proliferation. In our extensive collection of patients with type 3 neovascularization, some appear to have hyperfluorescence of a neovascular membrane that appears only with retinal arteriolar filling (Figs. 11.2, 11.3). This is suggestive of a retinal, rather than a choroidal origin for the neovascularization in these cases. The absence of cases of type 3 neovascularization developing from within the foveal avascular zone lends further support for a retinal origin. Finally, a clinical counterpart to intraretinal type 3 neovascularization can be found in macular telangiectasia type 2 (idiopathic perifoveal telangiectasia). In this condition, retinal vascular proliferation can occur in the deep capillary plexus with extension into the subretinal space. The neovascularization is believed to be purely retinal with no choroidal component. Unlike type 3 neovascularization, serous PED or CRA do not normally occur and the subsequent pathology and clinical presentation diverge after the initial stages. The belief that type 3 neovascularization develops from the retina led Yannuzzi et al. (20) to propose a three-step staging system in 2001 (Fig. 11.4).

Not all authors have accepted that type 3 neovascularization originates from the retina. In 2003, Gass et al. (21) retrospectively studied 24 eyes of 16 patients who presented with focal inner retinal hemorrhages and drusen. They presented clinical, angiographic, and histopathological evidence arguing that inner retinal

hemorrhages could be an early clinical sign of an ORCA developing at the site of occult CNV (Fig. 11.5). Costa et al. (22) used third-generation OCT to study 20 eyes of 11 patients who had CRA. Their findings were used to support the Gass hypothesis of occult CRA. Finally, Freund et al. (4) reported on five eyes of four patients in whom early RCA was visualized with multimodal imaging as small breaks in the Bruch's membrane/RPE complex *without* evidence of underlying occult type 1 neovascularization (either neurosensory or PED). This differs from previous reports of type 3 neovascularization in which RCA was described as an advanced phenomenon.

The debate over a retinal or choroidal origin for type 3 neovascularization continues. In an editorial by Yannuzzi in 2008 (20), the possibility of both origins, in different patients or even simultaneously in the same patient was raised (Fig. 11.6). This concept has support from a high resolution spectral-domain OCT (SD-OCT) study of type 3 neovascular lesions which showed isolated intraretinal neovascularization in some and a combined sub-RPE and sub-retinal neovascularization in another without a PED (23).

The use of the term "type 3 neovascularization" proposed by Freund et al. (3) avoids the controversy regarding the origin of the lesion by merely emphasizing its location (intraretinal) and distinguishes it from type 1 and type 2 neovascularization.

EPIDEMIOLOGY AND GENETICS

The prevalence of type 3 neovascularization has been estimated to be 20% of all occult CNV diagnosed by FA (24). In earlier fluorescein angiographic studies, CRA was estimated to occur in 21% (11) to 28% (25) of all occult CNV and 26.8% of all vascularized PEDs (9). Despite this, the introduction of SD-OCT with its greater ability to discriminate the level of neovascularization has led many to believe that the actual incidence is higher (3). Type 3 neovascularization is more common in elderly female patients, with a mean age at diagnosis of 80 years (8). It is seen almost exclusively in white patients and is reported rarely in Asians and to date it has not been seen in blacks (20). Approximately 50% of all patients present unilaterally (8). In a study by Gross et al., (26), 100% of patients with unilateral type 3 neovascularization developed fellow eye involvement (almost exclusively type 3 neovascularization) within three years of presentation. This is much higher than a 42% of five-year cumulative incidence of fellow eye involvement previously reported by the Macular Photocoagulation Study group for all types of neovascularization secondary to AMD (27). However, a separate study found only a 36% of three-year fellow eye involvement in patients with unilateral type 3 neovascularization (28). Several reasons were proposed for this discrepancy in rates: differences in population demographics, patients with aggressive disease presenting bilaterally from the outset, and a protective effect on the contralateral eye by unilateral anti-VEGF injections. Regardless of what the true rate is, a careful follow-up is recommended with particular attention to

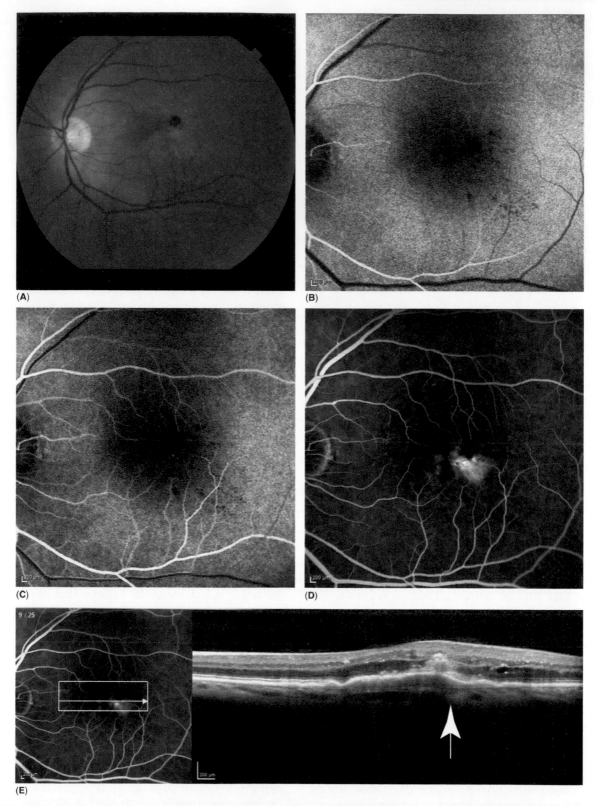

Figure 11.2 A 67-year-old white female presented with decreased vision and metamorphopsia in her left eye. Best-corrected visual acuities (BCVAs) were 20/20 OD and 20/60 OS. (**A**) Color fundus photograph (Topcon 50IA, Topcon Corporation, Paramus, New Jersey, USA) of the left eye demonstrates macular drusen and an intraretinal blot hemorrhage superotemporal to the fovea. Non-neovascular age-related macular degeneration was present in the right eye. (**B** and **C**) Early fluorescein angiography (Heidelberg Spectralis HRA + OCT, Heidelberg Engineering Inc., Heidelberg, Germany) demonstrates pinpoint hyperfluorescence just temporal to the fovea that developed during the arterial phase of filling. This suggests retinal rather than choroidal localization of the type 3 neovascular membrane. (**D**) Late FA demonstrates occult fluorescein leakage. (**E**) Spectral-domain optical coherence tomography (Heidelberg Spectralis HRA + OCT) demonstrates intraretinal hyper-reflectivity in the region of the type 3 neovascular membrane, retinal edema, and a pigment epithelial detachment with a possible break in the retinal pigment epithelium (arrow). The patient was treated with 4 monthly injections of intravitreal ranibizumab followed by an "OCT-guided PRN" regimen. Three months after the first injection, the BCVA improved to 20/25.

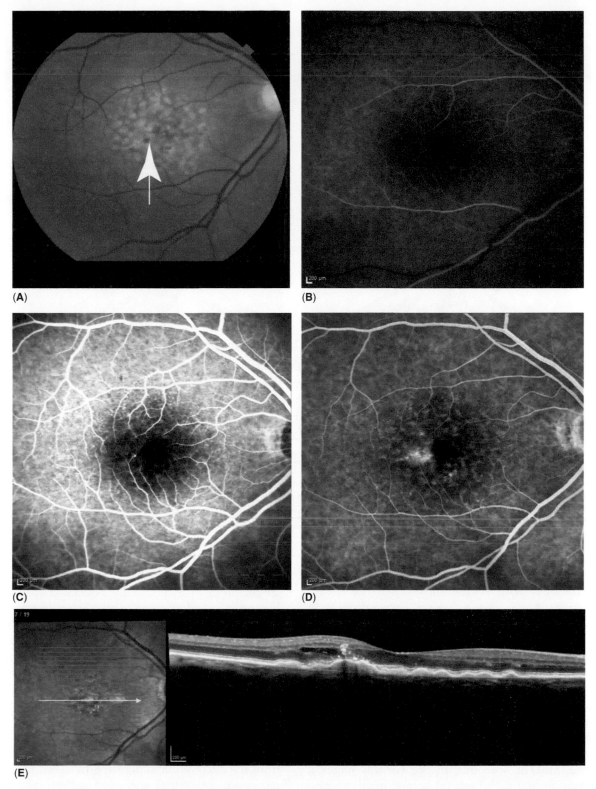

Figure 11.3 An 84-year-old white female presented with decreased vision and metamorphopsia in her right eye. Best-corrected visual acuities (BCVA) were 20/60 OD and 20/40 OS. (**A**) Color photograph (Topcon 50IA Topcon Corporation, Paramus, New Jersey, USA) of the right eye demonstrates confluent soft macular drusen and subtle intraretinal hemorrhage just inferotemporal to the fovea (arrow). Non-neovascular age-related macular degeneration was present in the left eye. (**B** and **C**) Early fluorescein angiography (FA; Heidelberg Spectralis HRA + OCT) demonstrates pinpoint hyperfluorescence just inferotemporal to the fovea that developed during the arterial phase of filling, suggestive of a retinal location of the type 3 neovascular membrane. (**D**) Late FA demonstrates occult fluorescein leakage. (**E**) Spectral-domain optical coherence tomography (Heidelberg Spectralis HRA + OCT) demonstrates intraretinal hyper-reflectivity in the region of the type 3 neovascular membrane, retinal edema, and a pigment epithelial detachment. The patient was treated with 2 monthly injections of intravitreal ranibizumab followed by an "OCT-guided PRN" regimen. Six months following initial therapy, the BCVA was 20/50 OD.

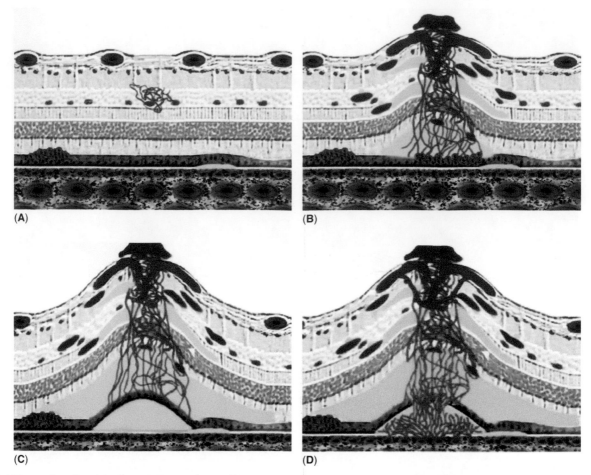

Figure 11.4 Yannuzzi et al.'s original retinal angiomatous proliferation staging system. (**A**) Stage I: intraretinal neovascularization. (**B**) Stage II: subretinal neovascularization with a retinal–retinal anastomosis. (**C**) Stage II: subretinal neovascularization with a serous pigment epithelial detachment. (**D**) Stage III: choroidal neovascularization with a vascularized pigment epithelial detachment and a retinal–choroidal anastomosis. *Source*: From Ref. 8.

detecting the subtle signs of early disease. Involvement in the second eye is frequently of the same morphology and location as in the first (20,28). In a study of 962 Japanese patients with AMD, those with the ARMS polymorphism A69S had a higher association with type 3 neovascularization, suggesting that patients with type 3 neovascularization may be a genetically distinct subgroup (29).

DIAGNOSIS
Funduscopic Findings and Staging
Most commonly, type 3 neovascularization presents with intraretinal hemorrhages and macular edema (20,30) associated with decreased visual acuity, metamorphopsia, and/or scotoma. In the earliest stages it may be asymptomatic. Subretinal hemorrhage can also occur, but only in advanced disease when there is extension of the intraretinal neovascularization into the subretinal space (20). The macular edema is often cystic and is greater than is often seen in other neovascular subtypes of AMD (20). Type 3 lesions have never been described as originating from within the foveal avascular zone. For reasons unknown, type 3 neovascularization has also never been reported to occur in the peripheral retina or peripapillary region (20).

Yannuzzi et al.'s 2001 paper on type 3 neovascularization, described three stages (Fig. 11.4) (8).

Stage I
The earliest manifestation of type 3 neovascularization is proliferation of the deep capillary plexus in the paramacular region (8). This is usually associated with intraretinal hemorrhage and macular edema. Dilated perfusing retinal arterioles and draining venules may develop. In approximately 30% of cases, a retinal–retinal anastomosis (RRA) may be evident clinically or on FA (8). At this stage, lesions may be confused with occult CNV on FA and present as a "hot spot" on indocyanine-green angiography (ICGA).

Stage II
Stage II disease is defined as the development of subretinal neovascularization. As the neovascularization extends from the deep retina to the superficial retina and subretinal space, preretinal and even subretinal hemorrhage can develop. Frequently, there is associated neurosensory retinal detachment and a serous PED (8). It is at this stage when type 3 neovascularization is most often diagnosed (8). The presence of a serous PED in type 3 neovascularization distinguishes it from macular telangiectasia.

Stage III
The development of CNV defines stage III disease. This distinction from stage II disease is often difficult to determine clinically with certainty. At this stage, a CRA can develop.

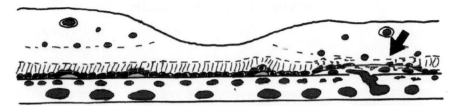

STAGE 1 - PRECLINICAL OCCULT TYPE 1 MEMBRANE

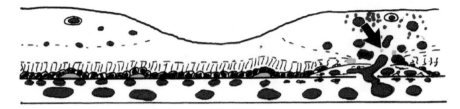

STAGE 2 - SUPERFICAL RETINAL HEMORRHAGE

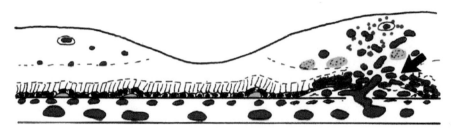

STAGE 3 - PIGGY - BACK TYPE 2 SSRN

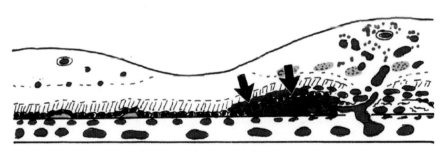

STAGE 4 - RPE DETACHMENT

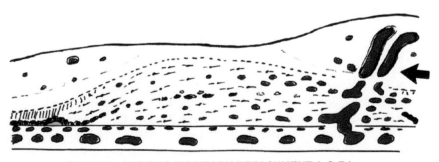

STAGE 5 - CHRONIC DISCIFORM DETACHMENT & C-RA

Figure 11.5 Gass et al.'s 2003 schema describing the presence of superficial retinal hemorrhages secondary to an occult type 1 neovascular membrane. *Source*: From Ref. 21.

Because of the ongoing controversy regarding a retinal or choroidal origin for type 3 neovascularization, in 2008 Yannuzzi et al. (20) expanded their staging to accommodate both these possibilities (Fig. 11.6). The 3 stages were still described, but were not necessarily considered a pathogenic sequence.

TYPE 3 NEOVASCULARIZATION (RAP)

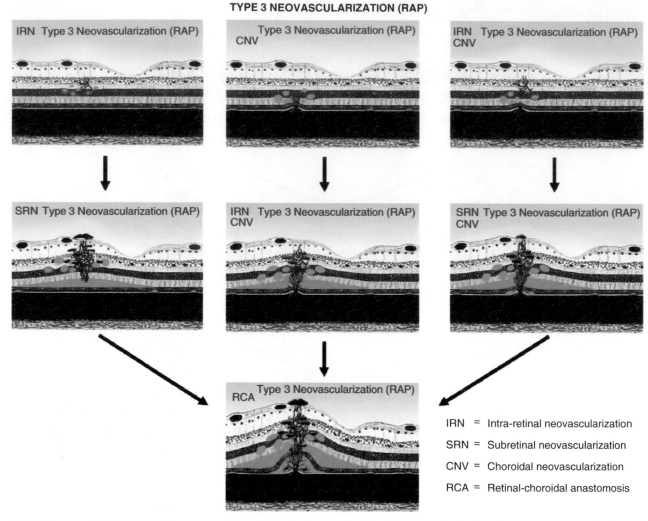

Figure 11.6 Yannuzzi et al.'s expanded representation of the development of type 3 neovascularization that accommodates both retinal and choroidal origin hypotheses. *Source*: From Ref. 20.

Given more findings from SD-OCT and clinicopathologic correlations of type 3 neovascularization, the utility of this staging system has been debated (3,21).

INVESTIGATIONS
Fluorescein Angiography

Type 3 neovascularization is best visualized during the transit phase of an FA (Figs. 11.2, 11.3, 11.7, 11.8) (30). A focal point of intraretinal neovascularization that may be accompanied by surrounding telangiectatic vessels is often seen. In the later phases, the fluorescein dye leaks from the neovascularization, filling any cystic intraretinal edema, neurosensory detachment and/or PED such that the intraretinal neovascularization often becomes difficult to distinguish from the surrounding occult leakage (20,30). This confusion was demonstrated in a study of 270 consecutive eyes with fluorescein angiographic diagnosis of occult neovascularization. Ten percent of patients diagnosed as a fibrovascular PED and 24% diagnosed as late leakage of undetermined source were subsequently reclassified as type 3 neovascularization by ICGA (24).

High-Speed Stereoscopic Indocyanine-Green Angiography

On ICGA, type 3 neovascularization may be seen as a "hot spot", a term that refers to intense focal hyperfluorescence of less than one disc area first visualized in the mid-phase of the angiogram and persistent in the very late phases when the dye has left the normal choroidal circulation (Fig. 11.8) (3). Dilated feeding arterioles, draining venules, and RRAs may also be visible. "Hot spots" are not specific to type 3 neovascularization. In a study of 34 eyes with "hot spots" by Fernandes et al., (30), 62% had polypoidal neovasculopathy, 30% had type 3 neovascularization, and 8% had focal occult CNV. In early-stage type 3 neovascularization, decreased choroidal filling is present in over 80% of eyes compared with only 50–60% in fellow eye controls (31). In contrast to FA, type 3 neovascularization is difficult to detect on ICGA in the early phases, particularly when the test is performed with a standard fundus camera rather than a scanning laser system. These lesions are better seen in the later phases of ICGA since the ICG molecule stains new vessels and becomes more prominent with time as the dye leaks intraretinally, often into associated cystoid

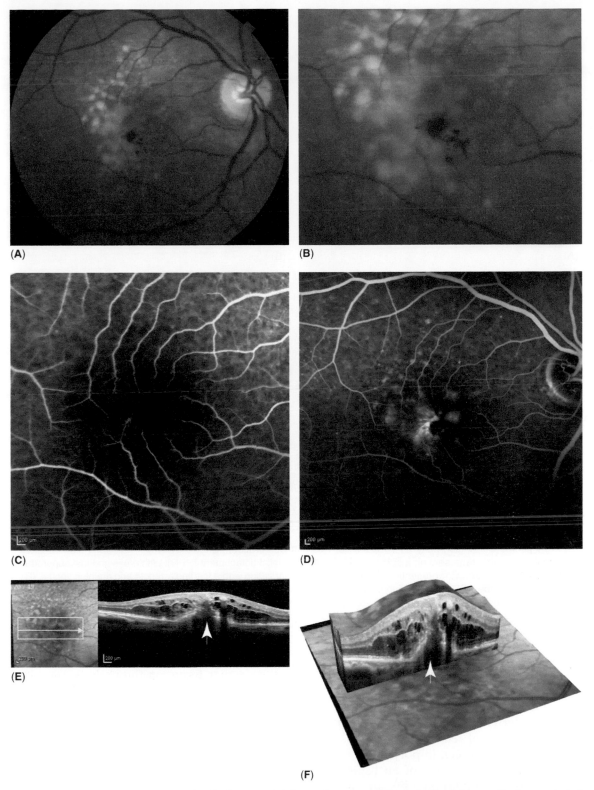

Figure 11.7 An 80-year-old white male presented with decreased vision and metamorphopsia in his right eye. Best-corrected visual acuities (BCVA) were 20/80 OD and 20/30 OS. (**A**) Color photograph (Topcon 50IA, Topcon Corporation, Paramus, NJ) demonstrates confluent soft macular drusen and intraretinal hemorrhages inferior to the fovea. (**B**) A magnified view of the right macula. Non-neovascular age-related macular degeneration was present in the left eye. (**C**) Early fluorescein angiography (FA, Heidelberg Spectralis HRA + OCT, Heidelberg Engineering Inc., Heidelberg, Germany) demonstrates pinpoint hyperfluorescence just inferotemporal to the fovea. (**D**) Late FA demonstrates occult fluorescein leakage and blockage from the intraretinal hemorrhage. (**E**) Spectral-domain optical coherence tomography (SD-OCT, Heidelberg Spectralis HRA + OCT, Heidelberg Engineering Inc., Heidelberg, Germany) is suggestive of a type 3 neovascular membrane with communication (retinal–choroidal anastomosis) to an underlying pigment epithelial detachment (arrow). Cystoid macular edema is present. (**F**) A 3-dimensional representation of the SD-OCT.

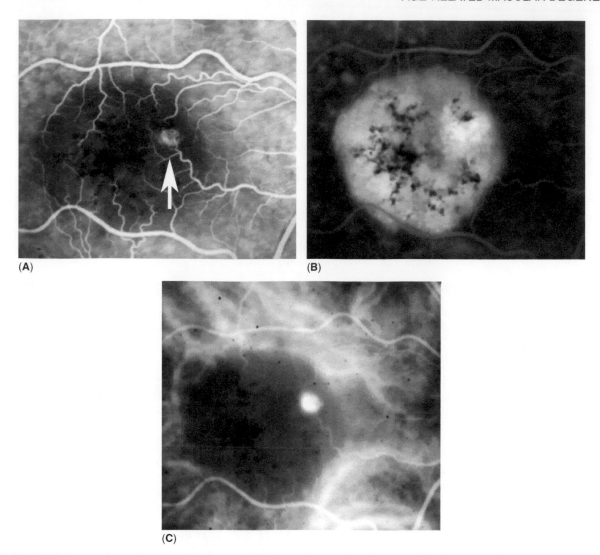

Figure 11.8 A, Early fluorescein angiography (FA, Topcon 50IA Topcon Corporation, Paramus, New Jersey, USA) demonstrates a well-circumscribed area of hypofluorescence representing a submacular pigment epithelial detachment (PED). Within this and just superonasal to the fovea, there is focal hyperfluorescence (arrow) representing intraretinal neovascularization with a feeding arteriole and draining venule. (**B**) In a late phase of the fluorescein angiogram, the PED fills with fluorescein dye simulating occult choroidal neovascularization. Within the staining PED there is hyperfluorescent leakage from the type 3 neovascular lesion. (**C**) Midphase indocyanine-green angiography (ICGA, Topcon 50IA) shows hypofluorescence of the PED and a hyperfluorescent "hot spot" corresponding to the type 3 neovascularization. *Source*: From Ref. 20.

macular edema (30). The ICG molecule has an affinity for fibrin, which may be present within intraretinal cystic spaces (20). Unlike fluorescein, ICG does not leak significantly into PEDs. A "hot spot" is most prominent when there is an underlying serous PED that produces a homogenous background of relative hypofluorescence. The "washout" of dye often seen in polypoidal neovascularization during the late phases of an ICGA is not seen in type 3 neovascularization (30). In advanced cases, an RCA may be visible (30).

Optical Coherence Tomography

OCT often shows intraretinal neovascularization as a focus of intraretinal hyper-reflectance extending from the outer plexiform and deeper layers (18,19,32). Intraretinal cysts are commonly seen, as are underlying serous PEDs. Occasionally, features suggesting a retinal to sub-RPE neovascularization (type 1 neovascularization) anastomosis or a CRA such as an RPE break, or even a vessel, may be identifiable on SD-OCT (Fig. 11.7) (33).

SD-OCT has allowed visualization of hyper-reflective neovascular tissue on the under-surface of a vascularized PED that could not previously be seen with time-domain OCT (3).

Management

Type 3 neovascularization rarely resolves spontaneously (4), and in most cases without treatment the natural history is poor. In a prospective study of 16 eyes of 14 patients followed for a mean of 20 months without treatment, the mean best-corrected visual acuity (BCVA) was 0.48 (20/42 Snellen equivalent) at baseline, decreasing to 0.23 (20/87 Snellen equivalent) after 6 months, and 0.19 (20/105 Snellen equivalent) at the final examination, with a mean decrease of 6 ETDRS lines from baseline (34). At final examination, BCVA had decreased to 0.1 (20/200 Snellen equivalent) or worse in 11 eyes (69%), and 5 of the 14 patients (36%) were legally blind.

The literature on management options for type 3 neovascularization is extensive. Better initial BCVA and earlier lesion stage are known to be associated with statistically significant better visual outcomes (35). The current standard of care is intravitreal anti-VEGF therapy with either ranibizumab or bevacizumab. In its early stages, type 3 neovascularization appears to be exquisitely sensitive to anti-VEGF therapy and resolution of neovascular manifestations can occur following a single injection (36). This may not be the case with more advanced lesions. Endothelial cells of type 3 neovascularization are known to test positive for VEGF and von Willebrand factor (vWF) on immunohistochemical staining (16). Many large clinical trials on intravitreal anti-VEGF therapy either excluded type 3 neovascularization or did not report subgroup analysis on this population (37,38). Thus, evidence is derived from smaller studies, some of which are conflicting.

Atmani et al. performed a prospective, nonrandomized study of 26 consecutive patients with treatment-naïve type 3 neovascularization treated with intravitreal ranibizumab and followed up for a minimum of 12 months (39). A loading dose of three monthly injections was followed by injections prescribed on a "pro re nata" (PRN) regimen guided by OCT with monthly follow-up. At month 12, 86% of patients had stabilization of their BCVA (loss of less than 15 letters), 69% maintained or improved vision, and 10% had improvement of 15 letters or more. Although these results supported the use of intravitreal ranibizumab for the treatment of type 3 neovascularization, they were worse than that which have been reported by MARINA and PrONTO study groups (Minimally Classic/Occult Trial of the Anti-VEGF Antibody Ranibizumab in the Treatment of Neovascular Age-Related Macular Degeneration (40) and the Prospective Optical coherence tomography imaging of patients with Neovascular AMD Treated with intra-Ocular ranibizumab study) (41). In the latter, 95% and 35% of patients had stabilization and improvement in BCVA (of 15 letters or more) at month 12. Comparable visual acuity results to those of MARINA and PrONTO were found in a prospective study of 31 eyes of 31 patients (42).

There is equal support for the use of intravitreal bevacizumab in the treatment of type 3 neovascularization. Meyerle et al. reported 17 eyes of patients who had 3-month follow-up: 5.9% had worse, 64.7% the same and 29.4% had improved visual acuity (36). Ghazi et al. described similar results (43). In a prospective study of 17 eyes of 16 patients by Gharbiya et al., 82.4% of eyes had stable vision and 17.7% improved 3 ETDRS lines or more at 12 months (44). To date there have been no head-to-head comparisons of intravitreal ranibizumab versus bevacizumab, specifically for the management of type 3 neovascularization. In a study by the Comparison of Age-Related Macular Degeneration Treatments Trials (CATT) research group, all lesion types including type 3 neovascularization were included (38). This study found equivalent effects on visual acuity at one year when administered according to the same schedule.

In general, the ocular and systemic side effects of intravitreal anti-VEGF for type 3 neovascularization are not thought to be any different from those for type 1 or 2

neovascularization secondary to AMD. However, a recent paper by McBain et al. (45). described a high rate (86%) of de novo RPE atrophy or enlargement of pre-existing RPE atrophy during a mean follow-up of 17 months in 66 eyes. All these eyes had received treatment with intravitreal anti-VEGF, intravitreal triamcinolone acetonide (IVTA), PDT, and/or laser. If this finding is replicated by future studies, the long-term visual prognosis of patients with type 3 neovascularization may be limited by geographic atrophy in addition to the damage secondary to the neovascular process. RPE tears have been reported to occur following treatment with both ranibizumab (42) and bevacizumab (46) for type 3 neovascularization. In both these cases a PED was present prior to the tear.

In an attempt to minimize the morbidity and cost of monthly dosing regimens, both "OCT-guided PRN" (39) and "Treat and Extend" (47) regimens for type 3 neovascularization have been described. With both regimens, treatment is given monthly until all clinical and OCT neovascular manifestations have fully resolved. In the PRN regimen, patients are seen monthly and reinjected if there is a decline in vision or recurrence of exudation clinically or by OCT imaging. In the study by Atmani et al., (39), a mean and standard deviation of 5.8 ± 1.7 injections were given in the first 12 months using this technique. With "Treat and Extend" dosing, treatment is given at each visit. However, if there is no evidence of recurrence, the follow-up period is sequentially extended to a maximum of 8–10 weeks. In the event of neovascular recurrence, the follow-up period is shortened until such time that the neovascular process is stabilized. Using this technique, Engelbert et al. (47) reported on 11 eyes of 10 consecutive patients with type 3 neovascularization treated with intravitreal ranibizumab and/or bevacizumab. All patients had a minimum of 12-months follow up. The mean baseline Snellen visual acuity was 20/80, improved to 20/40 at one month and maintained through a 36-month period (P < 0.04, paired t-test). The mean number of injections was 7 in the first year, 6 in the second year, and 7 in the third year.

Although intravitreal ranibizumab and/or bevacizumab monotherapy has been used with considerable success in the treatment of type 3 neovascularization (36,39,42–44,47,48), not all patients respond satisfactorily. Because of this, many other studies have looked at other therapies, either in isolation or in combination with anti-VEGF agents. These have included laser photocoagulation (49), photodynamic therapy (PDT) (50–59), transpupillary thermotherapy (60), anecortave acetate (61), periocular triamcinolone (54), IVTA (49–51,54,56,57,62,63), intravitreal pegaptanib (64), and submacular surgery (65). The most promising of these are PDT and IVTA. In a prospective trial by Rouvas et al., (56), 37 eyes of 37 patients were randomized to either: ranibizumab monotherapy (Group 1), ranibizumab plus a single session of PDT (Group 2), or a single IVTA injection plus a single session of PDT (Group 3). Re-treatment, with the same therapeutic regimen in each group, was considered in the event of

Table 11.1 Intravitreal and/or Photodynamic Therapies for Type 3 Neovascularization

Author	Year	Design	Eyes	Patients	Intervention	Duration	Outcomes
Ranibizumab Monotherapy							
Atmani et al.	2010	Prospective, consecutive patients	29	25	Ranibizumab	12 mos	86% of patients had stabilization of BCVA (loss of less than 15 letters), 69% maintained or improved vision and 10% had improvement of 15 letters or more
Konstantinidis et al.	2009	Prospective, consecutive patients	31	31	Ranibizumab	Mean 13.4 mos (last follow-up)	The mean logMAR BCVA improved significantly from baseline (0.72) to last follow-up (0.45) (P < 0.0001). The visual acuity (VA) improved by a mean of 2.7 lines (SD 2.5).
Bevacizumab Monotherapy							
Gharbiya et al.	2009	Prospective, consecutive patients	17	16	Bevacizumab	12 mos	Best-corrected visual acuity improved 3 ETDRS lines or more in 3 (17.7%) of 17 treated eyes, 14 (82.4%) eyes were stable, and 15 (88.2%) eyes gained 1 or more ETDRS lines.
Ghazi et al.	2008	Retrospective review	13	13	Bevacizumab	12 wks	Twelve eyes (92.3%) had stable or improved BCVA, and 8 eyes (61.5%) had at least 2 lines of vision improvement.
Meyerle et al.	2007	Retrospective review	23	23	Bevacizumab	12 wks	Of the 17 eyes available for 3-mo follow-up, 5 eyes (29.4%) had better visual acuity, 1 eye (5.9%) had worse acuity, and the remaining 11 (64.7%) had the same acuity.
Montero et al.	2009	Retrospective review	26	24	Bevacizumab	12 mos	Stage II (14 eyes): Mean BCVA 0.60 ± 0.24 (baseline), 0.62 ± 0.26 (6 mos), 0.63 ± 0.26 (12 mos) Stage III (12 eyes): Mean BCVA 1.13 ± 0.37 (baseline), 1.06 ± 0.37 (6 mos), 1.04 ± 0.37 (12 mos)
Intravitreal (Other than Anti-VEGF Monotherapy) and Photodynamic Therapies for Type 3 Neovascularization							
Freund et al.	2006	Prospective, consecutive patients	27	26	IVTA + PDT	12 mos	Visual acuity improved in 37% and was stable in 52% of eyes
Krebs et al.	2008	Prospective and retrospective cohort comparison	58	58	IVTA + PDT (Group 1: 27 patients prospective vs. PDT (Group 2: 27 patients retrospective)	12 mos	Distance BCVA decreased significantly over time (P < 0.0001) in both groups, from 65.6 ± 29.4 letters to 52.0 ± 26.0 after 12 mos in Group 1 and from 60.7 ± 28.2 letters to 44.0 ± 27.3 letters after 12 mos in Group 2. There were no significant differences in distance VA between groups at baseline or 12 mos (p = 0.76).
Lee et al.	2011	Prospective, consecutive patients	10	9	Ranibizumab + PDT	12 mos	At the 12-month visit, 7 eyes (78%) showed regression of the RAP lesions, of which 5 eyes (56%) required only a single session of combination treatment. The mean BCVA improved from 20/125 at baseline to 20/63 (P = 0.021).
Lo Giudice et al.	2009	Prospective, consecutive patients	8	8	PDT + Bevacizumab	9 mos	A significant improvement in the mean BCVA was observed at 1 mo, 3 mos, 6 mos, and 9 mos after combined treatment (P = 0.004). Visual acuity improved in 62.5% and was stable in 37.5% of cases.
Montero et al.	2008	Retrospective, non-randomized	79	68	PDT (42 eyes) vs. PeriocularTA + PDT (18 eyes) vs. IVTA + PDT (19 eyes)	12 mos	The mean (SD) initial CVA was 0.17 (0.19), 0.21 (0.20) and 0.20 (0.18), respectively. Mean BCVA was 0.12 (0.18), 0.10 (0.10) and 0.17 (0.26), respectively, at 12 mos (p = 0.12, 0.05 and 0.60, respectively, comparing vision at 12 mos with baseline.

(Continued)

Table 11.1 Intravitreal and/or Photodynamic Therapies for Type 3 Neovascularization (*Continued*)

Author	Year	Design	Eyes	Patients	Intervention	Duration	Outcomes
Rouvas et al.	2009	Prospective, randomized	37	37	Ranibizumab (Group 1: 13 eyes) *vs.* Ranibizumab + PDT (Group 2: 13 eyes) *vs.* IVTA + PDT (Group 3: 11 eyes)	Minimum 6 mos	A total of 61.5% patients in Group 1, 76.9% in Group 2, and all in Group 3 had the same or better visual acuity at the end of the follow-up (P = 0.0232).
Saito et al.	2010	Retrospective	25	22	IVTA + PDT (Group 1, 12 eyes) *vs.* Bevacizumab + PDT (Group 2, 13 eyes)	12 mos	In Group 1, the mean BCVA at baseline and 12 mos were 0.29 and 0.13, respectively with a significant decline (P < 0.05). In Group 2, the mean BCVA levels at baseline and 12 mos were 0.25 and 0.37 with a significant improvement (P < 0.05). At 12 mos, the difference in BCVA between the 2 groups was significant (P < 0.05).
Saito et al.	2010	Retrospective	11	10	Bevacizumab + PDT	6 mos	The mean BCVA levels at baseline and 6 mos after treatment were 0.16 and 0.29, respectively. A significant improvement in the mean BCVA was observed at 6 mos after intravitreal bevacizumab injection and PDT (P < 0.01). The mean improvement in BCVA 6 mos from baseline was 2.64 lines.
Viola et al.	2010	Prospective	21	18	Bevacizumab + PDT	9 mos	Mean visual acuity at baseline was 0.63 ± 0.25 logMAR. After treatment, BCVA showed no statistically significant differences between each visit (P = 0.10, ANOVA). At 9 mos, the BCVA improved by 3 or more lines in 3 eyes (14%), remained stable in 12 eyes (57%), and worsened in 6 eyes (29%).

Abbreviations: BCVA, best-corrected visual acuity; IVTA, Intravitreal Triamcinclone, mo/mos; PDT, photodynamic therapy; periocular TA, periocular triamciolone; mos, months.

persistent or recurrent subretinal or intraretinal fluid. All patients completed at least 6 months of follow-up. At the end of the follow-up, 61.5% patients in Group 1, 76.9% in Group 2, and 100% in Group 3 had the same or better visual acuity (P = 0.0232). In a study by Krebs et al., (51), of 57 eyes of 57 patients treated with either IVTA and PDT (Group 1, followed prospectively) or PDT alone (Group 2, reviewed retrospectively), no significant differences were found in the distance BCVA, retinal thickness, or lesion size between the groups at any time point up to month 12.

Due to the variable trial designs, sample sizes, interventions, durations, and outcome measures, it is difficult to compare these studies easily. Ultimately, the decision to add a therapy other than intravitreal anti-VEGF for persistent or recurrent exudation, or as initial combination therapy must be determined on a case-by-case basis. The findings of all known reviews of intravitreal and PDT therapies for type 3 neovascularization are summarized in Table 11.1.

Finally, in November 2011, the U.S. Food and Drug Administration approved the use of intravitreal aflibercept (*Eylea*, Regeneron Pharmaceuticals Inc.), a VEGF fusion protein, for the treatment of neovascular AMD. To date, no studies have been published on the efficacy of aflibercept for type 3 neovascularization, although its efficacy, like that for all types of neovascular AMD in two parallel phase 3 studies (VIEW 1 (66) and 2 (67)), is likely to be promising.

SUMMARY POINTS

- In summary, type 3 neovascularization is a distinct form of neovascularization present in a small subset of patients with AMD.
- It is distinguished by the presence of intraretinal proliferating vessels, although it can penetrate into the subretinal and sub-RPE layers, with development of RCA in advanced cases.
- The site of initiation remains debateable, with evidence for both choroidal and retinal origins. Indeed, both of these may be possible.
- It typically presents unilaterally in elderly white female patients, although involvement of the fellow eye is common.
- Typical clinical and OCT features include intraretinal hemorrhage, cystoid macular edema, and a serous PED. The lesion is most easily seen in the early phases of FA and the later phases of ICGA when a "hot spot" may be visible.
- Intravitreal anti-VEGF is currently the standard of care, although an alternative or adjunctive treatment may be considered on a case-by-case basis.

REFERENCES

1. Gass J. Stereoscopic Atlas of Macular Diseases, 4th edn. St.Louis: C.V. Mosby, 1997.
2. Freund KB, Yannuzzi LA, Sorenson JA. Age-related macular degeneration and choroidal neovascularization. Am J Ophthalmol 1993; 115: 786–91.
3. Freund KB, Zweifel SA, Engelbert M. Do we need a new classification for choroidal neovascularization in age-related macular degeneration? Retina 2010; 30: 1333–49. [Erratum appears in Retina. 2011 Jan;31(1):208]
4. Freund KB, Ho IV, Barbazetto IA, et al. Type 3 neovascularization: the expanded spectrum of retinal angiomatous proliferation. Retina 2008; 28: 201–11.
5. Hartnett ME, Weiter JJ, Garsd A, Jalkh AE. Classification of retinal pigment epithelial detachments associated with drusen. Graefes Arch Clin Exp Ophthalmol 1992; 230: 11–19.
6. Hartnett ME, Weiter JJ, Staurenghi G, Elsner AE. Deep retinal vascular anomalous complexes in advanced age-related macular degeneration. Ophthalmology 1996; 103: 2042–53.
7. Lafaut BA, Aisenbrey S, Vanden Broecke C, Bartz-Schmidt KU. Clinicopathological correlation of deep retinal vascular anomalous complex in age related macular degeneration. Br J Ophthalmol 2000; 84: 1269–74.
8. Yannuzzi LA, Negrao S, Iida T, et al. Retinal angiomatous proliferation in age-related macular degeneration. Retina 2001; 21: 416–34.
9. Kuhn D, Meunier I, Soubrane G, Coscas G. Imaging of chorioretinal anastomoses in vascularized retinal pigment epithelium detachments. Arch Ophthalmol 1995; 113: 1392–8.
10. Gass JD, Agarwal A, Lavina AM, Tawansy KA. Focal inner retinal hemorrhages in patients with drusen: an early sign of occult choroidal neovascularization and chorioretinal anastomosis. Retina 2003; 23: 741–51.
11. Slakter JS, Yannuzzi LA, Schneider U, et al. Retinal choroidal anastomoses and occult choroidal neovascularization in age-related macular degeneration. Ophthalmology 2000; 107: 742–53; discussion 53–4.
12. Scott AW, Bressler SB. Retinal angiomatous proliferation or retinal anastomosis to the lesion. Eye 2010; 24: 491–6.
13. Heckenlively JR, Hawes NL, Friedlander M, et al. Mouse model of subretinal neovascularization with choroidal anastomosis. Retina 2003; 23: 518–22.
14. Okamoto N, Tobe T, Hackett SF, et al. Transgenic mice with increased expression of vascular endothelial growth factor in the retina: a new model of intraretinal and subretinal neovascularization. Am J Pathol 1997; 151: 281–91.
15. Shimada H, Kawamura A, Mori R, Yuzawa M. Clinicopathological findings of retinal angiomatous proliferation. Graefes Arch Clin Exp Ophthalmol 2007; 245: 295–300.
16. Monson DM, Smith JR, Klein ML, Wilson DJ. Clinicopathologic correlation of retinal angiomatous proliferation. Arch Ophthalmol 2008; 126: 1664–8.
17. Klein ML, Wilson DJ. Clinicopathologic correlation of choroidal and retinal neovascular lesions in age-related macular degeneration. Am J Ophthalmol 2011; 151: 161–9.
18. Zacks DN, Johnson MW. Retinal angiomatous proliferation: optical coherence tomographic confirmation of an intraretinal lesion. Arch Ophthalmol 2004; 122: 932–3.
19. Brancato R, Introini U, Pierro L, et al. Optical coherence tomography (OCT) angiomatous proliferation (RAP) in retinal. Eur J Ophthalmol 2002; 12: 467–72.
20. Yannuzzi LA, Freund KB, Takahashi BS. Review of retinal angiomatous proliferation or type 3 neovascularization. Retina 2008; 28: 375–84.
21. Gass JDM, Agarwal A, Lavina AM, Tawansy KA. Focal inner retinal hemorrhages in patients with drusen: an early sign of occult choroidal neovascularization and chorioretinal anastomosis. Retina 2003; 23: 741–51.

22. Costa RA, Calucci D, Paccola L, et al. Occult chorioretinal anastomosis in age-related macular degeneration: a prospective study by optical coherence tomography. Am J Ophthalmol 2005; 140: 107–16.

23. Truong SN, Alam S, Zawadzki RJ, et al. High resolution fourier-domain optical coherence tomography of retinal angiomatous proliferation. Retina 2007; 27: 915–25.

24. Massacesi AL, Sacchi L, Bergamini F, Bottoni F. The prevalence of retinal angiomatous proliferation in age-related macular degeneration with occult choroidal neovascularization. Graefes Arch Clin Exp Ophthalmol 2008; 246: 89–92.

25. Axer-Siegel R, Bourla D, Priel E, Yassur Y, Weinberger D. Angiographic and flow patterns of retinal choroidal anastomoses in age-related macular degeneration with occult choroidal neovascularization. Ophthalmology 2002; 109: 1726–36.

26. Gross NE, Aizman A, Brucker A, Klancnik JM Jr, Yannuzzi LA. Nature and risk of neovascularization in the fellow eye of patients with unilateral retinal angiomatous proliferation. Retina 2005; 25: 713–18.

27. Macular Photocoagulation Study Group. Risk factors for choroidal neovascularization in the second eye of patients with juxtafoveal or subfoveal choroidal neovascularization secondary to age-related macular degeneration. Arch Ophthalmol 1997; 115: 741–7.

28. Campa C, Harding SP, Pearce IA, et al. Incidence of neovascularization in the fellow eye of patients with unilateral retinal angiomatous proliferation. Eye 2010; 24: 1585–9.

29. Hayashi H, Yamashiro K, Gotoh N, et al. CFH and ARMS2 variations in age-related macular degeneration, polypoidal choroidal vasculopathy, and retinal angiomatous proliferation. Invest Ophthalmol Vis Sci 2010; 51: 5914–19.

30. Fernandes LHS, Freund KB, Yannuzzi LA, et al. The nature of focal areas of hyperfluorescence or hot spots imaged with indocyanine green angiography. Retina 2002; 22: 557–68.

31. Koizumi H, Iida T, Saito M, Nagayama D, Maruko I. Choroidal circulatory disturbances associated with retinal angiomatous proliferation on indocyanine green angiography. Graefes Arch Clin Exp Ophthalmol 2008; 246: 515–20.

32. Matsumoto H, Sato T, Kishi S. Tomographic features of intraretinal neovascularization in retinal angiomatous proliferation. Retina 2010; 30: 425–30.

33. Krebs I, Glittenberg C, Hagen S, Haas P, Binder S. Retinal angiomatous proliferation: morphological changes assessed by stratus and cirrus OCT. Ophthalmic Surg Lasers Imaging 2009; 40: 285–9.

34. Viola F, Massacesi A, Orzalesi N, Ratiglia R, Staurenghi G. Retinal angiomatous proliferation: natural history and progression of visual loss. Retina 2009; 29: 732–9.

35. Bottoni F, Massacesi A, Cigada M, et al. Treatment of retinal angiomatous proliferation in age-related macular degeneration: a series of 104 cases of retinal angiomatous proliferation. Arch Ophthalmol 2005; 123: 1644–50.

36. Meyerle CB, Freund KB, Iturralde D, et al. Intravitreal bevacizumab (Avastin) for retinal angiomatous proliferation. Retina 2007; 27: 451–7.

37. Brown DM, Kaiser PK, Michels M, et al. Ranibizumab versus verteporfin for neovascular age-related macular degeneration. N Engl J Med 2006; 355: 1432–44.

38. Group CR, Martin DF, Maguire MG, et al. Ranibizumab and bevacizumab for neovascular age-related macular degeneration. N Engl J Med 2011; 364: 1897–908.

39. Atmani K, Voigt M, Le Tien V, et al. Ranibizumab for retinal angiomatous proliferation in age-related macular degeneration. Eye 2010; 24: 1193–8.

40. Rosenfeld PJ, Brown DM, Heier JS, et al. Ranibizumab for neovascular age-related macular degeneration. N Engl J Med 2006; 355: 1419–31.

41. Fung AE, Lalwani GA, Rosenfeld PJ, et al. An optical coherence tomography-guided, variable dosing regimen with intravitreal ranibizumab (Lucentis) for neovascular age-related macular degeneration. Am J Ophthalmol 2007; 143: 566–83.

42. Konstantinidis L, Mameletzi E, Mantel I, et al. Intravitreal ranibizumab (Lucentis) in the treatment of retinal angiomatous proliferation (RAP). Graefes Arch Clin Exp Ophthalmol 2009; 247: 1165–71.

43. Ghazi NG, Knape RM, Kirk TQ, Tiedeman JS, Conway BP. Intravitreal bevacizumab (Avastin) treatment of retinal angiomatous proliferation. Retina 2008; 28: 689–95.

44. Gharbiya M, Allievi F, Recupero V, et al. Intravitreal bevacizumab as primary treatment for retinal angiomatous proliferation: twelve-mo results. Retina 2009; 29: 740–9.

45. McBain VA, Kumari R, Townend J, Lois N. Geographic atrophy in retinal angiomatous proliferation. Retina 2011; 31: 1043–52.

46. Forooghian F, Cukras C, Chew EY. Retinal angiomatous proliferation complicated by pigment epithelial tear following intravitreal bevacizumab treatment. Can J Ophthalmol 2008; 43: 246–8.

47. Engelbert M, Zweifel SA, Freund KB. "Treat and extend" dosing of intravitreal antivascular endothelial growth factor therapy for type 3 neovascularization/retinal angiomatous proliferation. Retina 2009; 29: 1424–31.

48. Hemeida TS, Keane PA, Dustin L, Sadda SR, Fawzi AA. Long term visual and anatomical outcomes following anti-VEGF monotherapy for retinal angiomatous proliferation. Br J Ophthalmol 2010; 94: 701–5.

49. Mendis R, Leslie T, McBain V, Lois N. Combined therapy for retinal angiomatous proliferation with intravitreal triamcinolone and argon laser photocoagulation. Br J Ophthalmol 2008; 92: 1154–6.

50. Freund KB, Klais CM, Eandi CM, et al. Sequenced combined intravitreal triamcinolone and indocyanine green angiography-guided photodynamic therapy for retinal angiomatous proliferation. Arch Ophthalmol 2006; 124: 487–92.

51. Krebs I, Krepler K, Stolba U, Goll A, Binder S. Retinal angiomatous proliferation: combined therapy of intravitreal triamcinolone acetonide and PDT versus PDT alone. Graefes Arch Clin Exp Ophthalmol 2008; 246: 237–43.

52. Lee MY, Kim KS, Lee WK. Combination therapy of ranibizumab and photodynamic therapy for retinal angiomatous proliferation with serous pigment epithelial detachment in Korean patients: twelve-mo results. Retina 2011; 31: 65–73.

53. Lo Giudice G, Gismondi M, De Belvis V, et al. Single-session photodynamic therapy combined with intravitreal bevacizumab for retinal angiomatous proliferation. Retina 2009; 29: 949–55.

54. Montero JA, Ruiz-Moreno JM, Sanabria MR, Fernandez-Munoz M. Efficacy of intravitreal and periocular triamcinolone associated with photodynamic therapy for treatment of retinal angiomatous proliferation. Br J Ophthalmol 2009; 93: 166–70.

55. Nakata M, Yuzawa M, Kawamura A, Shimada H. Combining surgical ablation of retinal inflow and outflow vessels with photodynamic therapy for retinal angiomatous proliferation. Am J Ophthalmol 2006; 141: 968–70.

56. Rouvas AA, Papakostas TD, Vavvas D, et al. Intravitreal ranibizumab, intravitreal ranibizumab with PDT, and intravitreal triamcinolone with PDT for the treatment of retinal angiomatous proliferation: a prospective study. Retina 2009; 29: 536–44.

57. Saito M, Shiragami C, Shiraga F, Kano M, Iida T. Comparison of intravitreal triamcinolone acetonide with photodynamic therapy and intravitreal bevacizumab with photodynamic therapy for retinal angiomatous proliferation. Am J Ophthalmol 2010; 149: 472–81; e1.

58. Saito M, Shiragami C, Shiraga F, Nagayama D, Iida T. Combined intravitreal bevacizumab and photodynamic therapy for retinal angiomatous proliferation. Am J Ophthalmol 2008; 146: 935–41; e1.

59. Viola F, Mapelli C, Villani E, et al. Sequential combined treatment with intravitreal bevacizumab and photodynamic therapy for retinal angiomatous proliferation. Eye 2010; 24: 1344–51.

60. Kuroiwa S, Arai J, Gaun S, Iida T, Yoshimura N. Rapidly progressive scar formation after transpupillary thermotherapy in retinal angiomatous proliferation. Retina 2003; 23: 417–20.

61. Klais CM, Eandi CM, Ober MD, et al. Anecortave acetate treatment for retinal angiomatous proliferation: a pilot study. Retina 2006; 26: 773–9.

62. Bakri SJ, Ekdawi NS. Intravitreal triamcinolone and bevacizumab combination therapy for refractory choroidal neovascularization with retinal angiomatous proliferation. Eye 2008; 22: 978–80.

63. Sahu AK, Narayanan R. Intravitreal ranibizumab, intravitreal ranibizumab with photodynamic therapy (PDT), and intravitreal triamcinolone with PDT for the treatment of retinal angiomatous proliferation. Retina 2010; 30: 981; author reply.

64. Mahmood S, Kumar N, Lenfestey PM, et al. Early response of retinal angiomatous proliferation treated with intravitreal pegaptanib: a retrospective review. Eye 2009; 23: 530–5.

65. Krebs I, Binder S, Stolba U, et al. Subretinal surgery and transplantation of autologous pigment epithelial cells in retinal angiomatous proliferation. Acta Opthalmologica 2008; 86: 504–9.

66. A Randomized, Double-Masked Active Controlled Phase 3 Study of the Efficacy, Safety, and Tolerability of Repeated Doses of Intravitreal VEGF Trap-Eye in Subjects with Neovascular AMD. ClinicalTrials.gov identifier: NCT00509795. [Available from: http//clinicaltrials.gov/ct2/show/NCT00509795]

67. A Randomized, Double-Masked, Active Controlled, Phase 3 Study of the Efficacy, Safety, and Tolerability of Repeated Doses of Intravitreal VEGF Trap-Eye in Subjects With Neovascular AMD. ClinicalTrials.gov identifier: NCT00637377. [Available from: http://clinicaltrials.gov/ct2/show/NCT00637377]

12

Role of fluorescein angiography in the treatment of age-related macular degeneration

Jesse J. Jung, Quan V. Hoang, Irene A. Barbazetto, and Jason S. Slakter

OVERVIEW

Since its inception (1–3), fluorescein angiography (FA) has played a critical role in the diagnosis and management of numerous retinal vascular diseases. Various spatial and temporal patterns of FA hyper- and hypo-fluorescence have correlated well with specific diseases, disease states, and response to treatment modalities. In age-related macular degeneration (AMD), choroidal neovascularization (CNV) was classified by occult and classic patterns of fluorescein filling and leakage, which correlated with clinical outcomes and response to therapy in large randomized clinical trials employing thermal laser (4–9) and photodynamic therapy (PDT) (4,10–15). This chapter will summarize the basic principles underlying FA, its interpretation (specifically in the context of AMD), utility in guiding treatment in previous laser trials and developments in FA interpretation and application.

FLUORESCEIN ANGIOGRAPHY: BACKGROUND
Introduction

Fluorescein angiography is an important tool in diagnosing and following the treatment of retinal diseases. FA utilizes a molecule, sodium fluorescein, first synthesized by Baeyer in 1871 to create fluorescence (16). Combined with serial fundus photographs after intravenous injection of sodium fluorescein dye, one can study the retinal and choroidal circulation (1). Initially used in the human eye for differentiating between a choroidal melanoma and hemangioma (3), intravenous FA was further developed to study retinal vascular flow characteristics and circulation times, and as a powerful tool for diagnosing and classifying age-related macular degeneration (AMD).

Basic Principles of FA

The basic principles of fluorescence include luminescence, defined as emission of light from any source other than high temperature. Fluorescence is defined as luminescence that is maintained only by continuous excitation. When light energy is absorbed into a luminescent material, it excites free electrons into higher energy states. When the electrons spontaneously decay, energy is released as luminescent light in the visible spectrum (17).

Sodium fluorescein ($C_{20}H_{12}O_5Na$) is a hydrocarbon that absorbs light between 465–490 nm and will fluoresce at a wavelength of 520–530 nm (17,18). The excitation wavelength is in the blue spectrum. Once excited, these electrons spontaneously decay emitting a green-yellow wavelength (17). The fluorescence emitted is linked temporally with excitation and each quantum of stimulating light results in an almost immediate release of a quantum of fluorescent light (19). Sodium fluorescein weighs 375.27 Da and readily diffuses through fenestrated vessels of the choriocapillaris, but does not cross the blood–retina barrier, which is composed of the tight junctions between retinal pigment epithelium (RPE) or retinal vascular endothelium (18). Sodium fluorescein is highly soluble and has maximal fluorescence at the ideal human blood pH of 7.4 (20). The unbound molecule has few adverse side effects when delivered into the blood stream and remains relatively inert while most of the fluorescein molecules are bound to albumin and excreted renally (21). When injected intravenously, approximately 20% remains free in the bloodstream and are excited by blue light (emitted from the light source through a blue filter). Once the sodium fluorescein molecules are excited and subsequently decay, the camera receives the emitted yellow-green fluorescence. A barrier filter blocks the remaining reflected blue light and the image is recorded.

Fluorescein is eliminated by the liver and kidneys within 24 hours and due to its diffuse permeability, may result in a yellowish tinge of the urine and skin for a few hours post injection (17). Retention may increase if renal function is impaired and traces may be found in the body for up to a week after injection (17). Caution may be needed in patients with severe renal impairment. In a small series of diabetic patients, nine of the 22 study patients (20.5%) that underwent FA experienced an increase in serum creatinine within 72 hours of injection, but did not note any significant adverse effects (22). Nausea is the most frequent side effect of fluorescein injection, occurring in about 5% of patients, mostly in patients under 50 years of age or in whom fluorescein is injected rapidly (17). Vomiting occurs infrequently, affecting only 0.3–0.4% of patients (17). Symptoms of nausea and vomiting usually subside rapidly. Hives, unless very mild, are usually treated with antihistamines such as diphenhydramine (17,19). Vasovagal attacks occur much less frequently and are more likely due to patient anxiety rather than the actual injection (17). Anaphylaxis (defined as hypotension, tachycardia, bronchospasms, hives, and itching) is relatively rare given sodium fluorescein's relative minimal reactivity (17,19–24). Other potential serious side effects (1:1900) such as shock, flash pulmonary edema, delayed hypersensitivity reaction, laryngeal spasm, syncope, and even death (1:222,000) are fortunately rare (17,18,21). FA has been performed during pregnancy and although the molecule can cross the placenta, one survey has shown that fluorescein does not cause teratogenicity or complications (24,25). This same survey did report occurrence of a case of stillbirth, one therapeutic abortion related to complications of toxemia, one spontaneous abortion, and several babies born with low birth weights. Although thought to be unrelated to the use of fluorescein, caution should be utilized when performing FA during pregnancy (25).

FA Imaging Technology

Novotny and Alvis first utilized a modified Zeiss fundus camera in the 1960s to measure oxygen saturation levels in rabbit eyes (1). FA technologic advancements since that time include modification to the power pack, flash unit, dual camera backs, a motor drive for rapid and motionless film advancement, stereo separator, and the development of digital cameras which allow for even more efficient and higher-resolution image processing (1,18).

In addition, later developments such as utilizing scanning laser ophthalmoscopy (SLO) further enhanced FA photography (26). With SLO, argon and infrared laser illumination focuses laser light which is swept across the fundus in a raster pattern, detecting light only from a conjugate plane of interest and rejecting light from other planes, thereby enhancing contrast and allowing for higher temporal and spatial resolution (19). These optical properties also allow SLO to obtain images under low light intensity through a small pupil or media opacity (18). Additionally, video angiography using SLO-based imaging systems can record images in real time and a high frame rate, providing more information about the vascular filling patterns and abnormalities that may be associated with an area of choroidal neovascularization.

FA Filling Sequence

Common standardized photography sequences are composed of initial stereo color and red-free photographs of the macula. Rapid sequence photos are then taken of the eye with the macular pathology of greatest interest (primary macula) during the filling phase and followed by stereo pair of the primary macula at approximately 30, 40, 60, 90, and 180 seconds post injection. Late stereo photos are taken between 5–10 minutes post injections (17,18). Alternatively, a short video sequence (30–60 seconds) can be taken directly after injection of dye when using SLO-based imaging systems.

After injection, fluorescein dye first appears intraocularly within 10–12 seconds in young adults but may be delayed in older patients. As fluorescein molecules transit through the retinal and choroidal circulation, the angiographic sequence can be broken down into several defined phases.

The choroidal/early arterial phase occurs approximately 10–15 seconds post antecubital injection and is marked by patchy filling of the choriocapillaris vessels ("choroidal flush"). The choroid fills from a number of separate vessels simultaneously and dye diffuses through the choriocapillaris eventually staining Bruch's membrane but is blocked from forward diffusion into the retina by the tight junctions of the RPE. Once the choriocapillaris is completely filled, the central retinal artery is filled in the following two to three seconds.

Next, the arterial/early venous laminar phase occurs, which is marked by rapid filling of multiple branch arterioles, retinal capillary bed, and subsequently early laminar filling of the venous walls.

The full venous stage occurs approximately five to eight seconds later and is marked by complete filling of the arteries and the veins. The small capillary network surrounding the fovea is best demonstrated in this phase. The veins lead back to the optic nerve and coalesce into a single central retinal vein. Recirculation or late venous phases occurs over the next several minutes as the fluorescein dye transits through the eye circulation.

Late-stage photographs are completed in less than five minutes depending on the suspected pathology. This phase is characterized by staining of the lamina cribrosa and faint traces of dye remaining in the retinal vessels, choroid, and sclera.

FA of the macular area is unique due to its anatomy. Throughout all FA phases, the foveal area remains relatively darker than the surrounding areas for several reasons. The first is that the fovea itself is avascular and there is no capillary bed to fill with fluorescein. Another reason is that the macula contains high concentrations of xanthophyll pigment giving it a characteristic yellow hue. Xanthophyll also absorbs blue light thereby reducing the amount of excitation light stimulating the underlying fluorescein during FA. Additionally, RPE cells in the macular region are taller and contain large amounts of melanin pigment, which absorbs both the excitation blue light and emitted fluorescent light from the underlying choriocapillaris (19).

FA Interpretation

AMD has characteristic FA patterns that incorporate angiographic abnormalities such as increased fluorescence (hyperfluorescence) or decreased fluorescence (hypofluorescence) (18). Hypofluorescence may result from blockage of underlying fluorescence due to blood, turbid fluid/exudate, or thickened tissue layers or occur due to a filling defect within the vasculature. Hyperfluorescence in AMD can be due to a transmission defect secondary to loss of the normal barrier to background choroidal fluorescence, due to a pathological loss of melanin (in the choroid or RPE) or reduced xanthophyll pigment in the macula. Hyperfluorescence can also be due to staining of various lesions such as soft drusen, leakage of dye into a confined subretinal space (pooling), seen with serous RPE detachments, or leakage into an abnormal extravascular space due to neovascularization.

ANGIOGRAPHIC PATTERNS IN AMD
Angiographic Patterns in Non-Neovascular AMD

Drusen are classified based on their size and appearance. They may be large (>125 µm), intermediate (>63 µm), or small (<63 µm) (19). FA findings depend on the extent to which the overlying RPE has thinned and the histochemical composition of the drusen (19). Higher concentrations of phospholipids contribute to increased fluorescein staining, while neutral lipid accumulation does not (27).

There are several types of drusen that differ histopathologically and angiographically. Hard drusen (<63 µm) are accumulations of lipid and hyaline material in the inner and outer collagenous zones of Bruch's membrane and appear as round discrete deposits on ophthalmoscopy (28). FA often reveals a greater number of hard drusen than can be seen clinically (29) which appear as hyperfluorescent spots due to a transmission defect resulting from RPE thinning over the surface of hard drusen (19).

Cuticular or basal laminar drusen appear as innumerable, small, round, semitranslucent, and yellow lesions on fundus biomicroscopy (18). Histopathology reveals basal laminar drusen to be nodular elevations of a diffusely thickened inner Bruch's membrane (30). On FA, they appear as a "starry sky" with a multitude of tiny hyperfluorescent spots from multiple transmission defects (19).

Soft drusen on the other hand may coalesce forming a shallow elevation of the RPE (drusenoid RPE detachment) (31). During the early phase FA, there is a faint but increasing hyperfluorescence of the drusen with no signs of leakage. As time progresses, the fluorescence may continue to be apparent or decrease and fade. There is very little angiographic difference between large drusen and small pigment epithelial detachments (PEDs) (32). However, the FA pattern differs from larger serous PEDs with more turbid fluid, which appear hypo- or isofluorescent in the early FA phase followed by a slow increase of fluorescent dye ("pooling") within the detachment resulting in marked, uniform hyperfluorescence in the late phases (19).

Other manifestations of non-neovascular AMD include RPE abnormalities/pigmentary changes. Focal hyperpigmentation appears as blocked fluorescence on FA and histopathologically corresponds to focal RPE hypertrophy, detached pigment epithelial cells and pigment migration into the subretinal space and outer retina (19,33,34).

RPE atrophy commonly occurs in non-neovascular AMD. When the areas of atrophy are sharply defined, this is known as geographic atrophy (GA). When the borders are less defined and there are more granular regions of less severe atrophy, this is defined as non-geographic atrophy. Although both types of atrophy demonstrate RPE loss on histopathology, GA is more strongly associated with atrophy of the overlying retina and underlying choriocapillaris (18). On FA, GA does not hyperfluoresce in early phases due to loss of underlying choriocapillaris. Only larger choroidal vessels are apparent. In later phases, there is a well-defined hyperfluorescence from the staining of the exposed deep choroid and sclera without leakage (18). In comparison, non-GA typically appears as mottled early hyperfluorescence, which fades in the late phase consistent with a window defect and does not change in shape or size throughout the angiogram (18).

Angiographic Patterns in Neovascular AMD

The growth of abnormal blood vessels with serous or hemorrhagic detachment of the retina and retinal pigment epithelium, lipid exudation, subretinal fibrosis, or disciform scar formation defines neovascular AMD (18). CNV consists of abnormal blood vessels that grow from the choroid into Bruch's membrane, as well as under and into the neurosensory retina. The angiographic appearance of CNV is governed both by the density and maturity of the vessels and by the amount and character of the intervening tissue (19). CNV has been further subcategorized based on its location. Extrafoveal CNV lies greater than 200 µm from the foveal center; juxtafoveal CNV is located between 1 and 199 µm from the foveal center; and subfoveal CNV is located under the center of the fovea.

Classification of types of CNV has been determined based on FA filling and leakage patterns. Classic CNV (Fig. 12.1) is seen as a brightly hyperfluorescent lesion in the early phase of the angiogram, corresponding to choroidal filling. This early, almost immediate hyperfluorescence has well-demarcated boundaries but can also appear as an early lacy or cartwheel configuration. This hyperfluorescence corresponds to a relatively acute growth of vessels that break through Bruch's membrane and the RPE and then proliferate above the RPE in the subretinal space (35). These vessels show prominent leakage during the course of the angiogram and eventually the vessels and their borders become obscured by the overlying leakage (19). A variant of classic CNV has been described in which a new vessel filling is slower and the boundaries are not distinguished until approximately two minutes after dye injection. Eventually these boundaries become blurred in the later frames corresponding to classic abnormal vessel leakage (36).

Occult CNV (Fig. 12.2) differs from classic CNV in that the abnormal fibrovascular ingrowth is obscured by intervening tissue. It is typified by a fibrovascular PED in which abnormal vessels remain beneath intact RPE and can create an irregular elevation of the RPE (19,35). Based on the MPS study group findings, there are two fluorescein angiographic types of occult CNV differentiated upon the relative elevation of the leaking lesion (5). In one form of occult CNV, termed fibrovascular RPE detachment, the FA will show a fibrovascular PED slowly increasing in fluorescence often in a heterogeneous manner. This dye is retained in the fibrovascular PED late in the angiogram and leakage from the fibrovascular PED can result in the appearance of hyperfluorescence inside the fibrovascular elevation, subretinal space, or even into the retina (19). In the second form of occult CNV, known as late leakage of undetermined source, there is no early

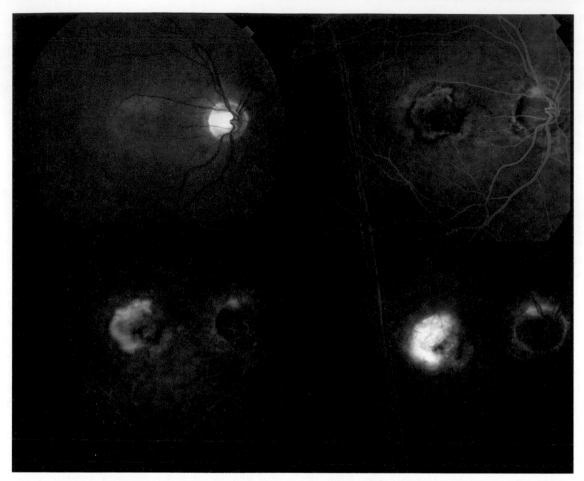

Figure 12.1 Color images of (*upper left panel*), early phase (*upper right panel*), mid-phase (*lower left panel*), and late phase fluorescein angiogram (*lower right panel*) of a patient with a classic choroidal neovascularization lesion. Note the brightly hyperfluorescent lesion in the early phase with well-demarcated boundaries with prominent leakage during the course of the angiogram with eventual blurring of the boundaries by the overlying leakage.

hyperfluorescence and during the late phase there is generalized leakage beneath the RPE often with mild to moderate stippled fluorescence, with minimal elevation of the fibrovascular PED (19).

Classic and occult forms of neovascularization can occur in the same lesion, thus demonstrating both leakage patterns on the FA. Interpretation of these mixed lesions and determining the components requires a careful analysis of all phases of the FA study. In some clinical trials, detailed characterization of these lesion components led to a classification system that has three main categories depending on the proportion of each type of CNV in the lesion. If the entire lesion (which is defined as all visible CNV and associated features that might obscure the underlying CNV, such as thick blood, serous PED, or elevated blocked fluorescence) is composed of 50% or more classic CNV, then it is termed "Predominantly Classic." If there is some classic CNV, but it accounts for less than 50% of the total lesion area, then it is termed "Minimally Classic". If no classic CNV is seen and there is only occult CNV noted on the FA, then it is termed "Occult with no Classic" (5,14,19).

These angiographic classifications of CNV were essential for treatment planning in the original Macular Photocoagulation Study (MPS), Treatment of AMD

with Photodynamic Therapy (TAP) Study, and the Verteporfin in Photodynamic Therapy (VIP) Study. Now with the development of additional imaging techniques such as indocyanine green (ICG) angiography and spectral domain optical coherence tomography (SD-OCT) and in conjunction with some histopathologic evidence, the original fluorescein CNV classification has been augmented. Gass (36) and subsequently Freund et al. (37) proposed a non-angiographic, more anatomic classification system of CNV. Type 1 CNV referred to vessels confined to the sub-RPE space, type 2 referred to vessels that have broken through Bruch's membrane and the RPE and proliferate above the RPE in the subneurosensory space, and type 3, also known as retinal angiomatous proliferation (RAP), referred to abnormal vessels located within retinal layers, originating either within the retina or from a choroidal source, which may also anastomose with subretinal CNV (36,37).

Other CNV Angiographic Patterns

The form of CNV referred to as RAP (Fig. 12.3) or type 3 CNV has been described in the Caucasian population, higher among women, and interestingly seen in those with focal RPE hyperpigmentation (19). RAP is a

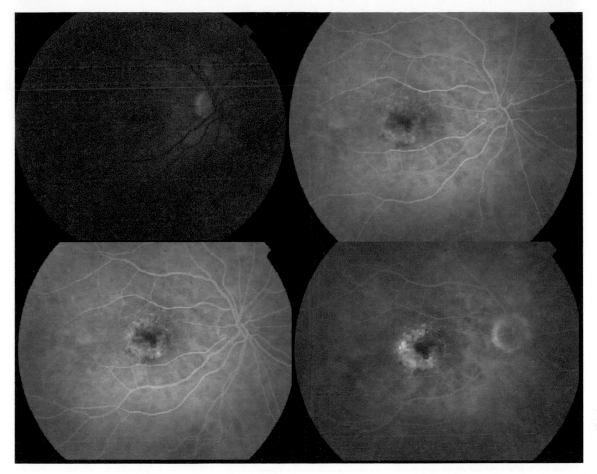

Figure 12.2 Color images of (*upper left panel*), early phase (*upper right panel*), mid-phase (*lower left panel*), and late phase fluorescein angiogram (*lower right panel*) of a patient with an occult choroidal neovascularization lesion. Note the lack of early hyperfluorescence and slowly increasing heterogeneous fluorescence with generalized leakage beneath the RPE and mild to moderate stippled fluorescence.

vasogenic process thought to proliferate within the retina (38–42). RAP was initially described in detail in 2001 by Yannuzzi et al. who proposed a three-stage evolution of RAP lesions based on clinical and angiographic observations (39). The first stage was thought to be an initial intraretinal neovascularization (IRN) with compensatory angiomatous proliferation of capillaries within the deep retinal layers producing intraretinal and superficial retinal hemorrhages (Stage 1). Then, the IRN was proposed to extend into the subneurosensory retinal space forming subretinal neovascularization, retinal–retinal anastomosis, and stimulating RPE hyperplasia (Stage 2). Eventually, the complex was felt to extend more posteriorly to form a serous RPE detachment and possibly a retinal–choroid anastomoses with an underlying type 1 sub-RPE CNV (Stage 3) (39,40). Other models have been proposed based on similar clinical and angiographic observations that speculate that the origin of neovascularization starts in the choroid followed by the choroidal–retinal anastomosis (40,41). Imaging with FA typically shows focal hypofluorescence from intraretinal hemorrhage, intraretinal leakage of fluorescein, cystoid macular edema, and an underlying drusenoid RPE detachment (40). Type 3 CNV also demonstrates an intraretinal hyperfluorescence similar to occult CNV and is difficult to distinguish, especially in later stage

type 3 CNV where the dye will stain the entire vascular and exudative process but not delineate the neovascularization (42). ICG and SD-OCT better characterizes the focal "hot spot" corresponding to the localized disruption of Bruch's membrane and RPE and chorioretinal anastomosis. However, without conclusive histopathological evidence, it remains unclear whether the initial neovascular process originates in the retinal or choroidal (39–42). It is possible that type 3 CNV can originate in either the retina or the choroid, with or without an underlying occult type 1 CNV (40).

Yannuzzi et al. described another type of CNV found in neovascular AMD, polypoidal choroidal vasculopathy (PCV) (Fig. 12.4), a variant of Type 1 CNV, which typically presents with a reddish-orange, spheroidal, thin-walled, choroidal polyp-like structure that can develop large serous and/or hemorrhagic PED (36,43). FA features of PCV depend on the pathological process of the disease and often show similar findings to that of occult CNV (43). Again, ICG is more effective in diagnosing the extent of the CNV because it is neither limited by melanin pigment in the RPE nor by the leakage into the cavity of the PED (19). It is important to distinguish PCV from the classic and occult CNV because these patients may be resistant to or show suboptimal response to anti-vascular

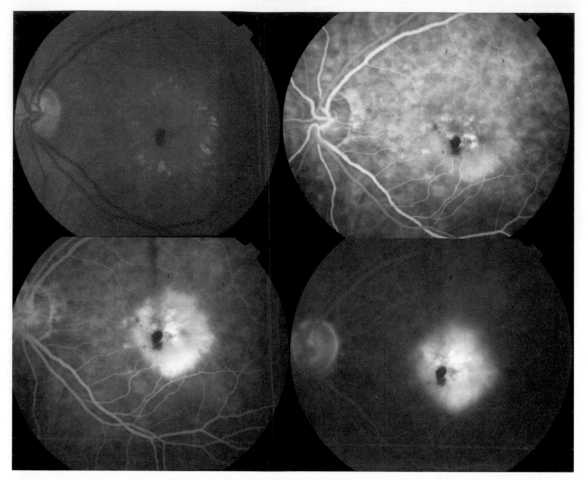

Figure 12.3 Color images of (*upper left panel*), early phase (*upper right panel*), mid-phase (*lower left panel*), and late phase fluorescein angiogram (*lower right panel*) of a patient with a retinal angiomatous proliferative (RAP) lesion. Note on the color photo there is central, superficial, and deep hemorrhage with overlying fluid and a ring of lipid exudation. On the early FA, there is a central blocked fluorescence from the blood and a focal area of hyperfluorescence associated with what appears to be anastomosing retinal vessels just temporal to the blood. There is early intraretinal and subretinal leakage from the lesion and an increasing marked leakage of the entire complex in the later phases of the angiogram.

endothelial growth factor (VEGF) therapy. In some, photodynamic therapy appears to have a more favorable outcome with PCV (44).

RPE detachments (PED) can occur in the context of neovascular AMD. As mentioned previously, a serous PED fills early in the early arteriovenous phase of the angiogram and reveals a progressive pooling of fluorescein and hyperfluorescence throughout the later frames (15,19). A notch or an irregular border usually indicates that occult CNV is present. A hemorrhagic PED has a dark, reddish-brown color on clinical examination, distinguishing it from the clear, translucent fluid of a serous PED (18). Due to the presence of the hemorrhage, which blocks fluorescence from the underlying structures, it is difficult to image and classify the type of CNV in a hemorrhagic PED (19).

RPE tears develop because of the persistent stress from the hydrostatic pressure within a PED and/or contracture of a neovascular membrane at the margin or undersurface of a PED. RPE tears can occur spontaneously or after treatment with laser, photodynamic therapy, or anti-VEGF injections. If a tear occurs, the RPE monolayer scrolls toward the neovascularization

leaving an exposed area of choroid (45). On FA, the exposed area becomes hyperfluorescent at an early stage, but typically does not leak in the later frames, thus distinguishing it from classic CNV. Occasionally in acute RPE tears, there may be leakage from the choroidal vessels making this distinction difficult. The scrolled RPE may appear particularly dark and block the underlying fluorescence (19).

Blockage from blood, exudative material, fibrous tissue, RPE hyperplasia, or RPE redundancy can obscure the boundaries of CNV and block fluorescence on fluorescein angiogram (18,19). In some of these situations, other imaging modalities such as ICG angiography can more effectively identify the extent of the CNV, providing useful information prior to initiation of treatment with thermal laser, PDT, or anti-VEGF therapy.

Eventually, chronic changes from the neovascular process may lead to a disciform scar. Invasion of fibroblasts and inflammatory cells leads to persistent exudation, bleeding, proliferation of abnormal vessels and hyperplasia of RPE. These changes eventually create a large, variable colored fibrous scar, devoid of actively

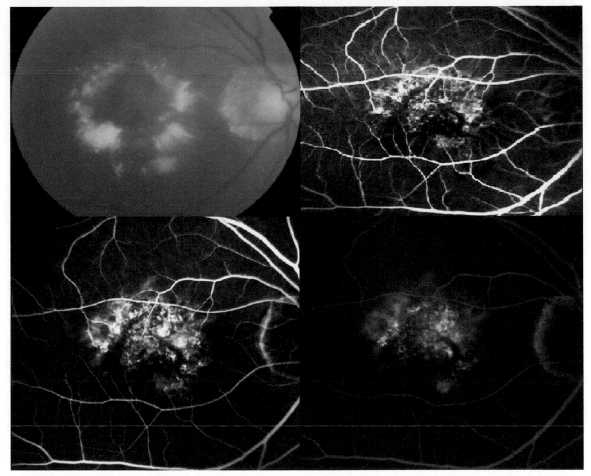

Figure 12.4 Color images of (*upper left panel*), early phase (*upper right panel*), midphase (*lower left panel*), and late phase fluorescein angiogram (*lower right panel*) of a patient with a polypoidal choroidal vasculopathy (PCV) lesion verified on indocyanine green angiography. There is extensive lipid exudation seen on the color image with irregular vascular changes at the level of the choroid on the fluorescein angiography. The lesions show slow leakage with mild blurring of the more peripheral parts of the PCV complex in the late phases.

proliferating vasculature. This end-stage manifestation on FA reveals blockage from RPE hyperplasia and blood, staining of the fibrous component, and mild to moderate leakage from any remaining chronic active CNV component (15,18).

CLINICAL APPLICATION OF FA IN AMD
FA in Previous Laser Clinical Trials

FA played a crucial role in past clinical trials utilizing thermal laser treatment both in guiding selection criteria and assessing response (detailed in chap. 18 of this book). The Macular Photocoagulation Study (MPS) (5–9) was a landmark trial that relied on FA to identify CNV location [with respect the center of the foveal avascular zone (FAZ)], CNV size, and CNV composition, and emphasized that CNV location affected the outcomes of response to laser photocoagulation. The MPS study randomly assigned patients to laser photocoagulation versus observation based on FA identification of CNV with treatment groups defined as: extrafoveal with vision better than 20/100, juxtafoveal with vision better than 20/400, subfoveal new with vision between 20/40 and 20/320, and subfoveal recurrent with previous laser treatment scar and vision between 20/40 and 20/320 (5). FA was also used to assess response of CNV to thermal

laser treatment in the MPS study. Well treated CNV membranes are evidenced on FA by early hypofluorescence in the area of treatment and later frames showing areas of staining or leakage within the area of staining (5–9). Recurrence of CNV was defined as visible leakage of fluorescein dye along the border of a laser treatment scar during FA 3 months or more after treatment (6,8). If the leakage was present at 2, 4, or 6 weeks after treatment, this was classified as CNV persistence and if the leakage was identified on a later angiogram, this was identified as a recurrence (6,9). Eyes that had recurrence (54% of treated eyes) had a poorer visual acuity outcome compared with those without recurrence after 5 years of follow-up (6,8,9).

In the TAP trial, which explored the utility of photodynamic therapy with verteporfin in controlling CNV due to AMD, patients included in the study had subfoveal CNV with a classic component, and a greatest linear dimension of <5400 µm (9 MPS disc areas) identified by FA and visual acuity of 20/40 to 20/200 (10–12). Patients were randomly assigned to verteporfin ocular photodynamic therapy (PDT) versus observation. Conclusions from the TAP trial reported that, although there were some differences depending on CNV composition, PDT treatment for predominantly classic lesions and even minimally classic CNV could prevent moderate to severe vision loss and reduce CNV leakage and the size of the lesion on FA in comparison to placebo.

In comparison, the VIP trial evaluated verteporfin ocular photodynamic therapy in the management of progressive subfoveal CNV that was not included in the TAP trial (specifically lesions comprised of occult CNV and no classic component and classic CNV with a best-corrected visual acuity of approximately 20/40 Snellen equivalents or better) (13,14). As demonstrated by the results of the VIP trial (detailed in chap. 23, "Photodynamic Therapy for Neovascular AMD"), FA was instrumental in following these patients over the entire study period and identifying the initial CNV lesion type as one of the main inclusion criteria for this study. Identifying CNV lesions on FA as defined by both the TAP and VIP study showed that the benefits of verteporfin therapy depended on both the lesion size and natural history of the lesion composition on presentation (15).

FA in the Era of OCT and Intravitreal Anti-VEGF
With the development and widespread use of OCT, the role of FA has diminished. Prior to anti-VEGF therapy, FA was required to localize CNV for laser treatment and later to classify, measure, and localize lesions to guide PDT. In the present era of spectral-domain OCT (see chap. 15 of this book) and intravitreal anti-VEGF injections, there is less emphasis on defining the exact location and type of CNV lesions.

Currently, FA may be useful in detecting CNV in instances where there is high suspicion, but CNV is undetectable by clinical examination alone. It is also helpful in patients with continued vision loss in spite of stable OCT findings. In general, OCT allows clinicians to quantifiably detect and track the amount of intraretinal or subretinal fluid. FA supplements this with qualitative information regarding the presence, location, and relative size of the CNV. It also aids in identifying areas of fibrosis, atrophy, and vascular changes that may affect visual outcomes.

QUANTITATIVE FLUORESCEIN ANGIOGRAPHY
Despite its qualitative nature, there has been a push toward quantitative FA measurements that are still being refined. In the past, there were attempts at defining CNV by two spatial, semiquantitative parameters (9). One parameter was the greatest linear dimension, which is the longest linear extent of the lesion as visualized on the FA expressed in millimeters (mm). The accuracy of this measurement depends on the ability of the clinician to correctly identify the borders and may be affected by subjective inter-observer variability (46). Another semiquantitative parameter that was used prior to the advent of digital imaging was an attempt to measure the area of the CNV by evaluating negative film strips and determining the number of disc areas the CNV encompassed. This was performed by utilizing a set of circle of predetermined size as defined in the MPS. Utilizing these circles, the lesion area was defined as the smallest circle which could completely encompass the lesion. Unfortunately, due to the broad categories in which CNV lesions were classified, lesions within a category could differ in size by as much as one unit disc area. These criteria were therefore insensitive to changes in a lesion of up to that size (46).

With advancing technology, more quantitative parameters have been utilized in the management and treatment of AMD. The development of digital fundus photography and high-resolution imaging, film scanners and high-speed computing software allow for more accurate, quantitative measurements of neovascular membrane size, which can aid in tracking therapeutic outcomes (46–48). Classification determination software programs can be quite objective and reproducible. Optimally, this process would incorporate software recognition of a fundus lesion that underwent prior manual delineation by a human grader and a database of comprehensive details of all known lesion types. Once defined by the clinician, classification can be based on pattern recognition. Descriptors such as size, shape, color, and edge strength can be created in an algorithm that the computer recognizes. Specifically, feature space is a pattern recognition description defined as the potential characteristics or parameters that define objects contained within it (46). Computer programs can recognize multiple dimensions that allow it to easily distinguish between the pixels that belong to vessels versus hemorrhages (49). FA provides multiple frames of information and dimensions of data that software can potentially accumulate to further define each pixel thereby providing accurate and objective interpretations (46).

SUMMARY
Fluorescein angiography (FA) has and continues to play an important role in managing patients with AMD. In the past, FA was crucial in identifying, localizing, and directing both laser and photodynamic therapies as well as monitoring outcomes of treatment. With the advent of anti-VEGF therapy, the focus has shifted to where FA is useful in confirming the cause of exudative findings and identifying features that may limit visual benefits from the therapy. As newer therapeutic approaches are developed that may more selectively target the subtypes and stages of neovascularization, FA may once again be a critical tool in patient selection for these interventions.

REFERENCES

1. Novotny HR, Alvis DL. A method of photographing fluorescence in circulating blood in the human retina. Circulation 1961; 24: 82–6.
2. Flocks M, Miller J, Chao P. Retinal circulation time with the aid of fundus cinephotography. Am J Ophthalmol 1959; 48: 3–10.
3. MacLean AL, Maumenee AE. Hemangioma of the choroid. Am J Ophthalmol 1960; 50: 3–11.
4. American Academy of Ophthalmology Preferred Practice Patterns Committee. Preferred Practice Pattern® Guidelines. Comprehensive Adult Medical Eye Evaluation. San Francisco, CA: American Academy of Ophthalmology, 2010. [Available from: www.aao.org/ppp]

5. Macular Photocoagulation Study Group. Manual of Procedures. Baltimore: MPS coordinating Center. US Dept of Commerce, 1991.

6. Macular Photocoagulation Study Group. Persistent and recurrent choroidal neovascularization after krypton laser photocoagulation for neovascular lesions of age-related macular degeneration. Arch Ophthalmol 1990; 108: 825–31.

7. Macular Photocoagulation Study Group. Laser photocoagulation of subfoveal neovascular lesions in age-related macular degeneration. updated findings from two clinical trials. Arch Ophthalmol 1993; 111: 1200–9.

8. Macular Photocoagulation Study Group. Argon laser photocoagulation for neovascular maculopathy. Five-year results from randomized clinical trials. Arch Ophthalmol 1991; 109: 109–14.

9. Macular Photocoagulation Study Group. Laser photocoagulation for juxtafoveal choroidal neovascularization. Five-year results from randomized clinical trials. Arch Ophthalmol 1993; 112: 500–9.

10. Treatment of Age-Related Macular Degeneration with Photodynamic Therapy (TAP) Study Group. Photodynamic therapy of subfoveal choroidal neovascularization in age-related macular degeneration with verteporfin: one-year results of 2 randomized clinical trials-TAP report 1. Arch Ophthalmol 1999; 117: 329–45.

11. Bressler NM. Photodynamic therapy of subfoveal choroidal neovascularization in age-related macular degeneration with verteporfin: two-year results of 2 randomized clinical trials-TAP report 2. Arch Ophthalmol 2001; 119: 198–207.

12. Bressler NM, Arnold J, Benchaboune M, et al. Verteporfin therapy of subfoveal choroidal neovascularization in patients with age-related macular degeneration: additional information regarding baseline lesion composition's impact on vision outcomes - TAP report no. 3. Arch Ophthalmol 2002; 120: 1443–54.

13. Verteporfin in Photodynamic Therapy (VIP) Study Group. Verteporfin therapy of subfoveal choroidal neovascularization in age-related macular degeneration: two-year results of a randomized clinical trial including lesions with occult with no classic choroidal neovascularization – verteporfin in photodynamic therapy report 2. Am J Ophthalmol 2001; 131: 541–60.

14. Treatment of Age-Related Macular Degeneration With Photodynamic Therapy (TAP) and Verteporfin in Photodynamic Therapy (VIP) Study Groups. Photodynamic therapy of subfoveal choroidal neovascularization with verteporfin: fluorescein angiographic guidelines for evaluation and treatment – TAP and VIP report no. 2. Arch Ophthalmol 2003; 121: 1253–68.

15. Treatment of Age-Related Macular Degeneration With Photodynamic Therapy and Verteporfin in Photodynamic Therapy Study Groups. Effect of lesion size, visual acuity, and lesion composition on visual acuity change with and without verteporfin therapy for choroidal neovascularization secondary to age-related macular degeneration: TAP and VIP report no. 1. Am J Ophthalmol 2003; 136: 407–18.

16. Ehrlich P. Uber provicierte fluoreszenzerscheinungen am auge. Dtsch Med Wochenschr 1882; 8: 8–21.

17. Johnson RN, McDonald HR, Ai E, et al. Fluorescein angiography: basic principles and interpretation. In: Ryan SJ, ed. Retina, 4th edn. Philadelphia: Elsevier Inc, 2012: 873–916.

18. Jumper JM, Fu AD, McDonald HR, et al. Fluorescein angiography. In: Alfaro DV III, Liggett PE, Mieler WF, Quiroz-Mercado H, Jager RD, Tano Y, eds. Age-Related Macular Degeneration. Philadelphia: Lippincot Williams & Wilkins, 2006: 86–100.

19. Spaide RF. Fundus angiography. In: Holz FG, Pauleikhoff D, Spaide RF, Bird AC, eds. Age-Related Macular Degeneration. Heidelberg: Springer-Verlag Berlin Heidelberg, 2004: 87–107.

20. Norton EW. Doyne memorial lecture, 1981. Fluorescein angiography. Twenty years later. Trans Ophthalmol Soc UK 1981; 101: 229–33.

21. Yannuzzi LA, Rohrer KT, Tindel LJ, et al. Fluorescein angiography complication survey. Ophthalmology 1986; 93: 611–17.

22. Alemzadeh-Ansari MJ, Beladi-Mousavi SS, Feghhei M. Effect of fluorescein on renal function among diabetic patients. Nefrologia 2011; 31: 612–13.

23. Kwiterovich KA, Maguire MG, Murphy RP, et al.; Results of a Prospective Study. Frequency of adverse systemic reactions after fluorescein angiography. Ophthalmology 1991; 98: 1139–42.

24. Kwan AS, Barry C, McAllister IL, Constable I. Fluorescein angiography and adverse drug reactions revisited: the lions eye experience. Clin Exp Ophthalmol 2006; 34: 33–8.

25. Halperin LS, Olk RJ, Soubrane G, et al. Safety of fluorescein angiography during pregnancy. Am J Ophthalmol 1990; 109: 563–6.

26. Gabel VP, Birngruber R, Nasemann J. The scanning laser ophthalmoscope and its use as a fluorescein angiography instrument. Fortschr Ophthalmol 1988; 85: 569–73.

27. Pauleikhoff D, Zuels S, Sheraidah GS, et al. Correlation between biochemical composition and fluorescein binding of deposits in Bruch's membrane. Ophthalmology 1992; 92: 1548–53.

28. Sarks SH, Council Lecture. Drusen and their relationship to senile macular degeneration. Aust J Ophthalmol 1980; 8: 117–30.

29. Bressler NM, Bressler SB, Fine SL. Age-related macular degeneration. Surv Ophthalmol 1988; 32: 375–413.

30. Gass JD, Jallow S, Davis B. Adult vitelliform macular detachment occurring in patients with basal laminar drusen. Am J Ophthalmol 1979; 88: 643–51.

31. Bressler NM, Silva JC, Bressler SB, et al. Clinicopathologic correlation of drusen and retinal pigment epithelial abnormalities in age-related macular degeneration. Retina 1994; 14: 130–42.

32. Schatz H, Burton TC, Yannuzzi LA, Rabb MF. Interpretation of Fundus Fluorescein Angiography. Saint Louis: CV Mosby, 1978.

33. Green WR, Key SN III. Senile macular degeneration: a histopathologic study. Trans Am Ophthalmol Soc 1977; 75: 180–254.

34. Spaide RF. Fundus autofluorescence and age-related macular degeneration. Ophthalmology 2003; 110: 392–9.

35. Chamberlin JA, Bressler NM, Bressler SB, et al.; The Macular Photocoagulation Study Group. The use of fundus photographs and fluorescein angiograms in the identification and treatment of choroidal neovascularization in the macular photocoagulation study. Ophthalmology 1989; 96: 526–34.

36. Gass JD. Biomicroscopic and histopathologic considerations regarding the feasibility of surgical excision of subfoveal neovascular membranes. Am J Ophthalmol 1994; 118: 258–98.

37. Freund KB, Zweifel SA, Engelbert M. Do we need a new classification for choroidal neovascularization in age-related macular degeneration. Retina 2010; 30: 1333–49.

38. Hartnett ME, Weiter JJ, Staurenghi G, et al. Deep retinal vascular anomalous complexes in advanced age-related macular degeneration. Ophthalmology 1996; 103: 2042–53.

39. Yannuzzi LA, Negrao S, Iida T, et al. Retinal angiomatous proliferation in age-related macular degeneration. Retina 2001; 21: 416–34.

40. Freund KB, Ho I-Van, Barbazetto IA, et al. Type 3 neovascularization the expanded spectrum of retinal angiomatous proliferation. Retina 2008; 27: 201–11.

41. Gass JDM, Agarwal A, Lavina A, et al. Focal inner retinal hemorrhages in patients with drusen: an early sign of occult choroidal neovascularization and chorioretinal anastomosis. Retina 2003; 23: 741–51.

42. Yannuzzi LA, Freund KB, Takahashi BS. Review of retinal angiomatous proliferation or type 3 neovascularization. Retina 2008; 28: 375–84.

43. Yannuzzi LA, Wong DWK, Sforzolini BS, et al. Polypoidal choroidal vasculopathy and neovascularized age-related macular degeneration. Arch Ophthalmol 1999; 117: 1503–10.

44. Spaide RF, Donsoff I, Lam DL, et al. Treatment of polypoidal choroidal vasculopathy with photodynamic therapy. Retina 2002; 22: 529–35.

45. Gass JD. Pathogenesis of tears of the retinal pigment epithelium. Br J Ophthalmol 1984; 104: 502–12.

46. Walsh AC, Updike PG, Sadda SR. Quantitative fluorescein angiography. In: Ryan SJ, ed. Retina, 4th edn. Philadelphia: Elsevier Inc, 2012: 917–48.

47. Esmaili DD, Ghafouri RH, Chakravarthy U, Lim JI. Quantitative retinal imaging. In: Lim JI, ed. Age-Related Macular Degeneration, 2nd edn. New York: Informa Healthcare USA, Inc, 2008: 185–8.

48. Goldbaum MH, Katz NP, Chaudhuri S, et al. Image understanding for automated retinal diagnosis. Proc IEEE Comp Soc Symp Comp Aided Med Care 1989: 756–60.

49. Chakravarthy U, Walsh AC, Muldrew A, et al. Quantitative fluorescein angiographic analysis of choroidal neovascular membranes: validation and correlation with visual function. Invest Ophthalmol Vis Sci 2007; 48: 349–54.

13

Use of indocyanine green angiography in the management of age-related macular degeneration

Lawrence A. Yannuzzi and Irene Barbazetto

INTRODUCTION

Fluorescein angiography (FA) has revolutionized the diagnosis of retinal disorders (1,2). However, there are certain limitations to this technique. Overlying hemorrhage, pigment, or serosanguineous fluid can block the underlying pathologic changes and prevent adequate visualization by FA. Indocyanine green (ICG) is a Food and Drug Administration-approved tricarbocyanine dye that has several advantageous properties over sodium fluorescein as a dye for ophthalmic angiography. The clinical usefulness of indocyanine green angiography (ICGA) in the past has been limited by our inability to produce high-resolution images. However, enhanced high-resolution ICG angiograms can now be obtained owing to the technological advance of coupling digital imaging systems to ICG cameras (3,4). Thus, digital ICGA finally allows the theoretical advantages of ICG as an ophthalmic dye to be realized.

SPECIAL PROPERTIES OF ICG

The ICG absorbs and fluoresces in the near-infrared range. Owing to the special characteristics of the dye, there is less blockage by the normal eye pigments, which allows enhanced imaging of the choroid and choroidal abnormalities. For example, Geeraets and Berry (5) have reported that the retinal pigment epithelium (RPE) and choroid absorb 59–75% of blue–green (500 nm) light, but only 21–38% of near-infrared (800 nm) light. The activity of ICG in the near-infrared range also allows visualization of pathologic conditions through overlying hemorrhage, serous fluid, lipid, and pigment that may block structures by FA. This property allows enhanced imaging of occult choroidal neovascularization (CNV) and pigment epithelial detachment (PED) in age-related macular degeneration (AMD) (4,6).

A second special property of ICG is that it is highly protein-bound (98%). Therefore, less dye escapes from the choroidal vasculature, which allows enhanced imaging of choroidal abnormalities.

HISTORICAL PERSPECTIVES

ICG dye was first used in medicine in the mid-1950s at the Mayo Clinic to obtain blood flow measurements (7). In 1956, ICG was used for determining cardiac output and characterizing cardiac valvular and septal defects. In 1964, studies of systemic arteriovenous fistulas and renal blood flow were reported. The finding that exclusively the liver excreted the dye soon led to the development of its application for measuring hepatic function. The use of real-time intraoperative ICGA provided information about vessel patency during neurosurgical aneurysm repair (8,9).

ICG first became attractive to ophthalmologists interested in better ways to image the choroidal circulation because of its safety and its particular optical and biophysical properties. Kogure and coworkers (10) in 1970 first performed choroidal absorption angiography in monkeys, using intra-arterial ICG injection. The first ICG angiogram in a human was performed by David (11) during carotid angiography.

In 1971, Hochheimer (12) described choroidal absorption angiography in cats using intravenous ICG injections and black-and-white infrared film instead of color film. One year later, Flower and Hochheimer performed intravenous absorption ICGA for the first time in a human (13,14). These same investigators then described the superior technique of ICG fluorescence angiography (15,16). Further technological improvements followed (17), and, in 1985, Bischoff and Flower (18) reported on their 10-year experience with ICGA, which included 500 angiograms of various disorders.

However, the sensitivity of infrared film was too low to adequately capture the low-intensity ICG fluorescence, as the fluorescence efficacy of ICG is only 4% of that of sodium fluorescein. The resolution of ICGA was improved in the mid-1980s by Hayashi and coworkers, who developed improved filter combinations and described ICG video angiography (19–21). However, their video system lacked freeze-frame image recording and possessed cumulative light toxicity potential due to its 300 W continuous halogen lamp illumination. In 1985, Destro and Puliafito (22) described a similar video system. In 1989, Scheider and Schroedel (23) reported the use of the scanning laser ophthalmoscope for ICG video angiography; refinements of their technique allowed for improved imaging of choroidal neovascular membranes (24,25).

In 1992, Guyer and coworkers (3) and Yannuzzi and associates (4) introduced the use of a 1024-line digital imaging system to produce high-resolution enhanced ICG images. These systems have improved the resolution of ICGA such that this technique is now of practical clinical value.

PHARMACOLOGY

ICG is a sterile, water-soluble tricarbocyanine dye, which is anhydro-3,3,3',3'-tetramethyl-1-1'-di-(4-sulfobutyl)-4,5,4',5-dibenzo indotricarbocyanine hydroxide sodium salt. Its empirical formula is $C_{43}H_{47}N_2NaO_6S_2$ and its molecular weight is 775 Da (26). It is highly protein-bound (98%). Although it has been thought that ICG is primarily bound to albumin in the serum (27), 80% of ICG in the blood is actually bound to globulins, such as alpha-1 lipoprotein (28).

ICG's spectral absorption is between 790 and 805 nm (28–30). The dye is excreted by the liver via bile. ICG is not reabsorbed from the liver, is not detected in cerebrospinal fluid (31,32), and does not cross the placenta (33).

TOXICITY

ICG is a relatively safe dye, with only a few side effects reported in clinical use (7,27,34–36). In our experience, it is safer than sodium fluorescein. In contrast to FA, nausea and vomiting are extremely uncommon during ICG angiography. We have observed two serious vasovagal-type reactions during ICGA.

No complications were reported in one study using intravenous ICG doses of 150–200 mg. No side effects were noted in another series of 700 procedures (18). In a study 1226 consecutive patients undergoing ICGA, there were three (0.15%) mild adverse reactions, four (0.2%) moderate reactions, one (0.05%) severe reaction, and no deaths (36).

ICGA should not be performed on patients allergic to iodide, since it contains approximately 5% iodide by weight. In addition, it should not be performed on patients who are uremic (18) or who have impaired hepatic clearance. Appropriate emergency equipment should be readily available, as with FA.

TECHNIQUE OF INJECTION

ICGA can be performed immediately before or after FA. We inject intravenously 25–50 mg of ICG (Cardio-Green: Hynson, Westcott & Dunning Products, Cockeysville, Maryland, USA) which has been diluted in the aqueous solvent supplied by the manufacturer. Rapid injection is essential and should be followed by a 5-mL normal saline flush. For wide angle angiography, the dosage is increased to 75 mg.

Bindewald and associates (37) tested the lower limits fluorescein and ICG dye doses for angiography. Using a confocal scanning laser ophthalmoscope (cSLO) (Heidelberg retina angiograph 2, Heidelberg Engineering, Dossenheim, Germany), they found that a fluorescein dose as low as 166 mg, and an ICG dose as low as 5 mg, allowed adequate resolution for diagnosis and management of neovascular AMD. Resolution was impaired, however, in late phase images, compared with standard doses.

DIGITAL IMAGING SYSTEMS

The coupling of a digital imaging system with an ICG camera allows production of enhanced high-resolution (1024-line) images, which are necessary for ICGA. The instantaneous images from these systems produce images which decrease patient waiting time and expedite treatment. Digital imaging systems also allow image archiving, hard-copy generation, and direct qualitative comparison between fluorescein and ICGA findings. These systems are useful for planning preoperative treatment strategies and for monitoring the adequacy of treatment postoperatively.

Imaging systems contain film, video, or digital cameras with special antireflective coatings and appropriate excitatory and barrier filters. Flash synchronization allows high-resolution image capture. The digitally charged coupling device camera captures the digitized images and transmits them to a digital imaging workstation. These images are captured at a speed of one frame per second, stored in buffer memory, and displayed on a high-contrast, high-resolution video monitor. The images can be printed to photographs or slides, transferred via a variety of storage media, or networked to other stations in treatment areas and in other offices.

INTERPRETATION OF ICGA FINDINGS IN AMD
Definitions

The terminology used to describe the angiographic manifestations of AMD corresponds, with certain exceptions described below, to definitions previously reported by the Macular Photocoagulation Study Group (38). Most relevant to the interpretation of ICGA in AMD are the definitions of serous pigment epithelium detachment (SPED), vascularized pigment epithelial detachment (VPED), classic CNV, and occult CNV (4,19,22,39).

Serous Pigment Epithelial Detachment

The SPED is an ovoid or circular detachment of the RPE. On FA study there is rapid filling with dye of the fluid in the sub-RPE space. This corresponds to early hyperfluorescence beneath the PED, which increases in intensity in the late phase of the study resulting in a bright and homogeneous well-demarcated pattern. ICGA reveals a variable, minimal blockage of normal choroidal vessels, more evident in the midphase of the angiogram. Thus, a SPED is bright (hyperfluorescent) on FA and dark (hypofluorescent) on ICG. This difference is caused by the fact that ICG molecules are larger and almost completely bound to plasma proteins, which prevents free passage of ICG dye throughout the fenestrated choriocapillaris in the sub-RPE space. Also, it is important to remember the difference of appearance on ICGA between a SPED in AMD and a SPED in central serous chorioretinopathy (CSC). In fact, in CSC there is increased permeability of the choriocapillaris that causes leakage of ICG molecules under the PED. As a result, a SPED in CSC appears bright (hyperfluorescent) with ICGA. Approximately 1.5% of newly diagnosed patients with neovascular AMD present with a pure SPED.

Choroidal Neovascularization

CNV is defined as a choroidal capillary proliferation through a break in the outer aspect of Bruch's membrane under the RPE and/or the neurosensory retina. CNV is divided into classic and occult based on the FA angiography appearance.

Classic CNV

Classic CNV is an area of bright, fairly uniform hyperfluorescence identified in the early phase of the FA. The fluorescence increases through the transit phase with leakage of dye obscuring the boundaries of this area by the late phase of the angiogram. With ICGA, a classic CNV has a similar appearance to that seen with FA angiography, but is usually less well delineated (Fig. 13.1) and exhibits little or no leakage in the late phases of the ICG study. Only 12% of newly diagnosed patients with neovascular AMD present with classic CNV.

Occult CNV

Occult CNV is characterized as either fibrovascular pigment epithelial detachment (FVPED) or late leakage of undetermined source (LLUS). FVPED consists of irregular elevation of the RPE consisting of stippled hyperfluorescence not as bright or discrete as classic CNV within one to two minutes after fluorescein injection, with persistence of fluorescence 10 minutes after injection. LLUS consists of areas of leakage at the level of the RPE in the late phase of the angiogram not corresponding to an area of classic CNV or FVPED discernible in the early or middle phase of the angiogram to account for the leakage. Also any area of blocked fluorescence contiguous to the CNV is considered occult CNV. More than 85% of newly diagnosed patients with neovascular AMD present with occult CNV (Fig. 13.2). Two main types of occult CNV are recognized on ICGA.

Without SPED

The first type of occult CNV is caused by sub-RPE CNV that is not associated with a PED. The early stages of the FA study reveal minimal subretinal hyperfluorescence of undetermined source that slowly increases over a period of several minutes to produce an irregular staining of the sub-RPE tissue. The ICG angiogram reveals early vascular hyperfluorescence and late staining of the abnormal vessels. If the ICG angiographic image has distinct margins, it is considered to be a well-defined CNV on ICGA. Two-thirds of newly diagnosed patients with an occult CNV present without an associated SPED.

With SPED

The second type of occult CNV is associated with a SPED of at least one-disc diameter in size. Combined CNV and SPED are called a VPED. This lesion is the

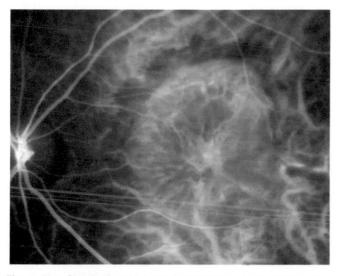

Figure 13.1 Classic choroidal neovascularization. Early phase indocyanine green angiogram shows a well-defined hyperfluorescent vascular network consistent with a classic choroidal neovascular membrane.

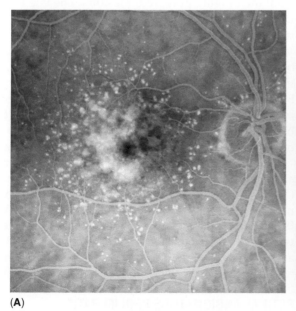

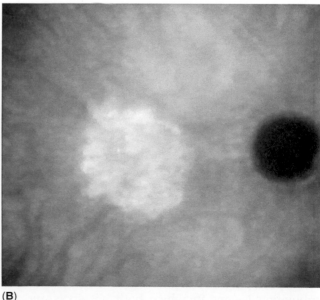

(A)   (B)

Figure 13.2 Occult choroidal neovascularization. Midphase fluorescein angiogram **(A)** demonstrates hyperfluorescent drusen, while the late phase indocyanine green angiogram **(B)** reveals a hyperfluorescent occult choroidal neovascular membrane.

result of sub-RPE neovascularization associated with a serous detachment of the RPE. One-third of newly diagnosed patients with AMD have an associated SPED. The determination of whether a SPED is present is best made on the basis of the FA study. FA may also demonstrate occult vessels as late, indistinct, subretinal hyperfluorescence beneath, or at the margin of the SPED. ICGA reveals early vascular hyperfluorescence and late staining of the CNV. The SPED, as noted previously, is comparatively hypofluorescent, because only minimal ICG leakage occurs beneath the serous detachment. ICG is more helpful than FA in differentiating between a SPED and a VPED. It also permits better identification of the vascularized and serous component of VPEDs. These differentiations between the vascularized and serous components are often not possible with FA alone because the serous and vascularized portions of a PED demonstrate late hyperfluorescence and leakage, respectively. Although fluorescein staining is more intense in the serous portion of the detachment than in the vascularized component, differences in intensity are often too minimal for accurate interpretation. However, the ICG angiographic findings are infinitely more reliable for this differentiation; the serous component of a PED is hypofluorescent and the vascularized component is hyperfluorescent.

Occult CNV is also subgrouped into two types, one with a solitary area of well-defined focal neovascularization (hot spot) and the other with a larger and delineated area of neovascularization (plaque).

Hot Spot (Focal CNV)

Focal CNV or a "hot spot" is an area of occult CNV that is both well delineated and no more than one-disc diameter in size on ICGA. Also a hot spot represents an area of actively proliferating and more highly permeable areas of neovascularization (active occult CNV). Chorioretinal anastomosis and polypoidal-type CNV may represent two subgroups of hot spots (see below).

Plaque

A plaque is an area of occult CNV larger than one-disc diameter in size. A plaque often is formed by late-staining vessels, which are more likely to be quiescent areas of neovascularization that are not associated with appreciable leakage (inactive occult CNV). Plaques of occult CNV seems to slowly grow in dimension with time. Well-defined and ill-defined plaques are recognized on ICG study. A well-defined plaque has distinct borders throughout the study and the full extent of the lesion can be assessed. An ill-defined plaque has indistinct margins or may be one in which any part of the neovascularization is blocked by blood.

In a review of our first 1000 patients with occult CNV by FA, which were imaged by ICGA, we categorized occult CNV into three morphologic categories: focal CNV or hot spots, plaques (well-defined and ill-defined), and combination lesions in which both hot spots and plaques were noted (39). The results of that study are discussed later in this chapter under clinical applications.

Two other forms of occult CNV are identified by ICGA: polypoidal choroidal vasculopathy (PCV) and retinal angiomatous proliferation (RAP).

POLYPOIDAL CHOROIDAL VASCULOPATHY

PCV is a primary abnormality of the choroidal circulation characterized by an inner choroidal vascular network of vessels ending in an aneurysmal bulge or outward projection, visible clinically as a reddish orange, spheroid, polyplike structure. The disorder is associated with multiple, recurrent, serosanguineous detachments of the RPE and neurosensory retina, secondary to leakage and bleeding from the peculiar choroidal vascular abnormality (40,41).

ICGA has been used to detect and characterize the PCV abnormality with enhanced sensitivity and specificity (Fig. 13.3) (42–55). In the initial phases of the ICG study, a distinct network of vessels within the choroid becomes visible. Optical coherence tomography (OCT) (Fig. 13.3C) delineates the polypoidal extensions of the choroidal vasculature. In patients with juxtapapillary involvement, the vascular channels extend in a radial, arching pattern and are interconnected with smaller spanning branches that become more evident and numerous at the edge of the PCV lesion (Fig. 13.4).

Early in the course of the ICG study, the larger vessels of PCV network start to fill before the retinal vessels, but the area within and surrounding the network is relatively hypofluorescent compared with the uninvolved choroid. The vessels of the network appear to fill more slowly than the retinal vessels. Shortly after the network can be identified on the ICG angiogram, small hyperfluorescent "polyps" become visible within the choroid.

These polypoidal structures correspond to the reddish, orange choroidal excrescence seen on clinical examination. They appear to leak slowly as the surrounding hypofluorescent area becomes increasingly hyperfluorescent. In the later phase of the angiogram there is a uniform disappearance of the dye ("washout") from the bulging polypoidal lesions. The late ICG staining characteristic of occult CNV is not seen in the PCV vascular abnormality.

While the first reports of PCV were in middle-aged black women, it is now recognized that PCV may be a variant of CNV seen in white patients with AMD, it may be localized in the macular area without any peripapillary component (Figs. 13.5 and 13.6), and it may be formed by a network of small branching vessels ending in polypoidal dilation difficult to image without ICGA (Fig. 13.6).

Ahuja and colleagues sought to determine the prevalence of PCV among British patients in their practice (50). Of the 40 consecutive patients with hemorrhagic or neovascular PEDs, PEDs were attributed to PCV in 34 (85%). Of those with PCV, 65% were female, the mean age was 65 years (range 44–88), 74% were white, 20% black, and 6% Asian. Eight had a history of hypertension. Sixty-eight percent of lesions were located in the macula.

RETINAL ANGIOMATOUS PROLIFERATION

RAP is a distinct subgroup of neovascular AMD, manifested by intraretinal neovascularization (IRN) that

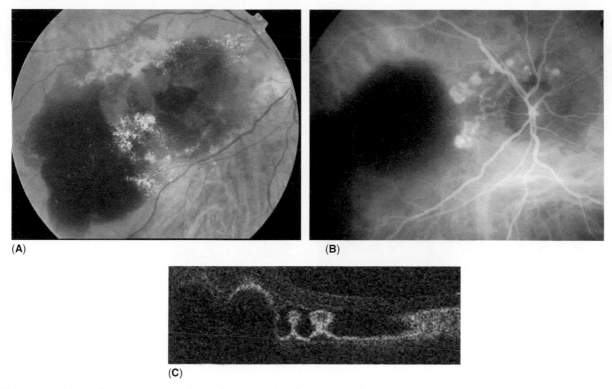

Figure 13.3 Polypoidal choroidal vasculopathy. Color photograph **(A)** demonstrates hemorrhagic detachment of the macula. Late phase indocyanine green study **(B)** reveals a peripapillary polyp-like vascular network. Note central hypofluorescence indicative of a pigment epithelial detachment. Optical coherence tomography **(C)** delineates the polypoidal extensions of the choroidal vasculature.

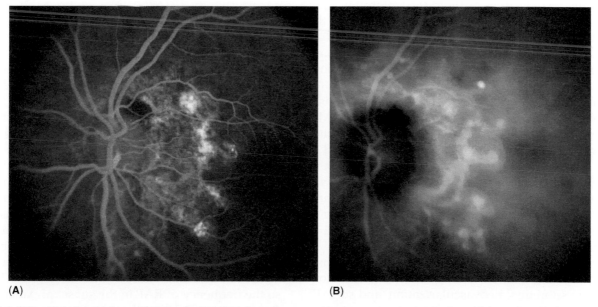

Figure 13.4 Polypoidal choroidal vasculopathy. Peripapillary hyperfluorescent lesions are apparent in the midphase fluorescein angiogram **(A)**; however, the indocyanine green **(B)** delineates a more extensive vascular network.

extends into the deep retinal, subretinal, and sub-RPE spaces.

Clinical evidence of pre-, intra-, or subretinal hemorrhage, sometimes with associated exudates or cystoid macular edema, in the setting of a PED suggests an RAP lesion. Often, dilated compensatory vessels perfuse and drain the neovascularization, forming a retinal–retinal anastomosis. Extension of the neovascular complex to the subretinal space may result in a retinochoroidal anastomosis (RCA).

On FA, indistinct RPE staining, often with associated PED, resembles occult CNV. Presence of active IRN extending into a PED is difficult to distinguish from a standard VPED. ICG allows better characterization of a

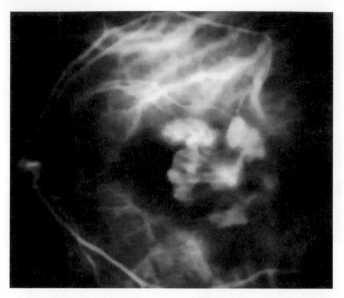

Figure 13.5 Macular polypoidal choroidal vasculopathy. Midphase indocyanine green angiogram demonstrates a prominent lesion of polypoidal channels in the macula.

VPED, revealing the neovascular hot spot contained within the hypofluorescent PED (Fig. 13.7A,B). The OCT (Fig. 13.7C) shows intraretinal cystic changes overlying a PED along with a hyper-reflective area suggestive of a RCA. Late intraretinal leakage may arise from the IRN. ICG permits visualization of the direct communication between the retinal and the choroidal components of the neovascularization as they form an RCA (Fig. 13.8) Lafaut and coworkers (56) documented the histopathology of an RCA, in which neovascularization grows out from the neuroretina into the subretinal space.

Kuhn et al. (57), in 1995, first identified RCA as a potential manifestation of this form of neovascular AMD in the setting of a VPED. With ICGA for enhanced choroidal imaging, this group found RCA in 50 of 186 (28%) patients with AMD and an associated VPED. Slakter et al. (58) detected RCA in 34 of 150 eyes (21%) with occult AMD and a focal hot spot in ICG. Fernandez and coworkers (59) reported a series of 190 patients with neovascular AMD in which ICGA revealed 34 eyes (16%) with RAP lesions.

Yannuzzi and colleagues (60) classified RAP into three stages: stage I involves IRN, stage II results from extension to subretinal neovascularization, and stage III occurs once CNV is documented.

Clinical knowledge and recognition of RAP are important because this form of neovascular AMD may have a natural course, visual prognosis, and response to treatment distinct from other forms of neovascular AMD. Different forms of treatment may be preferable for each stage of the disorder. For example, we have found that an uncomplicated focal area of IRN may be amenable to conventional thermal laser treatment; whereas, a more advanced stage involving a VPED and an RCA is less likely to respond to any form of currently available treatment.

Bottoni and colleagues (61) retrospectively reported results of 99 eyes of 81 patients with RAP treated with direct laser photocoagulation of the vascular lesion, laser photocoagulation of the feeder retinal arteriole, scatter grid-like laser photocoagulation, photodynamic therapy (PDT), or transpupillary thermotherapy. Complete obliteration was achieved in 24 (57%) cases of stage I lesions (73% closure from direct laser and 45% closure from PDT, 11 (26%) of stage II lesions (38% closure from scatter grid-like photocoagulation and 17% closure from direct photocoagulation of the vascular lesion), and only 3 (15%) of stage III lesions. The uncontrolled use of therapeutic interventions in this study makes it difficult to draw definitive conclusions about a superior treatment modality, but the study makes clear the difficulty in effectively treating more advanced stages of RAF."

Series using PDT alone or PDT with triamcinolone confirm the challenge in effectively treating RAP lesions. Boscia and colleagues (62) treated 21 eyes with stage II or III RAP using PDT alone and reported an overall decline in vision from 20 out of 80 to 20 out of 174, stabilization of vision in six eyes (29%), occlusion of RAP and PED flattening in three eyes (14%), and an RPE tear in four eyes (19%). Nicolo and colleagues (63) reported 10 eyes with stage II RAP treated with 20 mg of intravitreal triamcinolone acetonide (IVTA) followed one month later by PDT. All patients experienced flattening of the PED prior to PDT, six patients (60%) showed improved vision of at least three early treatment of diabetic retinopathy study (ETDRS) lines at three, six, and nine months while four patients (40%) maintained visual improvement at 12 months.

PDT with a photosensitizing dye such as verteporfin may have a different effect on RAP than on classic-CNV or occult-CNV lesions (64,65). Given the tendency for ICG dye to stain the retina in eyes with RAP, there is a possibility that similar staining may occur with the verteporfin molecule, theoretically predisposing the retina to photochemical damage when exposed to the excitatory light used in PDT. This possibility is speculative, since verteporfin has not yet been imaged successfully with good spatial and temporal definition in the human.

Because eyes with RAP are generally classified as pure occult CNV based on FA, it is possible that patients with RAP were actually treated in the treatment of age-related macular degeneration with photodynamic therapy (TAP) trial (65). ICGA was not used in the TAP trial, so the frequency of RAP in the subset of patients classified as occult CNV is unknown. Future studies of AMD that use ICG will be able to delineate between these two distinct forms of macular degeneration. Further details about RAP are given in chapter 11 (Variants of neovascular age-related macular degeneration: type 3 neovascularization (intraretinal neovascularization or retinal angiogmatous proliferation).

CLINICAL APPLICATION OF ICGA TO THE STUDY OF AMD

Patz and associates (26) were the first to study CNV by ICG video angiography. They could resolve only 2 of 25 CNVs with their early model. Bischoff and Flower (18)

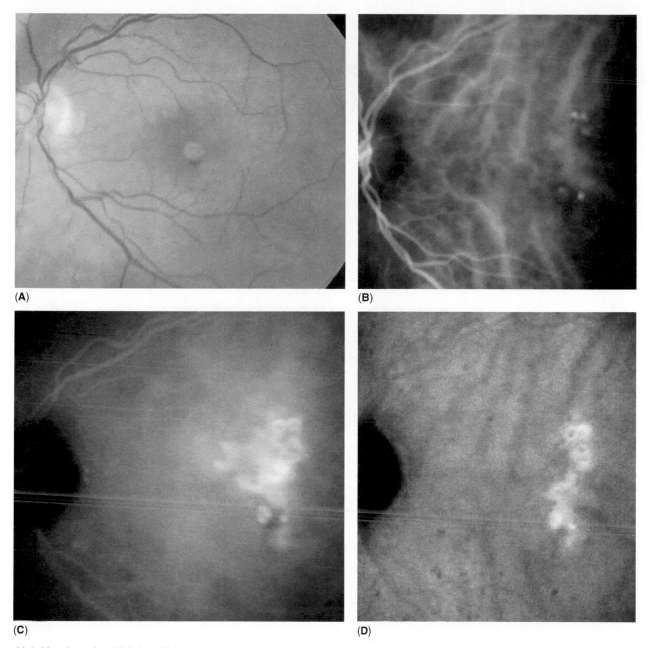

Figure 13.6 Macular polypoidal choroidal vasculopathy. Despite a fundus appearance **(A)** only of mild pigment epithelial change, the indocyanine green reveals progressive macular hyperfluorescence of polypoidal lesions in the early **(B)**, mid **(C)** and late **(D)** phases of the angiogram.

studied 100 ICG angiograms of patients with AMD. They found "delayed and/or irregular choroidal filling" in some patients. The significance of this finding is unclear, because these authors did not include an age-matched control group. Tortuous vessels and marked dilation of macular choroidal arteries, often with loop formation, were also observed.

Hayashi and associates (19,21) found that ICG video angiography was useful in the detection of CNV. ICG video angiography was able to confirm the fluorescein angiographic appearance of CNV in patients with well-defined CNV. It revealed a more well-defined neovascularization in 27 eyes with occult CNV by FA. In a subgroup of patients with poorly defined occult CNV, the ICG angiogram, but not the FA, imaged a well-defined CNV in 9 of 12 (75%) cases. ICG video angiography of the other three eyes revealed suspicious areas of

neovascularization. Hayashi and coworkers (19,21) were also the first to show that leakage from CNV with ICG was slow compared with the rapid leakage of sodium fluorescein. While the results of these investigators concerning ICG video angiographic imaging of occult CNV were promising, the spatial resolution that they could obtain was limited by the 512-line video monitor and analog tape of their ICG system.

Destro and Puliafito (22) reported that ICG video angiography was particularly useful in studying occult CNV with overlying hemorrhage and recurrent CNV. Guyer and coworkers (3) used a 1024-line digital imaging system to study patients with occult CNV. These authors reported that ICG video angiography was useful in imaging occult CNV and that this technique could allow photocoagulation of otherwise untreatable lesions. Scheider and co-investigators (25) have reported

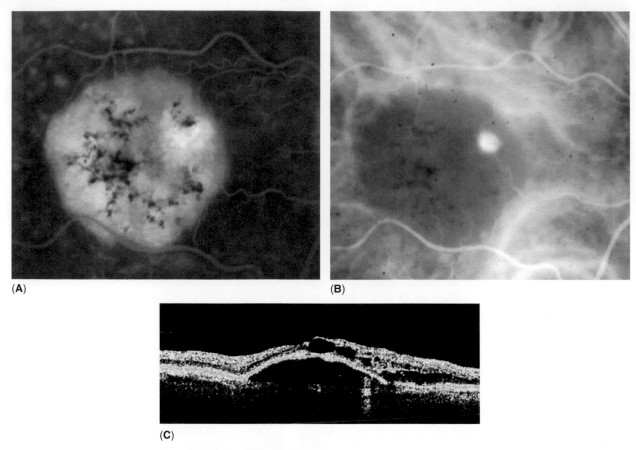

Figure 13.7 Retinal angiomatous proliferation. Fluorescein angiogram **(A)** indicates a pigment epithelial detachment, while the indocyanine green **(B)** reveals a focal area of hyperfluorescence adjacent to two retinal arterioles. The optical coherence tomography **(C)** shows intraretinal cystic changes overlying a pigment epithelial detachment along with a hyper-reflective area suggestive of a retinochoroidal anastomosis.

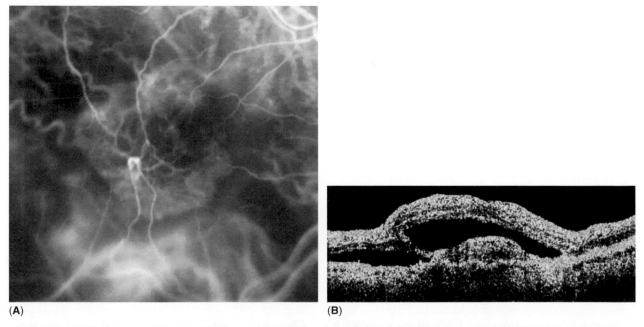

Figure 13.8 Retinal angiomatous proliferation (RAP) vasculature. Retinochoroidal anastomosis stands out in this indocyanine green angiogram **(A)** that reveals a larger underlying choroidal neovascularization. Optical coherence tomography **(B)** of this stage III RAP lesion demonstrates vessels from a low neurosensory detachment diving toward a subretinal choroidal neovascular membrane.

enhanced imaging of CNV in a study of 80 patients using the scanning laser ophthalmoscope with ICG video angiography.

Yannuzzi and associates (4) have shown that ICGA is extremely useful in reclassifying occult CNV into "well-defined CNV." In their study, 39% of 129 patients with occult CNV were reclassified as well-defined CNV based on information added by ICGA. Five of seven (72%) cases of occult CNV with SPED were reclassified as "well demarcated" CNV by ICG. In 17 of 38 (45%) VPED cases and in 11 of 19 (58%) combined VPED and SPED cases, ICGA allowed occult CNV to be reclassified as well-defined CNV. These authors concluded that ICGA was especially useful in identifying occult CNV in patients with SPED or with recurrent CNV.

Lim et al. found that ICG demonstrated well-demarcated hyperfluorescence in 50% of eyes thought to have occult CNV by FA and in 82% of eyes with PED (66). Baumal et al. found that ICG demonstrated underlying CNV in 19 of 23 eyes (83%) with an isolated PED and in 21 of 21 eyes (100%) with PED and occult CNV (67).

Yannuzzi and coworkers (68) studied with ICGA 235 consecutive AMD patients with occult CNV and associated VPED. These eyes were divided into two groups, depending on the size and delineation of the CNV. Of the 235 eyes 89 (38%) had a solitary area of neovascularization that was well delineated, no more than one-disc diameter in size, and defined as focal CNV. The other 146 (62%) eyes had a larger area of neovascularization, with variable delineation defined as a plaque CNV.

In a further report, 657 consecutive eyes with occult CNV determined by FA were studied with ICGA. Of the 413 eyes with occult CNV without pigment epithelium detachments, focal areas of neovascularization were noted in 89 (22%). Overall, 142 (34%) eyes had lesions that were potentially treatable by thermal laser photocoagulation based on additional information provided by ICGA. Of the 235 eyes with occult CNV and VPEDs, 98 (42%) were eligible for photocoagulation therapy based on ICGA findings. The authors calculated that ICGA enhances the treatment eligibility by approximately one-third (69).

In a expanded series (39) the same authors reported their results on ICGA study of 1000 consecutive eyes with occult CNV by FA. They recognized three morphologic types of CNV, which included focal spots, plaques (well defined and poorly defined), and combination lesions (in which both focal spots and plaques are noted). Combination lesions were further subdivided into marginal spots (focal spots at the edge of plaque of neovascularization), overlying spots (hot spots overlying plaques of neovascularization), or remote spots (a focal spot remote from a plaque of neovascularization).

The relative frequency of these lesions was as follows: focal spots 29%, plaques 61% consisting 27% of well-defined plaques and 34% of poorly defined plaques, and combination lesions 8%, consisting of 3% of marginal spots, 4% of overlying spots and 1% of remote spots (39). A follow-up study from the same authors of patients with newly diagnosed unilateral occult CNV secondary to AMD showed that the patients tended to develop the same morphologic type of CNV in the fellow eye (70).

Chang et al. (71) reported on the clinicopathologic correlation of AMD with CNV detected by ICGA. Histopathologic examination of the lesion revealed a thick sub-RPE CNV corresponding to the plaque-like lesion seen with ICGA.

Watzke and colleagues analyzed 104 consecutive AMD patients to determine the sensitivity of ICG in detecting lesions originally identified by FA (72). ICG hyperfluorescence was present in 87% of eyes with classic CNV and in 93% of eyes with fibrovascular pigment epithelium detachments (FVPEDs). Of eyes diagnosed with LLUS by FA, 50% were hyperfluorescent and 50% were isofluorescent by ICG. Additionally, three fellow eyes with dry AMD had hyperfluorescent lesions by ICG, but it is unknown whether these eyes progressed to neovascular AMD.

Finally, Lee et al. (73) reported on 15 eyes with surgically excised subfoveal CNV that underwent preoperative and postoperative ICGA. All excised membranes were examined by light microscopy, and all surgically excised ICG-imaged membranes corresponded to sub-RPE and subneurosensory CNV.

The above studies demonstrate that ICGA is an important adjunctive study to FA in the detection of CNV. FA is more sensitive than ICGA in imaging fine capillaries that connect larger vessels and capillaries at the proliferating edge of well-defined CNV. While FA images well-defined CNV better than ICGA in some cases, ICGA allows reclassification of FA-defined occult CNV into well-demarcated CNV eligible for ICG-guided thermal laser treatment in about 30% of cases (74).

The best imaging strategy to thoroughly classify CNV is the combination of FA and ICGA. Helbig et al. studied 502 patients using simultaneous FA and ICG to characterize AMD, and found that 3% of eyes had a hot spot within an occult lesion, 4% had plaques within an occult lesion, 9% had RAP, and 6% had PCV (75). Yanagi and colleagues (76) compared simultaneous fluorescein and ICG injection with FA-guided ICGA, in which FA was used to detect an area of leakage, allowing a lower dose ICG injection and focusing the ICG detector only on the lesion in question. Overall detection of feeder vessels (FVs) was similar between the simultaneous and FA-guided ICG groups, but the latter group required lower quantities of ICG and had shorter examination times. The benefits of simultaneous procedures, such as convenience and accurate diagnosis of treatable cases, must be weighed against the disadvantages of increased cost and adverse effects.

RECURRENT CNV IN AMD

Recurrent CNV following photocoagulation treatment is a major cause of treatment failure. Although most recurrences can be detected and imaged with clinical biomicroscopic examination and FA, a significant number of patients demonstrate new neovascular manifestations and visual symptoms without a clearly defined area of recurrent neovascularization identified by FA. These patients may exhibit diffuse staining and leakage at the site of previous treatment or may demonstrate no FA evidence of recurrence despite the new neovascular manifestations identified clinically. ICGA has proven to be often useful in detecting the recurrence.

Sorenson et al. (77) reported the use of ICG-guided laser treatment in 66 cases of recurrent occult CNV secondary to AMD. Only 29 (44%) were eligible for laser re-treatment, and of these 29 eyes 18 (62%) had anatomic success with an average follow-up of six months (54). Similar results were reported by Reichel et al., who reported 58 eyes with recurrent CNV from AMD (78). In 14 eyes (24%), a well-defined recurrent CNV could be identified by evaluating the fluorescein angiogram. In 6 (14%) of the remaining 44 eyes, a well-defined recurrent CNV was identifiable by ICGA.

However, clinical evidence of recurrence must accompany a hot spot detected by ICG. Chen and colleagues (79) performed ICGA two weeks after krypton laser treatment on 230 consecutive eyes with neovascular AMD. Forty patients (18%) developed ICG hot spots after treatment, and these hot spots spontaneously resolved without development of CNV in 31 patients. Recurrent CNV was present at the hot spot in four patients and away from the hot spot in five patients.

ICG-ASSOCIATED TREATMENT STRATEGIES FOR CNV IN AMD

In the past, patients were considered potentially eligible for laser photocoagulation therapy by ICG guidance if they had clinical and FA evidence of occult CNV. Of the two types of occult CNV identifiable by ICG study, hot spots and plaques, direct laser photocoagulation was recommended only to hot spots. In fact as mentioned above, hot spots represent areas of actively leaking neovascularization that can be obliterated by laser photocoagulation in attempt to eliminate the associated serosanguineous complications, and stabilize or improve the vision. On the contrary, plaques seem to represent a thin layer of neovascularization, which is not actively leaking, and which may benefit from PDT (80) or intravitreal anti-angiogenic agents (81–86).

In the case of a lesion comprised of a hot spot and a plaque, and in which the hot spot is at the margin of the plaque (that may extend under the fovea), laser photocoagulation to the extrafoveal hot spot spares the fovea. This treatment approach was successful in obliterating the CNV and stabilizing the vision in 56% of a consecutive series of AMD patients (74). On the contrary we have had poor success with direct laser treatment of hot spots overlying plaques, or confluent treatment of the entire plaque.

Slakter and associates (87) performed ICG-guided laser photocoagulation in 79 eyes with occult CNV. The occult CNV was successfully eliminated with stabilized or improved visual acuity in 29 (66%) of 44 eyes with occult CNV associated with neurosensory retinal elevations, and in 15 (43%) of 35 eyes with occult CNV associated with PED. This study demonstrated that in some cases ICGA imaging can successfully guide laser photocoagulation of occult CNV.

Another pilot study of ICG-guided laser treatment of occult CNV had similar results (88).

Guyer and coworkers (74) reported a pilot study with ICG-guided laser photocoagulation of 23 eyes with occult CNV secondary to AMD with focal spots at the edge of a neovascular plaque of the ICG study. ICG-guided laser photocoagulation was applied solely to the focal spot at the edge of the plaque. At 24 months of follow-up, anatomic success with resolution of the neovascular findings was obtained in six (37.5%) of 16 eyes. Importantly, these studies set the foundation for future prospective studies of ICG-guided laser treatment. In addition, they proved that the presence of a PED is a poor prognostic factor in the treatment of neovascular AMD.

Lim et al. reported the visual acuity outcome after ICGA-guided laser photocoagulation of CNV associated with PED in 20 eyes with AMD (89). At three months after laser photocoagulation, visual acuity had improved two or more Snellen lines in two eyes (10%), worsened by two or more lines in 10 (50%), and remained unchanged in eight of 20 (40%). At nine months after laser photocoagulation, visual acuity had improved by two or more lines in one eye (9%), worsened by two or more lines in nine (82%), and remained unchanged in one of 11 (9%). They concluded that ICG-guided laser photocoagulation may temporarily stabilize visual acuity in some eyes with CNV associated with PED, but final visual acuity decreases with time.

Da Pozzo and associates evaluated the efficacy of ICG-guided photocoagulation in 86 eyes with occult CNV and a hot spot on ICG (90). Of the 53 eyes without PED, 32 (60%) had stable or improved vision at one year, but 27 (51%) had recurrence of the CNV. Of the 33 eyes with PED, only five (15%) had stable or improved vision at one year and 23 (70%) had CNV recurrence.

Another potential therapeutic application using ICG is ICG dye-enhanced diode laser photocoagulation. The peak absorption of ICG (795 to 810 nm) is at a similar wavelength as the peak emission of the diode laser (805 nm). Thus, dye-enhanced laser photocoagulation may allow selective ablation of the ICG-containing CNV with relative sparing of the normal neighboring retina. However, leakage of ICG into the intraretinal space, which occurred in 11% of 149 eyes in a series reported by Ho and colleagues, may be a contraindication to ICG dye-enhanced diode photocoagulation (91).

A pilot study by Reichel and associates of 10 patients with poorly defined CNV resulted in closure of the CNV in all cases, but a severe immediate vision loss occurred in one patient (92). A larger series by Obana et al. studied 38 eyes with classic or occult CNV, and found that CNV occlusion was achieved in 92% of eyes, with and 18% recurrence rate over an average follow-up of 26 months (93). Ten eyes (26%) showed improved visual acuity, 16 (42%) showed no change, and 12 eyes (32%) worsened.

A pilot study by Arevalo et al. compared ICG dye-enhanced diode laser photocoagulation alone with dye-enhanced laser combined with IVTA (94). In their initial series of 19 eyes selected irrespective of lesion subtype, none of the 9 eyes receiving combination therapy required re-treatment at seven months, while 4 of 10 eyes receiving ICG dye-enhanced laser alone needed re-treatment. A follow-up paper by the same group reported 31 eyes treated with dye-enhanced laser and 4 mg of IVTA followed for a mean of nine months (95). Nineteen eyes (61%) showed stable vision, seven eyes (23%) improved, and five eyes (16%) worsened. In the occult subgroup, however, the proportion of patients who worsened was greater (33%). No severe acute vision loss was reported. Topically treatable glaucoma occurred in five eyes.

NEW TECHNIQUES IN ICG ANGIOGRAPHY

Advances in ICGA are real-time angiography, contrast enhancement ICGA, wide-angle angiography, digital subtraction-indocyanine green (DS-ICG) angiography, dynamic ICG-guided FV laser treatment of CNV, ICGA for dry AMD, and use of cSLO-ICG.

Contrast-Enhanced ICG Angiography

Contrast enhancement of ICG angiographic images using digital imaging software may enhance the diagnostic sensitivity and specificity of the study. Maberley and Cruess compared non-enhanced and contrast-enhanced ICG angiographic images of 50 consecutive patients with occult CNV from AMD (96). Only 36% of the non-enhanced images demonstrated well-defined membranes, whereas 58% were well defined with the contrast-enhanced images.

Real-Time ICGA

Real-time ICGA (97) uses a modified Topcon 50IA camera with a diode laser illumination system that has an output at 805 nm (Topcon 50IAL camera), can produce images at 30 frames per second, and allows continuous recording. The images can be acquired either as a video tape or as a single image at a frequency of 30 images per second. To make printed copies of these images single frames are digitized, but the resolution is limited to 640 by 480 pixels.

Wide-Angle ICGA

Wide-angle images of the fundus can be obtained by performing ICG video angiography with the aid of wide angle contact lenses. The contact lenses used are the Volk SuperQuad 160, the Volk Quadraspheric, or the Volk Transequator (Volk, Mentor OH). Because the image formed by these lenses lies about 1 cm in front of the lens, the fundus camera is set on A or + so that the camera is focused on the image plane of the contact lens.

This technique allows instantaneous imaging of a large area of the fundus. The combined use of the contact lens and of the laser illumination system in a high-speed digital fundus camera allows real-time imaging of 160° of field of view. Staurenghi and colleagues developed a combined contact and noncontact system to achieve wide-field images up to 150° with a cSLO ICG (98).

Digital Subtraction-Indocyanine Green Angiography

DS-ICGA uses DS of sequentially acquired ICG angiographic frames to image the progression of the dye front in the choroidal circulation (99,100). A method of pseudocolor imaging of the choroid allows differentiation and identification of choroidal arteries and veins. DS-ICGA allows imaging of occult CNV with greater detail and in a shorter period of time than with conventional ICGA.

Matsumoto et al. performed DS-ICGA on 20 patients with CNV accompanied by subretinal hemorrhage (101). In six of the 20 eyes, DS-ICGA distinguished hyperfluorescence due to a slowly expanding, poorly defined, large lesion from simple leakage with a well-defined lesion. The DS-ICGA technique made clear the expanding wave of hyperfluorescence from a more slowly filling, ill-defined lesion.

FV Therapy

Staurenghi et al. (102) considered a series of 15 patients with subfoveal CNVM in whom FVs could be clearly detected by means of dynamic ICGA but not necessarily with FA. Based on the pilot study, the authors simultaneously reported a second series of 16 patients with FVs smaller than 85 μm. FVs were treated with argon green laser. The ICGA was repeated immediately after treatment, and at 2, 7, and 30, and then every 3 months, to assess FV closure. An FV that remained patent was immediately re-treated, and the ICGA follow-up started again. In the pilot study, 40% of FVs were successfully occluded; this result was affected by the width and number of FVs. The occlusion success rate in the second series, with FVs under 85 μm, was 75%. The authors concluded that dynamic ICGA may detect small FVs that are more successfully occluded by argon photocoagulation.

ICG FOR DRY AMD

Hanutsaha et al. studied 432 patients by ICG with neovascular AMD in one eye and drusen without exudation in the fellow eye (103). Eighty-nine percent of eyes with drusen had normal fluorescence on ICG, while 11% of eyes with drusen had focal hot spots or hyperintense plaques. Over an average follow-up of 22 months, 27% of eyes with drusen and an abnormal ICG developed CNV, while only 10% of drusen eyes and a normal ICG developed neovascular AMD. The authors suggested that ICG may be a predictive indicator of future neovascular changes in eyes with drusen.

Patchy and slow choroidal filling on FA, in association with reduced choroidal fluorescence on ICGA, was associated by Pauleikoff and associates with early changes in AMD (104). One hundred eyes with early AMD were studied for the above characteristics, termed a prolonged choroidal filling phase (PCFP), which was associated with confluent drusen in the study eye, focal RPE atrophy in the study eye, and geographic atrophy in the fellow eye. The group postulated that PCFP was a clinical indicator of Bruch's membrane deposits and a predictor for geographic atrophy from AMD.

Ultra late phase ICGA, performed 24 hours after dye injection, demonstrates hypofluorescent geographic lesions in patients with both neovascular and dry AMD, as shown by Mori and associates. They demonstrated that 95% of AMD eyes with CNV had geographic hypofluorescent lesions, and that all CNV detectable by FA or ICG was contained within these lesions. In 73% of eyes without CNV, the same geographic areas were present, while age-matched normal subjects did not have the lesions. Mean fluorescence intensity was higher in a normal group older than 62 years, compared with normal subjects less than 36 years. The authors postulated that these geographic hypofluorescent areas may represent areas predisposed to CNV development.

CONFOCAL SCANNING LASER OPHTHALMOSCOPE ICG

With the availability of cSLO to perform ICG, many retinal physicians are choosing this modality over high-speed digital angiography because of the ability to use the cSLO for other functions, such as autofluorescence and FA. Geliskaen and colleagues simultaneously compared cSLO ICG with high-resolution fundus camera ICG in 100 eyes with occult CNV (105). Confocal SLO was superior in delineating vessel architecture of the neovascular lesion; however, fundus photography was much more sensitive than cSLO in detecting focal lesions (52% *vs.* 37%, respectively) and plaques (35% *vs.* 13%, respectively).

CONCLUSION

The role ICGA in the treatment of AMD is in evolution. As photocoagulation of extrafoveal CNV gave way to treatment of all types of CNV with PDT, ICG angiography has proven very useful in adding information to FA about lesion subtype. The ability of ICG to identify subtypes of occult CNV, such as VPED, hot spots, plaques, and RCA, allows targeted and sometimes effective therapy for these refractory types of CNV. Given that approximately 87% of new CNV from AMD is minimally classic or occult (106), many patients have derived some benefit from the additional information obtainable by ICGA.

The approval of pegaptanib sodium (Macugen) heralded a new era in AMD treatment (81). Shown to be equally efficacious for all lesion subtypes, pegaptanib was a departure from traditional laser-based, destructive procedures. Ranibizumab (Lucentis) has been shown to be even more efficacious and bevacizumab (Avastin) appears to show similar results as ranibizumab (82–85, 108,109). Eylea has also been shown to be efficacious and has been approved for treatment of neovasular AMD (110). Further research is necessary to determine whether a lesion subtype remains an important predictor of treatment response with these new modalities.

A systematic evidence-based review of the PubMed indexed literature in English or with an English abstract yielded a strong recommendation for the use of ICGA for the following conditions: PCV, occult CNV, neovascularization associated with PED, and recurrent choroidal neovascular membranes (107). The same review reported only modest evidence supporting the use of ICGA for

routine choroidal neovascular membranes and for identifying FVs in AMD. Future advances in ICGA, such as wide angle, real-time, and DS techniques may improve our diagnostic ability in AMD.

SUMMARY POINTS

- Indocyanine green angiography (ICGA) is a useful adjunctive technique to FA for the diagnosis of AMD. This is especially true in the presence of occult CNV. ICG allows better recognition of subtypes of occult choroidal neovascularization (CNV) such as vascularized pigment epithelial detachment, hot spots, plaques, and retinal-choroidal anastomosis.
- ICGA is useful in the diagnosis of polypoidal choroidal vasculopathy, retinal angiomatous proliferation, and recurrent choroidal neovascular membranes.
- Preliminary studies suggested that ICG-guided laser photocoagulation was beneficial in the treatment of CNV prior to the era of anti-vascular endothelial growth factor therapy.
- Further research is necessary to improve our understanding of all the information obtained by ICGA and its potential role in new therapeutic regimens.
- Real-time ICGA, wide-angle ICGA, and digital subtraction-ICGA may improve our diagnostic ability in AMD.

REFERENCES

1. Schatz H, Burton TC, Tannuzzi LA, Rabb MF. Interpretation of Fundus Fluorescein Angiograph. St. Louis: Mosby-Year Book, 1978.
2. Yannuzzi LA. Laser Photocoagulation of the Macula. Philadelphia, PA: JB Lippincott, 1989.
3. Guyer DR, Puliafito CA, Mones JM, et al. Digital indocyanine-green angiography in chorioretinal disorders. Ophthalmology 1992; 99: 287–91.
4. Yannuzzi LA, Slakter JS, Sorenson JA, Guyer DR, Orlock DA. Digital indocyanine green videoangiography and choroidal neovascularization. Retina 1992; 12: 191–223.
5. Geeraets WJ, Berry ER. Ocular spectral characteristics as related to hazards from lasers and other light sources. Am J Ophthalmol 1968; 66: 15–20.
6. Fox IJ, Wood EH. Applications of dilution curves recorded from the right side of the heart or venous circulation with the aid of a new indicator dye. Mayo Clin Proc 1957; 32: 541–50.
7. Fox IJ, Wood EH. Indocyanine green: physical and physiologic properties. Mayo Clin Proc 1960; 35: 732–44.
8. Kuroiwa T, Kajimoto Y, Ohta T. Development and clinical application of near-infrared surgical microscope: preliminary report. Minim Invasive Neurosurg 2001; 44: 240–2.
9. Raabe A, Nakaji P, Beck J, et al. Prospective evaluation of surgical microscope-integrated intraoperative near-infrared indocyanine green videoangiography during aneurysm surgery. J Neurosurg 2005; 103: 982–9.
10. Kogure K, David NJ, Yamanouchi U, Choromokos E. Infrared absorption angiography of the fundus circulation. Arch Ophthalmol 1970; 83: 209–14.

11. David NJ. Infrared absorption fundus angiography. In: Proceedings of the International Symposium on Fluorescein Angiography. Albi, France, 1969.

12. Hochheimer BF. Angiography of the retina with indocyanine green. Arch Ophthalmol 1971; 86: 564–5.

13. Flower RW, Hochheimer BF. Clinical infrared absorption angiography of the choroid. Am J Ophthalmol 1972; 73: 458–9.

14. Flower RW. Infrared absorption angiography of the choroid and some observations on the effects of high intraocular pressures. Am J Ophthalmol 1972; 74: 600–14.

15. Flower RW, Hochheimer BF. A clinical technique and apparatus for simultaneous angiography of the separate retinal and choroidal circulations. Invest Ophthalmol Vis Sci 1973; 12: 248–61.

16. Flower RW, Hochheimer BF. Indocyanine green dye fluorescence and infrared absorption choroidal angiography performed simultaneously with fluorescein angiography. Johns Hopkins Med J 1976; 138: 33–42.

17. Hyvarinen L, Flower RW. Indocyanine green fluorescence angiography. Acta Ophthalmol (Copenh) 1980; 58: 528–38.

18. Bischoff PM, Flower RW. Ten years experience with choroidal angiography using indocyanine green dye: a new routine examination or an epilogue? Doc Ophthalmol 1985; 60: 235–91.

19. Hayashi K, Hasegawa Y, Tazawa Y, de Laey JJ. Clinical application of indocyanine green angiography to choroidal neovascularization. Jpn J Ophthalmol 1989; 33: 57–65.

20. Hayashi K, Hasegawa Y, Tokoro T. Indocyanine green angiography of central serous chorioretinopathy. Int Ophthalmol 1986; 9: 37–41.

21. Hayashi K, de Laey JJ. Indocyanine green angiography of submacular choroidal vessels in the human eye. Ophthalmologica 1985; 190: 20–9.

22. Destro M, Puliafito CA. Indocyanine green videoangiography of choroidal neovascularization. Ophthalmology 1989; 96: 846–53.

23. Scheider A, Schroedel C. High resolution indocyanine green angiography with a scanning laser ophthalmoscope. Am J Ophthalmol 1989; 108: 458–9.

24. Scheider A. Indocyanine green angiography with an infrared scanning laser ophthalmoscope. Initial clinical experiences. Ophthalmologe 1992; 89: 27–33.

25. Scheider A, Kaboth A, Neuhauser L. Detection of subretinal neovascular membranes with indocyanine green and an infrared scanning laser ophthalmoscope. Am J Ophthalmol 1992; 113: 45–51.

26. Patz A, Flower RW, Klein ML, et al. Clinical applications of indocyanine green angiography. Doc Ophthalmol Proc Ser 1976; 9: 245–51.

27. Cherrick GR, Stein SW, Leevy CM, Davidson CS. Indocyanine green: observations on its physical properties, plasma decay, and hepatic extraction. J Clin Invest 1960; 39: 592–600.

28. Baker KJ. Binding of sulfobromophthalein (BSP) sodium and indocyanine green (ICG) by plasma alpha-1 lipoproteins. Proc Soc Exp Biol Med 1966; 122: 957–63.

29. Leevy CM, Bender J. Physiology of dye extraction by the liver: comparative studies of sulfobromophthalein and indocyanine green. Ann NY Acad Sci 1963; 111: 161–76.

30. Goresky CA. Initial distribution and rate of uptake of sulfobromophthalein in the liver. Am J Physiol 1964; 207: 13–26.

31. Ketterer SG, Weigand BD. The excretion of indocyanine green and its use in the estimation of hepatic blood flow. Clin Res 1959; 7: 71.

32. Ketterer SG, Weigand BD. Hepatic clearance of indocyanine green. Clin Res 1959; 7: 289.

33. Probst P, Paumgartner G, Caucig H, Frauolich H, Grabner G. Studies on clearance and placental transfer of indocyanine green during labor. Clin Chim Acta 1970; 29: 157.

34. Leevy CM, Smith F, Kiernan T. Liver function test. In: Bockus HL, ed. Gastroenterology, 3rd edn. Vol. 3. Philadelphia: PA: Saunders, 1976: 68.

35. Shabetai R, Adolph RJ. Principles of cardiac catheterization. In: Fowler NO, ed. Cardiac Diagnosis and Treatment, 3rd edn. Hagerstown, MD: Harper & Row, 1980: 117.

36. Hope-Ross M, Yannuzzi LA, Gragoudas ES, et al. Adverse reactions due to indocyanine green. Ophthalmology 1994; 101: 529–33.

37. Bindewald A, Stuhrmann O, Roth F, et al. Lower limits of fluorescein and indocyanine green dye for digital cSLO fluorescence angiography. Br J Ophthalmol 2005; 89: 1609–15.

38. Macular Photocoagulation Study Group. Occult choroidal neovascularization. Influence on visual outcome in patients with age-related macular degeneration. Arch Ophthalmol 1996; 114: 400–12.

39. Guyer DR, Yannuzzi LA, Slakter JS, et al. Classification of choroidal neovascularization by digital indocyanine green videoangiography. Ophthalmology 1996; 103: 2054–60.

40. Kleiner RC, Brucker AJ, Johnston RL. The posterior uveal bleeding syndrome. Retina 1990; 10: 9–17.

41. Yannuzzi LA, Sorenson J, Spaide RF, Lipson B. Idiopathic polypoidal choroidal vasculopathy (IPCV). Retina 1990; 10: 1–8.

42. Spaide RF, Yannuzzi LA, Slakter JS, Sorenson J, Orlach DA. Indocyanine green videoangiography of idiopathic polypoidal choroidal vasculopathy. Retina 1995; 15: 100–10.

43. Phillips WB II, Regillo CD, Maguire JI. Indocyanine green angiography of idiopathic polypoidal choroidal vasculopathy. Ophthalmic Surg Lasers 1996; 27: 467–70.

44. Yannuzzi LA, Ciardella A, Spaide RF, et al. The expanding clinical spectrum of idiopathic polypoidal choroidal vasculopathy. Arch Ophthalmol 1997; 115: 478–85.

45. Yannuzzi LA, Nogueira FB, Spaide RF, et al. Idiopathic polypoidal choroidal vasculopathy: a peripheral lesion. Arch Ophthalmol 1998; 116: 382–3.

46. Moorthy RS, Lyon AT, Rabb MF, et al. Idiopathic polypoidal choroidal vasculopathy of the macula. Ophthalmology 1998; 105: 1380–5.

47. Schneider U, Gelisken F, Kreissig I. Indocyanine green angiography and idiopathic polypoidal choroidal vasculopathy. Br J Ophthalmol 1998; 82: 98–9.

48. Yannuzzi LA, Wong DW, Sforzolini BS, et al. Polypoidal choroidal vasculopathy and neovascularized age-related macular degeneration. Arch Ophthalmol 1999; 117: 1503–10.

49. Yannuzzi LA, Freund KB, Goldbaum M, et al. Polypoidal choroidal vasculopathy masquerading as central serous chorioretinopathy. Ophthalmology 2000; 107: 767–77.

50. Ahuja RM, Stanga PE, Vingerling JR, Reck AC, Bird AC. Polypoidal choroidal vasculopathy in exudative and haemorrhagic pigment epithelial detachments. Br J Ophthalmol 2000; 84: 479–84.

51. Escano MF, Fujii S, Ishibashi K, Matsuo H, Yamamoto M. Indocyanine green videoangiography in macular variant of idiopathic polypoidal choroidal vasculopathy. Jpn J Ophthalmol 2000; 44: 313–16.

52. Uyama M, Wada M, Nagai Y, et al. Polypoidal choroidal vasculopathy: natural history. Am J Ophthalmol 2002; 133: 639–48.

53. Sho K, Takahashi K, Yamada H, et al. Polypoidal choroidal vasculopathy: incidence, demographic features, and clinical characteristics. Arch Ophthalmol 2003; 121: 1392–6.

54. Nishijima K, Takahashi M, Akita J, et al. Laser photocoagulation of indocyanine green angiographically identified feeder vessels to idiopathic polypoidal choroidal vasculopathy. Am J Ophthalmol 2004; 137: 770–3.

55. Nakajima M, Yuzawa M, Shimada H, Mori R. Correlation between indocyanine green angiographic findings and histopathology of polypoidal choroidal vasculopathy. Jpn J Ophthalmol 2004; 48: 249–55.

56. Lafaut BA, Aisenbrey S, Vanden Broecke C, Bartz-Schmidt KU. Clinicopathological correlation of deep retinal vascular anomalous complex in age related macular degeneration. Br J Ophthalmol 2000; 84: 1269–74.

57. Kuhn D, Meunier I, Soubrane G, Coscas G. Imaging of chorioretinal anastomoses in vascularized retinal pigment epithelium detachments. Arch Ophthalmol 1995; 113: 1392–8.

58. Slakter JS, Yannuzzi LA, Schneider U, et al. Retinal choroidal anastomoses and occult choroidal neovascularization in age-related macular degeneration. Ophthalmology 2000; 107: 742–53; discussion 753–44.

59. Fernandes LH, Freund KB, Yannuzzi LA, et al. The nature of focal areas of hyperfluorescence or hot spots imaged with indocyanine green angiography. Retina 2002; 22: 557–68.

60. Yannuzzi LA, Negrao S, Iida T, et al. Retinal angiomatous proliferation in age-related macular degeneration. Retina 2001; 21: 416–34.

61. Bottoni F, Massacesi A, Cigada M, et al. Treatment of retinal angiomatous proliferation in age-related macular degeneration: a series of 104 cases of retinal angiomatous proliferation. Arch Ophthalmol 2005; 123: 1644–50.

62. Boscia F, Parodi MB, Furino C, Reibaldi M, Sborgia C. Photodynamic therapy with verteporfin for retinal angiomatous proliferation. Graefes Arch Clin Exp Ophthalmol 2006; 244: 1224–32.

63. Nicolo M, Ghiglione D, Lai S, Calabria G. Retinal angiomatous proliferation treated by intravitreal triamcinolone and photodynamic therapy with verteporfin. Graefes Arch Clin Exp Ophthalmol 2006; 244: 1336–8.

64. Schmidt-Erfurth U, Hasan T. Mechanisms of action of photodynamic therapy with verteporfin for the treatment of age-related macular degeneration. Surv Ophthalmol 2000; 45: 195–214.

65. Treatment of age-related macular degeneration with photodynamic therapy (TAP) Study Group. Photodynamic therapy of subfoveal choroidal neovascularization in age-related macular degeneration with verteporfin: one-year results of 2 randomized clinical trials–TAP report. Arch Ophthalmol 1999; 117: 1329–45.

66. Lim JI, Sternberg P Jr, Capone A Jr, Aaberg TM Sr, Gilman JP. Selective use of indocyanine green angiography for occult choroidal neovascularization. Am J Ophthalmol 1995; 120: 75–82.

67. Baumal CR, Reichel E, Duker JS, Wong J, Puliafito CA. Indocyanine green hyperfluorescence associated with serous retinal pigment epithelial detachment in age-related macular degeneration. Ophthalmology 1997; 104: 761–9.

68. Yannuzzi LA, Hope-Ross M, Slakter JS, et al. Analysis of vascularized pigment epithelial detachments using indocyanine green videoangiography. Retina 1994; 14: 99–113.

69. Guyer DR, Yannuzzi LA, Slakter JS, et al. Digital indocyanine-green videoangiography of occult choroidal neovascularization. Ophthalmology 1994; 101: 1727–35; discussion 1735–7.

70. Chang B, Yannuzzi LA, Ladas ID, et al. Choroidal neovascularization in second eyes of patients with unilateral exudative age-related macular degeneration. Ophthalmology 1995; 102: 1380–6.

71. Chang TS, Freund KB, de la Cruz Z, Yannuzzi LA, Green WR. Clinicopathologic correlation of choroidal neovascularization demonstrated by indocyanine green angiography in a patient with retention of good vision for almost four years. Retina 1994; 14: 114–24.

72. Watzke RC, Klein ML, Hiner CJ, Chan BK, Kraemer DF. A comparison of stereoscopic fluorescein angiography with indocyanine green videoangiography in age-related macular degeneration. Ophthalmology 2000; 107: 1601–6.

73. Lee BL, Lim JI, Grossniklaus HE. Clinicopathologic features of indocyanine green angiography-imaged, surgically excised choroidal neovascular membranes. Retina 1996; 16: 64–9.

74. Guyer DR, Yannuzzi LA, Ladas I, et al. Indocyanine green-guided laser photocoagulation of focal spots at the edge of plaques of choroidal neovascularization. Arch Ophthalmol 1996; 114: 693–7.

75. Helbig H, Niederberger H, Valmaggia C, Bischoff P. Simultaneous fluorescein and indocyanine green angiography for exudative macular degencration. Klin Monatsbl Augenheilkd 2005; 222: 202–5.

76. Yanagi Y, Tamaki Y, Sekine H. Fluorescein angiography-guided indocyanine green angiography for the detection of feeder vessels in subfoveal choroidal neovascularization. Eye 2004; 18: 474–7.

77. Sorenson JA, Yannuzzi LA, Slakter JS, et al. A pilot study of digital indocyanine green videoangiography for recurrent occult choroidal neovascularization in age-related macular degeneration. Arch Ophthalmol 1994; 112: 473–9.

78. Reichel E, Pollock DA, Duker JS, Puliafito CA. Indocyanine green angiography for recurrent choroidal neovascularization in age-related macular degeneration. Ophthalmic Surg Lasers 1995; 26: 513–18.

79. Chen CJ, Chen LJ, Miller KR. Clinical significance of postlaser indocyanine green angiographic hot spots in age-related macular degeneration. Ophthalmology 1999; 106: 925–9; discussion 929–31.

80. Photodynamic Therapy Study Group. Verteporfin therapy of subfoveal choroidal neovascularization in age-related macular degeneration: two-year results of a randomized clinical trial including lesions with occult with no classic choroidal neovascularization-verteporfin in photodynamic therapy report 2. Am J Ophthalmol 2001; 131: 541–60.

81. Gragoudas ES, Adamis AP, Cunningham ET Jr, Feinsod M, Guyer DR. Pegaptanib for neovascular age-related macular degeneration. N Engl J Med 2004; 351: 2805–16.

82. Avery RL, Pieramici DJ, Rabena MD, et al. Intravitreal bevacizumab (Avastin) for neovascular age-related macular degeneration. Ophthalmology 2006; 113: 363–72; e5.

83. Michels S, Rosenfeld PJ, Puliafito CA, Marcus EN, Venkatraman AS. Systemic bevacizumab (Avastin) therapy for neovascular age-related macular degeneration twelve-week results of an uncontrolled open-label clinical study. Ophthalmology 2005; 112: 1035–47.

84. Spaide RF, Laud K, Fine HF, et al. Intravitreal bevacizumab treatment of choroidal neovascularization secondary to age-related macular degeneration. Retina 2006; 26: 383–90.

85. Heier JS, Antoszyk AN, Pavan PR, et al. Ranibizumab for treatment of neovascular age-related macular degeneration: a phase I/II multicenter, controlled, multidose study. Ophthalmology 2006; 113: 642; e1–4.

86. Rosenfeld PJ, Heier JS, Hantsbarger G, Shams N. Tolerability and efficacy of multiple escalating doses of ranibizumab (Lucentis) for neovascular age-related macular degeneration. Ophthalmology 2006; 113: 632; e1.

87. Slakter JS, Yannuzzi LA, Sorenson JA, et al. A pilot study of indocyanine green videoangiography-guided laser photocoagulation of occult choroidal neovascularization in age-related macular degeneration. Arch Ophthalmol 1994; 112: 465–72.

88. Regillo CD, Benson WE, Maguire JI, Annesley WH Jr. Indocyanine green angiography and occult choroidal neovascularization. Ophthalmology 1994; 101: 280–8.

89. Lim JI, Aaberg TM, Capone A Jr, Sternberg P Jr. Indocyanine green angiography-guided photocoagulation of choroidal neovascularization associated with retinal pigment epithelial detachment. Am J Ophthalmol 1997; 123: 524–32.

90. Da Pozzo S, Parodi MB, Ravalico G. A pilot study of ICG-guided laser photocoagulation for occult choroidal neovascularization presenting as a focal spot in age-related macular degeneration. Int Ophthalmol 2001; 24: 187–94.

91. Ho AC, Yannuzzi LA, Guyer DR, et al. Intraretinal leakage of indocyanine green dye. Ophthalmology 1994; 101: 534–41.

92. Reichel E, Puliafito CA, Duker JS, Guyer DR. Indocyanine green dye-enhanced diode laser photocoagulation of poorly defined subfoveal choroidal neovascularization. Ophthalmic Surg 1994; 25: 195–201.

93. Obana A, Gohto Y, Nishiguchi K, et al. A retrospective pilot study of indocyanine green enhanced diode laser photocoagulation for subfoveal choroidal neo-vascularization associated with age-related macular degeneration. Jpn J Ophthalmol 2000; 44: 668–76.

94. Arevalo JF, Mendoza AJ, Fernandez CF. Indocyanine green-mediated photothrombosis with and without intravitreal triamcinolone acetonide for subfoveal choroidal neovascularization in age-related macular degeneration: a pilot study. Retina 2005; 25: 719–26.

95. Arevalo JF, Garcia RA, Mendoza AJ. Indocyanine green-mediated photothrombosis with intravitreal triamcinolone acetonide for subfoveal choroidal neovascularization in age-related macular degeneration. Graefes Arch Clin Exp Ophthalmol 2005; 243: 1180–5.

96. Maberley DA, Cruess AF. Indocyanine green angiography: an evaluation of image enhancement for the identification of occult choroidal neovascular membranes. Retina 1999; 19: 37–44.

97. Spaide RF, Orlock DA, Herrmann-Delemazure B, et al. Wide-angle indocyanine green angiography. Retina 1998; 18: 44–9.

98. Staurenghi G, Viola F, Mainster MA, Graham RD, Harrington PG. Scanning laser ophthalmoscopy and angiography with a wide-field contact lens system. Arch Ophthalmol 2005; 123: 244–52.

99. Miki T, Shiraki K, Kohno T, Moriwaki M, Obana A. Computer assisted image analysis using the subtraction method in indocyanine green angiography. Eur J Ophthalmol 1996; 6: 30–8.

100. Spaide RF, Orlock D, Yannuzzi L, et al. Digital subtraction indocyanine green angiography of occult choroidal neovascularization. Ophthalmology 1998; 105: 680–8.

101. Matsumoto M, Shiraki K, Obana A. Detection of choroidal neovascularization by subtraction indocyanine green angiography. Osaka City Med J 2003; 49: 85–91.

102. Staurenghi G, Orzalesi N, La Capria A, Aschero M. Laser treatment of feeder vessels in subfoveal choroidal neovascular membranes: a revisitation using dynamic indocyanine green angiography. Ophthalmology 1998; 105: 2297–305.

103. Hanutsaha P, Guyer DR, Yannuzzi LA, et al. Indocyanine-green videoangiography of drusen as a possible predictive indicator of exudative maculopathy. Ophthalmology 1998; 105: 1632–6.

104. Pauleikhoff D, Spital G, Radermacher M, et al. A fluorescein and indocyanine green angiographic study of choriocapillaris in age-related macular disease. Arch Ophthalmol 1999; 117: 1353–8.

105. Gelisken F, Inhoffen W, Schneider U, Stroman GA, Kreissig I. Indocyanine green videoangiography of occult choroidal neovascularization: a comparison of scanning laser ophthalmoscope with high-resolution digital fundus camera. Retina 1998; 18: 37–43.

106. Freund KB, Yannuzzi LA, Sorenson JA. Age-related macular degeneration and choroidal neovascularization. Am J Ophthalmol 1993; 115: 786–91.

107. Stanga PE, Lim JI, Hamilton P. Indocyanine green angiography in chorioretinal diseases: indications and interpretation: an evidence-based update. Ophthalmology 2003; 110: 15–21; quiz 22–3.

108. CATT Research Group. Ranibizumab and bevacizumab for neovascular age-related macular degeneration. N Engl J Med 2011; 364: 1897–1908.

109. Comparison of Age-related Macular Degeneration Treatment Trials (CATT) Research Group. Ranibizumab and Bevacizumab for treatment of neovascular age-related macular degeneration two year results. Ophthalmology 2012; 119: 1388–98.

110. www.fda.gov/downloads/AdvisoryCommittees/…/UCM259143.pdf

14

Role of optical coherence tomography in the evaluation of age-related macular degeneration

Robin A. Vora, Caio V. Regatieri, and Elias Reichel

INTRODUCTION

Fourier spectral-domain optical coherence tomography (SD-OCT) systems provide clinicians with cross-sectional retinal images that closely resemble their histological counterparts. It has emerged as the most important ancillary examination for the evaluation and management of all types of age-related macular degeneration. In patients with dry macular degeneration, OCT is able to precisely and longitudinally track changes in drusen volume, drusen morphology, and geographic atrophy. Furthermore, OCT can either directly illustrate choroidal neovascularization or reveal subretinal fluid, cystoid macular edema, and other fine ultra-structural changes which implicitly suggest a transformation to wet macular degeneration. After initiation of pharmacological therapy, determination of the presence of subretinal fluid, intraretinal fluid or their combination and measurement of a change in fluid volume by OCT has become the most crucial feature in deciding whether to pursue additional treatment.

OCT IMAGING PRINCIPLES AND THE NORMAL OCT IMAGE

In a landmark paper nearly 20 years ago, OCT was introduced as a non-invasive technique to image the retina (1). Akin to B-scan ultrasonography, OCT image acquisition and resolution relies upon the differential reflective qualities of the tissue under investigation. However, instead of employing acoustic echoes, it uses light waves to obtain a reflective profile of the retina. The magnitude of the back-scattered and reflected light is measured and conveyed graphically as a two-dimensional cross-sectional image. The use of light results in a nearly 20-fold increase in the spatial resolution of OCT (5–10 μm) when compared with conventional ultrasonography (150 μm) (1,2).

The OCT 3000 (Stratus OCT; Carl Zeiss Meditec, Dublin, California, USA; 2002) was the first commercially-available OCT system. It relied on patented time-domain technology, and was able to achieve scan rates of 400 axial scans per second and an axial resolution of 10 μm. Although previously considered the gold standard of posterior segment tomography, it has now mostly been supplanted by spectral domain (SD) technology (2). With SD technology, low-coherence interferometry is used to detect light echoes and a high-speed spectrometer permits simultaneous measurement of all echoes of light.

This is in contrast to time-domain, where echoes of light are measured sequentially due to the need for a moving reference mirror. Instead, SD technology relies on the Fourier transformation to generate signal. As the reference mirror can remain in a fixed position, axial scanning speeds of greater than 20,000 A-scans per second can be achieved. This has led to dramatic signal-to-noise improvement and motion artifact reduction (3). Furthermore, by increasing acquisition speed, the amount of data which can reliably and reproducibly be measured has increased, permitting raster scanning of the entire macula. This makes volumetric analysis and three-dimensional imaging possible, and allows for exact image registration and more accurate inter-visit measurement comparisons.

With SD technology, axial resolution to the level of 3–7 μm is possible. Figure 14.1 depicts the OCT of a normal human retina. In general, layers of the retina that are hyper-reflective appear bright, whereas those that are hypo-reflective appear dark. When compared to in-vivo specimens, layers of relatively high reflectivity (i.e., bright layers) correspond to horizontally aligned retinal components (4). Thus, the nerve fiber layer, ganglion cell layer, and the plexiform layers all appear bright whereas the nuclear layers are dark. Henle's layer runs obliquely and is not clearly delineated with typical imaging protocols. However, it can be revealed with horizontal decentration of the incident light through the pupil (5).

The interpretation of inner retinal structures as seen in OCT seems to correlate well with histological specimens (6,7). However, the histological counterparts of outer retinal OCT anatomy remain controversial. There are four clear bands in the outer retina that can be resolved with spectral domain OCT. By convention, the first band has been attributed to the external limiting membrane (2). The second band has been ascribed to the boundary between the inner and outer photoreceptor segments (8). In the foveal area, this band bows anteriorly. This reflects the elongation of cones within the fovea, and has been termed the foveal bulge (9). The third band has been variously referred to as the cone outer segment tip line (COST) (9) or Verhoeff's membrane (10), and the fourth is felt to represent the retinal pigment epithelium (RPE)/Bruch's complex (11). A recent study compared representative SD-OCT scans to a well-researched and constructed scaled model drawing. The authors believed that the second band more likely represented the ellipsoid portion of photoreceptor inner segments and the third band corresponded to the contact cylinder of the RPE (12). Additional studies comparing in-vivo OCT with their histological correlations are ongoing, and this remains an area of active research and controversy.

OCT: DRY MACULAR DEGENERATION
Drusen

The presence of drusen is a hallmark feature of dry macular degeneration. Conventional high resolution fundus photography has been the traditional gold standard in the evaluation of patients with drusen, and the imaging modality chosen by reading centers to follow patients in large longitudinal, epidemiologic studies (13). However, interpretation of color photographs is subject to considerable variation and it is difficult to reproducibly outline indistinct drusen (14). Furthermore, stereoscopic images provide no direct information regarding drusen anatomy and their effect on surrounding retinal tissue and the RPE. Due to these limitations, OCT is gaining popularity in the evaluation of drusen (Fig. 14.2).

A descriptive study of drusen revealed 17 different types of OCT abnormalities (15). Inter-observer and intra-observer reliability was high. The most

Figure 14.1 High-definition B-scan optical coherence tomography image in a normal patient (Cirrus OCT; Carl Zeiss Meditec, Dublin, California, USA).

ILM: internal limiting membrane
GCL: ganglion cell layer
NFL: nerve fiber layer
IPL: inner plexiform layer
INL: inner nuclear layer
OPL: outer plexiform layer
ONL: outer nuclear layer

ELM: external limiting membrane
IS/OS: inner segment / outer segment junction
COST: cone outer segment tips
RPE: retinal pigment epithelium

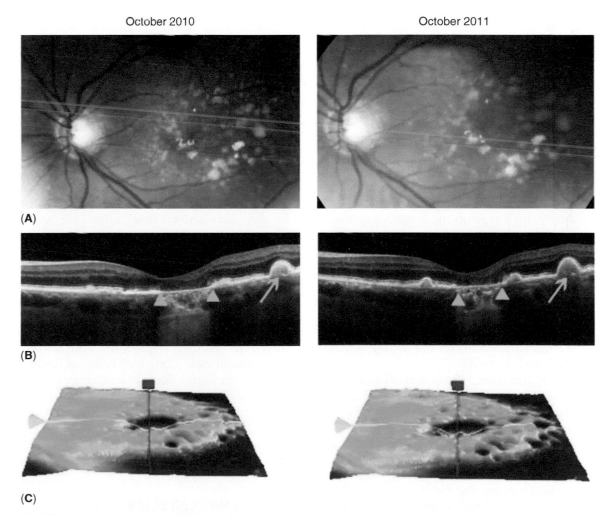

October 2010

October 2011

(A)

(B)

(C)

Figure 14.2 Evolution of drusen in this patient with age-related macular degeneration. (**A**) The color fundus photos show subtle changes in drusen morphology. (**B**) The high-definition optical coherence tomography (OCT) image illustrates drusen as homogeneous elevations of the retinal pigment epithelium with medium internal reflectivity (Cirrus OCT; Carl Zeiss Meditec)). There has been a slight increase in the volume and height of the larger drusen over the interval as seen on OCT B-scan image (green arrow) and the (**C**) OCT-generated elevation map. New, smaller drusen have also appeared. Arrowheads denote an area of geographic atrophy as illustrated by OCT. There is loss of the outer retina and RPE and increased transmission of light into the choroid.

common pattern revealed drusen as convex and homogenous with medium internal reflectivity. Also commonly noted are hyper-reflective foci overlying drusen, which are felt to be either RPE migration or pigment (16). Of interest, it was nearly impossible to predict the ultrastructural characteristics of drusen based on their photographic appearance (15). Other possible qualitative changes on OCT include disruption of the inner segment/outer segment junction and a hyper-reflective haze within the remaining outer nuclear layer, though this may simply be the unveiling of Henle's layer (5,17).

The photoreceptor layer overlying drusen also has been shown to be significantly thinned, with the degree of thinning directly correlated with the height of the drusen (18). It is unclear whether the anatomical changes in the outer retina are primary and precede drusen formation and RPE loss or are secondary and form as a result of alterations in their micro-environment from drusen or RPE dysfunction (18). It is also feasible that the observed retinal thinning, in some cases, is solely due to mechanical compression and that if the compressive forces are relieved, outer retinal anatomy could normalize (19). This has been demonstrated in a recent study of the natural history of drusen. Using SD-OCT and a novel segmentation algorithm, it was shown that drusen evolve dynamically over time, growing and shrinking with an overall tendency to increase in volume and area over time (19,20).

Geographic Atrophy

Geographic atrophy is the principal cause of visual loss in 20% of patients with age-related macular degeneration (AMD) (21). The gold standard in the assessment and evaluation of geographic atrophy has traditionally been conventional fundus photography. In the AREDS study, for example, high resolution stereoscopic images were taken yearly and ultimately used to develop a severity scale to predict progression toward advanced AMD (22). There are limitations to this approach, however. For one, there is the non-trivial degree of intra-observer and inter-observer variability in interpreting fundus photos (23). Standard photography also only renders a two-dimensional image of the retina, providing little direct information about the anatomy of the outer retina, RPE, and choroid.

Fundus autofluorescence (FAF) is another ancillary test useful in the evaluation of geographic atrophy. It relies on the fluorescent characteristics of the fluorophore lipofuscin, a toxic metabolite within the RPE. Areas of retinal pigment atrophy are devoid of lipofuscin and appear hypo-autofluorescent. A hyper-autofluorescent border may often be seen at the margins of the atrophic area. This is thought to represent swollen RPE cells filled with lipofuscin granules. These cells are at significant risk for necrosis, and this finding has been linked to progressive atrophy (24). Unfortunately, there are drawbacks to this imaging modality as well. FAF provides no direct information about the deeper retinal layers and choroid. Image quality degrades quickly in the presence

of significant media opacity. The main disadvantage, however, is the poor discrimination of atrophy in the foveal and parafoveal area. Central macular pigments absorb the excitation light—necessarily making this area hypo-autofluorescent. Thus, there is not enough contrast to clearly discriminate geographic atrophy as it approaches the fovea.

Because of these limitations, OCT has taken an expanding role in the assessment of geographic atrophy. OCT systems offer several complementary imaging protocols to illustrate the extent of geographic atrophy (Fig 14.2). Patients with geographic atrophy show attenuation of the outer retina with loss of the external limiting membrane and inner segment/outer segment junction. The outer nuclear layer is thinned, and there is a posterior bowing of the outer plexiform layer (25). At the margins of atrophy, two patterns have been described: smooth and irregular (26). Outer retinal and RPE structural changes are minimal in patients with the smooth margin pattern. These patients have corresponding normal auto-fluorescence signal at the border of atrophy. However, those patients with an irregular pattern have severe outer retinal abnormalities with significant RPE alterations at the margin. These patients have corresponding hyper-autofluorescent borders and are felt to be at risk for progressive atrophy.

Another key finding on OCT is the increased transmission of light through the retina and into the choroid. Atrophic pigment epithelium and choriocapillaris fail to scatter light, allowing deeper penetration of light into the choroid. This feature serves as the basis for the rendered OCT fundus image, which is an en-face compilation of reflected light from every A-scan. Because more light is transmitted through, areas of geographic atrophy appear bright on the virtual image. Studies have shown that geographic atrophy can be measured reproducibly with these images, and correlate well with measurements from FAF (27–29). Foveal sparing has been shown to be identified much more reliably and with more certainty than FAF (28). Based on OCT images, an enlargement rate of $1.2\,mm^2$ per year has been calculated (29).

The main advantage of OCT over other imaging modalities is that it provides both an en-face two-dimensional view along with cross-sectional images that allow direct visualization of outer retinal anatomy. Given that visual acuity is a poor indicator of progression of geographic atrophy and that FAF does not discriminately image parafoveal atrophy, OCT will likely become the ancillary test of choice in clinical trials involving pharmaceuticals designed to delay the progression of geographic atrophy.

OCT: WET MACULAR DEGENERATION

Neovascular AMD is characterized by the presence of choroidal neovascularization (CNV) and can be associated with retinal pigment epithelium detachment (PED), retinal pigment epithelium (RPE) tears, fibrovascular disciform scarring, and vitreous hemorrhage (30).

Neovascularization also may be localized predominantly within the retina. This is known as retinal angiomatous proliferation (31).

Historically, neovascularization associated with AMD has been classified in a number of ways. These classification schemes have been based upon either the technology available to detect the presence of neovascularization or the therapeutic options available to treat it. Fluorescein angiography (FA), which allows for the functional assessment of neovascularization, was used to develop a classification scheme within the context of treating CNV with photodynamic therapy (PDT) (32,33). Lesions were classified into "classic": early well-demarcated choroidal hyperfluorescence with progressive dye leakage; "minimally classic": those lesions with less than 50% classic component; or "occult": mottled hyperfluorescence in the midphase with associated late leakage or as late leakage of undetermined origin (34,35). Indocyanine green angiography (ICG) is an infrared dye-based imaging modality which is helpful in detecting and delineating the borders of occult neovascular membranes (36). ICG was instrumental in describing retinal angiomatous proliferation (36,37). Although fluorescein angiography is useful in determining the presence of leakage in neovascular AMD, this technique does not provide any three-dimensional anatomic information about the neurosensory retina, the RPE, or the choroid.

Using both biomicrosopic criteria and FA, Gass proposed a classification of CNV based on the location of the neovascular complex with respect to the RPE layer. Lesions were classified as type 1 when the vessels were confined under the RPE, or type 2, when the vessels proliferated in the subretinal space (38). Histopathological investigation of specimens from submacular surgery demonstrate that CNV due to

AMD is more likely to be below the RPE than CNV from other causes (39).

Freund et al. have proposed a more refined classification of CNV. It is not based on any single imaging modality but on the data gathered from a variety of imaging techniques, such as combined FA/SD-OCT, high-speed SD-OCT, and ICG (37). This new classification divides neovascularization into three types.

Type 1 neovascularization is characterized by vessels proliferating under the RPE. In regards to angiography, it would be described as occult or poorly defined CNV. With ICG angiography, it presents as low-intensity hyperfluorescence. On OCT (Fig. 14.3A–14.3B), it appears as a localized fusiform pigmented epithelial detachment (PED), which may be serous or fibrovascular in nature (2,12). Type 1 neovascularization is felt to represent fairly mature neovascular tissue, and as such may incompletely respond to anti-VEGF therapy (37). Polyploidal choroidal vasculopathy is included in this classification as a variant of type 1 neovascularization.

Type 2 neovascularization is characterized by the proliferation of neovascular tissue above the RPE, into the subretinal space. It represents classic CNV as seen on FA. In ICG angiography, it may be more difficult to identify due to the typical hyperfluorescence of the background choroidal circulation. SD-OCT localizes the vessels to the space between the RPE and the photoreceptor outer segments. Classic CNV on OCT (Fig. 14.3C) can present as a highly reflective fibrovascular tissue with irregular, yet defined, borders between the RPE and Bruch's membrane, or above the RPE (40). It may also present as a localized fusiform serous or fibrovascular PED (41). Disruption of the inner/outer photoreceptor junction and intraretinal cystic spaces are often observed. Type 2 vessels seem to respond better to anti-VEGF therapy (37).

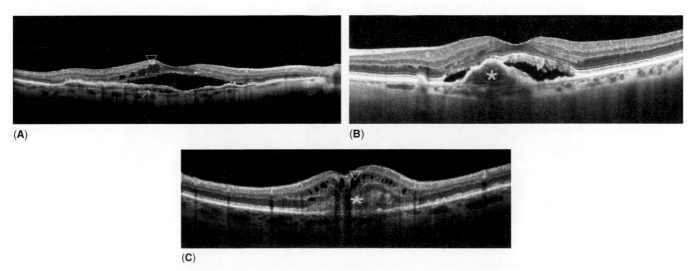

(A)   (B)

(C)

Figure 14.3 Cross-sectional optical coherence tomography images showing different types of choroidal neovascularization (CNV). (**A**) Cross-sectional image (Spectralis; Heidelberg Engineering, Heidelberg, Germany) depicting a thickened retinal pigment epithelium (RPE) raised by non-uniform moderately hyper-reflective type 1 CNV formation (green arrow) and the presence of subretinal and intraretinal fluid (green arrowhead). (**B**) Cross-sectional image (Spectralis) showing a fibrovascular pigment epithelium detachment, type 1 neovascularization (green asterisk), and the presence of subretinal fluid (green arrowhead). (**C**) Cross-sectional image (RTVue; Optovue, Inc., Fremont, California, USA) showing a classic CNV, type 2 neovascularization, delineated as a non-uniform moderately hyper-reflective formation above the RPE (green asterisk) and the presence of intraretinal cysts (green arrowhead).

Type 3 neovascularization, commonly referred to as retinal angiomatous proliferation, is characterized by intraretinal neovascularization. It has a distinct presentation on OCT. Imaging characteristics include sub-RPE CNV with intraretinal angiomatous change along with subretinal neovascularization and cystic change. These changes have been demonstrated to correlate well with clinical and angiographic findings and are hypothesized to be caused by aberrant retinal-choroidal anastomoses (42). Type 3 neovascularization appears to be sensitive to anti-VEGF therapy, if detected very early in its evolution (37).

In general, active CNV of any type is associated with presence of fluid (Fig. 14.4). This appears on OCT

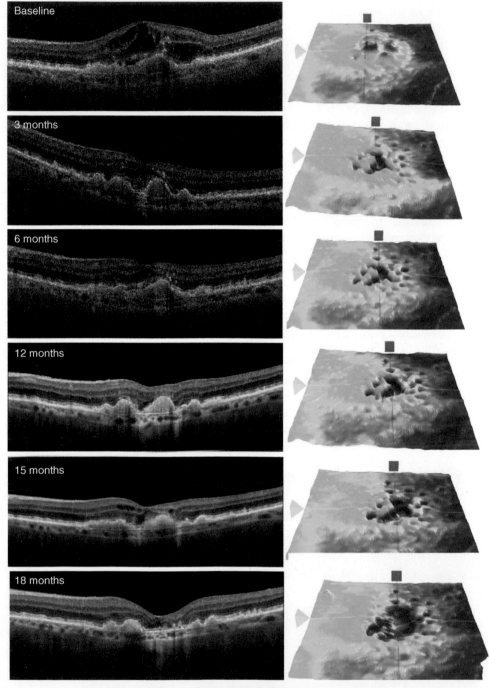

Figure 14.4 Sequential spectral-domain optical coherence tomography (OCT) scans (Cirrus OCT) of a 75-year-old woman with subfoveal choroidal neovascularization (CNV). A baseline scan depicted an elevation of the retinal pigment epithelium (RPE) layer, a localized fusiform thickening and duplication of the highly reflective external band (RPE/choriocapillaris complex), and intraretinal fluid corresponding to CNV. The patient was treated with intravitreous injection of ranibizumab at baseline, month 1, and month 2. Three months after the first injection, the OCT scan demonstrated improvement of macular architecture with mild intraretinal fluid. Additionally, the thickness map showed a significant decrease in the retinal thickness at the macular region. Between 3 and 12 months after treatment, three injections were administered due to the presence of discrete intraretinal fluid. It is important to note the better resolution of the 12-month scan due to image oversampling. The improvement in the resolution leads to a better visualization of retinal layers and it is possible to note the inner/outer segment junction interruption. At 15 months from the first injection, the patient again presented with intraretinal fluid and was treated with intravitreous ranibizumab. At 18 months of follow-up, no fluid was detected in the macular area, but diffuse retinal atrophy was noted as seen on the retinal thickness map.

as well-circumscribed hyporeflective spaces that distort the surrounding retinal architecture. The fluid can accumulate in the subretinal space, sub-RPE space, or between all layers of the inner retina and it can be quantitatively evaluated with OCT (31,43). Studies have demonstrated that SD-OCT is superior to TD-OCT in detecting subretinal, sub-RPE, and intraretinal fluid making it more suitable to detect CNV activity (44). SD-OCT devices have higher and earlier detection rates of CNV activity (45). For an average patient, earlier detection means a significant gain of vision, which may be equivalent to or better than the gain achieved with most CNV treatments (45).

An additional feature of neovascular AMD is RPE tears or rips. Rips may naturally occur or may come about after treatment is initiated. RPE rips are typically associated with the presence of a dome-shaped PED (46). On OCT, a tear in the RPE is characterized by a focal defect in the RPE with scrolling at the borders along with pleating of the adjacent, continuous RPE.

Recently, a new cystic structure, named outer retinal tubulation, was described in the outer retina of neovascular AMD patients (47,48). It is a hyporeflective area surrounded by a hyper-reflective ring (Fig. 14.5A). Outer retina tubulation may form as a result of sublethal injury to the photoreceptors. It is thought that, after photoreceptor injury, there is disruption of tight junctions with subsequent outward folding of the photoreceptor layer until the opposite sides of the fold establish contact and form a tubular structure (47). These structures do not respond to anti-VEGF therapy and are not indicative of active CNV. Another common OCT finding in AMD patients is the pseudocysts overlying an area of geographic atrophy (49). Nearly 25% of their study patients with geographic atrophy had these pseudocysts, and they were mainly found in the inner nuclear layer. These spaces are felt to be the sequelae of degenerated Muller cells, akin to the hyporeflective spaces seen in macular telangectasis type II. Like outer retinal tabulation, angiography failed to reveal any evidence of choroidal neovascularization, and the presence of pseudocysts overlying an area of geographic atrophy is not felt to represent active CNV.

The natural history of most untreated end-stage wet AMD is a fibrous, disciform scar. It can be visualized on OCT as a fibrotic scar consisting of hyper-reflective tissue in the same location as the inciting CNV. There is typically overlying outer retinal atrophy (31). Not infrequently, intraretinal cysts appear over these scars (Fig 14.5B). These too do not seem to represent active neovascular disease as they are typically not altered by anti-VEGF therapy (48).

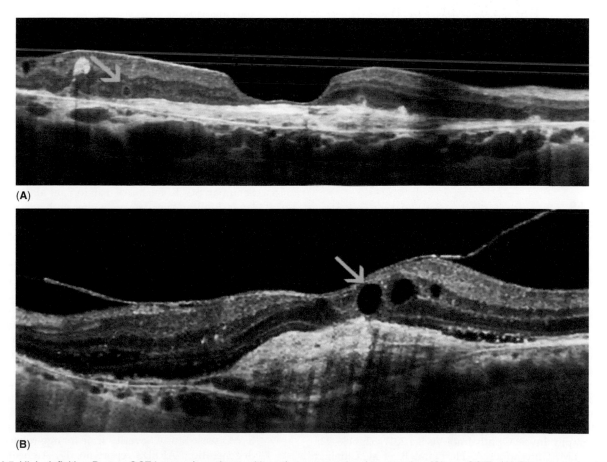

(A)

(B)

Figure 14.5 High-definition B-scan OCT images in patients with end-stage macular degeneration (Cirrus OCT). **(A)** There is a structure (green arrow) overlying an area of subretinal fibrosis that consists of a hyporeflective core and hyper-reflective border. This is an example of outer retinal tubulation. **(B)** In this patient with advanced macular degeneration and disciform scarring, there are cysts (green arrow) overlying an area of subretinal fibrosis. The presence of these types of cysts is not thought to represent active CNV.

OCT-GUIDED AMD TREATMENT

Monitoring response to therapy is one of the most important clinical uses of OCT. OCT can be used to quantify changes in central retinal thickness and volume as well as qualitatively evaluate subretinal fluid. These parameters are used in combination with visual acuity to critically analyze the response to therapy in neovascular AMD. In the PrONTO study, the authors used OCT to guide the treatment of neovascular AMD and demonstrated that OCT could detect the earliest signs of recurrent fluid in the macula after anti-VEGF injections were stopped (50). In a separate analysis of the study data, it was demonstrated that OCT findings alone predicted the need for re-treatment based upon features, such as appearance of macular cysts or subretinal fluid, and these signs were thought to represent the earliest manifestations of recurrent CNV. Other OCT-guided studies using ranibizumab (51,52) or bevacizumab (53) confirmed the visual outcomes reported by PrONTO using similar numbers of intravitreous injections. These studies will be discussed in more detail in other chapters of this textbook.

SUMMARY POINTS

- The only imaging modality that enables clinicians to directly visualize microscopic retinal structures is OCT.
- OCT can be used to reproducibly track drusen morphology, drusen volume, and geographic atrophy.
- Choroidal neovascular membranes can often be directly visualized with OCT. The presence of intraretinal fluid, subretinal fluid, or cystoid macular edema on OCT is highly suggestive of active neovascular tissue.
- Qualitative and quantitative information provided by OCT may serve as the most important criteria in re-treatment decisions.

REFERENCES

1. Huang D, Swanson EA, Lin CP, et al. Optical coherence tomography. Science 1991; 254: 1178–81.
2. Drexler W, Sattmann H, Hermann B, et al. Enhanced visualization of macular pathology with the use of ultrahigh-resolution optical coherence tomography. Arch Ophthalmol 2003; 121: 695–706.
3. Leitgeb R, Hitzenberger C, Fercher A. Performance of fourier domain vs. time domain optical coherence tomography. Opt Express 2003; 11: 889–94.
4. Toth CA, Narayan DG, Boppart SA, et al. A comparison of retinal morphology viewed by optical coherence tomography and by light microscopy. Arch Ophthalmol 1997; 115: 1425–8.
5. Lujan BJ, Roorda A, Knighton RW, Carroll J. Revealing Henle's fiber layer using spectral domain optical coherence tomography. Invest Ophthalmol Vis Sci 2011; 52: 1486–92.
6. Anger EM, Unterhuber A, Hermann B, et al. Ultrahigh resolution optical coherence tomography of the monkey fovea. Identification of retinal sublayers by correlation with semithin histology sections. Exp Eye Res 2004; 78: 1117–25.
7. Gloesmann M, Hermann B, Schubert C, et al. Histologic correlation of pig retina radial stratification with ultrahigh-resolution optical coherence tomography. Invest Ophthalmol Vis Sci 2003; 44: 1696–703.
8. Srinivasan VJ, Ko TH, Wojtkowski M, et al. Noninvasive volumetric imaging and morphometry of the rodent retina with high-speed, ultrahigh-resolution optical coherence tomography. Invest Ophthalmol Vis Sci 2006; 47: 5522–8.
9. Srinivasan VJ, Monson BK, Wojtkowski M, et al. Characterization of outer retinal morphology with high-speed, ultrahigh-resolution optical coherence tomography. Invest Ophthalmol Vis Sci 2008; 49: 1571–9.
10. Zawadzki RJ, Jones SM, Olivier SS, et al. Adaptive-optics optical coherence tomography for high-resolution and high-speed 3D retinal in vivo imaging. Opt Express 2005; 13: 8532–46.
11. Puliafito CA, Hee MR, Lin CP, et al. Imaging of macular diseases with optical coherence tomography. Ophthalmology 1995; 102: 217–29.
12. Spaide RF, Curcio CA. Anatomical correlates to the bands seen in the outer retina by optical coherence tomography: literature review and model. Retina 2011; 31: 1609–19.
13. The Age-Related Eye Disease Study. System for classifying age-related macular degeneration from stereoscopic color fundus photographs: the age-related eye disease study report number 6. Am J Ophthalmol 2001; 132: 668–81.
14. Klein R, Davis MD, Magli YL, et al. The Wisconsin age-related maculopathy grading system. Ophthalmology 1991; 98: 1128–34.
15. Khanifar AA, Koreishi AF, Izatt JA, Toth CA. Drusen ultrastructure imaging with spectral domain optical coherence tomography in age-related macular degeneration. Ophthalmology 2008; 115: 1883–90.
16. Pieroni CG, Witkin AJ, Ko TH, et al. Ultrahigh resolution optical coherence tomography in non-exudative age related macular degeneration. Br J Ophthalmol 2006; 90: 191–7.
17. Zarbin MA. Current concepts in the pathogenesis of age-related macular degeneration. Arch Ophthalmol 2004; 122: 598–614.
18. Schuman SG, Koreishi AF, Farsiu S, et al. Photoreceptor layer thinning over drusen in eyes with age-related macular degeneration imaged in vivo with spectral-domain optical coherence tomography. Ophthalmology 2009; 116: 488–96; e2.
19. Gregori G, Wang F, Rosenfeld PJ, et al. Spectral domain optical coherence tomography imaging of drusen in non-exudative age-related macular degeneration. Ophthalmology 2011; 118: 1373–9.
20. Yehoshua Z, Wang F, Rosenfeld PJ, et al. Natural history of drusen morphology in age-related macular degeneration using spectral domain optical coherence tomography. Ophthalmology 2011; 118: 2434–41.
21. Ferris FL 3rd, Fine SL, Hyman L. Age-related macular degeneration and blindness due to neovascular maculopathy. Arch Ophthalmol 1984; 102: 1640–2.
22. Davis MD, Gangnon RE, Lee LY, et al.; The Age-Related Eye Disease Study. Severity scale for age-related macular degeneration: AREDS report no. 17. Arch Ophthalmol 2005; 123: 1484–98.
23. Scholl HP, Peto T, Dandekar S, et al. Inter- and intra-observer variability in grading lesions of age-related

maculopathy and macular degeneration. Graefes Arch Clin Exp Ophthalmol 2003; 241: 39–47.

24. Holz FG, Bindewald-Wittich A, Fleckenstein M, et al. Progression of geographic atrophy and impact of fundus autofluorescence patterns in age-related macular degeneration. Am J Ophthalmol 2007; 143: 463–72.

25. Fleckenstein M, Schmitz-Valckenberg S, Adrion C, et al. Tracking progression with spectral-domain optical coherence tomography in geographic atrophy caused by age-related macular degeneration. Invest Ophthalmol Vis Sci 2010; 51: 3846–52.

26. Brar M, Kozak I, Cheng L, et al. Correlation between spectral-domain optical coherence tomography and fundus autofluorescence at the margins of geographic atrophy. Am J Ophthalmol 2009; 148: 439–44.

27. Lujan BJ, Rosenfeld PJ, Gregori G, et al. Spectral domain optical coherence tomographic imaging of geographic atrophy. Ophthalmic Surg Lasers Imaging 2009; 40: 96–101.

28. Sayegh RG, Simader C, Scheschy U, et al. A systematic comparison of spectral-domain optical coherence tomography and fundus autofluorescence in patients with geographic atrophy. Ophthalmology 2011; 118: 1844–51.

29. Yehoshua Z, Rosenfeld PJ, Gregori G, et al. Progression of geographic atrophy in age-related macular degeneration imaged with spectral domain optical coherence tomography. Ophthalmology 2011; 118: 679–86.

30. Bressler NM, Bressler SB, Fine SL. Age-related macular degeneration. Surv Ophthalmol 1988; 32: 375–413.

31. Castro LC. Exudative Age-Related Macular Degeneration. Imaging the Eye from Front to Back with RTVue Fourier-Domain Optical Coherence Tomography, 1st edn. Thorofare: Slack Inc, 2010: 137–53.

32. Macular Photocoagulation Study Group. Occult choroidal neovascularization influence on visual outcome in patients with age-related macular degeneration. Arch Ophthalmol 1996; 114: 400–12.

33. Macular Photocoagulation Study Group. Laser photocoagulation of subfoveal recurrent neovascular lesions in age-related macular degeneration. results of a randomized clinical trial. Arch Ophthalmol 1991; 109: 1232–41.

34. Macular Photocoagulation Study Group. Argon laser photocoagulation for neovascular maculopathy. five-year results from randomized clinical trials. Arch Ophthalmol 1991; 109: 1109–14.

35. Bressler NM, Arnold J, Benchaboune M, et al. Verteporfin therapy of subfoveal choroidal neovascularization in patients with age-related macular degeneration: additional information regarding baseline lesion composition's impact on vision outcomes-TAP report no. 3. Arch Ophthalmol 2002; 120: 1443–54.

36. Yannuzzi LA, Slakter JS, Sorenson JA, Guyer DR, Orlock DA. Digital indocyanine green videoangiography and choroidal neovascularization. Retina 1992; 12: 191–223.

37. Freund KB, Zweifel SA, Engelbert M. Do we need a new classification for choroidal neovascularization in age-related macular degeneration? Retina 2010; 30: 1333–49.

38. Gass JD. Biomicroscopic and histopathologic considerations regarding the feasibility of surgical excision of subfoveal neovascular membranes. Am J Ophthalmol 1994; 118: 285–98.

39. Grossniklaus HE, Green WR, Trials Research Group. Histopathologic and ultrastructural findings of surgically excised choroidal neovascularization. submacular surgery. Arch Ophthalmol 1998; 116: 745–9.

40. Giovannini A, Amato GP, Mariotti C, Scassellati-Sforzolini B. OCT imaging of choroidal neovascularisation and its role in the determination of patients' eligibility for surgery. Br J Ophthalmol 1999; 83: 438–42.

41. Ahlers C, Michels S, Beckendorf A, Birngruber R, Schmidt-Erfurth U. Three-dimensional imaging of pigment epithelial detachment in age-related macular degeneration using optical coherence tomography, retinal thickness analysis and topographic angiography. Graefes Arch Clin Exp Ophthalmol 2006; 244: 1233–9.

42. Truong SN, Alam S, Zawadzki RJ, et al. High resolution fourier-domain optical coherence tomography of retinal angiomatous proliferation. Retina 2007; 27: 915–25.

43. Chen Y, Vuong LN, Liu J, et al. Three-dimensional ultra-high resolution optical coherence tomography imaging of age-related macular degeneration. Opt Express 2009; 17: 4046–60.

44. Cukras C, Wang YD, Meyerle CB, et al. Optical coherence tomography-based decision making in exudative age-related macular degeneration: comparison of time- vs spectral-domain devices. Eye (Lond) 2010; 24: 775–83.

45. Loewenstein A. The significance of early detection of age-related macular degeneration: richard & hinda rosenthal foundation lecture, the macula society 29th annual meeting. Retina 2007; 27: 873–8.

46. Chang LK, Flaxel CJ, Lauer AK, Sarraf D. RPE tears after pegaptanib treatment in age-related macular degeneration. Retina 2007; 27: 857–63.

47. Zweifel SA, Engelbert M, Laud K, et al. Outer retinal tubulation: a novel optical coherence tomography finding. Arch Ophthalmol 2009; 127: 1596–602.

48. Wolff B, Maftouhi MQ, Mateo-Montoya A, Sahel JA, Mauget-Faysse M. Outer retinal cysts in age-related macular degeneration. Acta Ophthalmol 2011; 89: e496–9.

49. Cohen SY, Dubois L, Nghiem-Buffet S, et al. Retinal pseudocysts in age-related geographic atrophy. Am J Ophthalmol 2010; 150: 211–17; e1.

50. Fung AE, Lalwani GA, Rosenfeld PJ, et al. An optical coherence tomography-guided, variable dosing regimen with intravitreal ranibizumab (Lucentis) for neovascular age-related macular degeneration. Am J Ophthalmol 2007; 143: 566–83.

51. Rothenbuehler SP, Waeber D, Brinkmann CK, Wolf S, Wolf-Schnurrbusch UE. Effects of ranibizumab in patients with subfoveal choroidal neovascularization attributable to age-related macular degeneration. Am J Ophthalmol 2009; 147: 831–7.

52. Querques G, Azrya S, Martinelli D, et al. Ranibizumab for exudative age-related macular degeneration: 24-month outcomes from a single-centre institutional setting. Br J Ophthalmol 2010; 94: 292–6.

53. Leydolt C, Michels S, Prager F, et al. Effect of intravitreal bevacizumab (Avastin) in neovascular age-related macular degeneration using a treatment regimen based on optical coherence tomography: 6- and 12-month results. Acta Ophthalmol 2010; 88: 594–600.

15

How to analyze OCT images for management of neovascular age-related macular degeneration

Sebastian M. Waldstein, Bianca S. Gerendas, Markus Ritter, and Ursula Schmidt-Erfurth

INTRODUCTION

Neovascular age-related macular degeneration (nAMD) is one of the diseases that have derived the greatest benefit from progress in optical coherence tomography (OCT) imaging (1). Analysis of OCT scans by visualization and quantification of microstructural alterations in the specific anatomical compartments of the retina and surrounding tissues enables clinicians managing nAMD to assess its clinical features, trace its natural history, and document treatment response. An essential advantage of OCT as an imaging modality is the non-invasive and quick nature of the investigation which makes it appealing for both patients and physicians. Frequent follow-up examinations, which are necessary and valuable in a chronic progressive disease such as nAMD, are feasible with OCT by contrast to traditional fluorescein angiography (FA). In clinical practice today, OCT is used as the benchmark investigation for both primary diagnosis and follow-up of nAMD.

This chapter describes the clinically relevant alterations as visualized by spectral domain OCT (SD-OCT) and discusses the application of OCT in the current management of nAMD.

TECHNICAL ASPECTS
Current State of OCT Technology

The introduction of the new generation OCT, SD-OCT, has greatly advanced imaging technology. Novel SD-OCT devices perform scans with impressive speed (e.g., 50,000 A-scans per second), allowing systematic raster scanning patterns, and thus provide extensive morphologic insight (2,3). SD-OCT imaging systems achieve visualization at a high level of detail with axial resolutions of less than 5 μm. The inherently low signal-to-noise ratio in conventional OCT systems can also be overcome with SD-OCT by repeated acquisition of identical sections and subsequent scan averaging (4). As a result of its improved resolution and scanning speed, SD-OCT provides great advantages for imaging of nAMD, in particular preservation of retinal topography, a large field of view, and improved correlation of the image set to fundus features. The outer layers of the retina can also be analyzed due to the high resolution allowing assessment of structural changes affecting the photoreceptor layers and thereby providing information relevant for retinal function.

SD-OCT Image Acquisition in nAMD

Modern SD-OCT devices offer a wide range of scanning patterns with the option of numerous adjustments. A few points should be considered in order to choose optimal scan settings.

Central visual acuity is often compromised in nAMD patients, making stable foveal fixation difficult or impossible. Usage of large internal fixation targets and fast acquisition protocols is therefore beneficial. A wide scan area (e.g., 6 × 6 mm or more) can ensure imaging coverage of all structures of interest even when foveal fixation is lost. A dense spacing of B-scans preserves macular topography and is particularly useful when screening for subtle focal fluid accumulation (i.e., cysts). By contrast, scan patterns with only one or a few lines, for example, cross-hair patterns and radial scan patterns, are particularly problematic unless foveal fixation is extremely stable. Such scan patterns often miss the foveal center and can fail to detect important morphological detail in between the sections. Hence, these patterns should only be used for specific indications such as when particularly high resolution is required. The device operator should pay special care to manually ensure correct scan centering.

With the help of precise eye-tracking systems, B-scan averaging can be applied well in selected devices; however, it is important to balance achievable signal gain against lengthy acquisition times. Moreover, it should be kept in mind that B-scan averaging improves the signal-to-noise ratio, but also slightly blurs the image, which might lead to loss of detail.

Perspective: Future Developments in OCT Technology

Although SD-OCT has progressed enormously during the past years, there is still potential for further improvement of this technology. The areas of current research cover flow measurements (Doppler OCT), improvement of penetration depths (long wavelength OCT), tissue contrast (polarization sensitive OCT), speed (swept source OCT), and transverse resolution (adaptive optics).

Doppler OCT can highlight vascular networks and might be a future, non-invasive alternative to FA, with the most important limitation that Doppler OCT cannot currently visualize vascular leakage (5). OCT with light sources centered at a longer wavelength (e.g., 1050 nm) offer greatly improved depth penetration compared with conventional OCT (6). Fields of application in nAMD include visualization of the depth of choroidal neovascularization (CNV) lesions, as well as imaging of choroidal morphology including thickness and imaging in patients with media opacities.

Polarization-sensitive OCT (PS-OCT) measures the polarization state of back-scattered light, which is characteristically altered by specific ocular tissues (7). PS-OCT can thus provide tissue-specific contrast for birefringent tissues (e.g., retinal nerve fiber layer or fibrous tissue in CNV lesions) or polarization scrambling tissues [e.g., the retinal pigment epithelium (RPE)]. In nAMD, only PS-OCT is able to detect focal RPE defects indicating associated geographic atrophy and migration or reproliferation patterns during treatment (8). As the RPE is involved in the origin of the disease, PS-OCT imaging will contribute strongly to the pathophysiologic insight in nAMD. The birefringence of fibrous scars and fibrous tissue in CNV secondary to nAMD is subject to intensive research. The first series of PS-OCT instruments should soon be available on the commercial market and PS-OCT is likely to play an important role in both research and clinical practice.

SUBTYPES OF NEOVASCULAR AMD ON OCT

Before the era of OCT, neovascular lesions of the choroid were classified by FA only as classic CNV lesions or occult CNV lesions with subclassifications, for instance, minimally classic CNV lesions. This classification system was introduced based on the Macular Photocoagulation Study in the 1990s (9).

By FA standards, classic CNV lesions are marked by an area of early well-demarcated choroidal hyperfluorescence with a late phase progressive pooling of leakage in the subretinal space. The boundaries of the CNV are usually obscured by this leakage. On FA, the fluorescence is intense and the background is very dark. Classic CNV lesions are difficult to detect in indocyanine green angiography (ICGA) because of the intense fluorescence of the surrounding choroidal vasculature. Occult CNV lesions are characterized by two findings: One is a fibrovascular pigment epithelial detachment (PED), shown as stippled hyperfluorescence in the early phase, and persistent staining or leakage in the overlying subretinal space in the late phase. The other is late leakage of undetermined source, which is visible in FA as speckled hyperfluorescence lacking well-demarcated borders with fluid pooling in the overlying retinal tissue.

Uniformly recommended by retinal experts, the primary diagnosis of nAMD nowadays still requires an initial FA examination, as FA is the only modality imaging vascular features by definition such as neovascular networks and active leakage dynamics. However, over the last decade, the above-described FA-based classification had to be adapted to newly emerging examination modalities such as OCT and new treatment modalities such as anti-vascular endothelial growth factor (VEGF) therapy. OCT, on the other hand, images the morphologic features of CNV-related neurosensory destruction and allows a far more detailed structural evaluation

than FA (10). The original FA classification considers vascular filling and leakage as the strongest criterion for classification and does not describe the CNV lesions by their anatomical location and impact on the retinal architecture. The mechanisms of angiogenesis and the corresponding pathophysiologic pathways to nAMD cannot usually be classified by FA alone, added to which they are visible much earlier, and with more detail during disease progression, on OCT.

As early as 1994, Gass suggested that CNV lesions should be classified by their structure and anatomical location (11). His histopathology-based ideas were not well accepted because of the lack of appropriate imaging modalities for his classification. Even in the era of time-domain OCT, Gass' proposal was impracticable, because the resolution and speed of the devices were not adequate. Furthermore, OCT was not easily available everywhere. In the era of SD-OCT with high-resolution, high-speed scanning and the implementation of SD-OCT in most practices in the Western world, identification of disease activity in nAMD by SD-OCT is widely used and accepted. In 2010, a modified classification of Gass' approach based on OCT features was published which suggested a specific classification not only of type I and type II choroidal lesions but also of intraretinal neovascularization, the so-called retinal angiomatous proliferation (RAP), as type III neovascularization, abandoning the word "choroidal" in the classification context (10). Another, fourth subtype, polypoidal choroidal vasculopathy (PCV), which is believed to be a subtype of type I CNV, was added to this classification.

In summary, a combined classification taking SD-OCT, FA, and in some cases ICGA into consideration is useful for a comprehensive understanding of the pathophysiology of neovascular lesions in nAMD, while for monitoring disease activity, SD-OCT only is an established approach. In the following paragraphs, different types of lesions are described in the context of the relevance of SD-OCT for defining subtypes. Figure 15.1 provides representative SD-OCT images with angiographic correlates and annotations of typical pathomorphologic lesions.

Type I Lesions

Type I lesions are characterized by neovascularization underneath the RPE in the so-called "sub-RPE" compartment between the RPE and Bruch's membrane. This subtype is the most common form of neovascularization in nAMD. Type I neovascularization corresponds mainly to the "occult" CNV type of the FA classification, but it does not necessarily match the occult FA type in all cases. As in occult CNV, type I is visualized in FA as late phase leakage and fibrovascular PED with stippled hyperfluorescence. Type I is furthermore characterized by fibrovascular PED in SD-OCT and by plaques in ICGA (12). Type I lesions often remain clinically silent for a long time as the neurosensory retina is dry and preserved, underlining the importance of regular SD-OCT follow-up of high-risk patients in AMD screening

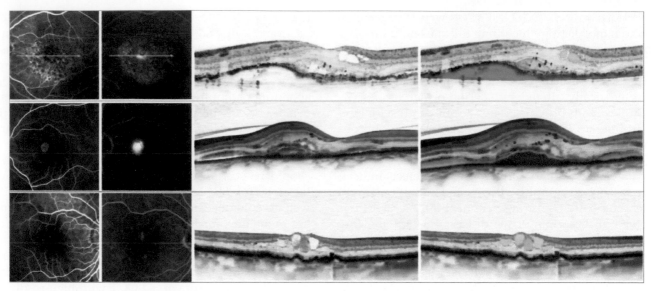

Figure 15.1 Typical appearance of type I, II, and III CNV on FA and SD-OCT. (Top row) Type I (occult) CNV typically produces fibrovascular PEDs (blue). Subretinal fluid (green), intraretinal cysts (light green) as well as intraretinal speckles (pink) indicate active leakage which is confirmed in FA. (*Middle row*) Type II (classic) CNV (red) is visible as hyper-reflective mass in the subretinal space. The inferior border is difficult to delineate in conventional SD-OCT due to limited depth penetration. Activity signs include subretinal fluid (green), intraretinal cysts (light green), and hyper-reflective speckles (pink). (*Bottom row*) Type III CNV (RAP) typically produces PEDs (not shown in this section) and cysts (light green). In this case, the central cyst shows higher reflectivity, indicating hemorrhage or exudation into the cyst. A branching lesion is visible at the RPE level (red).

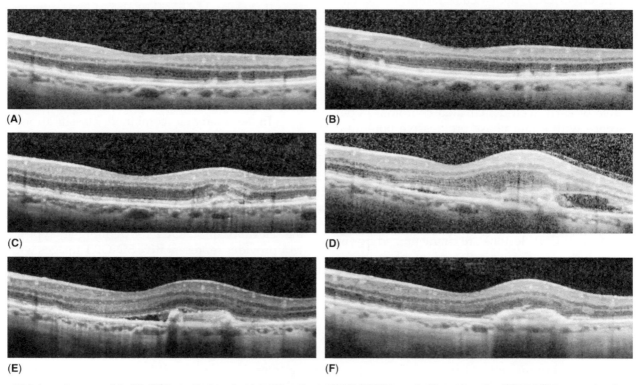

Figure 15.2 Long-term monthly SD-OCT monitoring of a high-risk patient. (**A**) Mild RPE irregularities at baseline; (**B** and **C**) progressive destruction of the RPE and invasion of the neurosensory retina; (**D**) active exudation and accumulation of subretinal fluid; anti-VEGF treatment was initiated; (**E** and **F**) CNV regression under continuous therapy.

(Fig. 15.2). In the early stages, fibrovascular PEDs are the defining feature on SD-OCT. When a type I lesion becomes clinically manifest, neovascular features, mostly subretinal fluid, can be seen on SD-OCT. Cystoid macular edema develops upon disease progression with advancing dysfunction of the blood–retinal barrier. Late stages of type I lesion are believed to have a worse prognosis for visual outcome than subretinal fluid alone

because of the advanced alteration of the RPE layer following disruption of tight junctions. Loss of the external limiting membrane (ELM) band on SD-OCT is an indicator for tight junction disruption (10).

PCV Lesions
PCV lesions were originally described as a choroidal disorder (13) but are now believed to be a subtype of

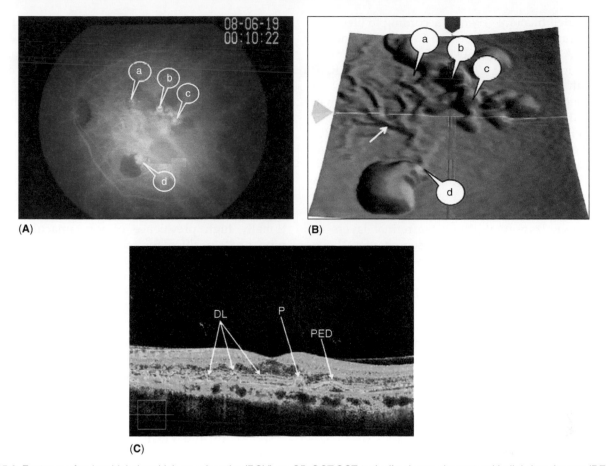

Figure 15.3 Features of polypoidal choroidal vasculopathy (PCV) on SD-OCT. OCT typically shows pigment epithelial detachment (PED) corresponding with the sites of polyps in indocyanine green angiography (ICGA). The en-face RPE map shows several PEDs intercommunicating through a branching network ("bola sign"). *Source*: From Ref. 51.

type I neovascularization (14). They have a comparatively high prevalence in Asian and African-American patients. Confirmation of the diagnosis is typically obtained from ICG angiography, which delineates the choroidal polyps.

On SD-OCT, PCV lesions are seen as sub-RPE proliferation accompanied by multiple smaller and larger PEDs, and branching communications (15,16). The topography of the lesion is best seen on en-face RPE maps, often showing the interconnecting branching network between polypoidal lesions ("bola sign", Fig. 15.3). B-scan sections typically demonstrate PEDs and sometimes "notch"-like type I CNV lesions in contact with the retina through surrounding subretinal fluid (SRF). Please see chapter 10 on PCV for more details on this disease.

Type II Lesions

Type II lesions consist of neovascular tissue that has penetrated the RPE layer and proliferates within the subretinal space. They usually represent the classic subtype of CNV by FA classification. Type II neovascularization does not usually appear in nAMD without a connection to a type I vessel within the choroidal bed (9). These connections are, however, so small that they cannot be seen on FA. Such lesions are therefore considered to be (classic) type II, only if evaluated on FA. The

consequence of type II neovascular infiltration seen on SD-OCT is the disruption of the inner outer segment junction (IS-OS) of the photoreceptor layer. Commonly, intraretinal fluid in the form of cysts is the first visible neovascular sign. Less SRF is seen compared with type I. FA is inadequate in the distinction of leakage into intraretinal cystic spaces compared with SD-OCT (10). SD-OCT is the modality of choice to detect even small intraretinal cysts as the first sign of incipient cystoid macular edema. Type II lesions are usually smaller, sensitive to anti-VEGF therapy, and can regress to type I lesions. RPE growth may lead to the envelopment of the vessels, subsidence of leakage, and restoration of the IS-OS layer on SD-OCT, indicating regained tissue function. However, if type II lesions are, left untreated, they often develop into subretinal fibrosis with accompanying progressive loss of photoreceptor layers and thinning of the outer nuclear layer. SD-OCT is again the modality of choice in the evaluation of such lesions, with its ability to quantify neurosensory damage and a reduced potential for recovery.

RAP/Type III Lesions

Type III lesions were first described by Hartnett et al., (17) as deep retinal vascular anomalous complexes and were later named RAP lesions by Yannuzzi (18). RAP lesions are often bilateral (19) and according to literature from angiographic studies appear in 10–15% of all newly diagnosed nAMD cases (20). SD-OCT seems to be a more sensitive imaging tool than FA for the detection of RAP lesions, with its typical feature demonstrating cystoid edema in conjunction with a PED (10). As yet it is unknown whether RAP lesions originate from retinal or choroidal vessels, but they usually form a retinal-choroidal anastomosis in the advanced stage. RAP lesions never appear within the foveal avascular zone (10).

Hypothetically, RAP may originate from drusen that might have been infiltrated by type I vessels. They can cause substantial photoreceptor loss and, in late stages, disorganization of the outer retinal layers as often observed on SD-OCT. Please see chapter 11 for more details on this disease.

RELEVANT MICROSTRUCTURAL FEATURES FOR SD-OCT ANALYSIS IN NEOVASCULAR AMD

The complex pathophysiologic mechanisms in nAMD affect several distinct anatomical compartments of the retina and its adjacent structures. Hence, each of the affected tissue components should be specifically considered and analyzed when evaluating SD-OCT scans in nAMD. In the following section, typical findings for the vitreomacular, intraretinal, subretinal, and sub-RPE compartments are discussed.

Vitreomacular Interface

With the availability of high-resolution raster scanning in SD-OCT, even very subtle changes at the vitreomacular interface can be detected by the discerning clinician

(Fig. 15.4). Evaluation of the vitreous configuration demands a thorough review of the entire SD-OCT volume stack, since vitreous attachments are often located extrafoveally or peripherally at the retinal vessel arcades and the optic disc.

With SD-OCT it is possible to distinguish between complete vitreous attachment, focal vitreomacular adhesion, detachment of the vitreous from the macula with vitreous adhesion at the optic disc or vessel arcades, and complete vitreous detachment.

Most patients in the typical AMD age-group (>50 years) show a complete posterior vitreous detachment (21). Eyes with CNV, however, exhibit a disproportionally high prevalence of **vitreomacular adhesion** with predisposition for focal adhesions at the site of CNV (22,23). Interestingly, OCT-based studies show equal progression rates of dry AMD to nAMD regardless of vitreomacular interface status, which makes a potential role of vitreomacular adhesion in the origin of nAMD rather unlikely (24). Researchers currently believe that neovascular processes at the retinal surface promote a tighter linkage between the retina and the vitreous cortex in CNV, secondarily leading to the high prevalence of vitreomacular adhesion observed in nAMD patients. Moreover, studies provide increasing evidence for a potential role of vitreous adhesion in the individual response to anti-VEGF treatment of CNV, with less favorable outcomes observed (25).

Apart from the three-dimensional aspect of vitreomacular adhesions, particular attention should be paid to the evaluation of frank **vitreomacular traction**, which can result in severe structural damage to the neurosensory

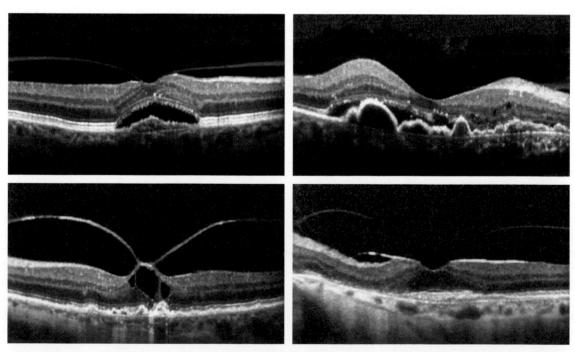

Figure 15.4 Common findings at the vitreomacular interface in nAMD. (*Top left*) Foveal vitreomacular adhesion without traction. Distortion of the retinal surface is not visible, and insertions and angulations of the vitreous membranes are flat. (*Bottom left*) Foveal vitreomacular traction with distortion of the retinal surface. Large cysts indicate structural damage following mechanical stress. Note the steep, angulated insertion of the vitreous membranes. (*Top right*) Complete attachment of the vitreous in the macular area with development of a posterior vitreous pocket. (*Bottom right*) Epiretinal membrane in a patient with long-standing CNV. The outline of the membrane is flat and displays a broad base in contact to the overlying angled adhesion of the posterior vitreous membrane.

retina (26). Tractional components of vitreomacular adhesions are best judged by an assessment of the retinal contour at the insertion sites of vitreous membranes and by considering the angle of the vitreous insertion. The angle is rather flat in concomitant disease, but presents a steep insertion in active traction syndrome where macular surgery is recommendable. It should however also be kept in mind that OCT images are (as standard device output) stretched in the z-direction; therefore angles appear generally steeper than in scale representations.

Epiretinal membranes are another frequent finding at the vitreomacular interface, although they are much less frequent in nAMD than, for instance, in diabetic maculopathy. The three-dimensional extent of the proliferation, its thickness, and the presence and severity of inner retinal folds can be easily assessed using SD-OCT (27).

Intraretinal Compartment

The neurosensory retina per se is severely affected in nAMD, most frequently secondary to exudation of fluid originating from the CNV, but also primarily through direct infiltration of type II neovascular lesions. Specific alterations in neurosensory microstructure can be visualized with high resolution and high reliability using SD-OCT. Cystic or diffuse swelling of the retina in nAMD is a common cause for increased retinal thickness in nAMD (28). However, direct qualitative assessment of the microanatomical lesions offers precise understanding of current pathophysiologic processes and should generally supplement quantitative retinal thickness assessment (29).

Intraretinal cysts are very commonly found in the direct vicinity of leaking CNV lesions and are strongly indicative for active disease (30). They are visualized as round or ovoid hyporeflective spaces with distinct borders. In some instances, cysts can show a slightly higher reflective signal intensity, which is believed to derive from high protein or particle concentrations in the fluid-filled cavity.

Cysts are often organized in one or two layers, with a focal predilection for the inner and outer nuclear layers. The topographic distribution in the retina is frequently rather focal in nAMD (in contrast to diffuse cystic edema secondary to diabetic maculopathy, uveitis, or retinal vein occlusion), which makes careful review of the entire stack of raster scans in SD-OCT necessary.

In contrast to their association with active CNV, intraretinal cysts are also often present above degenerated or scarred (thickened and hyper-reflective) RPE. In such cases, cysts indicate end-stage chronic tissue degeneration and frequently go hand in hand with a marked and irreversible reduction in visual acuity. It is important to distinguish between such **"degenerative cysts"** and "active leakage cysts," especially with regard to treatment and management options (Fig. 15.5). Usually, cystic degeneration of the retina overlies a thickened and irregular RPE band indicating RPE loss (which can be diagnosed with PS-OCT) and sub-RPE fibrosis. At the border of healthy RPE, a sharp demarcation is seen toward intact retinal layers without cystic changes.

In advanced disease, refractory cystic changes of degenerative origin with underlying RPE loss (based on PS-OCT diagnosis) are irreversible and should lead to treatment discontinuation.

Other common intraretinal SD-OCT findings are **hyper-reflective speckles**, which are dot-like lesions with strong signal intensity. Intraretinal speckles have been given the name "micro-exudates" in scientific studies, addressing their presumed origin as a conglomerate of precipitated proteins, cellular debris, and phagocytes (31). In nAMD, microexudates are often found in the direct vicinity of CNV lesions, indicating, as cysts do, disease activity (30).

With current SD-OCT systems, the achievable resolution in tissue is high enough to delineate several specific retinal layers, including aspects of the neurosensory photoreceptors and the glial components of the retina. Concerning the photoreceptors, layers such as the external limiting membrane (ELM), the IS-OS line, and the apical processes of the RPE invaginating the outer segments can be analyzed (32). Disruption of these signals (Fig. 15.6) is indicative for dysfunction or destruction of the photoreceptor cell (33,34). However, surrounding lesions in the retina (such as SRF and CNV lesions) often make it very difficult to comprehensively assess the condition of the photoreceptor layers, and care should be taken not to misinterpret imaging artifacts such as transmission or shadowing phenomena as structural damage. Although restoration of a previously lost photoreceptor signal upon treatment is sometimes seen, loss of the IS-OS and ELM signals on SD-OCT at baseline is suggestive of limited potential for recovery of function (35). Persistent disruption of the photoreceptors furthermore entails progressive atrophy of the glial and ganglion cell layers (ONL, INL, and GCL). Subsequent retinal thinning is a strong sign for irreversible loss of function.

Subretinal Compartment

The subretinal compartment, bordered by the neurosensory retina and the retinal pigment epithelium, is the primary growth site of type II and III neovascular lesions. Using SD-OCT, type II lesions can be directly visualized as an inhomogeneous, iso- or hyper-reflective mass with ill-defined borders (Fig. 15.6) (36,37). Follow-up examinations during a course of treatment can often directly show regression of CNV lesions with flattening of the mass, accompanied by a signal enhancement of the RPE band indicative of progressive fibrosis.

The neovascular processes in nAMD frequently lead to focal neurosensory detachments and an accumulation of **SRF**. SD-OCT can easily detect such fluid, which is visualized as homogeneous hyporeflective space between the retina and pigment epithelium. In the presence of a pigment epithelial detachment, SRF most often pools at the "knee" of the elevated pigment epithelium, showing a typical triangular shape. SRF is a strong activity sign, mostly of type I lesions, and should prompt treatment in most cases (38). The location,

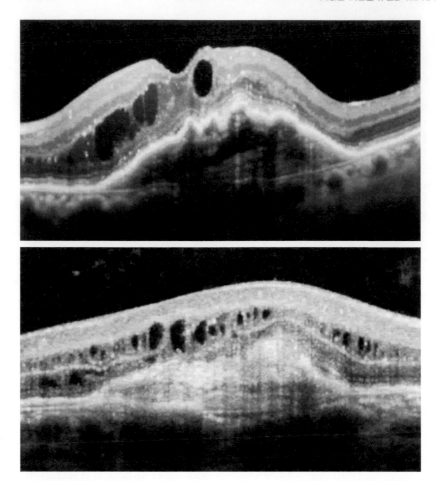

Figure 15.5 Comparison of intraretinal cysts caused by active leakage versus cystic degeneration. (*Top*) active leakage: Active type I CNV with fibrovascular PED. The cysts are distributed focally with a predilection for the outer nuclear layer. The photoreceptor layers appear mostly intact, suggesting preserved tissue viability. (*Bottom*) cystic degeneration: End-stage type I CNV. The fibrovascular PED has organized and now appears as a fibrous scar. Multiple diffuse small cysts are present overlying a degenerated RPE and associated wide-spread loss of the photoreceptor layers.

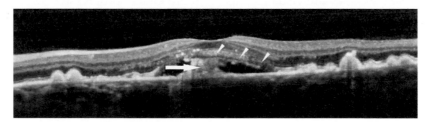

Figure 15.6 Type II CNV lesion with associated disruption of the photoreceptor layers. The neovascular infiltration imposes as a hyper-reflective, inhomogeneous mass with ill-defined borders (arrow). Overlying the lesion and associated subretinal fluid, the photoreceptor layers show pronounced signal loss (arrowheads), indicative for a reduction in visual function.

volume, height, and area of SRF are highly variable in the course of nAMD. When assessing disease severity or treatment response, the presence and extent of SRF should therefore be specifically studied in the complete stack of SD-OCT sections. Ideally, a volumetric measurement should be available, as macular function appears to correlate with the volume of SRF rather than with height or area alone (39). The pathologic impact of SRF likely consists of toxic components within the exudate more than the serous detachment per se, as the fluid reflectivity is higher in nAMD than, for example, in central serous chorioretinopathy, and a dense SRF signal correlates with a poor visual prognosis (40).

Sub-RPE Compartment

The anatomical compartment beneath the retinal pigment epithelium is the site of primary disease processes in early AMD. Proliferation of CNV underneath the RPE induces **PEDs** which separate the RPE from Bruch's membrane. PEDs vary greatly in size and configuration. Variables such as area, height, and content of PEDs should be considered when analyzing SD-OCT scans. Especially when CNV lesions contract under anti-VEGF therapy, very high PEDs with steep edges have a high risk for progression to **RPE rips**, often with devastating functional outcomes if the fovea is affected (41).

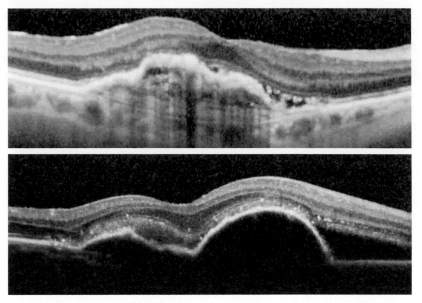

Figure 15.7 Comparison of fibrovascular versus serous PED. (*Top*) fibrovascular PED: The sub-RPE cavity is filled with inhomogeneous, hyperreflective material. (*Bottom*) serous PED: The sub-RPE cavity appears optically empty.

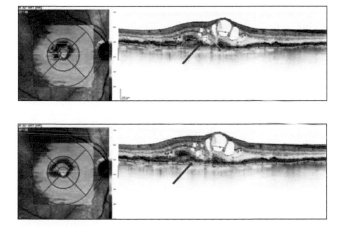

Figure 15.8 Assessment of retinal thickness. The color-coded map indicates macular edema (thickness above normal limits is shown as red or white). (*Top row*) Serial segmentation errors (arrow) lead to degradation of the thickness map. (*Bottom row*) Manual correction of the segmentation errors (arrow) is necessary to achieve reliable thickness information.

Based on their content, PEDs can be classified into predominantly **serous** or predominantly **fibrovascular** on SD-OCT (Fig. 15.7) (42). These two forms often coexist to varying degrees during the course of the disease. This is especially the case for chronic forms which gradually become organized. Predominantly serous PEDs are characterized by accumulation of fluid in the space between the RPE and Bruch's membrane. The PED is regular, dome shaped, and appears optically empty with a homogeneously hyporeflective content on SD-OCT. In fibrovascular PED (usually shaped irregularly), the cavity is filled with heterogeneous, moderately hyper-reflective material. Only part of the cavity appears to be optically empty. As long as the retina overlying the PED remains dry, function is not or only

minimally compromised. During the natural course of the disease and in about half of the eyes in response to treatment, the PED gradually collapses due to fluid resorption over an extended time period. The PED often becomes multilobed with its cavity organized and increasingly reflective, which suggests the development of fibrosis.

In general, it is impractical to distinguish between fibrovascular PEDs and **type I (occult) lesions** based on SD-OCT appearance. This distinction can be made with more confidence when other signs of CNV activity such as cysts and SRF are also present.

CRITERIA FOR DISEASE ACTIVITY AND PROGNOSIS
Macular Thickness
All common OCT devices can be used to calculate retinal thickness. The classic output of false-color coded **retinal thickness maps** (Fig. 15.8) provides a quick overview of macular topography and can be useful for initial rapid assessment. Instruments also deliver micrometer-scale thickness values, typically for each of the nine macular subfields introduced by the ETDRS Group (43). Derived **central macular thickness** (CMT, representing the average retinal thickness within a 1-mm diameter circular area centered on the fovea) has been heavily used both in practice and in research as an indicator of disease activity. Retinal thickness certainly shows a correlation with edematous swelling (44); however, it represents a mixture of multiple disease components and cannot accurately reflect the complicated pathomorphologic alterations in nAMD.

The correlation between CMT and retinal function in particular is not trivial (35,45). Many clinical trials on anti-VEGF therapy have used CMT changes to guide re-treatment decisions in a PRN regimen (e.g., PrONTO, SUSTAIN, MONT BLANC, DENALI, CATT, and VIEW); however, overall evidence suggests that re-treatment indications based solely on CMT are not practicable. A good correlation of CMT with visual acuity is found in the treatment-naïve baseline populations and during most of the treatment initiation phase with three consecutive monthly injections (38). With progressive disease (and especially with inadequate treatment), this correlation is lost over time, since resulting photoreceptor loss becomes irreversible despite a flattening retina (*Simader* et al., *submitted*). In advanced disease, CMT values are inconclusive regarding disease activity and visual prognosis as even small amounts of fluid may lead to substantial visual impairment, while a decrease in CMT may indicate progressive neurosensory atrophy. In consideration of the problematic interpretation of CMT, clinicians should in general prefer morphologic assessment over retinal thickness measurements when analyzing SD-OCT in nAMD.

Apart from the clinical limitations of CMT, it is critical to keep in mind that the **accuracy of thickness measurements** is dependent on several technical factors, including wide scan spacing, potentially erroneous layer segmentation, lack of patients' fixation, and incorrect ETDRS grid centering (46–48). In nAMD especially, failure in layer segmentation (Fig. 15.7) and unstable fixation frequently compromise the quality and reproducibility of thickness measurements. Numeric ETDRS subfield values are particularly unreliable in this context and should only be used after careful review of the scan set for segmentation accuracy and grid centering. In clinical trials, manual correction of segmentation errors and standardized grid plotting are usually performed by certified reading centers, which improves the validity of thickness measurements.

Microstructural Changes

A precise understanding of changes in different morphological variables in respect to visual acuity and time course of recurrence is essential to guide anti-VEGF treatment in nAMD, and to predict the potential overall benefit of treatment. In an era of personalized medicine, there is a strong trend toward **individualized anti-VEGF treatment** in patients with nAMD. However, most trials with a flexible "pro re nata" (PRN, as needed) regimen have shown functional outcomes that were inferior to those achieved by a fixed monthly treatment regimen. Clearly, a PRN regimen will only be viable if some prerequisites are achieved: First, definition of morphology-derived characteristics that stratify patients according to their individual risk for disease progression or recurrence; second, establishment of solid functionally relevant criteria for re-treatment; and third, prognosis of the potential treatment benefit. These goals are currently the subject of intensive research.

Several time-domain OCT-based studies have quantified the morphologic effects of intravitreal anti-VEGF therapy on the three "classic" morphologic alterations of central macular anatomy in eyes with nAMD, that is intraretinal cysts, SRF, and PED. Data from a compartment analysis during the loading phase of anti-VEGF therapy showed an immediate and intensive reduction in SRF volume which correlated well with an improvement in visual acuity in general, as well as with the characteristic time course of recovery of function (38). A subsequent study showed that a recurrence of disease, which could regularly be observed in a treatment arm using quarterly anti-VEGF injections, was predominantly reflected in the response of SRF rather than that of intraretinal fluid (40). With each discontinuation of intravitreal therapy, SRF volume values showed an immediate and pronounced response. More importantly, the morphologic changes were translated to an identical pattern of visual acuity fluctuations in a direct correlation of timing and intensity. Consecutively, SRF volume was suggested as an important variable when defining specific re-treatment criteria for individualized treatment regimens. Further studies identified intraretinal cysts at baseline as a negative prognostic feature for the overall achievable treatment benefit (*Simader* et al., *submitted*). The initial presence of such cysts was associated with lower baseline vision and poorer outcome alone and in combination with other signs of exudation such as SRF and PED. The association with poor outcome was particularly pronounced if cysts did not disappear during therapy.

The PrONTO trial (49) and the recent CATT trial (50) showed acceptable outcomes for PRN regimens with the application of "zero tolerance" re-treatment indications based on OCT, that is the presence of any intraretinal or SRF required prompt anti-VEGF treatment. However, CATT also showed substantial inconsistencies in the judgment of fluid on OCT images between the evaluating reading center and the investigators. While the reading center was very sensitive and graded even single cystic changes as "fluid," the investigators were generally less sensitive to activity signs on OCT. These discrepancies further underline the need for valid re-treatment criteria, ideally based on solid morphologic parameters on SD-OCT. To date, a fixed monthly treatment regimen has to be considered superior to any flexible treatment strategies. If a PRN regimen is suggested, strict monthly monitoring using professional SD-OCT analysis is the most important requirement, as recurrent fluid may unpredictably occur at any time, invariably leading to persistent visual loss if not treated in a timely fashion.

All prospective nAMD treatment trials so far have been based on conventional time-domain OCT technology which failed to reliably identify treatment-necessitating characteristics and which could not provide solid information on prognostic variables. Results of current prospective trials based on SD-OCT are expected to provide encouraging evidence and promise to identify valid criteria for PRN regimens in the future.

SUMMARY POINTS

- Morphologic assessment of optical coherence tomography (OCT) volume stacks should be preferred to the assessment of single foveal scans or **central macular thickness** measurements
- Intraretinal cysts, hyper-reflective speckles, and subretinal fluid are highly indicative for active choroidal neovascularization lesions. Care should be taken to distinguish neovascular from degenerative cysts
- Detection of even minimal fluid on OCT should prompt consideration of (re)treatment with anti-VEGF agents
- Alteration of photoreceptor-related reflectivity and intraretinal cysts at baseline has a negative prognostic implication
- The vitreomacular interface should always be considered as an additional disease factor

REFERENCES

1. Geitzenauer W, Hitzenberger CK, Schmidt-Erfurth UM. Retinal optical coherence tomography: past, present and future perspectives. Br J Ophthalmol 2011; 95: 171–7.
2. Wojtkowski M, Leitgeb R, Kowalczyk A, et al. In vivo human retinal imaging by fourier domain optical coherence tomography. J Biomed Opt 2002; 7: 457–63.
3. Ahlers C, Schmidt-Erfurth U. Three-dimensional high resolution OCT imaging of macular pathology. Opt Express 2009; 17: 4037–45.
4. Sakamoto A, Hangai M, Yoshimura N. Spectral-domain optical coherence tomography with multiple B-scan averaging for enhanced imaging of retinal diseases. Ophthalmology 2008; 115: 1071–8; e7.
5. Miura M, Makita S, Iwasaki T, et al. Three-dimensional visualization of ocular vascular pathology by optical coherence angiography in vivo. Invest Ophthalmol Vis Sci 2011. [Epub ahead of print]
6. de Bruin DM, Burnes DL, Loewenstein J, et al. In vivo three-dimensional imaging of neovascular age-related macular degeneration using optical frequency domain imaging at 1050nm. Invest Ophthalmol Vis Sci 2008; 49: 4545–52.
7. Pircher M, Hitzenberger CK, Schmidt-Erfurth U. Polarization sensitive optical coherence tomography in the human eye. Prog Retin Eye Res 2011; 30: 431–51.
8. Ahlers C, Götzinger E, Pircher M, et al. Imaging of the retinal pigment epithelium in age-related macular degeneration using polarization-sensitive optical coherence tomography. Invest Ophthalmol Vis Sci 2010; 51: 2149–57.
9. Freund KB, Yannuzzi LA, Sorenson JA. Age-related macular degeneration and choroidal neovascularization. Am J Ophthalmol 1993; 115: 786–91.
10. Freund KB, Zweifel SA, Engelbert M. Do we need a new classification for choroidal neovascularization in age-related macular degeneration? Retina 2010; 30: 1333–49.
11. Gass JD. Biomicroscopic and histopathologic considerations regarding the feasibility of surgical excision of subfoveal neovascular membranes. Am J Ophthalmol 1994; 118: 285–98.
12. Macular Photocoagulation Study Group. Five-year follow-up of fellow eyes of patients with age-related macular degeneration and unilateral extrafoveal choroidal neovascularization. Arch Ophthalmol 1993; 111: 1189–99.
13. Yannuzzi LA, Wong DW, Sforzolini BS, et al. Polypoidal choroidal vasculopathy and neovascularized age related macular degeneration. Arch Ophthalmol 1999; 117: 1503–10.
14. Imamura Y, Engelbert M, Iida T, et al. Polypoidal choroidal vasculopathy: a review. Surv Ophthalmol 2010; 55: 501–15.
15. Saito M, Iida T, Nagayama D. Cross-sectional and en face optical coherence tomographic features of polypoidal choroidal vasculopathy. Retina 2008; 28: 459–64.
16. Ozawa S, Ishikawa K, Ito Y, et al. Differences in macular morphology between polypoidal choroidal vasculopathy and exudative age-related macular degeneration detected by optical coherence tomography. Retina 2009; 29: 793–802.
17. Hartnett ME, Weiter JJ, Staurenghi G, et al. Deep retinal vascular anomalous complexes in advanced age-related macular degeneration. Ophthalmology 1996; 103: 2042–53.
18. Yannuzzi LA, Negrao S, Iida T, et al. Retinal angiomatous proliferation in age-related macular degeneration. Retina 2001; 21: 416–34.
19. Gross NE, Aizman A, Brucker A, et al. Nature and risk of neovascularization in the fellow eye of patients with unilateral retinal angiomatous proliferation. Retina 2005; 25: 713–18.
20. Slakter JS, Yannuzzi LA, Schneider U, et al. Retinal choroidal anastomoses and occult choroidal neovascularization in age-related macular degeneration. Ophthalmology 2000; 107: 742–53; discussion 53–4.
21. Yonemoto J, Ideta H, Sasaki K, et al. The age of onset of posterior vitreous detachment. Graefes Arch Clin Exp Ophthalmol 1994; 232: 67–70.
22. Krebs I, Brannath W, Glittenberg C, et al. Posterior vitreomacular adhesion: a potential risk factor for exudative age-related macular degeneration? Am J Ophthalmol 2007; 144: 741–6.
23. Lee SJ, Lee CS, Koh HJ. Posterior vitreomacular adhesion and risk of exudative age-related macular degeneration: paired eye study. Am J Ophthalmol 2009; 147: 621–6; e1.
24. Waldstein SM, Sponer U, Simader C, et al. Influence of vitreomacular adhesion on the development of exudative age-related macular degeneration: 4-Year results of a longitudinal study. Retina 2012; 32: 424–33.
25. Lee SJ, Koh HJ. Effects of vitreomacular adhesion on anti-vascular endothelial growth factor treatment for exudative age-related macular degeneration. Ophthalmology 2011; 118: 101–10.
26. Schulze S, Hoerle S, Mennel S, et al. Vitreomacular traction and exudative age-related macular degeneration. Acta Ophthalmol 2008; 86: 470–81.
27. Mirza RG, Johnson MW, Jampol LM. Optical coherence tomography use in evaluation of the vitreoretinal interface: a review. Surv Ophthalmol 2007; 52: 397–421.
28. Hee MR, Baumal CR, Puliafito CA, et al. Optical coherence tomography of age-related macular degeneration and choroidal neovascularization. Ophthalmology 1996; 103: 1260–70.
29. Charbel Issa P, Troeger E, Finger R, et al. Structure-function correlation of the human central retina. PLoS One 2010; 5: e12864.
30. Giani A, Luiselli C, Esmaili DD, et al. Spectral-domain optical coherence tomography as an indicator of fluorescein

angiography leakage from choroidal neovascularization. Invest Ophthalmol Vis Sci 2011; 52: 5579–86.

31. Bolz M, Schmidt-Erfurth U, Deak G, et al. Optical coherence tomographic hyperreflective foci: a morphologic sign of lipid extravasation in diabetic macular edema. Ophthalmology 2009; 116: 914–20.

32. Spaide RF, Curcio CA. Anatomical correlates to the bands seen in the outer retina by optical coherence tomography: literature review and model. Retina 2011; 31: 1609–19.

33. Yamauchi Y, Yagi H, Usui Y, et al. Biological activity is the likely origin of the intersection between the photoreceptor inner and outer segments of the rat retina as determined by optical coherence tomography. Clin Ophthalmol 2011; 5: 1649–53.

34. Yamauchi Y, Agawa T, Tsukahara R, et al. Correlation between high-resolution optical coherence tomography (OCT) images and histopathology in an iodoacetic acid-induced model of retinal degeneration in rabbits. Br J Ophthalmol 2011; 95: 1157–60.

35. Shin HJ, Chung H, Kim HC. Association between foveal microstructure and visual outcome in age-related macular degeneration. Retina 2011; 31: 1627–36.

36. Malamos P, Sacu S, Georgopoulos M, et al. Correlation of high-definition optical coherence tomography and fluorescein angiography imaging in neovascular macular degeneration. Invest Ophthalmol Vis Sci 2009; 50: 4926–33.

37. Sulzbacher F, Kiss C, Munk M, et al. Diagnostic evaluation of type 2 (Classic) choroidal neovascularization: optical coherence tomography, indocyanine green angiography, and fluorescein angiography. Am J Ophthalmol 2011; 152: 799–806, e1.

38. Bolz M, Simader C, Ritter M, et al. Morphological and functional analysis of the loading regimen with intravitreal ranibizumab in neovascular age-related macular degeneration. Br J Ophthalmol 2010; 94: 185–9.

39. Golbaz I, Ahlers C, Stock G, et al. Quantification of the therapeutic response of intraretinal, subretinal, and sub-pigment epithelial compartments in exudative AMD during Anti-VEGF therapy. Invest Ophthalmol Vis Sci 2011; 52: 1599–605.

40. Ahlers C, Golbaz I, Einwallner E, et al. Identification of optical density ratios in subretinal fluid as a clinically relevant biomarker in exudative macular disease. Invest Ophthalmol Vis Sci 2009; 50: 3417–24.

41. Barkmeier AJ, Carvounis PE. Retinal pigment epithelial tears and the management of exudative age-related macular degeneration. Semin Ophthalmol 2011; 26: 94–103.

42. Zayit-Soudry S, Moroz I, Loewenstein A. Retinal pigment epithelial detachment. Surv Ophthalmol 2007; 52: 227–43.

43. Early Treatment Diabetic Retinopathy Study Research Group. Photocoagulation for diabetic macular edema: early treatment diabetic retinopathy study report number 1. Arch Ophthalmol 1985; 103: 1796–806.

44. Hee MR, Puliafito CA, Wong C, et al. Quantitative assessment of macular edema with optical coherence tomography. Arch Ophthalmol 1995; 113: 1019–29.

45. Akagi-Kurashige Y, Tsujikawa A, Oishi A, et al. Relationship between retinal morphological findings and visual function in age-related macular degeneration. Graefe's Arch Clin Exp Ophthalmol 2012: 1–8. [Epub ahead of print].

46. Sadda SR, Wu Z, Walsh AC, et al. Errors in retinal thickness measurements obtained by optical coherence tomography. Ophthalmology 2006; 113: 285–93.

47. Parravano M, Oddone F, Boccassini B, et al. Reproducibility of macular thickness measurements using cirrus sd-oct in neovascular age-related macular degeneration. Invest Ophthalmol Vis Sci 2010; 51: 4788–91.

48. Han IC, Jaffe GJ. Evaluation of artifacts associated with macular spectral-domain optical coherence tomography. Ophthalmology 2010; 117: 1177–89; e4.

49. Fung AE, Lalwani GA, Rosenfeld PJ, et al. An optical coherence tomography-guided, variable dosing regimen with intravitreal ranibizumab (lucentis) for neovascular age-related macular degeneration. Am J Ophthalmol 2007; 143: 566–83; e2.

50. Martin DF, Maguire MG, Ying GS, et al. Ranibizumab and bevacizumab for neovascular age-related macular degeneration. N Engl J Med 2011; 364: 1897–908.

51. Abe S, Yamamoto T, Haneda S, et al. Three-dimensional features of polypoidal choroidal vasculopathy observed by spectral-domain OCT. Ophthalmic Surg Lasers Imaging 2011; 42: e1–e6.

16

Fundus autofluorescence imaging in age-related macular degeneration

Alex Yuan, Rishi P. Singh, and Peter K. Kaiser

INTRODUCTION

Autofluorescence (AF) is the emission of light by a natural substance (e.g., lipofuscin) after being stimulated by excitation energy. AF is distinguished from fluorescence that is the emission of light by an artificial molecule (e.g., fluorescein). Fundus AF was first recognized from control photographs taken prior to the injection of fluorescein dye during fluorescein angiography. The AF signal seen from normal patients was minimal, whereas increased AF was recognized from patients with abnormalities such as optic nerve drusen, Best's macular dystrophy, and Stargardt's disease (1). Fundus AF imaging was difficult with conventional photography due to the low levels of light emitted using the standard filter sets used for fluorescein angiography. The development of the fundus spectrophotometer allowed for the measurement of emission spectra from the fundus sampled in 2–3° diameter retinal fields (2). Fundus AF was found to be emitted in a broad spectrum between 500 and 750 nm with a maximum of approximately 630 nm. The optimal excitation wavelength was approximately 510 nm (2). The AF signal was highest at 7–15° from the fovea with a minimum at the fovea (2). Today, fundus AF imaging can be achieved with a scanning laser ophthalmoscope (SLO) or a modified fundus camera with special filter sets.

In this chapter, we will review the biology behind the fundus AF signal, the equipment used for fundus AF imaging, the patterns of fundus AF seen in different stages of age-related macular degeneration (AMD), and discuss the current and future use of AF imaging in the diagnosis and management of AMD.

Cellular Origin of the AF Signal

The predominant source of AF in the macula is lipofuscin, a complex mixture of fluorophores including A2E. Identified as the predominant fluorophore in retinal pigment epithelium (RPE) (3,4), A2E is named for its derivation from two molecules of vitamin A aldehyde and one molecule of ethanolamine (Fig. 16.1) (4,5). When RPE cells phagocytize the outer segments of photoreceptors, lipofuscin accumulates within lysosomes as an oxidative by-product (2,6,7). The intracellular lipofuscin content increases with age, occupying 1% of the cell volume during the first decade and increasing to almost 20% of the cell volume by the ninth decade (8,9).

In a normal retina, lipofuscin is most concentrated in the macula with the exception of the fovea and decreases toward the periphery (2,9,10). The highest lipofuscin level in the eye is found 7–13° away from the fovea, correlating with the area with the highest distribution of rod photoreceptors (11).

Fundus AF Imaging Systems

By evaluating fundus AF images that reflect lipofuscin accumulation, disturbances within the RPE can be readily detected. Three different imaging systems can be used to measure fundus AF; however, only two systems have clinical value. The fundus spectrophotometer is capable of quantitatively measuring excitation and emission spectra, but it is limited to a very small 2–3° field. The development of the fundus spectrophotometer allowed the ground-breaking work of Delori and colleagues (2). However, its limited field is not practical for recording AF in large patient populations in a clinical setting. The confocal scanning laser ophthalmoscope (cSLO) and modified fundus camera on the other hand, offer a wide field of view (55° and 50°, respectively) and rapid acquisition times. Both these systems are in clinical use for fundus AF imaging.

Confocal Scanning Laser Ophthalmoscope

The cSLO uses blue laser light at 488 nm for illumination and a 500 nm barrier filter to isolate autofluorescent light from other ocular structures such as the lens and cornea (12,13). The plane of the cSLO detection system is conjugate to the plane of the fundus, further reducing competing light signals (14). To improve the image quality limited by the low AF light intensity, several scans are averaged together to produce the final image. Compared with the modified fundus camera, cSLO images showed a higher reliability when evaluating single-patient images from one visit to the next (15). Although cSLO has significant advantages over the modified fundus camera, it requires the purchase of a new imaging device.

Modified Fundus Camera

Spaide has described an easy and inexpensive modification to pre-existing fundus cameras by adding a special filter set to optimize the AF signal while blocking the signal from the lens. A band-pass excitation filter with a range of 500–610 nm and a peak at 580 nm is used for the excitation light source and barrier filter with a range from 675 to 715 nm and a peak at 695 nm is used to detect the AF signal while blocking out the lower wavelength signals emitted by the lens (14). An updated filter set

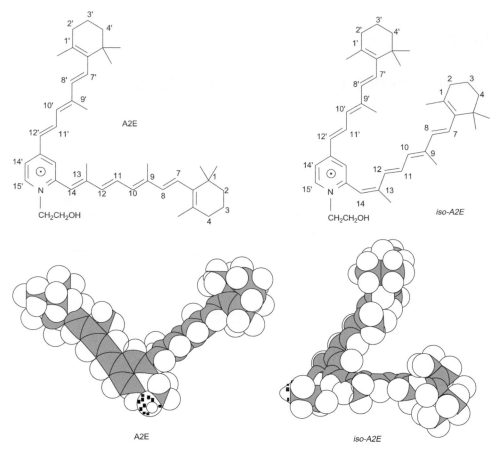

Figure 16.1 Structure of A2E and isomer iso-A2E from human retinal pigment epithelium. *Source*: From Ref. 58.

shifts the excitation filter to 535–580 nm, which is not within the absorption curve of fluorescein or indocyanine green so that AF images may be taken after angiography. This shift also minimizes the absorption from macular pigments and cataracts. The updated barrier filter has an expanded range of 615–715 nm, making the system more efficient (16).

AUTOFLUORESCENCE AND AGE-RELATED MACULAR DEGENERATION

The major fluorophore found in lipofuscin, A2E, has been shown to inhibit human RPE cell growth and induce apoptosis in vitro. It exhibits detergent-like activity, disrupting membrane-bound ATPase which maintains lysosomal pH (3,17,18). In mitochondria, A2E inhibits oxygen consumption synergistically with light by inhibiting cytochrome *c* oxidase (19). By mobilizing cytochrome *c* and apoptosis-inducing factor from mitochondria into the cytoplasm and nucleus, apoptosis is induced in RPE cells (20). A2E has also been shown to confer a dose-related sensitivity to blue light damage in RPE cells via oxidative mechanisms (21). Thus, an accumulation of A2E and lipofuscin may result in RPE cell injury or death and may play a role in the pathogenesis of AMD.

Several studies have found that the accumulation of lipofuscin over time may promote the development of AMD (Figs. 16.2 and 16.3). The age, spatial, and

racial distribution of lipofuscin correlates well with the AF patterns seen with AMD. Dorey and colleagues found significant correlation between photoreceptor loss and elevated lipofuscin levels in RPE within donor eyes of Caucasians over 50 years old. They hypothesized that lipofuscin accumulation may be indicative of increased phagocytic and metabolic stress on the RPE cells leading to photoreceptor death (22,23). Subsequent studies suggest that photo-oxidation of A2E and other bis-retinoid products found in lipofuscin could activate complement in vitro (24,25). Thus, the accumulation of lipofuscin may promote complement system dysregulation, which is thought to contribute to the pathogenesis of AMD as suggested by multiple genetic association studies (26–33).

Excessive lipofuscin accumulation may precede the development of geographic atrophy (GA) and the enlargement of pre-existing GA (34). Thus, AF imaging may be useful in evaluating the risk of AMD progression by mapping retinal AF and lipofuscin accumulation over extended periods. Previous work has shown a significant correlation in the amount of large, foveal, soft drusen and patterns of increased AF (15). Spaide reported greater levels of AF in fellow eyes of patients with neovascular AMD than in patients without a history of AMD (14). Delori and colleagues discovered that RPE overlying drusen have a central area of decreased

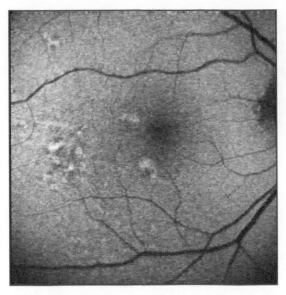
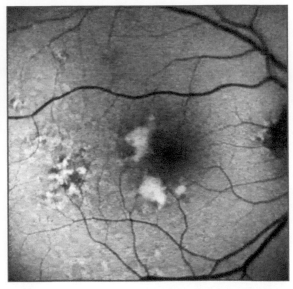

Figure 16.2 Lipofuscin accumulation in a 68–year-old patient over three years. *Source*: Photos courtesy of L. Yanuzzi, R. Spaide, and P. Bhatnagar.

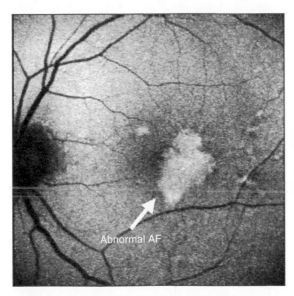
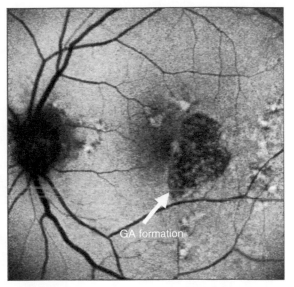

Figure 16.3 Progression to geographic atrophy over three years with abnormal autofluorescence. *Abbreviations*: AF, autofluorescence; GA, geographic atrophy. *Source*: Photos courtesy of L. Yanuzzi, R. Spaide, and P. Bhatnagar.

AF with a surrounding ring of increased AF, suggesting damage to RPE cells (7).

Autofluorescence Patterns with Normal Aging

The normal macular AF pattern is characterized by a homogeneous background AF with a gradual decrease in signal extending into the periphery and also centrally toward the fovea (Fig. 16.4A). The depressed AF signal at the center of the fovea is due to masking from macular pigments, as well as a decrease in lipofuscin in the fovea. The retinal vasculature appears dark due to absorption by blood. The optic nerve is also dark due to a lack of lipofuscin and other fluorescent pigments (12). With age, AF increases (2); however, due to limitations in the ability of cSLO and the modified fundus camera to quantitatively measure the AF signal, correlations between the absolute AF signal in patients of different ages cannot be easily obtained.

Autofluorescence Associated with Drusen

There have been numerous reports examining AF associated with drusen. Delori and associates identified a specific pattern of AF spatially associated with hard and soft drusen ranging between 60 and 175 µm in size. The pattern is characterized by a central area of decreased AF surrounded, in most cases, by an annulus of increased AF around the drusen (7). Delori hypothesizes that this AF pattern is due to RPE impairment with secondary accumulation of lipofuscin around drusen, with RPE atrophy overlying drusen. Spaide interprets the appearance of this pattern as secondary to thinner RPE cells on top of the drusen, and thicker RPE cells around the base (35). Soft drusen larger than 175 µm and confluent soft drusen show either a heterogenous distribution of AF or multifocal areas of decreased AF (7). Other studies have reported normal, hyper- or hypo-AF of the area overlying soft drusen

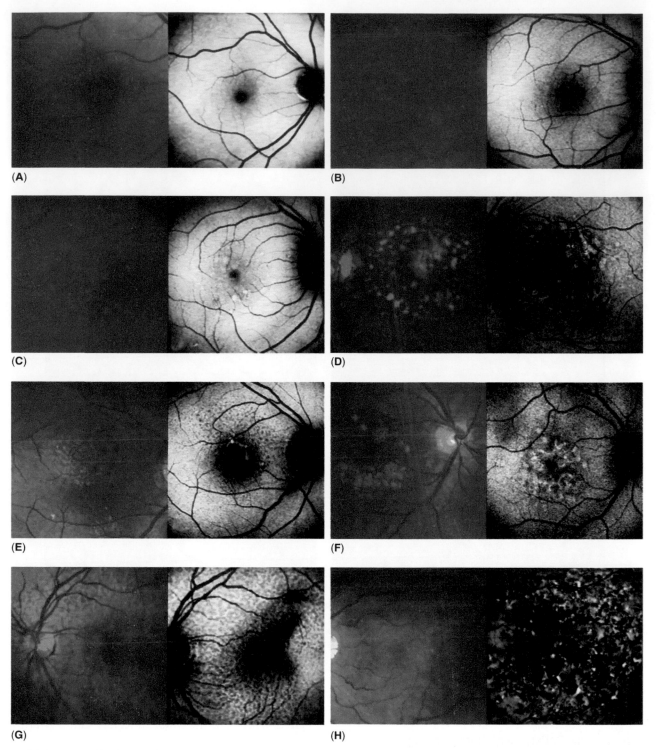

Figure 16.4 Patterns of fundus autofluorescence (AF) as established by IFAG. (**A**) Normal pattern; (**B**) minimal change pattern: very limited irregular increases or decreases of AF due to multiple small hard drusen; (**C**) focal increased pattern: several well-defined spots with markedly increased AF; (**D**) patchy pattern: multiple large areas of increased AF corresponding to multiple large soft drusen and/or hyperpigmentation in the fundus photograph; (**E**) linear pattern: at least one linear area with marked increased AF; (**F**) lace-like pattern: multiple branching linear structures of increased AF. (**G**) reticular pattern—multiple small areas of decreased AF with bright lines in between; (**H**) speckled pattern—presence of a variety of AF abnormalities, which extend beyond the macular area to the posterior pole.

with no proven biochemical explanation (13,15,36,37). These studies consistently showed that focal alterations in the normal fundus AF signal are not necessarily associated with corresponding areas of drusen or pigment identified by color fundus photo or angiographically. Thus, early changes in AF may reveal disease progression earlier than possible with color fundus photos or fluorescein angiography.

Autofluorescence Patterns in Early Age-Related Macular Degeneration

Abnormal AF patterns are seen in patients with AMD. The normal homogenous fundus appearance is altered with areas of either hyper or hypo-AF. Although it is generally accepted that lipofuscin is the dominant fluorophore in the macula, there is a lack of histologic correlation with AF images to confirm the origins of specific AF patterns.

Areas of reduced AF are believed to be due to a reduction in lipofuscin in RPE cells, whereas areas of increased AF are believed to be due to an accumulation of lipofuscin or other fluorescent molecules. Therefore, RPE atrophy and areas blocked by pigment or heme are usually seen as hypo-AF. Areas with increased lipofuscin or other fluorophores will result in hyper-AF patterns. To help standardize the patterns seen in AMD, an international group of clinicians established a classification system for fundus AF patterns seen in AMD (38,39).

The International Fundus Autofluorescence Classification Group (IFAG) described eight distinct patterns of AF in early AMD: normal pattern, minimal change pattern, focal increased pattern, patchy pattern, linear pattern, lace-like pattern, reticular pattern, and speckled pattern. Standardized photos of these AF patterns are shown in Figure 16.4 (38,39).

Normal Pattern

As described above, the normal AF pattern is characterized by a homogeneous background AF with a gradual decrease in signal converging at the fovea. The normal pattern may be seen in patients with drusen.

Minimal Change Pattern

The minimal change pattern is characterized by very small irregular increases or decreases of background AF without an obvious topographic pattern.

Focal Increased Pattern

Focal increased AF is described as the presence of at least one spot (less than 200 μm diameter) of markedly increased AF brighter than the surrounding fluorescence. The borders are well defined and some areas of focal increased AF may be surrounded by a darker-appearing halo. Visible alterations (focal hyperpigmentation or drusen) seen on color fundus photos may or may not correspond to areas of AF.

Patchy Pattern

Patchy AF is defined as at least one larger area (greater than 200 μm diameter) of markedly increased AF where the borders of the areas are typically less clearly defined than the previous pattern. There is a gradual increase in AF from the background to the patchy area. This pattern may also correspond to large drusen, soft drusen, and areas of hyperpigmentation seen on color photographs.

Linear Pattern

The linear pattern describes the presence of at least one linear area of markedly increased AF with well-demarcated borders and no gradual decrease in AF. These AF areas usually correspond to hyperpigmented lines on the color fundus photograph.

Lace-like Pattern

The lace-like pattern typically exhibits numerous branching linear structures of increased AF that form a lace pattern. The borders are poorly defined and a decline in AF is observed from the center of the AF areas to the surrounding areas. These lace-like areas can correspond to hyperpigmentation on the color image, but it may correspond to normal fundus areas as well.

Reticular Pattern

The reticular pattern is exemplified by the presence of multiple small areas (less than 200 μm diameter) of decreased AF with poorly defined borders. Funduscopically, there are usually visible small soft drusen, hard drusen, or areas with pigmentary changes overlying these areas, but the fundus can be normal as well.

Speckled Pattern

The speckled AF pattern has the simultaneous presence of a variety of AF abnormalities that extend beyond the macular area. There can be multiple, small areas of irregularly increased and decreased AF that appear punctate or resemble linear structures. Color fundus photographs may include corresponding hyper- and hypopigmentation and multiple subconfluent and confluent drusen.

Autofluorescence Patterns Associated with Geographic Atrophy

With loss of RPE containing lipofuscin, areas of GA appear dark, but AF imaging reveals distinctive patterns in the areas surrounding GA. Holz and colleagues found 83% of GA from AMD has increased AF at the border (40). This ring of elevated AF from lipofuscin bordering the GA supports the concept that excessive lipofuscin may be associated with RPE damage (41). In fact, the increased AF in the junctional zone around GA is thought to be characteristic for AMD since only 9% of geography atrophy from other causes exhibit similar findings (13,40). When tested with fundus perimetry, a significant degree of retinal sensitivity loss is found in the junctional area between the inner dark zone and ring of increased AF (42,43). Photopic and scotopic fine matrix mapping of these areas has shown a scotopic sensitivity loss demonstrating a preferential loss of rods (44). This correlation of AF abnormality to a loss of function may further suggest a relationship between GA progression and its increased AF border.

Manual measurement of GA is time consuming and results in significant inter-observer variability, whereas automated quantification and delineation of AF images is rapid and more accurate than fundus photography or fluorescein angiography in the delineation of GA (45,46). The quantitation of these lesions adds to the understanding of the natural history of GA formation and allows for the monitoring of future therapeutics to slow its progression.

To help standardize future studies, the Fundus Autofluorescence in age-related Macular degeneration (FAM) study group classified the AF patterns seen at the peripheral border of GA lesions. In the multicenter, prospective FAM study, 149 eyes from 107 patients (44 male, 63 female patients) with unilateral or bilateral GA were successfully characterized by fundus AF. In the peripheral zone of GA lesions, five patterns were described, including four additional subtypes:

Normal Pattern
No abnormal AF with a clearly defined border between GA and normal areas.

Focal Pattern
A single or multiple spots of increased AF are present at the margin of the GA lesion.

Banded Pattern
A continuous stippled band of increased AF surrounded the entire GA lesion.

Patchy Pattern
Nondistinct patchy areas of increased AF are present at the margin of the GA lesion. These areas were larger than the focal spots seen in the focal pattern.

Diffuse Pattern
An increased AF extending beyond the margins of the GA lesion, spreading into the posterior pole. These lesions were further subdivided into four patterns:

Reticular: radially oriented lines of increased AF.

Branching: a branching network of lines of increased AF.

Fine granular: a large area of increased AF with a granular appearance. The region of increased AF is clearly demarcated from the surrounding normal background AF.

Fine granular with peripheral punctate spots: Similar to the fine granular pattern except with additional small elongated spots scattered throughout the granular area.

The diffuse pattern was the most common (57%), followed by the banded, focal and normal patterns at about 12% per group. The patchy pattern was least common at about 2%. Within the diffuse pattern group, the most common were the branching (27.5%) and fine granular patterns (18.1%), with the other two subgroups encompassing less than 12% combined (38).

Longitudinal studies have demonstrated that AF is useful for the precise mapping and measurement of GA areas (Fig. 16.5) (34,47–49). Moreover, progression of increased AF from GA has been described in several studies (13,34,48,49). It has been noted that the rate of GA spread accelerates with expansion of GA, then levels off at five disc areas (50). A study from the FAM study group correlated the progression rates with the different patterns of GA seen on AF. Using the junctional zone patterns described above, the banded and diffuse patterns exhibited a significantly higher rate of

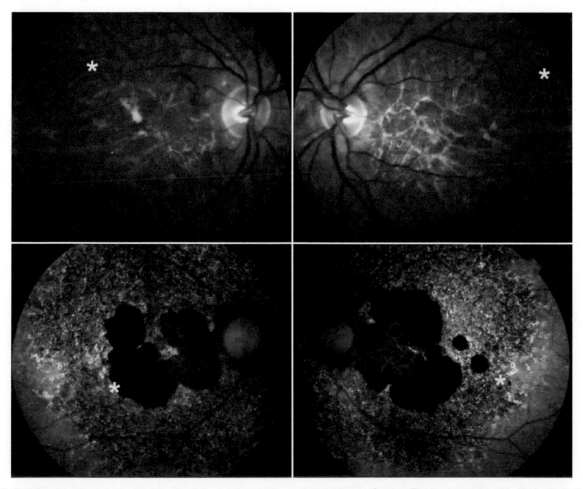

Figure 16.5 Precise mapping of geographic atrophy over time with autofluorescence. *Source*: Photos courtesy of L. Yanuzzi, R. Spaide, and P. Bhatnagar.

progression compared with the normal and focal patterns. They identified a fifth subgroup with a very rapid rate of progression, called the "diffuse trickling" subgroup. The patients in this new group resembled the diffuse branching or diffuse granular patterns but exhibited unique features. The atrophic areas appeared grayish rather than the dark black appearance typically seen with GA. In a vast majority of these eyes, there was also peripapillary atrophy and foveal sparing at baseline. There was increased AF at the margins of the atrophic areas with a diffuse trickling of AF signal toward the periphery (49). These studies suggest that different patterns of AF may help predict future expansion of GA.

In another study using AF photographs with different baseline patterns of AF, Hwang and colleagues found that only 34–50% of the new areas of GA fell into an area of increased AF. The positive predictive value for increased AF to form new GA was no better than chance (51). This study, however, was retrospective and small in size. More importantly, it utilized a special algorithm for quantitatively measuring AF signal. Quantitative measurements of AF signal using cSLO and the fundus camera are difficult and inconsistent as discussed previously. Due to these differences, direct comparisons between these studies cannot be made. Additional longitudinal studies using defined measurement criteria would be necessary to help settle this debate.

Autofluorescence Patterns Associated with Choroidal Neovascularization

While the majority of studies with AF in AMD have concentrated on the dry form, there has been limited work on determining a correlation between AF and choroidal neovascularization (CNV). Eyes with early CNV lesions show various patterns of increased AF (Fig. 16.6). Einbock and colleagues studied eyes with neovascular changes and found that 17% of eyes exhibited a "patchy" AF pattern, as well as some with "focal increased" plaque and "reticular" patterns. Other less intense patterns were not associated with progression to late AMD after 18 months of follow-up (52).

Dandekar and colleagues studied AF in 65 consecutive eyes with CNV secondary to AMD (53). Patients were stratified by the age of the CNV lesion. Eyes with recent-onset lesions (one to six months) showed no AF abnormalities, suggesting a healthy RPE. Older CNV lesions (greater than six months) exhibited decreased AF levels indicating RPE damage and photoreceptor loss. Eyes with better visual acuity were those with intact AF in early-onset lesions and others with intact AF through the fovea. Another study also correlated the CNV lesion types as defined by fluorescein angiography with fundus AF patterns. There was no correlation between the AF pattern and the type of CNV lesion, despite the hypothesis that classic CNV lesions would exhibit blockage of the AF signal from the RPE by the CNV complex (54). In this study, there was also a

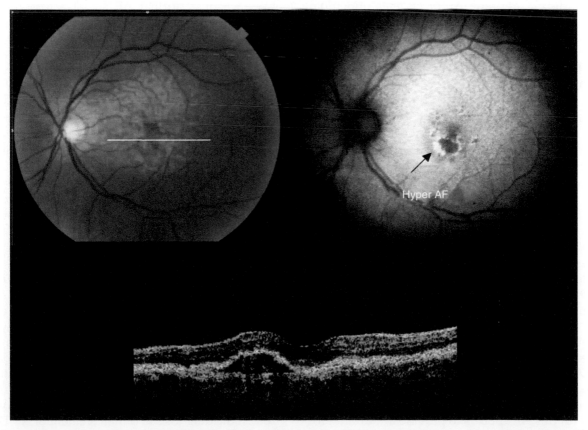

Figure 16.6 Fundus autofluorescence corresponding to subretinal fluid with choroidal neovascularization. *Abbreviations*: AF, autofluorescence. *Source*: Photos courtesy of L. Yanuzzi, R. Spaide, and P. Bhatnagar.

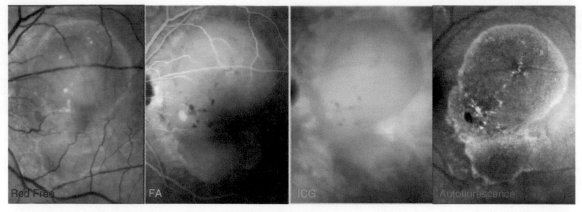

Figure 16.7 Serous pigment epithelial detachment imaged with various modalities. *Abbreviations*: FA, fluorescein angiography; ICG, indocyanine green. *Source*: Photos courtesy of L. Yanuzzi, R. Spaide, and P. Bhatnagar.

correlation between a normal AF pattern through the fovea with better vision (54).

In an observational case series examining pigment epithelial detachments (PEDs) associated with AMD, increased AF was seen in all serous PEDs regardless of whether there was an underlying CNV in the area of detachment (Fig. 16.7). The authors concluded that the increased AF seen with serous PEDs may be due to AF of sub-RPE fluid. In the case of a drusenoid PED, AF levels were dependent on pigment clumping with increased pigment correlating with lower AF levels. Larger numbers of patients are needed to verify these morphological features (55).

A few studies have attempted to classify CNV lesion type based on the AF pattern seen.

In a study examining AF of 68 eyes undergoing photodynamic therapy (PDT) treatment, Framme found 79% of the untreated classic lesions were associated with decreased AF and a junctional zone of increased or normal AF. In untreated occult membranes, a normal or mottled AF pattern with foci of hyper- and hypo-AF was seen. After PDT treatment, 90% of the classic CNV lesions showed decreased AF signal. There appeared to be no AF change in occult portions of CNV lesions after PDT (56). These baseline AF patterns were also described by McBain and colleagues in patients with neovascular AMD. Low AF signal at the site of classic CNV was detected in 90% of neovascular AMD lesions. While multiple foci of low AF was seen in half of occult CNV lesions, focally increased AF was rarely seen with CNV lesions (57). Contrary to these two studies, Vaclavik and colleagues failed to show a correlation between the type of CNV lesion and AF pattern. Additional studies, perhaps with the inclusion of optical coherence tomography, are necessary to settle this debate.

Use of Autofluorescence in the Clinical Setting

Widespread use of fundus AF in patients with neovascular AMD has not been adopted by most retina specialists owing to its limitations with its inability to identify CNV lesions compared with other imaging modalities. Although fundus AF appears to provide important prognostic information in non-neovascular AMD patients, its use in this setting is also limited because there are no studies suggesting a change in management (e.g., closer

follow-up interval) based on fundus AF findings results in improved outcomes for patients. For now, fundus AF largely remains a research tool and may be useful in identifying the borders of GA in AMD patients with new-onset vision loss without obvious neovascular changes.

The Future of Autofluorescence in Managing AMD

One area of active research is the development of therapies for non-neovascular AMD. Due to the slow progression of non-neovascular AMD, novel methods to assess the efficacy of new treatments must be developed. Fundus AF may emerge as one of the imaging modalities that can be used to measure and compare the effectiveness of various non-neovascular AMD treatments. Furthermore, as suggested by Vaclavik and Dandekar, the presence of a normal AF signal across the fovea in patients with neovascular AMD may portend a better prognosis and future non-neovascular AMD treatment trials may benefit from incorporating fundus AF data to further evaluate its predictive value. In patients with an unknown duration of symptoms, fundus AF may give valuable information regarding the visual potential. This information will be helpful in management decisions including the decision to terminate anti-VEGF therapy.

Finally, stem cell therapies are on the horizon for the treatment of various macular diseases including AMD. The ability of fundus AF to assess the health of RPE cells and photoreceptors in a noninvasive manner could be an important research tool to monitor the effectiveness of these therapies.

LIMITATIONS

There are several limitations in the use of AF in the evaluation of patients for AMD. AF detection is limited in patients with significant media opacities such as cataract and vitreous hemorrhage. Furthermore, the comparative quantification of AF images cannot occur between patients. Rather, only images from the same patient can be compared to determine changes in intensities of AF seen over time. Thus, the use of AF is still in its infancy and further studies need to be performed to evaluate its role in the diagnosis and management of AMD.

Reports on the use of AF in the diagnosis and management of AMD are preliminary at best and sometimes conflicting. There remains a need for further data to clarify the relationship of AF patterns in the formation and expansion of GA. More information is needed to substantiate the relationship between AF patterns and risk of CNV. There is a lack of studies identifying AF criteria useful in the classification of CNV subtype. The current literature consists mostly of nonrandomized small case series limiting its applicability in the general population. To address these limitations, the FAM study group, a multicenter study is currently under way, and continuing to make progress. The goal of the group is to investigate the correlation between fundus AF and the natural history of AMD. The group also intends to identify high-risk AF characteristics that can predict patients who will progress to late AMD (52).

SUMMARY POINTS

- The predominant source of autofluorescence (AF) in the macula is lipofuscin, a complex mixture of fluorophores
- The pigment within lipofuscin that causes this fluorescence is A2E (named for its derivation from two molecules of vitamin A aldehyde and one molecule of ethanolamine)
- Fundus AF is a useful modality to image lipofuscin in retinal pigment epithelium (RPE) cells and is a unique way to assess RPE function in age-related macular regeneration (AMD)
- In geographic atrophy (GA), automated imaging analysis by AF has been shown superior to fundus photography or fluorescein angiography in assessing the extent of atrophy. Increased AF, especially at the edge of GA area, may predict GA expansion
- AF has been helpful in assessing RPE health in neovascular AMD, and can consistently visualize serous pigment epithelial detachments
- Larger randomized controlled studies using AF are needed to further assess its potential in the detection and management of AMD
- Fundus AF is a useful research tool to help validate and measure the efficacy of novel treatments for non-neovascular AMD

REFERENCES

1. Miller SA. Fluorescence in best's vitelliform dystrophy, lipofuscin, and fundus flavimaculatus. Br J Ophthalmol 1978; 62: 256–60.
2. Delori FC, Dorey CK, Staurenghi G, et al. In vivo fluorescence of the ocular fundus exhibits retinal pigment epithelium lipofuscin characteristics. Invest Ophthalmol Vis Sci 1995; 36: 718–29.
3. Eldred GE, Lasky MR. Retinal age pigments generated by self-assembling lysosomotropic detergents. Nature 1993; 361: 724–6.
4. Eldred GE. Age pigment structure. Nature 1993; 364: 396.
5. Sakai N, Decatur J, Nakanishi K, Eldred GE. Ocular age pigment "A2E": an unprecedented pyridinium bisretinoid. J Am Chem Soc 1996; 118: 1559–60.
6. Gaillard ER, Atherton SJ, Eldred G, Dillon J. Photophysical studies on human retinal lipofuscin. Photochem Photobiol 1995; 61: 448–53.
7. Delori FC, Fleckner MR, Goger DG, Weiter JJ, Dorey CK. Autofluorescence distribution associated with drusen in age-related macular degeneration. Invest Ophthalmol Vis Sci 2000; 41: 496–504.
8. Kennedy CJ, Rakoczy PE, Constable IJ. Lipofuscin of the retinal pigment epithelium: a review. Eye (Lond) 1995: 9(Pt 6): 763–71.
9. Feeney-Burns L, Hilderbrand ES, Eldridge S. Aging human RPE: morphometric analysis of macular, equatorial, and peripheral cells. Invest Ophthalmol Vis Sci 1984; 25: 195–200.
10. Wing GL, Blanchard GC, Weiter JJ. The topography and age relationship of lipofuscin concentration in the retinal pigment epithelium. Invest Ophthalmol Vis Sci 1978; 17: 601–7.
11. Delori FC, Goger DG, Dorey CK. Age-related accumulation and spatial distribution of lipofuscin in RPE of normal subjects. Invest Ophthalmol Vis Sci 2001; 42: 1855–66.
12. von Ruckmann A, Fitzke FW, Bird AC. Distribution of fundus autofluorescence with a scanning laser ophthalmoscope. Br J Ophthalmol 1995; 79: 407–12.
13. von Ruckmann A, Fitzke FW, Bird AC. Fundus autofluorescence in age-related macular disease imaged with a laser scanning ophthalmoscope. Invest Ophthalmol Vis Sci 1997; 38: 478–86.
14. Spaide RF. Fundus autofluorescence and age-related macular degeneration. Ophthalmology 2003; 110: 392–9.
15. Lois N, Owens SL, Coco R, et al. Fundus autofluorescence in patients with age-related macular degeneration and high risk of visual loss. Am J Ophthalmol 2002; 133: 341–9.
16. Spaide RF. Optimized filters for fundus autofluorescence imaging. Retina Today 2009; 79–81.
17. Mellman I, Fuchs R, Helenius A. Acidification of the endocytic and exocytic pathways. Annu Rev Biochem 1986; 55: 663–700.
18. Sparrow JR, Parish CA, Hashimoto M, Nakanishi K. A2E, a lipofuscin fluorophore, in human retinal pigmented epithelial cells in culture. Invest Ophthalmol Vis Sci 1999; 40: 2988–95.
19. Shaban H, Gazzotti P, Richter C. Cytochrome c oxidase inhibition by N-retinyl-N-retinylidene ethanolamine, a compound suspected to cause age-related macula degeneration. Arch Biochem Biophys 2001; 394: 111–16.
20. Suter M, Reme C, Grimm C, et al. Age-related macular degeneration. the lipofusion component N-retinyl-N-retinylidene ethanolamine detaches proapoptotic proteins from mitochondria and induces apoptosis in mammalian retinal pigment epithelial cells. J Biol Chem 2000; 275: 39625–30.
21. Nilsson SE, Sundelin SP, Wihlmark U, Brunk UT. Aging of cultured retinal pigment epithelial cells: oxidative reactions, lipofuscin formation and blue light damage. Doc Ophthalmol 2003; 106: 13–16.
22. Dorey CK, Wu G, Ebenstein D, Garsd A, Weiter JJ. Cell loss in the aging retina. Relationship to lipofuscin accumulation and macular degeneration. Invest Ophthalmol Vis Sci 1989; 30: 1691–9.
23. Dorey CK, Staurenghi G, Delori FC. Lipofuscin in age and ARMD eyes. In: Hollyfield JG, ed. Retinal Degeneration. New York: Plenum Pub Corp, 1993: 3–14.
24. Zhou J, Jang YP, Kim SR, Sparrow JR. Complement activation by photooxidation products of A2E, a lipofuscin constituent of the retinal pigment epithelium. Proc Natl Acad Sci U S A 2006; 103: 16182–7.
25. Zhou J, Kim SR, Westlund BS, Sparrow JR. Complement activation by bisretinoid constituents of RPE lipofuscin. Invest Ophthalmol Vis Sci 2009; 50: 1392–9.

26. Conley YP, Thalamuthu A, Jakobsdottir J, et al. Candidate gene analysis suggests a role for fatty acid biosynthesis and regulation of the complement system in the etiology of age-related maculopathy. Hum Mol Genet 2005; 14: 1991–2002.

27. Edwards AO, Ritter R 3rd, Abel KJ, et al. Complement factor H polymorphism and age-related macular degeneration. Science 2005; 308: 421–4.

28. Hageman GS, Anderson DH, Johnson LV, et al. A common haplotype in the complement regulatory gene factor H (HF1/CFH) predisposes individuals to age-related macular degeneration. Proc Natl Acad Sci U S A 2005; 102: 7227–32.

29. Haines JL, Hauser MA, Schmidt S, et al. Complement factor H variant increases the risk of age-related macular degeneration. Science 2005; 308: 419–21.

30. Klein RJ, Zeiss C, Chew EY, et al. Complement factor H polymorphism in age-related macular degeneration. Science 2005; 308: 385–9.

31. Zareparsi S, Branham KE, Li M, et al. Strong association of the Y402H variant in complement factor H at 1q32 with susceptibility to age-related macular degeneration. Am J Hum Genet 2005; 77: 149–53.

32. Gold B, Merriam JE, Zernant J, et al. Variation in factor B (BF) and complement component 2 (C2) genes is associated with age-related macular degeneration. Nat Genet 2006; 38: 458–62.

33. Yates JR, Sepp T, Matharu BK, et al. Complement C3 variant and the risk of age-related macular degeneration. N Engl J Med 2007; 357: 553–61.

34. Holz FG, Bellman C, Staudt S, Schutt F, Volcker HE. Fundus autofluorescence and development of geographic atrophy in age-related macular degeneration. Invest Ophthalmol Vis Sci 2001; 42: 1051–6.

35. Spaide RF, Curcio CA. Drusen characterization with multimodal imaging. Retina 2010; 30: 1441–54.

36. Solbach U, Keilhauer C, Knabben H, Wolf S. Imaging of retinal autofluorescence in patients with age-related macular degeneration. Retina 1997; 17: 385–9.

37. Sunness JS, Ziegler MD, Applegate CA. Issues in quantifying atrophic macular disease using retinal autofluorescence. Retina 2006; 26: 666–72.

38. Bindewald A, Schmitz-Valckenberg S, Jorzik JJ, et al. Classification of abnormal fundus autofluorescence patterns in the junctional zone of geographic atrophy in patients with age related macular degeneration. Br J Ophthalmol 2005; 89: 874–8.

39. Bindewald A, Bird AC, Dandekar SS, et al. Classification of fundus autofluorescence patterns in early age-related macular disease. Invest Ophthalmol Vis Sci 2005; 46: 3309–14.

40. Holz FG, Bellmann C, Margaritidis M, et al. Patterns of increased in vivo fundus autofluorescence in the junctional zone of geographic atrophy of the retinal pigment epithelium associated with age-related macular degeneration. Graefes Arch Clin Exp Ophthalmol 1999; 237: 145–52.

41. Robson AG, Moreland JD, Pauleikhoff D, et al. Macular pigment density and distribution: comparison of fundus autofluorescence with minimum motion photometry. Vision Res 2003; 43: 1765–75.

42. Schmitz-Valckenberg S, Bultmann S, Dreyhaupt J, et al. Fundus autofluorescence and fundus perimetry in the junctional zone of geographic atrophy in patients with age-related macular degeneration. Invest Ophthalmol Vis Sci 2004; 45: 4470–6.

43. Meleth AD, Mettu P, Agron E, et al. Changes in retinal sensitivity in geographic atrophy progression as measured by microperimetry. Invest Ophthalmol Vis Sci 2011; 52: 1119–26.

44. Scholl HP, Bellmann C, Dandekar SS, Bird AC, Fitzke FW. Photopic and scotopic fine matrix mapping of retinal areas of increased fundus autofluorescence in patients with age-related maculopathy. Invest Ophthalmol Vis Sci 2004; 45: 574–83.

45. Schmitz-Valckenberg S, Jorzik J, Unnebrink K, Holz FG; FAM Study Group. Analysis of digital scanning laser ophthalmoscopy fundus autofluorescence images of geographic atrophy in advanced age-related macular degeneration. Graefes Arch Clin Exp Ophthalmol 2002; 240: 73–8.

46. Deckert A, Schmitz-Valckenberg S, Jorzik J, et al. Automated analysis of digital fundus autofluorescence images of geographic atrophy in advanced age-related macular degeneration using confocal scanning laser ophthalmoscopy (cSLO). BMC Ophthalmol 2005; 5: 8.

47. Dreyhaupt J, Mansmann U, Pritsch M, et al. Modelling the natural history of geographic atrophy in patients with age-related macular degeneration. Ophthalmic Epidemiol 2005; 12: 353–62.

48. Schmitz-Valckenberg S, Bindewald-Wittich A, Dolar-Szczasny J, et al. Correlation between the area of increased autofluorescence surrounding geographic atrophy and disease progression in patients with AMD. Invest Ophthalmol Vis Sci 2006; 47: 2648–54.

49. Holz FG, Bindewald-Wittich A, Fleckenstein M, et al. Progression of geographic atrophy and impact of fundus autofluorescence patterns in age-related macular degeneration. Am J Ophthalmol 2007; 143: 463–72.

50. Schatz H, McDonald HR. Atrophic macular degeneration. Rate of spread of geographic atrophy and visual loss. Ophthalmology 1989; 96: 1541–51.

51. Hwang JC, Chan JW, Chang S, Smith RT. Predictive value of fundus autofluorescence for development of geographic atrophy in age-related macular degeneration. Invest Ophthalmol Vis Sci 2006; 47: 2655–61.

52. Einbock W, Moessner A, Schnurrbusch UF, Holz FG, Wolf S; FAM Study Group. Changes in fundus autofluorescence in patients with age-related maculopathy. Correlation to visual function: a prospective study. Graefes Arch Clin Exp Ophthalmol 2005; 243: 300–5.

53. Dandekar SS, Jenkins SA, Peto T, et al. Autofluorescence imaging of choroidal neovascularization due to age-related macular degeneration. Arch Ophthalmol 2005; 123: 1507–13.

54. Vaclavik V, Vujosevic S, Dandekar SS, et al. Autofluorescence imaging in age-related macular degeneration complicated by choroidal neovascularization: a prospective study. Ophthalmology 2008; 115: 342–6.

55. Karadimas P, Bouzas EA. Fundus autofluorescence imaging in serous and drusenoid pigment epithelial detachments associated with age-related macular degeneration. Am J Ophthalmol 2005; 140: 1163–5.

56. Framme C, Bunse A, Sofroni R, et al. Fundus autofluorescence before and after photodynamic therapy for choroidal neovascularization secondary to age-related macular degeneration. Ophthalmic Surg Lasers Imaging 2006; 37: 406–14.

57. McBain VA, Townend J, Lois N. Fundus autofluorescence in exudative age-related macular degeneration. Br J Ophthalmol 2007; 91: 491–6.

58. Parish CA, Hashimoto M, Nakanishi K, Dillon J, Sparrow J. Isolation and one-step preparation of A2E and iso-A2E, fluorophores from human retinal pigment epithelium. Proc Natl Acad Sci U S A 1998; 95: 14609–13.

Microperimetry and psychophysical testing to aid in the determination of progression of age-related macular degeneration

Dinah Zur, Oded Ohana, and Anat Loewenstein

INTRODUCTION

Early detection and treatment of choroidal neovascularization (CNV) is crucial for achieving better visual outcomes and avoiding permanent vision loss. This fact was shown for all currently employed treatment strategies (1–4). A subgroup analysis of 24-month data from the MARINA study found initial visual acuity and CNV lesion size to be important predictors for final visual acuity (5). The development of highly effective anti-VEGF therapies made early detection of neovascular lesions even more important.

Visual acuity testing is still considered the gold standard for visual testing in clinical practice. However, it does not represent all qualities of visual function and notably misses parameters causing impairments in daily life, such as difficulties in reading caused by (para)central scotomas. A complete evaluation, rather, includes a combination of visual acuity, contrast sensitivity, dark adaptation, perimetry, and microperimetry. Conventional visual field testing is inadequate in evaluating macular disease as it requires foveal and stable fixation in order to achieve accurate results. In the case of extrafoveal fixation, fixation losses will be registered but the map will not be adapted to the real fixation. During testing, eye movements due to instable fixation can cause difficulty in finding the correct scotoma size and location.

Patient self-assessment for progression of AMD is usually done with an Amsler grid. However, an Amsler grid has low specificity and sensitivity and often fails to recognize disease progression from non-neovascular to neovascular AMD (6). Preferential hyperacuity perimetry (PHP) presents a promising alternative for patient self-monitoring (7–9).

Microperimetry (or fundus perimetry) offers a reliable method of visual field testing in patients with unstable or eccentric fixation due to macular disorders (10). It provides correlation between retinal pathologies and functional defects (11). Accurate examination conditions are given even for patients with small retinal or choroidal lesions and poor fixation.

MICROPERIMETRY: TECHNICAL DEVELOPMENT, INSTRUMENTS, AND APPLICATION IN AMD

The technique of microperimetry is based on the testing of retinal sensitivity. Different thresholds for light sensitivity are determined and integrated in the fundus display.

Furthermore, characteristics of fixation are measured, by defining the exact position and stability of fixation location and size, as well as the location of scotomas. These parameters make it a useful tool for follow-up and evaluation of therapeutic success.

Scanning Laser Ophthalmoscope

The scanning laser ophthalmoscope (SLO) was the first instrument which combined static perimetry testing with simultaneous fundus control. SLO measures the reflectance of light at individual successive points on the fundus, scanned by a laser in a raster pattern over an area of $33°$ by $21°$. A helium neon laser beam (632.8 nm) and an infrared diode laser (780 nm) are simultaneously projected on the fundus. Background and stimulus illuminations are adjusted. Images of different size and stimulus are projected on the retina while the fundus image is captured. The result is a card of sensitivity in decibels (dB) or colors including data about fixation area and characteristics and retinal threshold. The original SLO is no longer available, mainly because it did not support automated examinations which are needed for comparison with follow-up examinations (12).

SLO Microperimetry

Rohrschneider et al. developed an advanced software which allows for automated static threshold fundus perimetry and kinetic perimetry based on the SLO technique (13). Examination time was markedly reduced. Sunness et al. proposed a landmark-driven SLO microperimeter which provides an accurate and repeatable examination of retinal sensitivity at specific locations (14).

Assisted by landmark settings, a stimulus is projected at a predefined point on the retina. Stimulus size, time, and intensity can be varied. The test is started with supra-threshold values in order to shorten the examination time; intensity is then adapted relative to the surrounding threshold (15). A normative database is available, showing that light sensitivity and stability of fixation decrease with age even in healthy subjects (16).

In cases of small pathologic macular findings with reduced stability of fixation, manual microperimetry provides more accurate detection of scotoma borders (17). The stimulus is moved by the technician until recognized by the patient; the fundus image is then digitized. An automated kinetic perimetry is performed in a centrifugal and centripetal direction. It is less exact in patients with decreased fixation stability as there is no correction of eye movements (15).

SLO microperimetry is a helpful tool in the detection of AMD progression. An initial mild decrease in central retinal sensitivity can be noticed before deterioration of visual acuity, followed by progressive instability of fixation and finally formation of an absolute central scotoma with eccentric fixation.

MP1 Microperimeter

The MP1 Microperimeter (Nidek, Gamagori, Japan) is another fully automated microperimeter which combines objective fundus imaging with subjective computerized perimetry. The fundus image is observed with an infrared fundus camera; perimetry is performed using a liquid crystal display. Size and intensity of the stimulus can be varied. The stimulus is presented for 100–200 milliseconds. If the stimulus is not seen even with brightest intensity, an absolute scotoma is present. A relative scotoma goes along with reduced threshold for light sensitivity.

The MP1 microperimeter allows for a fast, accurate, reliable functional fundus examination. Its main advantage is its automatic eye tracking under real-time conditions, which enables exact presentation of the stimulus at the predefined retinal location. MP1 has good reliability, allowing examiner-independent measurements in healthy patients as well as in patients with impaired fixation due to AMD (18). Midena et al. showed significantly higher thresholds with MP1 testing compared with standard perimetry and a low mean standard deviation (SD) of intraindividual variation (19). A comparison revealed comparable results between MP1 and SLO perimetry in the detection of central sensitivity loss and fixation behavior. Yet, MP1 microperimetry facilitated examination and allowed testing in a larger area ($36° \times 44°$) (20). Precise automated follow-up is possible, irrespective of baseline fixation. At the end of the examination the clinician receives a fundus image with the integrated functional results.

MP1 microperimetry also provides an option for automated kinetic perimetry. The stimulus moves centripetally or centrifugally until seen by the patient or until it reaches a maximum extent of eccentricity. As with SLO, there is no correction for eye movements in the kinetic program which impairs its accuracy.

AMD progression with development of subfoveal CNV can be reliably detected by MP1 microperimetry. A progressive deterioration of retinal fixation and sensitivity is recorded, followed by the development of extrafoveal fixation and the formation of a dense scotoma. These changes are functionally more limiting for the patient than visual acuity deterioration.

Microperimetry: Performance and Analysis

In both instruments the course of examination is similar: First, a stimulus is projected on the blind spot in predefined intervals in order to test patient reliability. The scanning field should be defined in a manner that

allows identification of even small scotoma but without using unnecessary test points. The baseline situation should be recorded for follow-up purposes. In most cases, automated threshold techniques are preferred. However, extensive scotoma can be recorded by kinetic testing with short examination times. Results are displayed in dB or as interpolated color maps as shown in Figures 17.1 and 17.2.

Evaluation of fixation provides valuable information about macular function. In the clinic, direct ophthalmoscopy is an available modality for subjective testing of fixation but lacks the option of documentation. Modified fundus cameras have little clinical value for this purpose as they use high illumination levels (21). Microperimetry provides information about fixation location and stability over time. The location of fixation is defined as fixation position in relation to the center of the foveal avascular zone (FAZ). Fixation stability is the ability of the eye to retain fixation in a "referred retinal location" (PRL). The patient is asked to look at a fixation point which is projected on a background for a certain time

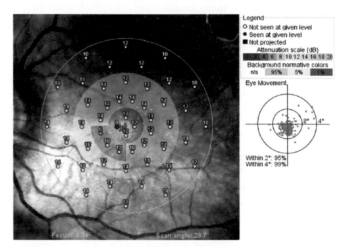

Figure 17.1 SLO microperimetry of the left eye from a 63 year-old AMD patient with stable fixation (>75% of fixation points lie within the central 2° around the center of fixation) and reduced central retinal sensitivity.

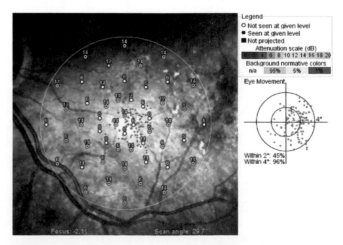

Figure 17.2 Microperimetry of the left eye from a 64 year-old AMD patient. Fixation is relative instable (<75% of fixation points lie within the central 2° but >75% lie within the central 4° around the centre of fixation).

(usually 60 seconds) under mesopic light levels. A standardized circular fixation area of 2° (700 μm) diameter is used to determine the location of fixation (22). Shifting of fundus details in comparison to the initial reference fundus image is detected by a tracking system. Hence, fixation position and stability are recorded over time. In case of deep or absolute central scotoma, patients will shift the location of fixation and develop a new extrafoveal PRL. Alternating fixation can be observed during the process of developing a PRL (23).

Fixation location is classified into predominantly central fixation, poor central fixation, and predominantly eccentric fixation (i.e., >50%, >25–50%, and <25% of preferred fixation points lie within the central fixation, respectively). Fixation stability is classified into stable fixation (>75% of fixation points lie within the central 2° around the center of fixation), relative instable fixation (<75% of fixation points lie within the central 2° but >75% lie within the central 4° around the center of fixation), and instable fixation (<75% of fixation points lie within the central 4° around the center of fixation) (22).

"Bivariate contour ellipse calculated area" (BCEA) allows quantification of fixation stability. X and y values reflecting the horizontal and vertical eye positions are obtained and used to calculate the BCEA in minutes of arc. A two-dimensional ellipse is created and represents the portion of retinal surface which is within the center of the targeted imaged at least 68% of the time. Follow-up examinations provide accurate localization of prior tested retinal points—independent of changed fixation.

Integration of different retinal imaging modalities into the MP1 microperimeter is possible and enables exact and congruent display between threshold maps and fixation parameters on the original image.

Microperimetry and AMD Progression

Neovascular AMD is associated with deteriorating retinal fixation and retinal sensitivity. Only later in the course of the disease is decreased visual acuity detected. Microperimetry is able to detect a decline in fixation stability, loss of central fixation, and impaired retinal sensitivity. In an early stage of the disease—before even advanced imaging modalities are able to display neovascular changes—the macula is already frequently unable to sustain foveal fixation. Development of eccentric fixation appears relatively early with neovascular AMD and is distinguishable from other etiologies (12). Midena et al. tested 118 AMD eyes with subfoveal CNV with the MP1 microperimeter. In this study, 63% had eccentric fixation, 15% had poor central fixation, and 22% had central fixation. In 63% a dense central scotoma was found. There was no relation between lesion type and fixation pattern (10). Fuji et al. found better results regarding fixation patterns in 179 eyes with subfoveal CNV using the SLO (24). 89% of eyes with less than 3 months of symptoms had predominantly central fixation versus 41% of eyes with more than 6 months of symptoms. In 15 eyes of patients who chose not to receive treatment and were followed up for 18 months, central fixation deteriorated during the course of follow-up. The development of retinal sensitivity loss

was heterogeneous. Even with profound loss of parafoveal retinal sensitivity up to an absolute dense scotoma, a preserved small island of foveal sensitivity allowed preservation of central fixation. On the other hand, an absolute foveal scotoma even with good parafoveal sensitivity resulted in eccentric and unstable fixation. However, eccentric location of fixation can still present with relatively stable fixation. Early morphologic changes explain patient's symptoms such as metamorphopsia and blurred vision due to subfoveal CNV. These changes are related to impaired photoreceptor function. The finding in the work of Fuji, that the subgroup of eyes with symptoms for less than three months presented mostly with preserved fixation characteristics, suggests viable foveal photoreceptors in the early course of CNV formation. The persistence of those morphologic changes results in progressive and irreversible damage, observable as development of a new extrafoveal PRL. After longer duration of symptoms, eccentric fixation becomes stable (10). This observation implies that the establishment of stable eccentric fixation needs time and requires cortical adaptation.

SELF-ASSESSMENT OF MACULAR FUNCTION
Amsler Grid

Although its role in the detection of AMD progression has been questioned many times, the Amsler grid is in routine use. The Amsler grid, introduced in 1947, was the first method for patient self-monitoring of the central visual field in macular diseases (25). The test uses a suprathreshold stimulus and evaluates 10° of visual field surrounding the fixation. Its main clinical application was to detect the possible appearance of CNV in non-neovascular AMD. Yet, many patients fail to identify disease progression (6). The two main reasons why Amsler grid fails are noncompliance and the subjective nature of the test. The ability to assess scotomas and metamorphopsia psychophysically is limited (26). Patients are frequently not aware of small visual field defects outside of central vision. This can be partly explained by perceptual completion which leads to imperfect filling-in of scotomas which is a dynamic and fluctuating process (27). Unstable and eccentric fixation may add to poor test performance (28). The crowding effect decreases test sensitivity and reduces its reliability (29). Furthermore, the non-interactive nature of the test makes it unsuitable for monitoring, because the quality of test performance and reliability cannot be controlled. Patient compliance to perform the Amsler grid at home on a regular basis is low (30).

Compared with SLO microperimetry, Schuchard et al. found that Amsler grid fails to detect about half of the existing scotomas (31). For scotomas of 6° or less in diameter, up to 87% of threshold scotomas were not detected by Amsler grid testing.

Modified Amsler Grid

A number of alternatives have been developed in an effort to either improve or replace the Amsler grid. However, Augustin et al. showed that the sensitivity of the original Amsler grid (white lines on a black background) is significantly better than that of a modified version (black lines on a white background) in the detection of visual disturbances in AMD patients (32). The sensitivity of the original Amsler grid can be improved by lowering the contrast of the printed charts which helps detect central field defects (33). Viewing the test through a cross-polarizing filter which creates low luminance conditions increases both the number of defects found and the total area of these defects by approximately a factor of 5 (34). A three-dimensional (3D) computer-automated version of the Amsler grid is available. Patients are instructed to trace the area of the scotoma with their finger on an Amsler grid raster with different contrast levels displayed on a touch-screen monitor. The clinician receives a 3D display of the visual field showing the extent of the scotoma and retinal contrast sensitivity (35). A study examined 41 eyes of 25 patients with neovascular and non-neovascular AMD with the 3D computerized Amsler grid. Visual fields depicted central scotomas with scallop-shaped borders and step-like patterns. Non-neovascular AMD eyes showed rather steep slopes, whereas neovascular eyes showed shallow slopes (36).

Still, all of these tests are limited by the characteristics of the original Amsler grid which have been discussed in detail.

Preferential Hyperacuity Perimetry

The preferential hyperacuity perimetry (PHP, Notal Vision Ltd., Tel Aviv, Israel) is a computerized psychophysical test which was developed for monitoring of non-neovascular AMD patients to achieve early diagnosis of CNV by detection and quantification of metamorphopsia. PHP uses hyperacuity stimuli based on the principle of Vernier acuity, that is the human ability to perceive minute differences in the relative spatial localization of two objects in space (7). The technology has been described in detail elsewhere (37,38), but in principle it is based on the phenomenon of hyperacuity.

Briefly, the patient is presented with a pattern of dotted lines projected for 160 milliseconds to the central 14° of the visual field. In each line there is an artificial distortion of different extent. If a line is presented at a location corresponding to a CNV lesion, the patient perceives a pathologic distortion. The artificial distortion then serves as a competitive stimulus to the pathologic distortion (hyperacuity defect), and attention competition between the artificial and the pathologic distortion takes place in the patient's brain. When there is a larger stimulus present, the brain ignores the smaller one. Using this phenomenon, PHP assesses the extent of the pathologic distortion by varying sizes of the artificial distortion and analyzing the patient's response. The test takes between three to four minutes per eye. At the end of the test, a visual field map is generated, analyzed, and compared with normative data; the probability of the presence of CNV is calculated.

The PHP has been shown to have much potential in the early detection of CNV in AMD patients. The first PHP study, published in 2003, compared the PHP with an Amsler grid in the detection of AMD under

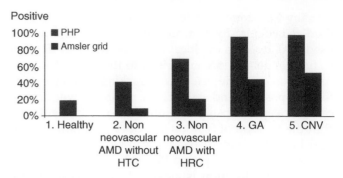

Figure 17.3 Comparison of detection rate between the Amsler grid and the PHP for detecting various categories of AMD.

supervised conditions in the office. One hundred and eight AMD patients and 51 age-matched control patients without retinal disease underwent PHP testing. Patients with different AMD disease stages ranging from early AMD to CNV and GA were included. Of the 32 patients with CNV (37), 30 (94%) had positive findings on the PHP compared with 11 (34%) on the Amsler grid.

A multicenter study was conducted in order to confirm these positive results (39). This study included 150 patients in five groups: healthy eyes, non-neovascular AMD without high-risk characteristics (HRC), non-neovascular AMD with HRC, geographic atrophy, and CNV. For PHP, a sensitivity of 68% and specificity of 81% were found for differentiating patients with healthy retina from those with AMD, significantly greater than that of Amsler grid (p < 0.001). As displayed in Figure 17.3, a similar significant difference was found when analyzing each group separately. The high sensitivity of the test apparently contributed to the relatively high rate of false-positive results for individuals with healthy retina.

Hence, the algorithm was amended and the device was further refined to differentiate between patients with intermediate AMD (i.e., at risk for developing CNV) and those with a recent-onset of CNV. In a study to valuate whether the PHP (PreView PHP®, Carl Zeiss Meditec, Dublin, California, USA) can be used as a tool for monitoring patients at risk for developing CNV (38), 122 patients (57 with intermediate AMD and 65 with untreated neovascular AMD diagnosed within the last 60 days) were enrolled. Using PHP, the sensitivity to detect newly diagnosed CNV was 82%, whereas the specificity to differentiate newly diagnosed CNV from intermediate AMD was 88%.

In these prior studies, PHP was performed in a clinical setting under supervision that ensures optimal conditions (fixed distance from display, single-eye test, adjusted refraction, and illumination). In order to make the device suitable for unsupervised home-monitoring and testing by elderly patients, a number of modifications were required. The ForeseeHome® (Notal Vision) was specifically developed for this purpose (Fig. 17.4). A multicenter study tested this device in patients with intermediate AMD and recent-onset neovascular AMD (40).

Results showed that the home device could distinguish between patients with newly diagnosed CNV and

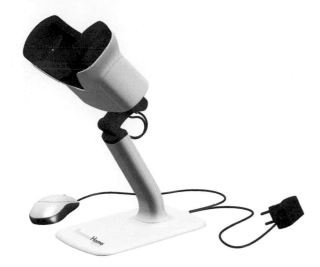

Figure 17.4 The PHP home device (ForeseeHome).

intermediate AMD with an average sensitivity and specificity of 85%. This accuracy is comparable with that obtained with the professional device used under supervised conditions in the office. Moreover, it was shown that specific lesion characteristics had no effect on the specificity of the test.

This home monitor is unique and promises reliable early detection of disease progression. Still, there are some limitations. A false-positive rate of 15% means that the patient will be alerted by a false alarm if the test is frequently performed. The false-positive rate can be decreased by lowering the sensitivity at the expense of true-positive results. Lowering the sensitivity can also increase detection time—still acceptable when held within an adequate time frame. Another limitation is the prerequisite of experience with a computer mouse in the elderly population.

Especially in situations when ophthalmoscopic examination of AMD patients is troublesome this home monitor turns out to be a helpful tool. The use of such a device in growing numbers will most probably lead to better detection rates, earlier referral to therapy, and better treatment outcomes for neovascular AMD patients.

ADDITIONAL PSYCHOPHYSICAL TEST IN AMD

The currently available therapeutic interventions for AMD mainly reside in nutritional supplements for intermediate AMD with the goal of delaying progression of the disease and in the treatment of neovascular AMD - currently by anti-VEGF therapies. Final visual outcome after long-term therapy was shown to be better with higher baseline VA (41,42). Therefore efforts are made to detect the transformation to neovascular AMD as early as possible.

Early macular changes in non-neovascular AMD are associated with only a modest decrease in VA which is not easily detectable (43). Visual deterioration associated with advanced AMD is frequently the result of extensive photoreceptor dysfunction, rather than a progressive process, an observation that can be explained by the

sampling theorem and the Nyquist frequency (44). The sampling theorem states that a signal can be reconstructed without loss of information as long as the signal has no frequencies above half the sampling frequency. Therefore, a 50% decrease in VA actually represents a sampling density decrease of 75%, meaning that the majority of photoreceptors in the fovea must become dysfunctional before significant loss of VA is evident. This observation may explain why the value of VA as a tool for detecting disease progression in AMD is limited.

Several psychophysical tests reflect visual deterioration in the early stages of AMD. Contrast sensitivity, visual adaptation, central visual field, and color discrimination were shown to predict progression of early and intermediate to advanced AMD (45).

Non-Neovascular AMD

While there is no currently available treatment for non-neovascular AMD patients, early detection of progression of the disease is crucial for preserving visual function. Several psychophysical and microperimetric tests were found beneficial in monitoring progression.

Low contrast visual acuity (LCVA) is assessed using low or variable contrast letter charts. The letters are presented at relatively low contrast, with letter size decreasing down the chart. LCVA has been shown to deteriorate with age. Still, the deterioration is larger in AMD patients. There is a significant change in LCVA scores between AMD patients and controls. One study reported an inverse correlation between number of letters read correctly and drusen size (46).

Contrast sensitivity (CS) measures the amount of difference needed by the patient to visualize a light-dark transition. The threshold is defined as the smallest difference between shades of gray detected by the patient. The CS is the reciprocal of the threshold. Data suggest a reduction in CS in AMD with association between disease severity and deteriorating CS function; AMD patients with focal hyperpigmentation and RPE atrophy have significantly worse CS function. However, this test fails to recognize disease progression to neovascular AMD (47). Still, the test holds great value in detecting visual disturbances that interfere with a patient's vision-related quality of life. Cummings et al. found that a decrease in CS is associated with an increased risk of hip fractures in women over the age of 65 years (48). Therefore, CS function is still a valuable tool in the evaluation of AMD patients and may be helpful in order to refer patients to obtain vision aids at the proper time.

Flicker contrast sensitivity tests assess the patient's response to a flickering stimulus. These tests are considerably robust to the refractive status of the patient and to the spatial features of the stimulus. A recent study which evaluated psychophysical testing in early AMD patients versus controls found that 14 Hz flicker coupled with a photostress recovery test detected 71% of early AMD (49). Flickering perimetry exposes foveal defects in intermediate AMD better than do static targets with high sensitivity and specificity (50).

Because of the impairment of the central visual field in AMD, **motion perception** of objects in the near periphery is of great importance in these patients, especially for the assessment of driving ability. Motion contrast sensitivity was shown to be reduced in early AMD patients, not only in the macula but up to 20° eccentric to the fovea compared with age-matched controls (51).

Progression to Neovascular AMD

Since AMD treatments mainly target neovascular AMD, an extensive effort has been made to detect such disease progression as early as possible. Several psychophysical tests are available for detection of disease progression with varying sensitivity and specificity.

Mayer et al. showed that **flicker modulation sensitivity** at two frequencies discriminated fellow non-affected eyes from both patients with neovascular AMD and from healthy older eyes with 100% accuracy. Seven of 16 eyes of the AMD group converted to the neovascular stage during follow-up. These two groups could also be discriminated with 100% accuracy, while fundus appearance assessed with a grading system did not reach an accuracy at better than chance levels (52).

Several studies examined **dark adaptation** (DA) patterns in AMD patients. A prolongation of DA time and a decrease in DA sensitivity were observed in AMD patients compared with age-matched controls. Sunness et al. found that DA sensitivity was a good predictor for AMD progression to geographic atrophy, RPE detachment, and CNV in a cohort of 18 patients (53). The degree of loss of foveal dark-adapted sensitivity predicted which patients developed advanced AMD with 100% sensitivity and 92% specificity. In contrast, the presence of high-risk drusen as a predictor had a sensitivity of 100% but only 55% specificity. In a later work, Sunness et al. found a high association between functional foveal compromise (especially slow rates of dark adaptation) and high-risk fundus characteristics in eyes whose fellow eyes had neovascular AMD. Still, the authors emphasize that this association does not imply that these functional tests can themselves be adapted for prognostic use. Prospective studies are necessary to determine their utility (54).

CONCLUSION

Microperimetry and a number of self-monitoring tests are available for identifying AMD progression. Ongoing development of modern technologies allows detection of more subtle defects, quantitative analysis, and accurate follow-up. Application of these tools in clinical practice and patient's everyday life raises hope for earlier detection of disease progression and hereby better chances to preserve vision.

SUMMARY POINTS

- Early detection and treatment of choroidal neovascularization is crucial for achieving better visual outcomes and avoiding permanent vision loss.

- Microperimetry offers a reliable method of visual field testing in patients with unstable or eccentric fixation due to macular disorders and provides correlation between retinal pathologies and functional defects.
- Self-assessment with an Amsler grid frequently fails to identify disease progression.
- The preferential hyperacuity perimeter is highly specific and sensitive in identifying new choroidal neovascularization.
- A device suitable for unsupervised home-monitoring has been developed.
- The value of further psychophysical tests in the recognition of AMD progression is discussed.

REFERENCES

1. Macular Photocoagulation Study Group. Visual outcome after laser photocoagulation for subfoveal choroidal neovascularization secondary to age-related macular degeneration. Arch Ophthalmol 1994; 112: 480–8.
2. The Treatment of Age-related Macular Degeneration with Photodynamic Therapy Study Group. Verteporfin in photodynamic therapy study group. effect of lesion size, visual acuity, and lesion composition on visual acuity change with and without verteporfin therapy for choroidal neovascularization secondary to age-related macular degeneration: TAP and VIP report No. 1. Am J Ophthalmol 2003; 136: 407–18.
3. The VEGF Inhibition Study in Ocular Neovascularization Clinical Trial Group. Enhanced efficacy associated with early treatment of neovascular age-related macular degeneration with pegaptanib sodium: an exploratory analysis. Retina 2005; 25: 815–27.
4. The MARINA Study Group. Subgroup analysis of the MARINA study of ranibizumab in neovascular age-related macular degeneration. Ophthalmology 2007; 114: 246–52.
5. The MARINA Study Group. Improved vision-related function after ranibizumab treatment of neovascular agerelated macular degeneration: results of a randomized clinical trial. Arch Ophthalmol 2007; 125: 1460–9.
6. Zaidi FH, Cheong-Leen R, Gair EJ, et al. The Amsler chart is of doubtful value in retinal screening for early laser therapy of subretinal membranes: the West London Survey. Eye 2004; 18: 503–8.
7. Goldstein M, Loewenstein A, Barak A, et al. Preferential Hyperacuity Perimeter Research Group. Results of a multicenter clinical trial to evaluate the preferential hyperacuity perimeter for detection of age-related macular degeneration. Retina 2005; 25: 296–303.
8. Loewenstein A, Malach R, Goldstein M, et al. Replacing the amsler grid: a new method for monitoring patients with age-related macular degeneration. Ophthalmology 2003; 110: 966–70.
9. The Preferential Hyperacuity Perimeter Research Group. Results of a multicenter clinical trial to evaluate the preferential hyperacuity perimeter for detection of age-related macular degeneration. Retina 2005; 25: 296–303.
10. Midena E, Radin PP, Pilotto E, et al. Fixation pattern and macular sensitivity in eyes with subfoveal choroidal

neovascularization secondary to age-related macular degeneration. a microperimetry study. Sem Ophthalmol 2004; 19: 55–61.

11. Timberlake GT, Mainster MA, Webb RH, et al. Retinal localization of scotomata by scanning laser ophthalmoscopy. Invest Ophthalmol Vis Sci 1982; 22: 91–7.

12. Midena E, Pilotto E. Microperimetry. In: Holz FG, Pauleikhoff D, Spaide RF, et al. eds. Age-Related Macular Degeneration. Berlin Heidelberg: Springer, 2011: 178–92.

13. Rohrschneider K, Fendrich T, Becker M, et al. Static fundus perimetry using the scanning laser ophthalmoscope with an automated threshold strategy. Graefe's Arch Clin Exp Ophthalmol 1995; 233: 743–9.

14. Sunness JS, Schuchard RA, Shan N, et al. Landmark-driven fundus perimetry. using the scanning laser ophthalmoscope. Invest Ophthalmol Vis Sci 1995; 36: 1863–74.

15. Rohrschneider K. Microperimetry in macular disease. In: Holz FG, Spaide RF, eds. Medical Retina. Berlin Heidelberg: Springer, 2007: 1–20.

16. Rohrschneider K, Becker M, Schumacher N, et al. Normal values for fundus perimetry with the scanning laser ophthalmoscope. Am J Ophthalmol 1998; 126: 52–8.

17. Rohrschneider K, Becker M, Fendrich T, et al. Kinetische funduskontrollierte perimetrie mit dem scanning-laser-ophthalmoskop. Klin Monatsbl Augenheilkd 1995; 207: 102–10.

18. Weingessel B, Sacu S, Vecsei-Marlovits PV, et al. Interexaminer and intraexaminer reliability of the microperimeter MP-1. Eye 2009; 23: 1052–8.

19. Midena E, Radin PP, Convento E, et al. Macular automatic fundus perimetry threshold versus standard perimetry threshold. Eur J Ophthalmol 2007; 17: 63–8.

20. Rohrschneider K, Springer C, Bueltmann S, et al. Microperimetry – comparison between the microperimeter 1 and scanning laser ophthalmoscope-fundus perimetry. Am J Ophthalmol 2005; 139: 125–34.

21. Crone RA. Fundus television in the study of fixation disturbances. Ophthalmologica 1975; 171: 51–2.

22. Fujii Gy, De Juan E Jr, Humayun MS, et al. Characteristics of visual loss by scanning laser opthalmoscope microperimetry in eyes with subfoveal choroidal neovascularization secondary to age-related macular degeneration. Am J Ophthalmol 2003; 136: 1067–78.

23. Sunness JS, Applegate CA, Haselwood D, et al. Fixation patterns and reading rates in eyes with central scotomas from advanced atrophic age-related macular degeneration and Stargardt's disease. Ophthalmology 1996; 103: 1458–66.

24. Fujii GY, De Juan E, Humayun MS, et al. Characteristics of visual loss by scanning laser opthalmoscope microperimetry in eyes with subfoveal choroidal neovascularization secondary to age-related macular degeneration. Am J Ophthalmol 2003; 136: 1067–78.

25. Marmor MF. A brief history of macular grids: From Thomas Reis to Edward Munch and Marc Amsler. Surv Ophthalmol 2000; 44: 343–53.

26. Fine AM, Elman MJ, Ebert JE, et al. Earliest symptoms caused by neovascular membranes in the macula. Arch Ophthalmol 1986; 104: 513–14.

27. Achard OA, Safran AB, Duret FC, et al. Role of the completion phenomenon in the evaluation of amsler grid results. Am J Ophthalmol 1995; 120: 322–9.

28. Crossland MD, Culham LE, Kabanarou SA, et al. Preferred retinal locus development in patients with macular disease. Ophthalmology 2005; 112: 1579–85.

29. Parkes L, Lund J, Angelucci A. Compulsory averaging of crowded orientation signals in human vision. Nat Neurosci 2001; 4: 739–44.

30. Fine AM, Elman MJ, Ebert JE, et al. Earliest symptoms caused by neovascular membranes in the macula. Arch Ophthalmol 1986; 104: 513–14.

31. Schuchard RA. Validity and interpretation of amsler grid reports. Arch Ophthalmol 1993; 111: 776–80.

32. Augustin AJ, Offermann JL, Lutz J, et al. Comparsion of the original amsler grid with the modified amsler grid results for patients with age-related macular degeneration. Retina 2005; 25: 443–5.

33. Cheng AS, Vingrys AJ. Visual losses in early age-related maculopathy. Optom Vis Sci 1993; 70: 89–96.

34. Wall M, Sadun AA. Threshold amsler grid testing: cross polarizing lenses enhance yield. Arch Ophthalmol 1986; 104: 520–3.

35. Fink W, Sadun A. Three-dimensional computerautomated threshold amsler grid test. J Biomed Opt 2004; 9: 149–53.

36. Nazemi PP, Fink W, Lim JI, et al. Scotomas of age-related macular degeneration detected and characterized by means of a novel three-dimensional computer-automated visual field test. Retina 2005; 25: 446–53.

37. Loewenstein A, Malach R, Goldstein M, et al. Replacing the amsler grid: a new method for monitoring patients with age-related macular degeneration. Ophthalmology 2003; 110: 966–70.

38. Alster Y, Bressler NM, Bressler SB, et al.; Preferential Hyperacuity Perimetry Research Group. Preferential hyperacuity perimeter for detecting choroidal neovascularization study. Ophthalmology 2005; 112: 1758–65.

39. Loewenstein A, Ferencz JR, Lang Y, et al. Toward earlier detection of choroidal neovascularization secondary to age-related macular degeneration: multicenter evaluation of a preferential hyperacuity perimeter designed as a home device. Retina 2010; 30: 1058–64.

40. Goldstein M, Loewenstein A, Barak A, et al. Results of a multicenter clinical trial to evaluate the preferential hyperacuity perimeter for detection of age-related macular degeneration. Retina 2005; 25: 296–303.

41. Kaiser PK, Brown DM, Zhang K, et al. Ranibizumab for predominantly classic neovascular age-related macular degeneration: subgroup analysis of first-year ANCHOR results. Am J Ophthalmol 2007; 144: 850–7.

42. Boyer DS, Antoszyk AN, Awh CC, et al. Subgroup analysis of the MARINA study of ranibizumab in neovascular age-related macular degeneration. Ophthalmology 2007; 114: 246–52.

43. Lamoureux EL, Mitchell P, Rees G, et al. Impact of early and late age-related macular degeneration on vision-specific functioning. Br J Ophthalmol 2011; 95: 666–70.

44. Geller AM, Sieving PA, Green DG. Effect on grating identification of sampling with degenerate arrays. J Opt Soc Am A Opt Image Sci 1992; 9: 472–7.

45. Neelam K, Nolan J, Chakravarthy U, Beatty S. Psychophysical function in age-related maculopathy. Surv Ophthalmol 2009; 54: 167–210.

46. Kleiner RC, Enger C, Alexander MF, Fine SL. Contrast sensitivity in age-related macular degeneration. Arch Ophthalmol 1988; 106: 55–7.

47. Midena E, Degli Angeli C, Blarzino MC, Valenti M, Segato T. Macular function impairment in eyes with early age-related macular degeneration. Invest Ophthalmol Vis Sci 1997; 38: 469–77.

48. Cummings SR, Nevitt MC, Browner WS. Study of osteoporotic fractures research group. risk factors for hip fracture in white women. N Engl J Med 1995; 332: 767–73.

49. Dimitrov PN, Robman LD, Varsamidis M, et al. Visual function tests as potential biomarkers in age-related macular degeneration. Invest Ophthalmol Vis Sci 2011; 52: 9457–69.

50. Phipps JA, Dang TM, Vingrys AJ, et al. Flicker perimetry losses in age-related macular degeneration. Invest Ophthalmol Vis Sci 2004; 5: 3355–60.

51. Eisenbarth W, MacKeben M, Poggel DA, et al. Characteristics of dynamic processing in the visual field of patients with age-related maculopathy. Graefes Arch Clin Exp Ophthalmol 2008; 246: 27–37.

52. Mayer MJ, Ward B, Klein R, et al. Flicker sensitivity and fundus appearance in pre-exudative age-related maculopathy. Invest Ophthalmol Vis Sci 1994; 35: 1138–49.

53. Sunness JS, Massof RW, Johnson MA, et al. Diminished foveal sensitivity may predict the development of advanced age-related macular degeneration. Ophthalmology 1989; 96: 375–81.

54. Eisner A, Stoumbos VD, Klein ML, et al. Relations between fundus appearance and function. Eyes whose fellow eye has exudative age-related macular degeneration. Invest Ophthalmol Vis Sci 1991; 32: 8–20.

18

Laser photocoagulation for choroidal neovascularization

Catherine A. Cukras

INTRODUCTION

Until the initial Macular Photocoagulation Study (MPS) outcome data were published in June 1982, there were no reported treatments of proven benefit for patients with choroidal neovascularization (CNV) secondary to age-related macular degeneration (AMD). The MPS trials conducted from 1979 to 1994 showed that laser photocoagulation was preferable to observation for several categories of well-defined CNV based on the fluorescein angiographic location of the CNV with respect to the geometric center of the fovea, that is, extrafoveal, juxtafoveal, and subfoveal (1–5). The MPS publications also described the factors which limited the utility of laser photocoagulation treatment.

1. Only a small proportion of symptomatic AMD eyes met MPS eligibility criteria as being appropriate for laser treatment (6,7).
2. There was a high rate of persistent and recurrent leakage even after initial successful closure of the CNV (8,9).
3. Laser photocoagulation caused immediate and permanent damage to the retina in the area treated and this damage typically resulted in an immediate decrease in visual acuity (VA) (2).
4. Treated as well as untreated eyes continued to lose central vision over time, despite initial closure of the CNV in laser-treated eyes.

In addition, because laser photocoagulation is a focal treatment, there is no expected beneficial effect beyond the area of laser application. With the advent of safe and effective antiangiogenic therapies, it would appear that laser photocoagulation will have an extremely limited role in the management of CNV secondary to AMD. Thus, the following narrative is presented primarily for a historical perspective on how treatment for CNV secondary to AMD developed over the last quarter century.

EPIDEMIOLOGY AND NATURAL HISTORY

AMD is a leading cause of severe and irreversible central vision loss in the developed world among people over the age of 55 (10–13). Up to 90% of the severe vision loss in AMD is caused by CNV (14–16).

Before the MPS was initiated in 1979, there were several natural history studies which documented the unfavorable visual prognosis of eyes with untreated CNV secondary to both AMD and ocular histoplasmosis (17,18). These natural history data were substantiated by the visual outcomes of untreated eyes among participants in the MPS. In the MPS trial of juxtafoveal CNV, 65% of untreated eyes lost six or more lines of acuity after five years' follow-up, and 93% progressed from juxtafoveal to subfoveal CNV (4,19).

The initial component of the MPS evaluated argon laser photocoagulation in patients with extrafoveal CNV secondary to AMD. At the time, this trial was known as the Senile Macular Degeneration Study (SMDS). Eyes with extrafoveal CNV were assigned randomly to immediate argon laser treatment or to observation. By 18 months after enrollment, 60% of untreated eyes had lost six or more lines of VA. By one year after enrollment, fluorescein angiography showed that 73% of untreated eyes had progressed from extrafoveal to subfoveal CNV (20).

In 1985, Guyer et al. reported that among 92 AMD patients with subfoveal neovascular lesions, 64% lost six or more lines of vision within two years (18). In the MPS trial of subfoveal lesions, 30% of untreated eyes lost six or more lines of VA at 12 months follow-up, and 39% lost six or more lines of vision by two years (2).

The MPS Trials

The MPS documented that the visual outcome of laser treatment for eyes with extrafoveal CNV was better than the natural history (21–23). In fact, recruitment into the argon laser trial of extrafoveal CNV (SMDS) was halted early because 18 months after enrollment, only 25% of laser treated eyes compared with 60% of observed eyes had lost six or more lines of VA (21). Although laser treatment did not reverse or stop progression of vision loss, laser-treated eyes continued to have better vision than untreated eyes even after five years of follow-up (5). Trials of similar design conducted at Moorfields Eye Hospital in London, England and by Coscas and Soubrane in Creteil, France also demonstrated a benefit of laser treatment versus observation in AMD patients with selected CNV lesions (24,25). Several MPS trials reported that the difference in vision loss between laser-treated and untreated eyes was maintained over a four to five years' course of follow-up. The patient eligibility criteria defining the study population as well as the results from the key trials are summarized in Tables 18.1 and 18.2 (1–5,27).

Decreased Vision After Laser Treatment

The studies which showed a benefit of laser treatment compared with observation for eyes with study-eligible CNV lesions also documented that laser treatment did

Table 18.1 Summary of the Major Results of the MPS

MPS study lesion type	CNV description	Location	Size	Age	VA	Exclusion
Extrafoveal (5)	Angiographic evidence of leaking CNV with "well-demarcated borders"	200–2500 µm from the center of FAZ		>50 yrs	>20/100	VA <20/400, prior laser, other ocular disease, systemic steroids
Juxtafoveal—AM DS-K (4)	Angiographic evidence of leaking CNV with "well-demarcated borders"	1–199 µm from the center of FAZ or >200 µm from FAZ if adjacent blood or pigment extended to within 200 µm		>50 yrs	>20/100	VA <20/400, prior laser, other ocular disease
New subfoveal CNV (1,2)	FA within 96 hrs of randomization; leaking CNV with "well-demarcated borders"; most of lesion either classic or occult	New vessels under FAZ center	<3.5 MPS standard disc area (1 MPS standard area=1.77 mm²); some area within 2 disc diameters of retina must be able to be left untreated	>50 yrs	20/40–20/320 inclusive	Prior laser, other ocular disease, systemic steroids
Recurrent subfoveal CNV (1,3)	FA within 96 hrs of randomization; leaking CNV with "well-demarcated borders"; contiguous to the scar from earlier treatment	New vessels under FAZ center or CNV within 150 µm of FAZ scar under FAZ center	Area of treatment plus scar <6 MPS disc areas (10.6 mm²) and some portion of retina within 1-disc diameter (1.5 mm) of FAZ must remain untreated			Previous treatment directly to the center of the FAZ, other ocular disease, systemic steroids

Abbreviations: AMDS-K, age-related macular degeneration study-krypton laser; CNV, choroidal neovascularization; FA, fluorescein angiography; FAZ, foveal avascular zone; MPS, Macular Photocoagulation Study; VA, visual acuity.
Source: From Ref. 26. Courtesy of Lippincott Williams and Wilkins.

Table 18.2 Percentage Progressing to Severe Vision Loss Defined as Loss of More than Six Lines of Visual Acuity

MPS AMD study	One year		Two years		Three years for all (except four years "subfoveal new")		Five years	
	Treated (%)	Control (%)	Treated (%)	Control (%)	Treated (%)	Control (%)	Treated (%)	Control (%)
Extrafoveal CNV (5)	24	41	33[b]	51[b]	45	63	46	64
Juxtafoveal CNV (4)	31	45	45	54	51	61	55	65
Subfoveal CNV (new) (1)	24 (20)[a]	30 (11)[a]	23	39	23	45		
Subfoveal CNV (recurrent) (1)	11	29	9	28	17	3		

[a] 3 months.
[b] 18 months.
Abbreviations: AMD, age-related macular degeneration; CNV, choroidal neovascularization; MPS, Macular Photocoagulation Study.
Source: From Ref. 27. Courtesy of Routledge/Taylor & Francis Group, LLC.

not prevent the progressive vision loss associated with CNV. Significant vision loss occurred over time in most treated eyes. Follow-up also showed that persistent and recurrent CNV were responsible for the progressive loss of vision. For example, 24 months after laser treatment of extrafoveal CNV lesions, 52% of eyes showed evidence of recurrence (28). Even for subfoveal lesions, after three

years of follow-up, nearly half the treated eyes had persistent or recurrent CNV (9). One MPS trial reported that eyes with recurrent CNV had less vision loss with laser treatment than with observation (Table 18.2) (3).

It must be noted that in eyes with subfoveal lesions and relatively good VA, there is greater loss of vision in laser-treated versus untreated eyes within the first three months after laser treatment (3). This observation documents the immediate harmful effects of laser treatment to the fovea. However, when patients with subfoveal CNV were followed for longer periods, it became evident that lase-treated eyes had less vision loss than observed eyes, indicating some long-term benefit of laser treatment even when applied to subfoveal CNV (3). This benefit was maintained over the three years' course of follow-up.

As indicated in the opening paragraphs, this review and the accompanying tables are provided for historical perspective. At present, anti-vascular endothelial growth factor (anti-VEGF) therapy is the first-line treatment for all subtypes of subfoveal CNV secondary to AMD (29–31). The reasons include that anti-VEGF therapy is not associated with immediate loss of vision due to destruction of visual elements in the retina, and that anti-VEGF is more effective than laser photocoagulation or photodynamic therapy (20,32–38). As randomized controlled clinical trials with anti-VEGF agents use center-involved exudation as inclusion criterion, there is still a potential role for thermal laser treatment in eyes with extrafoveal CNV lesions as defined by the MPS (5,31). However, many clinicians extrapolate the data from these studies to consider intravitreal injections of anti-VEGF agents for most of all forms of CNV secondary to AMD (29–31).

SUMMARY POINTS

- The Macular Photocoagulation Study (MPS) trials were conducted from 1979 to 1994 and showed that laser photocoagulation was a preferable therapy to observation for several categories of well-defined choroidal neovascularization (CNV) based on the fluorescein angiographic location of the CNV with respect to the geometric center of the fovea, that is, extrafoveal, juxtafoveal, and subfoveal.
- The MPS studies also documented that laser treatment did not prevent the progressive vision loss associated with CNV.
- A significant vision loss occurred over time in most treated eyes.

REFERENCES

1. Macular Photocoagulation Study Group. Laser photocoagulation of subfoveal neovascular lesions of age-related macular degeneration. Updated findings from two clinical trials. Arch Ophthalmol 1993; 111: 1200–9.
2. Macular Photocoagulation Study Group. Laser photocoagulation of subfoveal neovascular lesions in age-related macular degeneration. Results of a randomized clinical trial. Arch Ophthalmol 1991; 109: 1220–31.
3. Macular Photocoagulation Study Group. Laser photocoagulation of subfoveal recurrent neovascular lesions in age-related macular degeneration. Results of a randomized clinical trial. Arch Ophthalmol 1991; 109: 1232–41.
4. Macular Photocoagulation Study Group. Laser photocoagulation for juxtafoveal choroidal neovascularization. Five-year results from randomized clinical trials. Arch Ophthalmol 1994; 112: 500–9.
5. Macular Photocoagulation Study Group. Argon laser photocoagulation for neovascular maculopathy. Five-year results from randomized clinical trials. Arch Ophthalmol 1991; 109: 1109–14.
6. Ciulla TA, Danis RP, Harris A. Age-related macular degeneration: a review of experimental treatments. Surv Ophthalmol 1998; 43: 134–46.
7. Freund KB, Yannuzzi LA, Sorenson JA. Age-related macular denegeration and choroidal neovascularization. Am J Ophthalmol 1993; 115: 786–91.
8. Macular Photocoagulation Study Group. Persistent and recurrent neovascularization after krypton laser photocogulation for neovascular lesions of age-related macular degeneration. Arch Ophthalmol 1990; 108: 825–31.
9. Macular Photocoagulation Study Group. Persistent and recurrent neovascularization after laser photocoagulation for subfoveal choroidal neovascularization of age-related macular degeneration. Arch Ophthalmol 1994; 112: 489–99.
10. Fine SL, Berger JW, Maguire MG, Ho AC. Age-related macular degeneration. N Engl J Med 2000; 342: 483–92.
11. Evans J, Wormald R. Is the incidence of registrable age-related macular degeneration increasing? Br J Ophthalmol 1996; 80: 9–14.
12. Vingerling JR, Dielemans I, Hofman A, et al. The prevalence of age-related maculopathy in the Rotterdam Study. Ophthalmology 1995; 102: 205–10.
13. Klein R, Klein BE, Jensen SC, Meuer SM. The five-year incidence and progression of age-related maculopathy: the beaver dam eye study. Ophthalmology 1997; 104: 7–21.
14. Leibowitz HM, Krueger DE, Maunder LR, et al. The framingham eye study monograph: an ophthalmological and epidemiological study of cataract, glaucoma, diabetic retinopathy, macular degeneration, and visual acuity in a general population of 2631 adults, 1973–1975. Surv Ophthalmol 1980; 24: 335–610.
15. Ferris FL III, Fine SL, Hyman L. Age-related macular degeneration and blindness due to neovascular maculopathy. Arch Ophthalmol 1984; 102: 1640–2.
16. Hyman LG, Lilienfeld AM, Ferris FL III, Fine SL. Senile macular degeneration: a case-control study. Am J Epidemiol 1983; 118: 213–27.
17. Bressler SB, Bressler NM, Fine SL, et al. Natural course of choroidal neovascular membranes within the foveal avascular zone in senile macular degeneration. Am J Ophthalmol 1982; 93: 157–63.
18. Guyer DR, Fine SL, Maguire MG, et al. Subfoveal choroidal neovascular membranes in age-related macular degeneration. Visual prognosis in eyes with relatively good initial visual acuity. Arch Ophthalmol 1986; 104: 702–5.
19. Macular Photocoagulation Study Group. Krypton laser photocoagulation for idiopathic neovascular lesions. Results of a randomized clinical trial. Arch Ophthalmol 1990; 108: 832–7.
20. Barbazetto I, Burdan A, Bressler NM, et al. Photodynamic therapy of subfoveal choroidal neovascularization with verteporfin: fluorescein angiographic guidelines for evaluation and treatment—TAP and VIP Report No. 2. Arch Ophthalmol 2003; 121: 1253–68.
21. Macular Photocoagulation Study Group. Argon laser photocogulation for senile macular degeneration. Results of a randomized clinical trial. Arch Ophthalmol 1982; 100: 912–8.

22. Macular Photocoagulation Study Group. Argon laser photocogulation for ocular histoplasmosis. Results of a randomized clinical trial. Arch Ophthalmol 1983; 101: 1347–57.

23. Macular Photocoagulation Study Group. Argon laser photocogulation for idiopathic neovascularization. Results of a randomized clinical trial. Arch Ophthalmol 1983; 101: 1358–61.

24. The Moorfields Macular Study Group. Treatment of senile disciform macular degeneration: a single-blind randomised trial by argon laser photocoagulation. Br J Ophthalmol 1982; 66: 745–53.

25. Coscas G, Soubrane G. Argon laser photocoagulation of subretinal neovascularization in senile macular degeneration. Results of a randomized study of 60 cases. Bull Mem Soc Fr Ophtalmol 1982; 94: 149–54.

26. Cukras C, Fine SL. Thermal laser treatment in AMD: therapeutic and prophylactic. Int Ophthalmol Clin 2007; 47: 75–93.

27. Yoken J, Duncan JL, Berger JW, et al. Laser photocoagulation for choroidal neovascularization in age-related macular degeneration. In: Lim JI, ed. Age-Related Macular Degeneration. New York: Marcel Dekker, 2002: 181–201.

28. Macular Photocoagulation Study Group. Recurrent choroidal neovascularization after argon laser photocoagulation for neovascular maculopathy. Arch Ophthalmol 1986; 104: 503–12.

29. Brown DM, Kaiser PK, Michels M, et al. Ranibizumab versus verteporfin for neovascular age-related macular degeneration. N Engl J Med 2006; 355: 1432–44.

30. Rosenfeld PJ, Brown DM, Heier JS, et al. Ranibizumab for neovascular age-related macular degeneration. N Engl J Med 2006; 355: 1419–31.

31. Rosenfeld PJ, Rich RM, Lalwani GA. Ranibizumab: phase III clinical trial results. Ophthalmol Clin North Am 2006; 19: 361–72.

32. Ferrara N, Damico L, Shams N, et al. Development of ranibizumab, an anti-vascular endothelial growth factor antigen binding fragment, as therapy for neovascular age-related macular degeneration. Retina 2006; 26: 859–70.

33. Ferrara N. Role of vascular endothelial growth factor in physiologic and pathologic angiogenesis: therapeutic implications. Semin Oncol 2002; 29: 10–14.

34. Brown DM, Michels M, Kaiser PK, et al. Ranibizumab versus verteporfin photodynamic therapy for neovascular age-related macular degeneration: two-year results of the ANCHOR study. Ophthalmology 2009; 116: 57–65; e5.

35. Abraham P, Yue H, Wilson L. Randomized double-masked, sham-controlled trial of ranibizumab for neovascular age-related macular degeneration: PIER study year 2. Am J Ophthalmol 2010; 150: 315 e1–324 e1.

36. Ip MS, Scott IU, Brown GC, et al. American academy of ophthalmology. anti-vascular endothelial growth factor pharmacotherapy for age-related macular degeneration: a report by the american academy of ophthalmology. Ophthalmology 2008; 115: 1837–46.

37. CATT Research Group. Martin DF, Maguire MG, Ying GS, et al. Ranibizumab and bevacizumab for neovascular age-related macular degeneration. N Engl J Med 2011; 364: 1897–908.

38. American Academy of Ophthalmology Retina Panel. Preferred Practice Pattern® Guidelines. Age-Related Macular Degeneration. San Francisco, CA: American Academy of Ophthalmology, 2008. [Available from: www.aao.org/ppp]

19

Anti-VEGF drugs and clinical trials

Clement C. Chow, Jennifer I. Lim, Dimple Modi, Todd R. Klesert, and Philip J. Rosenfeld

INTRODUCTION

In 1989, Ferrara and Henzel (1) isolated a diffusible protein from bovine pituitary follicular cells that showed cell-specific mitogenic activity for vascular endothelium. They named this protein vascular endothelial growth factor (VEGF). Further research showed that VEGF was in fact Michelson's factor X, which was the postulated diffusible angiogenesis factor (2). VEGF was then shown to have a major role in choroidal neovascularization (CNV) (3,4).

The human VEGF-A gene, located on chromosome 6p21.3, consists of eight exons and seven introns. Alternative splicing produces mRNA transcripts that code for at least six different protein isoforms: 121, 145, 165, 183, 189, and 206 amino acids in length (5). These different isoforms vary in their affinity for heparin binding, and as such, in their affinity for the extracellular matrix. The larger isoforms, such as $VEGF_{189}$ and $VEGF_{206}$, bind heparin with high affinity, and are therefore almost completely sequestered in the extracellular matrix. The smaller isoform, $VEGF_{121}$, does not bind heparin and is freely diffusible. All VEGF isoforms contain a plasmin cleavage site. Cleavage at this site creates a freely diffusible, 110 kDa, bioactive form of VEGF ($VEGF_{110}$). Plasmin-mediated extracellular proteolysis may therefore be an important regulator of VEGF bioavailability (6). Further details on VEGF pathways in neovascular AMD can be found in chapter 4.

CURRENT ANTI-VEGF THERAPIES
Aptamers: Pegaptanib Sodium

The first anti-VEGF therapy to undergo clinical testing was a VEGF aptamer. Approved by the Food and Drug Administration (FDA) in 2004, Pegaptanib (Macugen—Eyetech Pharmaceuticals and Pfizer Inc., New York, USA) was the first anti-VEGF agent with proven efficacy for the treatment of CNV secondary to age-related macular degeneration (AMD). Pegaptanib is an aptamer—a short single-stranded oligonucleotide sequence that functions as a high affinity inhibitor of a specific protein target. Aptamers are created by a form of in-vitro evolution called systematic evolution of ligands by exponential enrichment (SELEX) (7).

Pegaptanib is a 28-base RNA oligonucleotide that is covalently linked to two 20 kDa polyethylene glycol moieties to extend the half-life. Pegaptanib selectively binds to the heparin-binding domain of $VEGF_{165}$ and larger isoforms, preventing ligand-receptor binding. The smaller VEGF isoforms and proteolytic fragments are therefore not inhibited by pegaptanib (7).

Safety and efficacy of pegaptanib for the treatment of neovascular AMD was established through the VEGF Inhibition Study in Ocular Neovascularization (VISION) study (8). VISION consisted of two phase III prospective, multicenter, randomized, controlled, double-masked trials comparing intravitreal injections of pegaptanib with sham injections. Patients (1186 in total) were randomized to receive pegaptanib (at a dose of 0.3, 1.0, or 3.0 mg) or sham injection (usual care), every six weeks for a total of 54 weeks. The primary end point of the study was the number of patients losing less than 15 letters of Early Treatment Diabetic Retinopathy Study (ETDRS) visual acuity at 54 weeks. Patients with all CNV lesion subtypes with sizes up to and including 12 disc areas in size were included. Concomitant photodynamic therapy (PDT) with verteporfin (Visudyne®, Novartis, East Hanover, New Jersey, USA) was allowed at the physician's discretion. Twenty-five percent of the VISION patients received PDT during the study period.

In the pooled analysis, efficacy was demonstrated for all three doses, without a dose–response relationship. Seventy percent of pegaptanib-treated patients lost less than 15 letters, compared with 55% of usual care patients. More pegaptanib-treated patients maintained or gained visual acuity (33%) at 54 weeks than usual care patients (23%). In addition, the usual care group was twice as likely to experience severe vision loss (30 or more letters) during the study period than pegaptanib-treated patients. However, only 6% of pegaptanib-treated patients in the study gained 15 or more letters at 54 weeks (compared with 2% of usual care controls), and as a group, the pegaptanib-treated patients lost an average of eight letters over the study period (compared with 15 letters in the usual care group). Adverse ocular events in the VISION trial resulted in severe vision loss in 0.1% of patients. These adverse events included endophthalmitis (1.3%), traumatic lens injury (0.6%), and retinal detachment (0.6%).

In year 2 of the VISION study, patients were re-randomized to the treatment and usual care arms (9). The results indicated that those patients continuing with pegaptanib treatment for a second year did better than those reassigned to the usual care control arm at 54 weeks, and better than those assigned to the usual care arm for the entire two years. The percentage of pegaptanib-treated patients who progressed to moderate visual loss (from baseline) during the second year of treatment was half (7%) that of those reassigned to the control group at 54 weeks (14%), and those who continued in the control group for the second year (14%). Of note, however, patients who had benefited from their year 1 treatment assignment (defined as less than or equal to zero letters of vision loss from baseline), and who subsequently lost 10 or more letters of vision after re-randomization at 54 weeks, were allowed to receive "salvage therapy" (a reassignment back to their original year 1 treatment arm). Year-2 safety data continue to show that pegaptanib is a relatively safe drug. Nonocular hemorrhagic events were not significantly different from the usual care group (10).

Studies with pegaptanib continued. The Verteporfin Intravitreal Triamcinolone Acetonide Study (VERITAS) was a phase III prospective, multicenter, randomized, double-masked trial comparing PDT combined with one of two doses of intravitreal triamcinolone (1 mg, 4 mg) versus PDT combined with 0.3 mg of intravitreal pegaptanib. One hundred eleven patients were enrolled in the study, which included all CNV lesion subtypes (11). Patients in the pegaptanib group received 0.3 mg dose every 1.5 months while those in the triamcinolone groups received 1 or 4 mg dose every 3 months and sham injection in the 1.5, 4.5, 7.5, and 10.5 month visit. All patients received PDT at baseline and every 3 months up to month 9 only if leakage was detected on fluorescein angiogram. At 12 months, 59.4%, 63.4%, and 71.1% of patients lost less than 15 ETDRS letters in the 1 mg triamcinolone, 4 mg triamcinolone, and 0.3 mg pegaptanib groups, respectively (primary outcome measure); 6.3%, 0%, and 13.2% gained 15 or more letters, respectively. In terms of ocular adverse events, cataract developed in 25% and 24.4% of patients in the triamcinolone groups but only 5.3% in the pegaptanib group. The incidence of increased intraocular pressure was not reported.

Studies are also ongoing at OSI/Eyetech to create a sustained-release form of pegaptanib, with the goal of reducing the frequency of intravitreal injections required for treatment, and thereby reducing the risk of serious adverse events associated with intravitreal injections, such as endophthalmitis and retinal detachment. Preliminary animal work with poly(lactic-co-glycolic) acid (PLGA)-based microsphere encapsulation suggests that sustained-release of pegaptanib for greater than six months is possible with a single intravitreal injection (12). However, subsequent data noted that microspheres could not achieve a duration more than about three to four months (personal communication).

Monoclonal Antibodies: Ranibizumab (Lucentis®)

In June 2006, ranibizumab (Lucentis, Genentech, South San Francisco, California, USA) became the second VEGF inhibitor approved by the FDA for use in the treatment of CNV secondary to AMD. Ranibizumab is a humanized, affinity-maturated Fab fragment of a murine monoclonal antibody directed against human VEGF-A. Ranibizumab is a potent, nonselective inhibitor of all VEGF-A isoforms and bioactive proteolytic products. Ranibizumab was specifically designed as a molecule smaller than its parent full-size precursor

anti-VEGF antibody, because it was felt that the full-sized antibody was unable to cross the inner retina and choroid, as suggested by a histologic study of the Herceptin antibody (13). A histologic analysis of bevacizumab in rabbits by Sharar et al. (14) however, suggests that a full-length antibody such as bevacizumab could penetrate all layers of the retina quite effectively. Because ranibizumab is missing the Fc region, it is believed that it is less likely to incite an immune response, as it can no longer bind to complement C1q or Fc gamma receptors (15).

Efficacy and safety of ranibizumab have thus far been established through two large prospective, multicenter, randomized, double-masked, controlled clinical trials: Minimally Classic/Occult Trial of Anti-VEGF Antibody Ranibizumab in the Treatment of Neovascular Age-Related Macular Degeneration (MARINA) (16) and Anti-VEGF Antibody for the Treatment of Predominantly Classic CNV in AMD (ANCHOR) (17). The MARINA trial was limited to patients with subfoveal occult or minimally classic CNV, either primary or recurrent, with evidence of recent disease progression. In MARINA, 716 patients were randomized 1:1:1 to receive monthly intravitreal injections of ranibizumab (either 0.3 or 0.5 mg) or sham injections. The primary outcome measure was the proportion of patients losing less than 15 ETDRS letters at 12 months; 94.5% of patients assigned to the 0.3 mg group and 94.6% of patients assigned to the 0.5 mg ranibizumab treatment arms, compared with 62.2% in the sham-treatment arm, met this end point. More eyes gained 15 or more letters of visual acuity by month 12 in the ranibizumab treatment arms than the control arms: 24.8% in the 0.3 mg group, 33.8% in the 0.5 mg group, and 5.0% in the sham-treated group. Mean visual acuity increased by 6.5 letters in the 0.3 mg group and 7.2 letters in the 0.5 mg group at 12 months. In contrast, mean visual acuity dropped by 10.4 letters in the sham-treated group. In general, vision gains were maintained throughout year 2 of the MARINA trial in ranibizumab-treated patients, whereas vision continued to decline in the sham-treated patients; mean loss was 14.9 letters in the sham group.

There was also a difference in the lesion size outcomes between the ranibizumab and control groups. While lesion size on average remained stable in the ranibizumab-treated patients, lesion size increased by about 50% in the sham-treated patients at 12 months. The area of leakage in the ranibizumab-treated lesions decreased on average by approximately 50%.

Adverse ocular events in ranibizumab-treated patients in the MARINA trial over 24 months included presumed endophthalmitis in 1.0% of patients and serious uveitis in 1.3% of patients. No retinal detachments were observed in the ranibizumab-treated patients, although retinal tears were identified in two patients (0.4%). Lens damage as a result of intravitreal injection was seen in one patient (0.2%). No statistically significant difference in serious systemic adverse events was observed between the treatment and control arms of the study, although there was a trend toward the increased rate of serious (1.3% in 0.3 mg group; 2.1% in 0.5 mg group; 0.8% in sham group) and nonserious (9.2% in 0.3 mg group; 8.8% in 0.5 mg group; 5.5% in sham group) non-ocular hemorrhages.

The ANCHOR trial has likewise demonstrated the efficacy of ranibizumab for the treatment of predominantly classic CNV lesions secondary to AMD. ANCHOR was designed as a head-to-head comparison between ranibizumab and PDT with verteporfin (Visudyne), which was then the standard of care for subfoveal CNV at that time. In ANCHOR, 423 patients were randomized in a 1:1:1 fashion to receive monthly intravitreal injections with ranibizumab 0.3 mg and sham PDT, ranibizumab 0.5 mg with sham PDT or monthly sham injections plus active verteporfin PDT. The primary end point was the number of patients losing fewer than 15 letters of baseline visual acuity at 12 months. This end point was achieved in 94.3% of the patients receiving 0.3 mg ranibizumab and 96.4% of patients receiving 0.5 mg ranibizumab versus 64.3% of the verteporfin group. The percentage of patients experiencing an improvement over baseline visual acuity of at least 15 letters was 35.7% and 40.3% respectively, in the ranibizumab-treated patients, versus only 5.6% in the verteporfin-treated patients. Mean visual acuity increased by 8.5 letters in the 0.3 mg ranibizumab group and 11.3 letters in the 0.5 mg ranibizumab group at 12 months. In contrast, mean visual acuity dropped by 9.5 letters in the verteporfin PDT group at 12 months.

Measurement of CNV lesion size throughout the ANCHOR study revealed positive morphologic effects similar to those observed in the MARINA study. In general, average total lesion size remained relatively stable in the ranibizumab-treated patients over one year, while increasing significantly in the verteporfin-treated patients. Moreover, the average total area of leakage and the average total area of classic CNV leakage, both decreased significantly at one year in the ranibizumab-treated patients, while they increased in the verteporfin-treated group.

No statistically significant difference in serious systemic adverse events was observed between the ranibizumab and verteporfin arms of the study, but as in the MARINA trial, there was a trend toward an increased rate of serious (1.5% in 0.3 mg group; 2.1% in 0.5 mg group; 0% in PDT group) and non-serious (5.1% in 0.3 mg group; 6.4% in 0.5 mg group; 2.1% in PDT group) non-ocular hemorrhages. Serious adverse ocular events in the ranibizumab-treated ANCHOR trial patients over 12 months included presumed endophthalmitis in 0.7% of patients and significant uveitis in 0.4% of patients. One patient each developed a retinal detachment (0.4%) or vitreous hemorrhage (0.4%). There were no cases of lens damage as a result of the intravitreal injection. The most common adverse event (12% patients) was mild post-injection inflammation.

The PIER (A Phase IIIb, Multicenter, Randomized, Double Masked, Sham Injection Controlled Study of the Efficacy and Safety of Ranibizumab in Subjects with Subfoveal Choroidal Neovascularization (CNV) with or without Classic CNV Secondary to Age-Related Macular Degeneration) study was a phase IIIb, prospective, multicenter, randomized, double-masked, controlled study of 184 patients with predominantly classic or occult CNV randomized to receive ranibizumab 0.3 or 0.5 mg or sham injections monthly for the first three months, followed by an injection once every three months for a total of 24 months (18,19). The purpose of PIER was to help determine the optimal dosing schedule for ranibizumab. At three months of monthly treatment, there was a mean gain in visual acuity by +2.9 letters in the 0.3 mg group and by +4.3 letters in the 0.5 mg group. By the end of one year, the mean change in visual acuity (primary outcome measure) was −1.6 letters in the 0.3 mg ranibizumab group, −0.2 letters in the 0.5 mg group, and −16.3 letters in the sham group (p ≤ 0.0001). At one year, 83% (0.3 mg) and 90% (0.5 mg) of ranibizumab-treated eyes lost less than 15 letters of visual acuity, compared with 49% of sham eyes. However, the percentage of eyes improving 15 or more letters was only 12% (0.3 mg) and 13% (0.5 mg) in ranibizumab-treated eyes, compared with 10% of sham eyes. Therefore, the effect of the drug declined with quarterly dosing. In the second year of the study, all eligible patients rolled over to the 0.5 mg treatment group and there was improvement in visual acuity during the first three months but this gain was not sustained when treatment was extended to quarterly. Overall though, there was a gain of 16 letters in the 0.5 mg ranibizumab-treated group over the sham group ($P < 0.0001$). At 24 months, the visual acuity decreased by a mean of 2.2 letters in the 0.3 mg group, 2.3 letters in the 0.5 mg group, and 21.4 letters in the sham group ($P < 0.0001$). Of the sham patients who crossed over to the 0.5 mg ranibizumab group in the second year, there was only a mean loss of 3.5 letters at 10 months after the switch. Of those in the 0.3 mg and 0.5 mg ranibizumab groups that switched to monthly treatment, there was a mean gain of 2.2 and 4.1 letters, respectively, at four months after the cross-over. Therefore, there appeared to be an additional benefit to switching over to monthly dosing after being treated with ranibizumab quarterly, but not in patients who started receiving ranibizumab after greater than 14 months of sham injections.

The EXCITE (Efficacy and Safety of Monthly Versus Quarterly Ranibizumab Treatment in Neovascular Age-related Macular Degeneration) study, similar to PIER, was also a phase IIIb prospective, multicenter double-masked, randomized controlled study which enrolled 353 patients with classic or occult CNV lesions secondary to AMD (20). This study was designed to demonstrate non-inferiority of intravitreal ranibizumab given quarterly versus intravitreal ranibizumab given monthly. Patients were randomized 1:1:1 to receive either 0.3 mg quarterly, 0.5 mg quarterly, or 0.3 monthly (through month 11). The quarterly-dosed eyes initially received monthly injections for the first three months and then injections at months 5, 8, and 11. The primary end point outcome measure was the mean change in best corrected visual acuity at month 12 compared with baseline. Visual acuity gain was greater in the monthly-treated group than the quarterly groups. The 0.3 mg quarterly group gained 4.9 letters, the 0.5 mg quarterly group gained 3.8 letters, and the 0.5 mg monthly group gained 8.3 letters. Central retinal thickness was reduced by 96 μm in the 0.3 mg quarterly group, 105.6 μm in the 0.5 mg quarterly group, and 105.3 in the 0.3 mg monthly group. Non-inferiority of quarterly dosing to monthly was not achieved with the now commonly accepted margin of less than or equal to 5 letters .

The SUSTAIN (Study of Ranibizumab in Patients With Subfoveal Choroidal Neovascularization Secondary to Age-Related Macular) trial was also a phase III, multi-center, open-label, single arm, 12-month study (21). In SUSTAIN, 513 patients with CNV secondary to AMD were treatment naïve with respect to anti-VEGF drugs and a smaller subset (18 patients) had previously been enrolled in ANCHOR. The ANCHOR-SUSTAIN patients were not included in the primary analysis of the data. Patients received a monthly intravitreal ranibizumab injection for the first three months and then were re-treated pro re nata (PRN) based on re-treatment criteria. (Re-treament criteria included a loss of visual acuity of more than five letters or an increase in the central retinal thickness (CRT) by more than 100 μm on optical coherence tomography (OCT)). Re-treatment could be deferred if the visual acuity was 79 or more letters or if the CRT was less than or equal to 225 μm. After the first three injections, the re-treatment criteria did not require continued treatment until the macula was dry. The investigators were given the discretion to stop treatment if the visual acuity was better than 79 letters or the central retinal thickness was less than 225 μm. After the initial three injections, patients on average needed 2.7 injections for the remaining nine months. There was an initial gain of 5.8 letters after the three monthly treatments; this decreased to 2.2 letters over the next two to three months, and resulted in a net gain of 3.6 letters at 12 months. Similarly, the central retinal thickness decreased by 101.1 μm in the first three months and by 91.5 μm at 12 months. This study showed that a PRN dosing regimen was reasonable. The authors concluded that their re-treatment criteria, which allowed for some undertreatment, could be tightened to improve the visual acuity outcomes. They specifically stated that the 100 μm or more increase in CRT should be decreased to 50 μm. This study was one of the first that evaluated individualized anti-VEGF therapy.

Another phase IIIb study, the SAILOR (Safety Assessment of Intravitreous Lucentis for AMD) study, compared the safety and efficacy of the 0.3 mg ranibizumab dose versus the 0.5 mg dose (22). The patients were randomized 1:1 to receive three loading doses (monthly injections) of either dose and then treated on pre-established re-treatment criteria. Patients were only scheduled to return every three months, but could receive treatment earlier if needed. There was evidence of adverse effects in this study, although not statistically significant. Overall, 0.7% of patients in the 0.3 mg group versus 1.2% in the 0.5 mg group reported an incidence of cerebrovascular stroke. There were eight deaths in study patients. Nineteen patients suffered arterial thromboembolic events, and five patients had serious ocular events. The most frequent ocular side effect after injection reported was decreased visual acuity in 18.5%, retinal hemorrhage in 7.2%, increased intraocular pressure in 7.0%, and subconjunctival hemorrhage in 5.5%.

The long-term safety and efficacy of ranibizumab were studied in the HORIZON, an open-label, multi-center, extension study (23). In this study, patients who completed the controlled treatment phase of MARINA, ANCHOR, or FOCUS clinical trials were eligible for enrollment. Analyses were performed for three groups: (i) patients treated with ranibizumab in the initial study ($n = 600$); (ii) patients randomized to control who crossed over to receive ranibizumab ($n = 190$); and (iii) ranibizumab-naïve patients ($n = 63$). Ranibizumab 0.5 mg was administered at the investigator's discretion. The patients were followed every three months, but could receive treatments more frequently if deemed appropriate by the investigator. In terms of safety, there was one occurrence of mild endophthalmitis per 3552 injections. There were no serious adverse events such as lens damage, retinal tears, or rhegmatogenous retinal detachments in the study eyes. The proportion of patients with glaucoma was 3.2%, 4.2%, and 3.2% in the ranibizumab-treated initial, ranibizumab-treated cross-over, and ranibizumab-naïve groups, respectively. Cataract formation was less frequent in the ranibizumab-untreated group: 6.3% versus 12.5% and 12.1% in the ranibizumab-treated initial and ranibizumab-treated cross-over groups, respectively. The proportion of patients with arterial thromboembolic events was 5.3% in the ranibizumab-treated initial and ranibizumab-treated cross-over groups, and 3.2% in the ranibizumab-untreated group. At month 48 (2 years of HORIZON), the mean change in BCVA relative to the initial study baseline was +2.0 in the ranibizumab-treated initial group versus −11.8 in the pooled ranibizumab treated-cross over and ranibizumab-untreated groups. This study shows that multiple ranibizumab injections were well tolerated for greater than four years. However, less frequent follow-up and treatment lead to in incremental decline of the visual acuity gains achieved with monthly treatment.

All of the above phase III studies demonstrate that monthly injections provide for sustained improvement in visual acuity and decreased central retinal thickness than quarterly or PRN dosing. Overall, ocular and systemic adverse events were statistically nonsignificant and the improvements in vision outweigh the risks associated with intravitreal injection of ranibizumab.

PRospective Optical coherence tomography imaging of patients with Neovascular AMD Treated with intra-Ocular ranibizumab (PRONTO) was a two-year, single site, open-label, uncontrolled study of 40 patients designed to evaluate the durability of response to ranibizumab and whether OCT could be used to guide treatment of neovascular AMD (24). As in the PIER study, patients received monthly injections of ranibizumab for the first three months. Thereafter, re-treatment with ranibizumab is performed if one of the following changes were observed between visits: a loss of five letters in vision in conjunction with fluid on OCT, increase in OCT CRT of at least 100 µm, new-onset classic CNV, new macular hemorrhage, or persistent macular fluid detected by OCT at least one month after the previous injection of ranibizumab. At 12 months, mean visual acuity improved by 9.3 letters ($P < 0.001$) and the mean OCT CRT decreased by 178 µm ($P < 0.001$). Visual acuity improved to 15 or more letters in 35% of patients. These visual acuity and OCT outcomes were achieved with an average of 5.6 injections over 12 months. Once a fluid-free macula was achieved, the mean injection-free interval was 4.5 months before another reinjection was necessary. Unlike the PIER study, visits were monthly and visual acuity gains did occur despite the less frequent dosing scheme. In the second year of the study, 37 of the 40 patients completed the two-year trial (25). Re-treatment criteria were modified to allow re-treatment if any fluid was detected in the macula. At the end of 24 months, there was a gain of 11.1 letters and 43% of patients gained 15 or more letters. There was a decrease in CRT by 212 µm. The average number of injections needed over the 24-month period was 9.9. PRONTO outcomes suggested that OCT could be useful for guiding re-treatment with intravitreal ranibizumab in neovascular AMD, and that the use of an OCT-guided variable-dosing regimen could decrease the injection burden without sacrificing improvements in visual acuity.

The HARBOR (A Study of Ranibizumab Administered Monthly or on an As-Needed Basis in Patients With Subfoveal Neovascular Age-Related Macular Degeneration) study was a two-year, phase III, multicenter, randomized trial investigating the efficacy and safety of high dose ranibizumab (2.0 mg) administered monthly or as needed (26). In HARBOR, 1097 patients with neovascular AMD were randomized to receive 2.0 mg or 0.5 mg ranibizumab intravitreally dosed monthly or PRN after three loading doses. At month 12, BCVA for the four treatment groups were +10.1 letters for 0.5 mg monthly, +9.2 letters for 2.0 mg monthly, 8.2 letters for 0.5 mg PRN, and +8.6 letters for 2.0 mg PRN. The PRN groups did not meet the pre-specified noninferiority criteria (margin of 4 letters) as compared to ranibizumab 0.5 mg monthly. The proportion of patients who lost less than 15 letters from baseline at month 12 were similar in all groups (97.8%, 93.4%, 94.5%, and 94.9%, respectively). Mean change from baseline in OCT central foveal thickness was −172.0 µm, −163.3 µm, −161.2 µm, and −172.4 µm, respectively. The number of injections required for the PRN groups were 7.7 and 6.9 in the 0.5 and 2.0 mg group respectively. The incidence of ocular and systemic adverse events were similar in all groups. The investigators concluded that high-dose ranibizumab (2.0 mg) did not provide superior results to 0.5 mg dosing at 12 months and that PRN dosing was inferior to monthly dosing.

Monoclonal Antibodies: Bevacizumab (Avastin®)

Bevacizumab (Avastin, Genentech, South San Francisco, California, USA) is a full-length humanized murine monoclonal antibody directed against human VEGF-A. It was FDA approved in 2004 for the intravenous treatment of metastatic colorectal cancer. Its potential for use in the treatment of CNV was first tested by Michels et al. (27) via intravenous infusion in a 12-week open-label uncontrolled study. Striking results were observed with improvement in visual acuity, reduction of CRT on OCT, and decreased leakage of the neovascular lesion on fluorescein angiography. However, patients experienced a mean increase of 12 mmHg in systolic blood pressure, which was felt to be a deterrent to its common use. This systemic side effect, combined with the promising visual and anatomic results from the intravenous infusion of bevacizumab, led investigators to consider use of an intravitreal injection of bevacizumab (28). Since then, several retrospective, uncontrolled, open-label case series detailing the visual and anatomic results of intravitreal bevacizumab for treatment of CNV secondary to AMD (29–32) have been published. As with ranibizumab, the effect of bevacizumab has been impressive.

Avery and colleagues (29) treated 79 patients with 1.25 mg of intravitreal bevacizumab monthly and reported the early results at three months of follow-up. Many of these patients had failed prior treatment with verteporfin or pegaptanib. At three months, median Snellen visual acuity improved from 20/200 at baseline to 20/80. Mean CRT on OCT decreased by 67 µm at three months. No ocular or systemic adverse events were observed.

Spaide and colleagues treated (30) 266 patients with 1.25 mg of intravitreal bevacizumab monthly. By three months, Snellen visual acuity improved from a mean of 20/184 at baseline to 20/109, with 38.3% of patients experiencing some improvement in visual acuity. Mean CRT on OCT improved from 340 µm at baseline to 213 µm at 3 months. Again, no adverse ocular or systemic adverse events were observed.

In contrast to the intravenous administration of bevacizumab, intravitreal injection of bevacizumab did not result in the systemic side effect of hypertension in any of these studies. The systemic concentration of bevacizumab when given intravenously is obviously several times larger than the systemic concentrations seen after intravitreal injections. No elevation in blood pressure has yet been reported in patients treated with intravitreal bevacizumab.

Animal and in-vitro studies published thus far have failed to identify any specific toxicity associated with bevacizumab use. Luthra et al. (33) demonstrated that viability of human RPE cells, rat neurosensory cells, and human microvascular endothelial cells in culture was normal after exposure to bevacizumab at concentrations of up to 1 mg/mL. Rabbit studies by Manzano et al. (34) found no changes in the electroretinogram (ERG) patterns of eyes injected with intravitreal bevacizumab at doses up to 5.0 mg. Mild vitreous inflammation was seen at a dose of 5.0 mg, but not at lower doses. Bakri et al. (35) looked at retinal histology of rabbit eyes injected with bevacizumab, and again found no histologic changes compared with control eyes.

One important aspect in which ranibizumab and bevacizumab may differ is their pharmacokinetics. Because of its larger molecular weight, it was assumed that bevacizumab had a significantly longer half-life in the vitreous, and possibly a longer systemic half-life as well. While a longer intravitreal half-life may allow for less frequent injections to achieve the same biologic effect, the lower affinity of bevacizumab for VEGF results in similar VEGF binding characteristics in the eye when compared with ranibizumab (36).

The National Eye Institute sponsored a multicenter, non-inferiority trial comparing bevacizumab with ranibizumab in AMD patients with subfoveal CNV. This study, the Comparison of Treatment Trial (CATT) study, randomized 1208 patients into one of four treatment arms: monthly intravitreal injection of ranibizumab, monthly injection of bevacizumab, monthly injection of ranibizumab followed by as-needed treatment, and monthly injection of bevacizumab followed by as-needed treatment (37). The primary outcome was the mean change in visual acuity between baseline and one year. The noninferiority limit for the difference among study groups was five letters (one line on the ETDRS visual acuity chart). At one year, visual acuity improved in all four groups, ranging from 5.9 ± 1.0 letters in the bevacizumab as-needed group to 8.5 ± 0.8 letters in the ranibizumab monthly group. Bevacizumab was equivalent to ranibizumab (99.2% confidence interval) both when the drugs were given monthly and when the drugs were given as needed. Ranibizumab given as needed was equivalent to ranibizumab or bevacizumab given monthly. However, the comparisons between bevacizumab given as needed and ranibizumab or bevacizumab given monthly were inconclusive (did not meet the noninferiority limit). In the secondary outcome measures, the mean decrease in thickness at the foveal center ranged from $152 \pm 178\,\mu m$ in the group given bevacizumab as needed to $196 \pm 176\,\mu m$ in the group given ranibizumab monthly ($P = 0.03$). The mean number of injections was 6.9 ± 3.0 for ranibizumab given as needed and 7.7 ± 3.5 for bevacizumab given as needed ($P = 0.003$). The average cost of a study drug per patient for the first year was $23,400 in the ranibizumab-monthly group, $13,800 in the ranibizumab-as-needed group, $595 in the bevacizumab-monthly group, and $385 in the bevacizumab-as-needed group. There were no significant difference in death rates, arterial thrombotic events, or venous thrombotic events. The rate of serious systemic adverse events was higher among bevacizumab-treated patients than ranibizumab-treated patients (24.1% vs. 19.0%, $P = 0.04$). Endophthalmitis rates were low and similar in both bevacizumab (0.07%) and ranibizumab (0.04%) ($P = 0.49$). The results of the CATT study suggested that bevacizumab is an attractive treatment option given its clinical equivalence to and its cost advantage over ranibizumab, especially for those patients without drug insurance coverage or with large drug co-payment requirements.

The two-year CATT study group has reported not only the visual and anatomic results for each regimen at two years, but have also described the visual and anatomic results of switching to as-needed treatment after one year of monthly treatment (38). At one year, patients initially assigned to monthly treatment were reassigned randomly to monthly or as-needed treatment, without changing the drug assignment. Among patients following the same regimen for two years, the mean increase in letters of visual acuity from baseline was 8.8 in the ranibizumab-monthly group, 7.8 in the bevacizumab monthly group, 6.7 in the ranibizumab-as-needed group, and 5.0 in the bevacizumab-as-needed group (drug, $P = 0.21$; regimen, $P = 0.046$). The proportion without fluid ranged from 13.9% in the bevacizumab-as-needed group to 45.5% in the ranibizumab monthly group (drug, $P = 0.0003$; regimen, $P < 0.0001$). Switching from monthly to as-needed treatment resulted in greater mean decrease in vision during year 2 (-2.2 letters; $P = 0.03$) and a lower proportion without fluid (-19%; $P < 0.0001$). Rates of death and arterial thrombotic events were similar for both drugs ($P > 0.60$). The proportion of patients with one or more systemic serious adverse events was higher with bevacizumab than ranibizumab (39.9% vs. 31.7%; adjusted risk ratio, 1.30; $P = 0.009$). Most of the excess events have not been associated previously with systemic therapy targeting VEGF. The conclusion of this study was that ranibizumab and bevacizumab had similar effects on visual acuity over a two-year period. Treatment as needed resulted in less gain in visual acuity, whether instituted at enrollment or after one year of monthly treatment. When instituted after one year of monthly treatment, as-needed treatment resulted in a loss of vision that was indistinguishable from the group given as-needed treatment from baseline.

Similar to CATT, IVAN (A Randomised Controlled Trial of Alternative Treatments to Inhibit VEGF in Age-related Choroidal Neovascularisation) was a two-year multicenter, noninferiority trial conducted in the United Kingdom and compared the efficacy and safety of ranibizumab with bevacizumab in eyes with neovascular AMD (39). In IVAN, 610 patients were randomized to one of four regimens: ranibizumab or bevacizumab, given either monthly or as needed with monthly office visits for all groups. The primary outcome measures were visual acuity at distance and arterial thrombotic events or heart failure at two years. At one year, the comparison by drug was inconclusive; bevacizumab was neither inferior nor equivalent to ranibizumab using the predetermined 3.5 non-inferiority letter limit. As-needed treatment was found to be equivalent to monthly treatment. Fewer patients receiving bevacizumab had an arterial thrombotic event or heart failure ($P = 0.03$) and there was no difference between drugs in the proportion having a serious systemic adverse event ($P = 0.25$). In terms of structural outcomes (secondary measures), OCT total foveal thickness did not differ by drug, but was 9% less with monthly treatment ($P = 0.005$). Fewer patients in the monthly treatment group had fluid on OCT and dye leakage on fluorescein angiography at one year but no difference was found between drugs.

Serum VEGF levels were measured at baseline, visits 1, 11, and 12. Median serum VEGF concentrations at one year were lower than at baseline in all groups, but were significantly lower at one year for bevacizumab than ranibizumab and higher for the as-needed than monthly regimen. On average, the as-needed groups received seven injections in the first year. As expected, bevacizumab was less costly for both treatment regimen ($P < 0.0001$). The investigators concluded that the one-year visual acuity comparison between bevacizumab and ranibizumab was inclusive but that monthly and as-needed treatment regimens were equivalent. The safety profile was similar in both drugs. Two-year data are pending at this time.

Bevacizumab was FDA approved only for the intravenous treatment of metastatic colon cancer, thus an intravitreal injection of bevacizumab is an off-label use based on its altered route of administration and the fact that it has never been FDA-approved for intravitreal injection for neovascular AMD. This makes documentation of the informed consent process especially important when using bevacizumab. While obtaining informed consent, the physician should explain to patients that the safety and efficacy of bevacizumab have not been established with certainty, and that there may be unknown risks with its use. A bevacizumab-specific consent form is recommended, and can be found on the website of the Ophthalmic Mutual Insurance Company (OMIC) (40,41).

Bevacizumab comes in preservative-free 100 mg vials, containing 4 cc of a 25 mg/cc solution, intended for one-time use only for treatment of a single cancer patient. A single vial can theoretically be aliquoted out to provide up to eighty individual 0.05 cc intravitreal doses in 1 cc tuberculin syringes. The pharmacy should confirm the dose and sterility, provide proper storage instructions, and mark all aliquots with an expiration date. Although bevacizumab is a very stable drug with a shelf-life of many months, compounded aliquots will usually have an expiration date due to sterility concerns.

VEGF Trap-Eye: Aflibercept (Eylea®)

Pegaptanib, ranibizumab, and bevacizumab all inhibit VEGF-A; they do not bind other members of the VEGF family. VEGF Trap-Eye ("VEGF Trap") or aflibercept (Eylea, Regeneron, Tarrytown, New York, USA and Bayer, Basel, Switzerland) is a drug designed to inhibit all members of the VEGF family: VEGF-A, -B, -C, -D, and placental growth factors (PlGF-1 and PlGF-2). VEGF Trap is a recombinant chimeric VEGF receptor fusion protein in which the binding domains of VEGF receptors 1 and 2 are combined with the Fc portion of immunoglobulin G to create a stable, soluble, high-affinity inhibitor. VEGF Trap also binds VEGF-A with higher affinity (kDa < 1 pmol/L) than any of the currently available anti-VEGF drugs (42).

The CLEAR-AMD 1 study was a randomized, multicenter, placebo-controlled, dose-escalation study designed to assess the safety, tolerability, and bioactivity of intravenously administered VEGF Trap (42). The study enrolled 25 patients with CNV secondary to AMD with lesions ≤12 disc areas in size and with ≥50% active leakage, and with ETDRS visual acuity of 20/40 or worse. Patients were randomized to receive either placebo or one of three doses of VEGF Trap (0.3, 1.0, or 3.0 mg/kg). The VEGF Trap was given as a single intravenous dose, followed by a four-week observation period, followed by three additional doses two weeks apart. Dose-limiting toxicity was observed for two of the five patients treated with the 3.0 mg/kg dose: one patient developed grade 4 hypertension and the other developed grade 2 proteinuria. Although reduced leakage on fluorescein angiography and reduced retinal thickening on OCT was observed in the treated patients, there was no corresponding reduction in CNV lesion size or improvement in visual acuity observed in these patients over the short 71-day study period. It was concluded that the maximum tolerated IV dose of VEGF Trap was 1.0 mg/kg.

The CLEAR-IT 1 study was similarly designed to assess the safety, tolerability, and bioactivity of VEGF Trap through an intravitreal route of administration (43). The study enrolled 21 patients using the same inclusion criteria as CLEAR-AMD 1, and randomized them to receive one of six doses of VEGF Trap as single intravitreal injection: 0.05, 0.15, 0.5, 1.0, 2.0, or 4.0 mg. After 43 days of follow-up, no adverse ocular or systemic events were observed. Mean decrease in excess foveal thickness for all patients was 72%. The mean increase in ETDRS visual acuity was 4.75 letters and visual acuity remained stable or improved in 95% of patients. Notably, three of six patients treated with the higher doses (2.0 or 4.0 mg) gained three or more lines of visual acuity by day 43. Clearly, VEGF Trap given intravitreally showed promise as a novel treatment for CNV in AMD patients. Phase 2 study (CLEAR-IT 2) showed that repeated dosing with VEGF Trap was well tolerated over 52 weeks of treatment (44). These studies laid the groundwork for the phase three multicenter trials evaluating the safety and efficacy or aflibercept.

The pivotal trials that led to aflibercept's FDA approval were the VIEW 1 and VIEW 2 trials (VEGF trap-eye: Investigation of Efficacy and safety in Wet AMD) (45,46). VIEW 1 enrolled 1217 wet AMD patients in the USA and Canada while VIEW 2 enrolled 1240 patients in the EU, Asia Pacific, Japan, and Latin America. In each study, patients were randomly assigned in a 1:1:1:1 ratio to one of four treatment regimens: (i) Aflibercept 2 mg every eight weeks following three initial monthly doses; (ii) aflibercept 2 mg every four weeks; (iii) aflibercept 0.5 mg every four weeks; and (iv) ranibizumab administered 0.5 mg every four weeks. The primary outcome measure was the proportion of patients who maintained vision, defined as losing fewer than 15 letters on the ETDRS chart. At 52 weeks, the VIEW 1 study showed that in the aflibercept groups, vision was maintained in 96% of patients receiving 0.5 mg monthly, 95% of patients receiving 2 mg monthly, and 95% of patients receiving 2 mg every 2 months. In the group receiving ranibizumab 0.5 mg monthly, 94% of patients maintained vision. In VIEW 2, vision was maintained in 96% of patients in all three aflibercept groups and in 94% of patients in the ranibizumab group at 52 weeks. Both studies showed clinical equivalence among all treatment groups and demonstrated excellent safety. Aflibercept was approved by the FDA on November 18, 2011. The approved dose and regimen were 2 mg every eight weeks following three initial monthly loading doses. The two-year data are pending at this time.

COMBINATION THERAPIES

There have been several clinical trials that have evaluated the efficacy and safety of combination therapy for neovascular AMD. The rationale behind combination therapy is to use agents which possess different mechanisms of action in order to better attack the CNV lesion. The sought improvement in outcomes include better visual acuity and anatomic results as well as a decreased need for re-treatment with anti-VEGF drugs. Further details on combination therapy can be found in chapter 22. The following focuses upon clinical trials that use agents in combination with anti-VEGF therapies.

Combination Therapy with PDT

The RhuFab V2 Ocular Treatment Combining the Use of VISUDYNE® to Evaluate Safety (FOCUS) study (47) was a two-year, phase I/II, multicenter, randomized, single-masked, controlled study of 162 patients with predominantly classic CNV. FOCUS compared the safety and efficacy of intravitreal ranibizumab (0.5 mg) combined with verteporfin PDT versus verteporfin PDT alone (combined with sham injection). Patients received monthly ranibizumab (0.5 mg) ($n = 106$) or sham ($n = 56$) injections. The PDT was performed seven days before initial ranibizumab or sham treatment and then quarterly as needed. The primary outcome measure was the proportion of patients who lost fewer than 15 letters from baseline at 12 months. At 12 months, 90.5% of the ranibizumab-treated patients and 67.9% of the control patients lost fewer than 15 letters ($P < 0.001$).

The most frequent ranibizumab-associated serious ocular adverse events were intraocular inflammation (11.4%) and endophthalmitis (1.9%; 4.8% if including presumed cases). On average, patients with serious inflammation had better visual acuity outcomes at 12 months than did controls. Key serious non-ocular adverse events included myocardial infarctions in the PDT-alone group (3.6%) and cerebrovascular accidents in the ranibizumab-treated group (3.8%). Notably, ranibizumab-treated patients experiencing intraocular inflammation still had better visual acuity outcomes at 12 months than the control patients. Thus, ranibizumab combined with PDT was more efficacious than PDT alone for treating neovascular AMD. In addition, the FOCUS study showed that despite a history of prior PDT therapy, a significant proportion of these patients were able to gain visual acuity when treated with ranibizumab and PDT. The need for additional PDT was 27.6% for the combined group but 91.1% for the PDT group. A difference in the rate of PDT re-treatment was seen

by the three-month follow-up period and maintained for the study. The FOCUS study, however, did not compare the ranibizumab plus PDT combination to ranibizumab alone.

The SUMMIT clinical program, which included the DENALI (United States and Canada) (48) and MONT BLANC (Europe) (49) studies, was designed to evaluate the efficacy and safety of PDT plus ranibizumab compared with ranibizumab alone. In the DENALI study, 321 patients with neovascular AMD were randomized to either monthly ranibizumab 0.5 mg monotherapy, standard fluence (SF) verteporfin PDT combination therapy (three initial ranibizumab loading doses followed by as-needed PDT and ranibizumab), or reduced fluence (RF) verteporfin PDT combination therapy. Mean BCVA change at 12 months was 5.3 and 4.4 letters with verteporfin SF ($n = 103$) or verteporfin RF ($n = 105$) plus ranibizumab, respectively, compared with 8.1 letters with monthly ranibizumab monotherapy. Noninferiority (7-letter margin) of either combination regimen to monthly ranibizumab monotherapy was not demonstrated (primary end point). A ranibizumab treatment-free interval of three months or longer was achieved in 92.6% and 83.5% of the patients randomized to verteporfin SF or verteporfin RF groups, respectively. These patients received a mean of 5.1 and 5.7 ranibizumab injections, respectively, while patients in the ranibizumab monotherapy arm received 10.5 injections. No new safety issues were noted and the combination therapy was well tolerated in all three regimens. In DENALI, although both monotherapy and combination therapy improved BCVA at month 12, noninferiority was not reached for either combination therapy regimen. In addition, reduced fluence verteporfin PDT did not confer clinical benefits over SF verteporfin PDT. Two-year data are pending at this time.

In the MONT BLANC study, 255 wet AMD patients were randomized 1:1 to as-needed combination therapy (initial SF verteporfin PDT and three initial monthly 0.5 mg ranibizumab doses followed by as-needed PDT and/or ranibizumab) or as-needed 0.5 mg ranibizumab monotherapy after three initial monthly doses. The mean change in BCVA at month 12 was 2.5 and 4.4 letters in the combination and monotherapy groups, respectively. Noninferiority with a margin of seven letters (95% confidence interval) was achieved in this study. The proportion of patients with a treatment-free interval of three months at any time-point after month two was high (combination, 96%; monotherapy, 92%), but did not show a clinically relevant difference between the treatment groups. Secondary efficacy endpoints included the mean number of ranibizumab re-treatments after month 2 (combination, 1.9; monotherapy, 2.2). The time to first ranibizumab re-treatment after month 2 was delayed by 34 days with combination (month 6) *vs.* monotherapy (month 5). The mean number of verteporfin/sham PDT treatments was comparable in the two groups (combination, 1.7; monotherapy, 1.9). The safety profiles of the two groups were comparable, with a low incidence of ocular serious adverse events. Thus, the combination as-needed treatment regimen with verteporfin PDT and ranibizumab was effective in achieving BCVA gain comparable with as-needed ranibizumab monotherapy; however, the study did not show benefits with respect to reducing the number of ranibizumab re-treatment over 12 months. Two-year data are still pending at this time. Further information on the combination of anti-VEGF and PDT is available in chapter 23 of this book.

Combination Therapy with Brachytherapy

The rationale for radiation therapy was based on the known effects of radiation therapy on tumor microvasculature and its ability to prevent proliferation of vascular tissue by inhibiting neovascularization (50). The Macular Epiretinal Brachytherapy in Treated Age-related Macular Degeneration (MERITAGE) Trial is a three-year prospective interventional trial to assess whether epimacular brachytherapy (EMB) is a safe and effective treatment method for neovascular AMD (51). In particular, the MERITAGE trial targeted patients who required frequent injections of anti-VEGF therapy to treat their disease, because they had the most to gain from a treatment that may reduce neovascular activity. Fifty-three eyes of 53 participants were enrolled in this study. On average, these patients had received 12.5 anti-VEGF injections prior to enrollment. Each patient underwent pars plana vitrectomy during which a single 24-Gy dose of EMB was delivered using an intraocular, handheld, 20-gauge device containing a strontium 90/yttrium 90 source positioned over the active lesion. Using predefined re-treatment criteria, participants were re-treated with ranibizumab administered monthly as needed. Primary outcomes at 12 months included the proportion of participants with stable vision (losing less than 15 ETDRS letters) and mean number of anti-VEGF re-treatments. After a single treatment with EMB, 81% maintained stable vision, with a mean of 3.49 anti-VEGF re-treatments at 12 months. Mean change in visual acuity was –4.0 +/– 15.1 ETDRS letters. Mean OCT CRT increased by 50 +/–179 μm. Common adverse events included conjunctival hemorrhage ($n = 38$), cataract ($n = 16$), vitreous hemorrhage ($n = 6$), and eye pain ($n = 5$). The investigators concluded that epimacular brachytherapy produced stable visual acuity in most participants with previously treated, active disease and may reduce the need for frequent anti-VEGF re-treatment. Further details on radiation therapy are available in chapter 21 of this book.

Safety Considerations

The observation that injection of intravitreal bevacizumab (52) or pegaptanib (53) for the treatment of proliferative diabetic retinopathy results in the regression of neovascularization in the fellow eye provides compelling evidence that these molecules are indeed absorbed systemically to levels that are clinically relevant. Although no serious systemic concerns were raised by the MARINA, ANCHOR, VISION or VIEW studies, it should be remembered that studies of this size are powered to detect only relatively large differences in rare events between the study groups. A modest increase in the risk of heart attack or stroke, for example, might not be detected by these studies. In this regard, both the MARINA (16) and ANCHOR (17) trials revealed a non-statistically significant trend toward an increased risk of serious systemic hemorrhage. In MARINA, the incidence of such events was 1.3% in 0.3 mg group, 2.1% in 0.5 mg group, versus 0.8% in sham group at 24 months. In ANCHOR, the incidence of such events was 1.5% in 0.3 mg group, 2.1% in 0.5 mg group, versus 0% in sham group at 12 months. A similar trend was observed for nonserious systemic hemorrhages. No such trend was observed in the VISION trial (10) of pegaptanib, in which the incidence of serious systemic hemorrhage was 0.5% in the treatment arm, versus 1.9% in the sham arm. Subsequent trials including PIER, EXCITE, SUSTAIN, SAILOR, HORIZON, PrONTO, CATT, and IVAN demonstrated that intravitreal ranibizumab is well tolerated and has a very low rate of adverse ocular or systemic side effects. As mentioned previously, bevacizumab was associated with a higher overall rate of systemic adverse events in the CATT trial, but most of the excess events have not been associated previously with systemic anti-VEGF therapy. These data simply underscore the fact that anti-VEGF agents are potent drugs, and they should always be used with due caution and consideration.

Intravitreal Injection Technique

It appears that the greatest risks associated with the use of current anti-VEGF therapies for the treatment of AMD (endophthalmitis, retinal detachment, and lens trauma) stem from the intravitreal injection itself. Therefore, proper injection technique and careful antiseptic practices are important.

Supplies that are recommended for prepping the eye include 5% povidine-iodine solution, povidine-iodine sticks, and a sterile lid speculum. At one of our centers, we use sterile gloves, a sterile drape, and an empty sterile 1 cc tuberculin syringe to mark the sclera. Alternatively, one can use a caliper to mark the location for the injection procedure. For ranibizumab and aflibercept, the drug is drawn from the drug vial using a filtered needle attached to a tuberculin syringe. The needle is then changed to a sterile 30-gauge needle prior to the injection. For bevacizumab, the drug is packaged in syringes and a sterile 30-gauge needle is affixed to the tuberculin syringe. Preinjection prophylactic antibiotic drops may also be used, although no benefit of antibiotic prophylaxis has been established.

Adequate anesthesia is a necessity to ensure patient comfort and perhaps future compliance with intravitreal injection regimens needed to treat neovascular AMD. In our hands, topical administration of anesthesia appears to result in anesthesia similar to subconjunctival injection of lidocaine, but either method can be used. For topical anesthesia, a cotton tip applicator is soaked with tetracaine or lidocaine and placed under the upper or lower eyelid in the conjunctival fornix, so that it rests against the superotemporal or inferotemporal bulbar conjunctiva at the site where the injection is planned. The patient should be instructed to look in the opposite direction and remain that way, so as not to scratch the cornea on the cotton tip applicator. After three to five minutes, the applicator can be removed. Another strategy is to apply direct pressure on the globe with the cotton tip applicator for a few minutes to both anesthetize the site of injection and soften the globe to minimize the intraocular pressure increase after injection. The eye is then prepped with 5% povidine-iodine solution placed directly on the globe, and 5% povidine sticks used to clean the eyelids, lashes, and periocular skin. Gloves are worn and a sterile lid speculum is inserted between the eyelids. A sterile drape may be used over the eye if desired, but is not necessary. The patient is then asked to fix his or her gaze in the direction opposite to where the injection is planned, so as to provide the best possible exposure of the injection site. Providing the patients with an object to fixate upon, such as their own raised thumb, can improve the stability of the eye during the injection.

A sterile 1 cc syringe hub or a sterile caliper can be used to mark the site of injection. The safest point of injection in phakic patients is 4 mm posterior to the limbus; the round tip of the tuberculin 1 cc syringe is 4 mm in diameter. Alternatively one can use a sterile caliper to mark the site. The drug is then injected into the vitreous cavity through the pars plana using a 30- or 32 gauge needle (0.05 cc total volume in the case of ranibizumab, bevacizumab, aflibercept or 0.1 cc total volume in the case of pegaptanib). The needle is withdrawn and a dry cotton tip applicator is immediately applied over the injection site for a few seconds to help prevent prolapse and incarceration of vitreous in the wound, which can serve as a possible wick for the introduction of bacteria into the eye. Antibiotic drops can be placed on the eye, but the use of prophylactic antibiotic drops after injection has been fallen out of favor due to lack of evidence of efficacy in the prevention of endophthalmitis as well as the increased risk of increased bacterial resistance (54,55). The lid speculum is then removed. We usually monitor the intraocular pressure following the injection to confirm that it returns to normal. Alternatively, some physicians prefer to document the presence of vision in the injected eye or confirm that the central retinal artery is perfused via an indirect ophthalmoscopic examination.

Most compliant patients do not need to be rechecked in the clinic until they are due for their next injection usually four weeks later, presuming they have received clear instructions on the signs and symptoms of infection or retinal detachment and the need to return immediately should those occur. Povidine iodine can be quite irritating to the corneal epithelium. It is therefore normal for patients to have some degree of irritation, burning, and tearing following their injection, in addition to varying amounts of subconjunctival hemorrhage. The wise physician will warn their patients of these possibilities at the time of injection. However, any antiseptic-associated discomfort should resolve by the following day. Therefore, any pain or decreased vision reported by the patient on post-injection day 1 or later should be taken very seriously.

FUTURE ANTI-VEGF THERAPIES
Soluble Fusion Protein
KH902 (Chengdu Kanghong Biotechnology, Chengdu, China) is a soluble fusion protein that combines ligand-binding elements taken from the extracellular components of VEGF receptors 1 and 2 fused to the Fc portion of IgG1 (56). The difference between KH902 and aflibercept is that there is an extra extracellular domain 4 of VEGF receptor 2, KDRd4, that may help increase the efficacy of stabilizing the molecular structure. This domain may increase the half-life of KH902 and increase the affinity for VEGF.

Animal studies in rhesus monkey have shown intravitreal injection of KH902 could inhibit CNV growth and leakage at doses as high as 300–500 µg without showing signs of toxicity (57). Phase I studies done in 28 humans at doses of 3.0 mg were also tolerated without toxicity noted (58). And 42 days after injection there was an improvement of 19.6 letters. No patient lost more than one letter and 57% of patients gained 15 letters or more from baseline. The area of CNV on fluorescein angiography decreased by 12.6% and the central retinal thickness improved by 77.2 µm. No adverse effects were noted after the patients received one injection and currently a phase III trial is taking place in China.

Small Interfering RNAs
The therapeutic potential of RNA interference was born in 1998, when Fire and Mello (59) discovered that injection of gene-specific double-stranded RNA into cells resulted in potent silencing of that gene's expression. They had discovered one of the fundamental mechanisms by which the cell regulates gene expression and protects itself against viral infection: RNA interference. Fire and Mello were awarded the Nobel Prize in Physiology and Medicine for 2006.

The components of the RNA interference machinery have since been identified. Double-stranded RNA binds to a protein complex called Dicer, which cleaves it into multiple smaller fragments. A second protein complex called RNA induced silencing complex (RISC) then binds these RNA fragments and eliminates one of the strands. The remaining strand stays bound to RISC, and serves as a probe that recognizes the corresponding messenger RNA transcript in the cell. When the RISC complex finds a complementary messenger RNA transcript, the transcript is cleaved and degraded, thus silencing that gene's expression (60).

Small interfering RNAs (siRNAs) have quickly become important tools in genetic research, and their potential as therapeutic agents is being explored in many areas of medicine. Reich and Tolentino (60,61) were the first to apply siRNA technology for the treatment of CNV. Bevasiranib/Cand5 (Acuity Pharmaceuticals, Philadelphia, Pennsylvania, USA) is an siRNA inhibitor of VEGF, which is given as an intravitreal injection. A phase I, open-label, dose-escalation study of 15 patients revealed no serious ocular or systemic adverse effects at a dose up to 3.0 mg.

The CARE study (Cand5 Anti-VEGF RNA: Evaluation) is a phase II multicenter, randomized, double-masked trial of bevasiranib/Cand5 in patients with CNV secondary to AMD (62). A hundred and twenty seven patients with predominantly classic, minimally classic, or retinal angiomatous proliferation lesions (occult no classic lesions excluded) were randomized to receive one of the three doses of the drug (0.2, 1.5, and 3.0 mg) at baseline and at six weeks. The primary end point was the mean change in ETDRS visual acuity from baseline at 12 weeks, which was 4 letters (0.2 mg), 7 letters (1.5 mg), and 6 letters (3.0 mg). The authors have theorized that these disappointing results stem from the fact that bevasiranib/Cand5 only blocks the production of new VEGF; VEGF already present at the time of injection was not inhibited. The investigators postulated that a baseline combination treatment with a VEGF protein blocker may be required to "mop up" the pre-existing VEGF load. However, the half-life of VEGF is short and it does not explain why the results are not seen by 12 weeks time point with siRNA treatment. Efficacy for the proposed treatment combination remains to be shown. A phase III, randomized, double-masked study of intravitreal bevasiranib sodium, administered every 8 or 12 weeks as maintenance therapy following three injections of ranibizumab compared with ranibizumab monotherapy every 4 weeks in patients with wet AMD (COBALT) has completed enrollment. The results of this study is still pending at this time. The investigators envision a role of bevasiranib/Cand5 as a long-term "maintenance" drug. The CARE trial raised no safety concerns, with only one patient developing uveitis. Other therapeutic targets for siRNAs are being investigated. siRNAs directed against the VEGFR-1 receptor have shown promise in a mouse model of CNV (63), and are currently in clinical development (Sirna-027, Sirna Therapeutics, Boulder, Colorado, USA). A prospective, open-label, single dose, dose-escalation phase I study was conducted in 26 patients with wet AMD (64). Intravitreal injection of a single dose of Sirna-027 from 100 to 1600 µg was well tolerated in patients with AMD, with no dose-limiting toxicity found. Adverse events were mild to moderate in severity. Adjusted mean foveal thickness decreased within two weeks after study treatment. This phase I study demonstrates that a single dose of siRNA can be administered safely by intravitreal injection and shows that Sirna-027 may have some biological activity. However, a phase II trial comparing monthly intravitreal Sirna-027 (aka AGN211745) at doses of 100, 500, and 1000 µg with monthly ranibizumab was terminated early by Allergan not related to safety issues.

Subsequent studies suggest that non-specific siRNAs of any sequence of 21 nucleotide or longer can suppress CNV via activation of Toll-like receptor-3 (TLR3) (65). However, there is also evidence that TLR3 activation can induce cell death in human and mouse RPE cells, depending on the TLR3 genotype (66). Therefore, siRNA therapeutics might increase the risk of patients to geographic atrophy depending on the TLR3 genotype. Further studies involving chemical modifications to siRNA that abolish TLR3 activation may enhance their therapeutic specificity. Chapter 4 presents further information in this area.

Receptor Tyrosine Kinase Inhibitors

Non-RNA inhibitors of VEGF receptor tyrosine kinase activity have been identified, and their anti-angiogenic properties are being investigated for use in the treatment of systemic malignancy, as well as CNV. One advantage of this class of drugs over those discussed thus far in this chapter is the possibility of an oral route of administration, thereby avoiding the ocular complications associated with frequent intravitreal injections.

One promising compound is PTK787, which is a nonselective inhibitor of all known VEGF receptors (67). PTK787 has been shown to inhibit retinal neovascularization in a hypoxic mouse model (68,69). Phase I/II clinical trials of PTK787 (Vatalanib, Novartis, East Hanover, New Jersey, USA) have been done in patients with solid malignancies, hematologic malignancies, and wet AMD. The ADVANCE study is a randomized, double-masked, multicenter, phase I/II study of the safety of vatalanib administered in conjunction with photodynamic therapy with verteporfin to patients with predominantly classic, minimally classic, or occult with no classic subfoveal CNV secondary to AMD (70). Fifty patients with all CNV lesion types received PDT with Visudyne at baseline, and were randomized to receive concurrent treatment with either 500 or 1000 mg of oral PTK787/Vatalanib or placebo, once daily for three months. ADVANCE is designed to assess the safety and efficacy of the drug but no results have been published to date.

Pazopanib (GW786034) is a second-generation multitargeted tyrosine kinase inhibitor against all VEGFR, PDGFRa, PDGFRb, and c-kit (71). A phase I clinical trial using pazopanib as eye drops in 38 healthy volunteers has successfully demonstrated its safety and tolerability. Subsequently, a phase II trial to evaluate its pharmacodynamics, pharmacokinetics, and safety has completed enrollment (70 patients) although no results have been published to date. A phase I trial involving oral pazopanib is also underway.

TG100801 (TargeGen Inc., San Diego, California, USA) is a potent tyrosine kinase inhibitor and a prodrug of TG100572, which binds and inhibits the activities of VEGFR and PDGFR (72). To minimize systemic exposure, this drug was delivered topically as an eye drop. Data have suggested that substantial levels were achieved in the choroid and retina yet undetectable in the plasma. It was shown that topical TG100801 significantly suppressed laser-induced CNV in mice. A phase I trial was completed using low and high doses applied topically twice daily for 14 days in 44 healthy volunteers, which showed good tolerance.

However, a phase II randomized study was terminated prior to completion. No published results are available at this time.

Anti-VEGF treatment has enabled a sizeable proportion of treated patients to attain significant visual improvement or to maintain vision. Several novel classes of anti-angiogenesis targets are currently under investigation for the treatment of various cancers and their use could potentially be expanded for ocular indications such as AMD. These include sunitinib (SU11248), sorafenib (BAY 43-9006), AEE 788, axitinib (AG 013736), vandetanib (Zactima, ZD 6474), tivozanib (AV-951, KRN 951) , and motesanib (AMG706) (73). Future research will hopefully continue to build on these advances and make restoration of vision a reality for the majority of these patients.

SUMMARY POINTS

- Three anti-VEGF agents are currently approved by the FDA for treatment of neovascular AMD: pegaptanib (Macugen), ranibizumab (Lucentis), and aflibercept (Eylea).
- Pegaptanib, an aptamer (short oligonucleotide) that specifically binds and inhibits VEGF isoforms containing at least 165 amino acids, was shown to delay the rate of vision loss in a large, prospective, randomized clinical trial. Visual acuity results however are limited.
- Ranibizumab, an antigen-binding fragment of a humanized monoclonal antibody directed against all the biologically active forms of VEGF-A, including the known active proteolytic breakdown products, effectively slows down the rate of vision loss and can improve vision as shown in prospective, randomized clinical trials. Monthly injections provide superior sustained improvement in visual acuity and decreased central retinal thickness as compared with quarterly or as-needed dosing. Overall, intravitreal ranibizumab is well tolerated and has a low rate of adverse ocular or systemic side effects.
- Bevacizumab is a full-sized humanized monoclonal antibody with VEGF binding characteristics similar to ranibizumab; is approved by the FDA for systemic treatment of metastatic colorectal cancer and lung cancer, but is an off-label treatment for neovascular AMD.
- A large, prospective, randomized clinical trial (CATT) showed that the visual outcome of bevacizumab was noninferior to ranibizumab. However, the as-needed therapy resulted in less visual gain than the monthly therapy of either drug. Bevacizumab was associated with a higher overall rate of systemic adverse events in the CATT trial, but most of the excess events have not been associated previously with systemic anti-VEGF therapy.

- Aflibercept is a recombinant chimeric VEGF receptor fusion protein that inhibits all VEGF isoforms and placental growth factors and binds VEGF-A with high affinity. The FDA-approved dosing regimen—three monthly injections followed by injections every two months—has been shown to have clinical equivalent effects as monthly ranibizumab in two large, prospective, randomized controlled trials.
- Additional anti-VEGF drugs are in development.

REFERENCES

1. Ferrara N, Henzel WJ. Pituitary follicular cells secrete a novel heparin-binding growth factor specific for vascular endothelial cells. Biochem Biophys Res Commun 1989; 161: 851–8.
2. Michaelson IC. The mode of development of the vascular system of the retina with some observations on its significance for certain retinal disorders. Trans Ophthalmol Soc UK 1948; 68: 137–80.
3. Kvanta A, Algvere PV, Berglin L, et al. Subfoveal fibrovascular membranes in age-related macular degeneration express vascular endothelial growth factor. Invest Ophthalmol Vis Sci 1996; 37: 1929–34.
4. Wells JA, Murthy R, Chibber R, et al. Levels of vascular endothelial growth factor are elevated in the vitreous of patients with subretinal neovascularisation. Br J Ophthalmol 1996; 80: 363–6.
5. Robinson C, Stinger S. The splice variants of vascular endothelial growth factor (VEGF) and their receptors. J Cell Sci 1991; 114: 853–65.
6. Keyt BA, Berleau LT, Nguyen HV, et al. The carboxylterminal domain (111–165) of vascular endothelial growth factor is critical for its mitogenic potency. J Biol Chem 1996; 271: 7788–95.
7. Ng EW, Shima DT, Calias P, et al. Pegaptanib, a targeted anti-VEGF aptamer for ocular vascular disease. Nat Rev Drug Discov 2006; 5: 123–32.
8. Gragoudas ES, Adamis AP, Cunningham ET Jr, et al. Pegaptanib for neovascular age-related macular degeneration. N Engl J Med 2004; 351: 2805–16.
9. Chakravarthy U, Adamis AP, Cunningham ET Jr, et al. Year 2 efficacy results of 2 randomized controlled clinical trials of pegaptanib for neovascular age-related macular degeneration. Ophthalmology 2006; 113: 1508–21.
10. D'Amico DJ, Masonson HN, Patel M, et al. Pegaptanib sodium for neovascular age related macular degeneration: two-year safety results of the two prospective, multicenter, controlled clinical trials. Ophthalmology 2006; 113: 992–1001.
11. A safety and efficacy study comparing the combination treatments of verteporfin therapy plus one of two different doses of intravitreal triamcinolone acetonide and the verteporfin therapy plus intravitreal pegaptanib (VERITAS). 2005. [Available from: http://clinicaltrials.gov/ct2/show/NCT00242580] (Last accessed 17 May 2012)
12. Adamis AP, Cook G, Shima D, et al. Abstract of Papers, Combined Meeting of Club Jules Gonin and The Retina Society. Cape Town, South Africa, 15–20 October, 2006.
13. Mordenti J, Cuthbertson RA, Ferrara N, et al. Comparisons of the intraocular tissue distribution, pharmacokinetics, and safety of 125I-labeled full-length and fab

antibodies in rhesus monkeys following intravitreal administration. Toxicol Pathol 1999; 27: 536–44.

14. Shahar J, Avery RL, Heilweil G, et al. Electrophysiologic and retinal penetration studies following intravitreal injection of bevacizumab (Avastin). Retina 2006; 26: 262–9.

15. Kaiser PK. Antivascular endothelial growth factor agents and their development: therapeutic implications in ocular diseases. Am J Ophthalmol 2006; 142: 660e1–10.

16. Rosenfeld PJ, Brown DM, Heier JS, et al. Ranibizumab for neovascular age-related macular degeneration. N Engl J Med 2006; 355: 1419–31.

17. Brown DM, Kaiser PK, Michels M, et al. Ranibizumab versus verteporfin for neovascular age-related macular degeneration. N Engl J Med 2006; 355: 1432–44.

18. Regillo CD, Brown DM, Abraham P, et al. Randomized, double-masked, sham-controlled trial of ranibizumab for neovascular age-related macular degeneration: PIER study year 1. Am J Ophthalmol 2008; 145: 239–48.

19. Abraham P, Yue H, Wilson L. Randomized, double-masked, sham-controlled trial of ranibizumab for neovascular age-related macular degeneration: PIER study year 2. Am J Ophthalmol 2010; 150: 315–24.

20. Schmidt-Erfurth U, Eldem B, Guymer R, et al.; EXCITE Study Group. Efficacy and safety of monthly versus quarterly ranibizumab treatment in neovascular age-related macular degeneration: the EXCITE study. Ophthalmology 2011; 118: 831–9.

21. Holz FG, Amoaku W, Donate J, et al.; SUSTAIN Study Group. Safety and efficacy of a flexible dosing regimen of ranibizumab in neovascular age-related macular degeneration: the SUSTAIN study. Ophthalmology 2011; 118: 663–71.

22. Boyer DS, Heier JS, Brown DM, et al. A Phase IIIb study to evaluate the safety of ranibizumab in subjects with neovascular age-related macular degeneration. Ophthalmology 2009; 116: 1731–9.

23. Singer MA, Awh CC, Sadda S, et al. HORIZON: an open-label extension trial of ranibizumab for choroidal neovascularization secondary to age-related macular degeneration. Ophthalmology 2012; 119: 1175–83.

24. Fung AE, Lalwani GA, Rosenfeld PJ, et al. An OCT guided, variable dosing regimen with intravitreal ranibizumab (Lucentis) for Neovascular age-related macular degeneration. Am J Ophthalmol 2007; 143: 566–83.

25. Lalwani GA, Rosenfeld PJ, Fung AE, et al. A variable-dosing regimen with intravitreal ranibizumab for neovascular age-related macular degeneration: year 2 of the PrONTO study. Am J Ophthalmol 2009; 148: 43–58; e1.

26. Suner IJ, Yau L, Lai P. HARBOR study: one-year results of efficacy and safety of 2.0 mg versus 0.5 mg ranibizumab in patients with subfoveal choroidal neovascularization secondary to age-related macular degeneration. Invest Ophthalmol Vis Sci 2012: 3677.

27. Michels S, Rosenfeld JR, Puliafito CA, et al. Systemic bevacizumab (Avastin) therapy for neovascular age-related macular degeneration: twelve-week results of an uncontrolled open-label clinical study. Ophthalmology 2005; 112: 1035–47.

28. Rosenfeld PJ, Moshfeghi AA, Puliafito CA. Optical coherence tomography findings after an intravitreal injection of bevacizumab (Avastin) for neovascular age-related macular degeneration. Ophthalmic Surg Lasers Imaging 2005; 36: 331–5.

29. Avery RL, Pieramici DJ, Rabena MD, et al. Intravitreal bevacizumab (Avastin) for neovascular age-related macular degeneration. Ophthalmology 2006; 113: 363–72.

30. Spaide RF, Laud K, Fine HF, et al. Intravitreal bevacizumab treatment of choroidal neovascularization secondary to age-related macular degeneration. Retina 2006; 26: 383–90.

31. Rich RM, Rosenfeld PJ, Puliafito CA, et al. Short-term safety and efficacy of intravitreal bevacizumab (Avastin) for neovascular age-related macular degeneration. Retina 2006; 26: 495–511.

32. Bashshur ZF, Bazarbachi A, Schakal A, et al. Intravitreal bevacizumab for the management of choroidal neovascularization in age-related macular degeneration. Am J Ophthalmol 2006; 142: 1–9.

33. Luthra S, Narayanan R, Marques LE, et al. Evaluation of in vitro effects of bevacizumab (Avastin) on retinal pigment epithelial, neurosensory retinal, and microvascular endothelial cells. Retina 2006; 26: 512–18.

34. Manzano RP, Peyman GA, Khan P, et al. Testing intravitreal toxicity of bevacizumab (Avastin). Retina 2006; 26: 257–61.

35. Bakri SJ, Cameron JD, McCannel CA, et al. Absence of histologic retinal toxicity of intravitreal bevacizumab in a rabbit model. Am J Ophthalmol 2006; 142: 162–4.

36. Stewart MW, Rosenfeld PJ, Penha FM, et al. Pharmacokinetic rationale for dosing every 2 weeks versus 4 weeks with intravitreal ranibizumab, bevacizumab, and aflibercept (vascular endothelial growth factor Trap-eye). Retina 2012; 32: 434–57.

37. Martin DF, Maguire MG, Ying GS, et al.; CATT Research Group. Ranibizumab and bevacizumab for neovascular age-related macular degeneration. N Engl J Med 2011; 364:1897–908.

38. Martin DF, Maguire MG, Fine SL, et al.; CATT Research Group. Ranibizumab and bevacizumab for treatment of neovascular age-related macular degeneration: two-year results. Ophthalmology 2012; 119: 1388–98.

39. Chakravarthy U, Harding SP, Rogers CA, et al.; The IVAN Study Investigators Writing Committee. Ranibizumab versus bevacizumab to treat neovascular age-related macular degeneration: one-year findings from the IVAN Randomized trial. Ophthalmology 2012; 119: 1399–1411.

40. [Available from: www.omic.com] (Accessed on June 4, 2012).

41. Klesert TR. So you want to try intravitreal avastin. Retina Times 2006; 14: 18–21.

42. Nguyen QD, Shah SM, Hafiz G, et al. A phase I trial of an IV-administered vascular endothelial growth factor trap for treatment in patients with choroidal neovascularization due to age-related macular degeneration. Ophthalmology 2006; 113: 1522–38.

43. Nguyen QD, Shah SM, Browning DJ, et al. A phase I study of intravitreal vascular endothelial growth factor trap-eye in patients with neovascular age-related macular degeneration. Ophthalmology 2009; 116: 2141–8.

44. Heier JS, Boyer D, Nguyen QD, et al.; CLEAR-IT 2 Investigators. the 1-year results of CLEAR-IT 2, a phase 2 study of vascular endothelial growth factor trap-eye dosed as-needed after 12-week fixed dosing. Ophthalmology 2011; 118: 1098–106.

45. Vascular endothelial growth factor (VEGF) trap-eye: investigation of efficacy and safety in wet age-related

macular degeneration (VIEW1). 2011, updated 13 April 2012. [Available from: http://clinicaltrials.gov/ct2/show/NCT00509795] (Last accessed 23 April 2012).

46. Vascular endothelial growth factor (VEGF) trap-eye: investigation of efficacy and safety in wet age-related macular degeneration (VIEW2). 2011, updated 27 February 2012. [Available from: http://clinicaltrials.gov/ct2/show/NCT00637377] (Last accessed 23 April 2012).

47. Heier JS, Boyer DS, Ciulla TA, et al. Ranibizumab combined with verteporfin photodynamic therapy in neovascular age-related macular degeneration: year 1 results of the FOCUS study. Arch Ophthalmol 2006; 124: 1532–42.

48. Kaiser PK, Boyer DS, Cruess AF, et al.; DENALI Study Group. Verteporfin plus ranibizumab for choroidal neovascularization in age-related macular degeneration: twelve-month results of the DENALI Study. Ophthalmology 2012; 119: 1001–10.

49. Larsen M, Schmidt-Erfurth U, Lanzetta P, et al.; MONT BLANC Study Group. Verteporfin plus ranibizumab for choroidal neovascularization in age-related macular degeneration: twelve-month MONT BLANC study results. Ophthalmology 2012; 119: 992–1000.

50. Hosoi Y, Yamamoto M, Ono T, Sakamoto K. Prostacyclin production in cultured endothelial cells is highly sensitive to low doses of ionizing radiation. Int J Radiat Biol 1993; 63: 631–8.

51. Dugel PU, Petrarca R, Bennett M, et al. Macular epiretinal brachytherapy in treated age-related macular degeneration: meritage study: twelve-month safety and efficacy results. Ophthalmology 2012; 119: 1425–31.

52. Cheung CS, Wong AW, Lui A, et al. Incidence of endophthalmitis and use of antibiotic prophylaxis after intravitreal injections. Ophthalmology 2012. [Epub ahead of print].

53. Milder E, Vander J, Shah C, Garg S. Changes in antibiotic resistance patterns of conjunctival flora due to repeated use of topical antibiotics after intravitreal injection. Ophthalmology 2012; 119: 1420–4.

54. Avery RL, Pearlman J, Pieramici DJ, et al. Intravitreal bevacizumab (Avastin) in the treatment of proliferative diabetic retinopathy. Ophthalmology 2006; 113: 1695e1–15.

55. Adamis AP, Altaweel M, Bressler NM, et al. Changes in retinal neovascularization after pegaptanib (Macugen) therapy in diabetic individuals. Ophthalmology 2006; 113: 23–8.

56. Zhang M, Yu D, Yang C, et al. The pharmacology study of a new recombinant human VEGF receptor-fc fusion protein on experimental choroidal neovascularization. Pharm Res 2009; 26: 204–10.

57. Zhang M, Zhang J, Yan M, et al. Recombinant anti-vascular endothelial growth factor fusion protein efficiently suppresses choridal neovasularization in monkeys. Mol Vis 2008; 14: 37–49.

58. Zhang M, Zhang J, Yan M, et al.; KH902 Phase 1 Study Group. A phase 1 study of KH902, a vascular endothelial growth factor receptor decoy, for exudative age-related macular degeneration. Ophthalmology 2011; 118: 672–8.

59. Fire A, Xu S, Montgomery MK, et al. Potent and specific genetic interference by double-stranded RNA in Caenorhabditis elegans. Nature 1998; 391: 806–11.

60. Reich SJ, Fosnot J, Kuroki A, et al. Small interfering RNA (siRNA) targeting VEGF effectively inhibits ocular neovascularization in a mouse model. Mol Vis 2003; 9: 210–16.

61. Tolentino MJ, Brucker AJ, Fosnot J, et al. Intravitreal injection of vascular endothelial growth factor small interfering RNA inhibits growth and leakage in a nonhuman primate, laser-induced model of choroidal neovascularization. Retina 2004; 24: 132–8.

62. Brucker AJ, The Cand5 Study Group. Abstract of Papers, Combined Meeting of Club Jules Gonin and The Retina Society. Cape Town, South Africa, 15–20, October, 2006.

63. Shen J, Samul R, Silva RL, et al. Suppression of ocular neovascularization with siRNA targeting VEGF receptor 1. Gene Ther 2006; 13: 225–34.

64. Kaiser PK, Symons RC, Shah SM, et al. Sirna-027 Study Investigators. RNAi-based treatment for neovascular age-related macular degeneration by Sirna-027. Am J Ophthalmol 2010; 150: 33–9.

65. Kleinman ME, Yamada K, Takeda A, et al. Sequence- and target-independent angiogenesis suppression by siRNA via TLR3. Nature 2008; 452: 591–7.

66. Yang Z, Stratton C, Francis PJ, et al. Toll-like receptor 3 and geographic atrophy in age-related macular degeneration. N Engl J Med 2008; 359: 1456–63.

67. Wood JM, Bold G, Buchdunger E, et al. PTK787/ZK 222584, a novel and potent inhibitor of vascular endothelial growth factor receptor tyrosine kinases, impairs vascular endothelial growth factor-induced responses and tumor growth after oral administration. Cancer Res 2000; 60: 2178–89.

68. Maier P, Unsoeld AS, Junker B, et al. Intravitreal injection of specific receptor tyrosine kinase inhibitor PTK787/ ZK222 584 improves ischemia-induced retinopathy in mice. Graefes Arch Clin Exp Ophthalmol 2005; 243: 593–6.

69. Ozaki H, Seo MS, Ozaki K, et al. Blockade of vascular endothelial cell growth factor receptor signaling is sufficient to completely prevent retinal neovascularization. Am J Pathol 2000; 156: 697–707.

70. Safety and Efficacy of Oral PTK787 in Patients With Subfoveal Choroidal Neovascularization Secondary to Age-Related Macular Degeneration (AMD) (ADVANCE). 2005.updated 12 November 2008 [Available from: http://clinicaltrials.gov/ct2/show/NCT00138632] (Last accessed 4 June 2012).

71. Sonpavde G, Hutson TE, Sternberg CN. Pazopanib, a potent orally administered small molecule multitargeted tyrosine kinase inhibitor for renal cell carcinoma. Expert Opin Investig Drugs 2008; 17: 253–61.

72. Doukas J, Mahesh S, Umeda N, et al. Topical administration of multi-targeted kinase inhibitor suppresses choroidal neovascularization and retinal edema. J Cell Physiol 2008; 216: 29–37.

73. Mousa SA, Mousa SS. Current status of vascular endothelial growth factor inhibition in age-related macular degeneration. BioDrugs 2010; 24: 183–94.

20

Non-VEGF related antiangiogenesis pathways for treatment of age-related macular degeneration

Anthony B. Daniels, Ivana K. Kim, Joan W. Miller, and Demetrios G. Vavvas

INTRODUCTION

The biggest breakthrough in the treatment of neovascular age-related macular degeneration (AMD) in the past decade was the development and widespread adoption of therapies that specifically target vascular endothelial growth factor (VEGF). Ranibizumab intravitreal injection set a new therapeutic standard, with only 5% of ranibizumab-treated eyes losing 15 letters of visual acuity, and 34–40% of patients gaining at least 15 letters of visual acuity (1,2). However, despite the success of anti-VEGF treatment, significant room for improvement remains. Most patients (60%) still do not experience significant improvement of vision, and the first long-term results (>= 4 years of treatment) show a loss of the vision gained in the first two years (3).

In addition, monthly injections can be burdensome. Several studies have looked at alternative dosing, either less frequently (4), on an "as needed" basis (PRN) (5), or with successive extension of the inter-injection interval ("treat-and-extend") usually with somewhat decreased efficacy (6,7).

The reasons that certain patients treated with anti-VEGF monotherapy fail to regain a significant amount of vision fall into several categories. Either the subretinal and intraretinal edema persists (nonresponse), or, despite cessation of leakage, patients develop either subretinal fibrosis or photoreceptor atrophy overlying the choroidal neovascular membrane (CNVM), leading to irreversible vision loss. Because of these limitations, interest is again shifting toward other treatments that, either alone or in combination with anti-VEGF agents, might improve visual outcomes by (i) making CNVMs more responsive to anti-VEGF agents, (ii) decreasing the development of subretinal fibrosis, or (iii) preventing the loss of photoreceptors (neuroprotection). Thus, several other molecular pathways important in angiogenesis are being explored as therapeutic targets. Some of these emerging therapies modulate VEGF signaling, some mediate VEGF escape from therapy, and some are completely independent of the VEGF pathway.

This chapter explores what is known about these various molecular pathways and their roles in angiogenesis; it also reviews the clinical and preclinical evidence that targeting these pathways might decrease choroidal neovascularization (CNV) in patients with AMD.

Fibroblast Growth Factor

The fibroblast growth factor (FGF) family of proteins comprises 22 different proteins in mammals, and is involved in a plethora of different functions, including organogenesis and wound response. Most of these proteins, including those acting in the eye, function in a paracrine fashion, exerting their effect over cells and tissues located adjacent to their source. FGFs all share a homologous core region of ~120 amino acids that are arranged into 12 antiparallel β-pleated sheets, with variation in the sequence at the amino and carboxy termini conferring the different biology of the various FGF ligands (8). There are four FGF receptor (FGFR) genes, which, through variable splicing, encode seven different functional receptors (9).

FGF signaling involves a ternary complex formed by FGF, FGFR, and heparin sulfate proteoglycan (HSPG), which form a 1:1:1 complex, and facilitates receptor dimerization in a 2:2:2 fashion (9). Interactions of this complex or its various constituents with other molecules (e.g., fibronectin) in the extracellular matrix (ECM) also regulate receptor function and could serve as potential antiangiogenic targets (10). Binding of FGFR to its ligand FGF and to HSPG induces FGFR dimerization and subsequent autophosphorylation of the receptors. This in turn activates the mitogen-activated protein kinase (MAPK) and phosphoinositide 3-kinase (PI3K)-AKT pathways via fibroblast growth factor receptor substrate 2-alfa [FRS2α], and the protein kinase C (PKC) pathway via protein lipase C (PLC), thereby transducing the receptor's intracellular signal (9,11).

FGF2 has been implicated in various aspects of angiogenesis. FGF2 induces the production of proteases, stimulates endothelial cell proliferation and migration, and maintains vascular integrity by annealing adherens junctions (12). In fact, *in vitro* studies in choriocapillary endothelial cells have demonstrated that FGF2 is a stronger inducer of endothelial cell proliferation than VEGF (13), and the effects of FGF2 and VEGF are additive (14,15). In retinal pigment epithelial (RPE) cells from CNVMs, transcription of FGF2 is upregulated compared with normal RPE (16). FGFR is expressed on the surface of inner choroidal cells, and FGF/FGFR complexes have been demonstrated, consistent with paracrine stimulation (17). FGF2 lacks a secretion signaling peptide that is required for conventional golgi-mediated exocytosis (9). However, several studies have demonstrated an unconventional direct transmembrane pathway for protein secretion (18), and that cellular injury also causes release of intracellular FGF, consistent with its function as a wound response growth factor (19–21).

There is evidence that targeting both VEGF and FGF is superior to targeting VEGF alone. In RPE cells derived from CNVMs, targeting VEGF alone at concentrations that completely inactivated all VEGF was still insufficient to completely inhibit endothelial cell sprouting, whereas combined anti-VEGF and anti-FGF antibody inhibition completely blocked all endothelial cell sprouting (15). There are several potential molecules that can be used to inhibit the FGF pathway, most of which were devised initially as anticancer agents. Suramin is a heparin mimic that binds and disrupts the FGF/FGFR complex, and has been used as an angiogenesis inhibitor in clinical trials for the treatment of several cancers (9). However, this molecule is associated with coagulopathy as a side effect. Interestingly, a new heparinoid derived from shrimp has been found to also have anti-FGF properties, but without the associated coagulopathy and hemorrhage (22). Sunitinib is a nonspecific tyrosine kinase inhibitor that targets FGFR in addition to several other receptor tyrosine kinases, and has also been used in clinical trials for various cancers (23). Lastly, thalidomide has been shown to interfere with FGF2-induced thrombosis, and has been found to be effective in several phase 2 clinical trials for various types of cancer (9). The fact that most patients with AMD are beyond child-bearing age would obviate many of the teratogenic concerns associated with thalidomide.

Pigment Epithelium-Derived Factor

Pigment epithelium-derived factor (PEDF) is a member of the serine protease inhibitor (serpin) family of proteins, yet does not exhibit their typical inhibitory activity. In contrast, it plays a role in many other processes, including neurotropism, neuroprotection, antiangiogenesis, and anti-vasopermeability (24). Although it is transcribed predominantly in the RPE and retinal ganglion cells in the retina (25), PEDF protein is predominantly localized to the vitreous and the interphotoreceptor matrix in the eye (26), because of the binding affinity of PEDF for extracellular matrix components such as glycosaminoglycans and collagen. In fact, ECM products such as heparin sulfate may play a role in modulating ligand-receptor interactions (24,26).

PEDF is one of the most potent natural inhibitors of angiogenesis (27), and the molecular mechanisms of the antiangiogenic properties of PEDF are beginning to be elucidated. PEDF functions as a VEGF pathway antagonist by inhibiting VEGF-mediated VEGFR-1 phosphorylation (28), as well as by regulated intramembrane proteolysis of VEGFR-1 in a γ-secretase-dependent fashion (28,29). Independent of the VEGF pathway, PEDF induces apoptosis of neovascular endothelial cells. Interestingly, PEDF appears to induce apoptosis in its antiangiogenic capacity, and block apoptosis in its neuroprotective capacity. Likewise, neovascular vessels are affected, but existing vessels are unaffected. This specificity for apoptotic activity in neovascular endothelial cells appears to occur via a Fas–FasL interaction, as PEDF has been shown to upregulate FasL on endothelial cells, while its interacting partner, Fas, is expressed at low levels on quiescent mature vessels, but is induced by the process of angiogenesis (30).

There is also evidence for the involvement of PEDF in pathologic ocular neovascularization. PEDF expression has been detected in RPE cellular components of experimental laser-induced CNV long after VEGF expression has ceased (25). In human AMD-associated CNVM harvested at the time of submacular surgical membranectomy, PEDF was co-expressed with VEGF in RPE cells throughout the membrane, but was only expressed in vascular endothelial cells in areas where the membrane was active, and not in areas where fibrosis was present (31). It appears that the PEDF–VEGF balance is modulated by hypoxia and oxidative stress. In areas with decreased PEDF levels, a permissive environment for angiogenesis is created (32). Interestingly, nicotine increases the VEGF/PEDF ratio *in vitro*, which might partially explain the association between smoking and AMD progression (33). These findings are consistent with *in vivo* evidence from humans, where vitreous levels of PEDF were significantly lower in patients with AMD and CNV than in control patients (34). Further corroborating this association between PEDF and AMD-associated angiogenesis is the fact that certain PEDF gene polymorphisms are associated with the development of neovascular AMD (35).

Given the strong natural antiangiogenic capacity of PEDF and the angiogenic permissiveness of low PEDF levels, it will be beneficial to be able to modulate the PEDF-VEGF ratio by increasing PEDF levels in patients with neovascular AMD. It is known that the normally occurring level of PEDF in the vitreous of patients without pathologic neovascularization is sufficient to inhibit endothelial cell migration, even in the presence of a concentration of VEGF as high as that found in the vitreous of patients with proliferative diabetic retinopathy (27). Thus, increasing the low PEDF levels found in patients with neovascular AMD might be sufficient to block angiogenesis in patients with AMD, even in the presence of elevated levels of VEGF in these patients. As a proof of this concept, Mori and associates (2002) (36) have demonstrated that virus-mediated PEDF gene transfer can decrease the size of CNV in a mouse model of laser-induced CNV. A phase I clinical trial of an intravitreally injected replication-deficient adenovirus expressing PEDF [AdGVPEDF.11D (GenVec)] for the treatment of severe neovascular AMD with extensive fibrotic scarring has been completed, and reported no serious adverse events or dose-limiting toxicities (37).

Notch

The Notch family of receptors comprise four single-transmembrane receptors (Notch1–4) that have five single-transmembrane ligands in mammals (Jagged1, Jagged2, Delta-like ligand [Dll]-1, Dll-3, and Dll-4) (38–40). With respect to the ocular vasculature, Notch1 and Notch3 are expressed by the endothelium, and Notch3 functions in the smooth muscle (38). Binding of Notch by its ligands activates sequential receptor cleavage. First, the extracellular domain is cleaved by a disintegrin and metalloproteinase (ADAM), causing release of the extracellular domain with its bound ligand, which can be endocytosed by adjacent cells and influence signaling (41). Subsequently, γ-secretase cleaves the membrane portion of the receptor, releasing the Notch intracellular domain (NICD), which translocates to the nucleus, displaces a co-repressor complex, and thus activates transcription factors [C Promoter-Binding Factor 1 (CBF-1), Su(H), Lag-1]-type transcription factors (CSL) (known as recombination signal-binding protein for immunoglobulin kappa J region (RBP-J) in rodents) and CBP (39,40). This leads to a transcription of downstream gene targets, including Hey1, Hey2, and Hes1, which are expressed in vessels.

The Notch pathway is involved in several aspects of both normal and pathologic angiogenesis. In the formation of a vascular sprout, the "tip" cell migrates and dictates the direction of growth, whereas the "stalk" cells proliferate and form the body of the new vessel. Notch signaling is important in tip and stalk cell selection, specifically by restricting tip cell selection. Dll4 is upregulated in tip cells in response to VEGF (42,43), and paracrine stimulation of adjacent endothelial cells via their Notch receptors leads to an inhibition of the tip cell phenotype and expression of the stalk cell phenotype (44). Via the Notch network, the tip cell reacts with enhanced migration and decreased proliferation in response to a VEGF gradient, while the stalk cells respond to the VEGF signal with increased proliferation (45). Notch signaling is also important in pericyte recruitment as part of normal vessel maturation (46), in arterial fate specification (47,48), in vessel homeostasis, and in maintaining endothelial cell quiescence (49).

Thus, Notch serves as an overall check to excessive VEGF signaling, and dysfunction or deregulation of the Notch pathway leads to deregulation of angiogenesis. While VEGF/VEGFR signaling leads to Dll4 upregulation, Notch signaling counteracts this by upregulating VEGFR-1 and downregulating VEGFR-2, VEGFR-3 (43,45), and PlGF (50). In the eye, disruption of RBP-J downstream to Notch induces retinal and corneal neovascularization (49) and loss of Notch1 causes corneal neovascularization in addition to widespread systemic vascular tumors and lethal hemorrhage (51).

Since Notch signaling is so intimately involved with modulating VEGF signaling, it is not surprising to find that the manipulation of the Notch signal can be used to alter angiogenesis. In a laser-induced CNV mouse model, abrogation of Notch signaling enhanced the angiogenic response (49). Similarly, activation of Notch with Jag1 peptide reduced CNV volume, while inhibition of the pathway with a γ-secretase inhibitor promoted CNV growth—thereby preventing the formation of the NICD complex. The NICD translocates to the nucleus, where it forms a complex with the DNA binding protein CSL, displacing a histone deacetylase (HDAc)-co-repressor (CoR) complex from CSL. Components of an activation complex, such as Mastermind-like protein 1 (MAML1) and histone acetyltransferases (HATs), are recruited to the NICD–CSL complex, leading

to the transcriptional activation of Notch target genes (52).

Platelet-Derived Growth Factor

The four platelet-derived growth factor (PDGF) isoforms (PDGF-A, PDGF-B, PDGF-C, and PDGF-D) exist as homodimers (namely, PDGF-AA, PDGF-BB, PDGF-CC, and PDGF-DD) and as a PDGF-AB heterodimer. There are two receptors, PDGFR-α and PDGFR-β, which are both receptor tyrosine kinases.

PDGF-B plays an important role in vessel maturation and pericyte recruitment. PDGF-B is secreted by proliferating endothelial cells, and is highest in the tip cells (53). The adjacent undifferentiated mesenchymal cells express PDGFR-β, and are thereby induced to proliferate and migrate to the maturing vessels by this PDGF-B signal (12,38). Therefore, mice lacking PDGF-B or PDGFR-β develop incompetent vessels devoid of pericytes and smooth muscle cells, develop microaneurysms (54), display blood–brain barrier defects from insufficient pericyte coverage (55), and succumb to generalized edema during embryogenesis (56).

Recently, the role of the PDGF-CC homodimer has been explored and elucidated. Not only does PDGF-C play a similar role in pericyte recruitment and vessel wall maturation, but also seems to be involved in many other steps of neovascularization, such as in the proliferation, survival, and migration of fibroblasts and macrophages, and in the survival of vascular endothelial cells (57). Unlike PDGF-B, which signals via PDGFR-β, PDGF-C transduces its signal via PDGFR-α. In fact, PDGF-C appears to be the major angiogenic ligand of this receptor, as antibody-mediated neutralization of PDGF-C inhibits CNV to the same extent as antibody-mediated neutralization of PDGFR-α (57). In addition, PDGF-C upregulates the expression of PDGF-B and PDGFR-β, as well as of VEGF (57).

Therapies that target VEGF are more efficient at destroying immature vessels devoid of pericytes than they are at destroying mature vessels (58), and immature vessels are selectively destroyed by VEGF inhibition (59). Thus, targeting PDGF to prevent pericyte coating of new vessels should render anti-VEGF strategies more effective. While specific targeting of PDGF-B in conjunction with VEGF did not improve the efficacy of VEGF inhibition in tumor models of angiogenesis (60), in models of ocular neovascularization, concurrent inhibition of PDGF-B did enhance the efficacy of anti-VEGF therapies (61). This possible synergy underlies a phase I clinical trial of E10030 (Ophthotech, New York, USA), a pegylated aptamer against PDGF-B. When delivered intravitreally in conjunction with ranibizumab, 100% of patients showed neovascular regression, with an average of 14 ETDRS (Early Treatment Diabetic Retinopathy Study) letters gained at 12 weeks, and with 59% of patients achieving a 15-letter or greater gain in vision (ARVO Ft Lauderdale 2009 Program 1260 Combined Inhibition of Platelet Derived (PDGF) and Vascular Endothelial (VEGF) Growth Factors for the Treatment of Neovascular Age-Related Macular Degeneration (NV-AMD) - Results of a Phase 1 Study). A phase II study is currently underway.

Transforming Growth Factor-β

There are many proteins in the transforming growth factor-β (TGFβ) family, including the TGFβs themselves (TGFβ1, TGFβ2, and TGFβ3), the BMPs (bone morphogenic proteins), activins and inhibins, which all play a variety of roles in different processes, including in immunity and angiogenesis (62). The two main receptor classes for these ligands are the TGFβ receptor 1 class (TGFβR1) and TGFβ receptor 2 class (TGFβR2), each comprising multiple specific receptors. Interaction of a TGFβ family ligand with TGFβR1 signals via phosphorylation and nuclear translocation of the (Sma [small] and MAD [mothers against decapentaplegia], an intracellular mediator of the TGF superfamily of receptors) family of proteins to affect transcription of target genes. The TGFβR2 class of receptors transmit their signal upon ligand binding by their interaction with, and activation of, TGFβR1 (43).

The role of TGFβ signaling in angiogenesis is not completely clear, with some studies demonstrating angiogenic properties while others show an antiangiogenic effect of TGFβ signaling. It is known that TGFβ signaling is important in vessel maturation, and plays a role in mural cell differentiation, proliferation, and migration, as well as in the production of ECM (63). In mouse models, loss of TGFβ receptor signaling leads to vessel fragility, and in humans, mutation of certain TGFβ receptor genes leads to hereditary hemorrhagic telangiectasia, a disease characterized by abnormal vessels with abnormal vessel walls (63). In the process of ocular neovascularization, it is known that inhibition of the TGFβ pathway decreases laser-induced CNV in a rat model, thus indicating that TGFβ promotes pathologic angiogenesis (64). This effect might be at least in part mediated via the interplay with VEGF, as TGFβ induces the expression of $VEGF_{121}$, $VEGF_{165}$, and $VEGF_{189}$ in human RPE cells, via a MAPK-mediated pathway (65). Polymorphisms in the HTRA1 gene promoter are associated with AMD, and HTRA1 seems to signal via the TGFβ family member, GDF6 (66).

Angiopoietin and Tie

Tie1 and Tie2 are receptor tyrosine kinases expressed on endothelial cells as well as on many other cell types. Angiopoietin (Ang)-1, Ang-2, Ang-3, and Ang-4 are glycoproteins that serve as specific ligands of Tie2. Ang-1 and Ang-4 are activators of Tie2 signaling (67), whereas Ang-2 and Ang-3 bind Tie2 but transduce a weak signal, and thus function predominantly as antagonists (68,69). However, under hypoxic conditions, when levels of Ang-2 predominate, and in the presence of VEGF, Ang-2 can nonetheless serve as a Tie2 agonist (68). A specific ligand for Tie1 is not known, and phosphorylation of Tie1 is dependent on concomitant activation of Tie2 in a heterodimeric complex (70). With regard to angiogenesis, Tie2 is the important receptor in this family, and Ang-1 and Ang-2 are the important ligands, sharing and competing with equal affinity for the exact same binding site on Tie2 (68). Ang-1 is secreted, forms multimers of varying sizes, and is stored in the extracellular matrix, while Ang-2 is stored in the cytoplasm of endothelial cells and secreted when needed (71). Ang-1 binding leads to Tie2 dimerization and autophosphorylation, and subsequent downstream activation of the PI3K-Akt pathway and of the Ras-Raf-MAPK pathway, overall leading to cellular survival, chemotaxis, and migration (71,72). Ang-1/Tie2 signaling via the Akt pathway induces Dll4 and thus maintains vascular quiescence by augmenting Notch signaling (see above) (73). Ang-1 or Tie2 null mice die during embryogenesis from disrupted vessel structures and defective mural cell coverage, leading to edema and hemorrhage, and this is phenocopied in mice overexpressing Ang-2 (38,74).

Ang-1/Tie2 signaling appears to cause two seemingly paradoxical responses. When Tie2-expressing endothelial cells are associated in *trans* with other endothelial cells, Ang-1 signaling leads to further vascular stabilization and quiescence. However, when Tie2-expressing cells are stimulated by ECM-bound Ang-1, MAPK/ERK-mediated cellular migration and proliferation ensue, leading to angiogenesis (75). In ocular neovascularization, the former role in vessel stabilization is better characterized, and in this regard Ang-1 plays two related roles: in pericyte and mural cell recruitment for vessel wall stabilization, and in maintenance of mature vessel quiescence. Ang-1 is secreted by pericytes and smooth muscle cells and activates Tie2 on endothelial cells, thus leading to pericyte adhesion, tight endothelial junctions, and the formation of stable, mature vessel walls, which are relatively resistant to VEGF-mediated permeability and angiogenic signaling (12). In contrast, Ang-2 antagonizes these effects, leading to mural cell dissociation, and in the presence of VEGF, these destabilized vessels are more susceptible to VEGF-mediated sprouting angiogenesis (38).

Clinical and *in vitro* studies have corroborated these roles in ocular neovascularization. In the corneal micropocket assay, addition of Ang-2 to the VEGF stimulus led to increased length and extent of corneal neovascularization, consistent with increased angiogenesis, whereas addition of Ang-1 to the VEGF stimulation led to increased vessel diameter and perfusion without increasing vessel length, consistent with vessel maturation (76). In the retina, Ang-2 mRNA levels are increased during pathologic angiogenesis in a mouse model of ischemic retinopathy (77). In surgically excised human CNVMs, Tie2 is expressed on almost all vascular structures. Ang-1 and Ang-2 are also expressed, but Ang-2 immunoreactivity is higher in the highly vascularized regions of the CNVM, with a localization similar to that of VEGF (78). Interestingly, VEGF upregulates Ang-1 (but not Ang-2) mRNA levels by stabilizing Ang-1 mRNA without increasing Ang-1 gene transcription, and also increases Ang-1 protein secretion (79). This suggests that within VEGF stimulation lies the seed to its own termination, by creating a negative feedback loop through Ang-1-mediated vessel maturation, which leads to relative resilience of the vessels to further VEGF stimulation.

Since Ang-1-mediated Tie2 signaling can inhibit VEGF-mediated neovascularization, this pathway may serve as an antiangiogenic target in AMD. Increased expression of Ang-1 in mouse models of retinal ischemia or laser-induced CNV significantly suppressed the development of retinal or choroidal neovascularization, and also reduced vascular permeability in response to VEGF (80). Similarly, a single intramuscular injection of an adenoviral vector expressing the extracellular domain of Tie2 reduced retinal neovascularization in a mouse model of retinal ischemia by 47%, reduced laser-induced CNV size by 45%, and reduced the incidence of CNV fluorescein leakage by 52% (81). Neutralizing antibodies against Ang-2 (or an antibody directed against both Ang-1 and Ang-2) inhibited retinal neovascularization and laser-induced CNV to the same degree as did anti-VEGF antibody (82). A small molecule inhibitor of Tie2 was developed, and significantly diminished aberrant vessel growth in an *in vitro* model of CNV (83). Thus, there appear to be many potential ways to target the Ang-1/Ang-2/Tie2 signaling system to inhibit ocular neovascularization.

Matrix Metalloproteinases

There are at least 23 different matrix metalloproteinase (MMP) proteins in humans and all have certain characteristics in common: (i) they contain a secretory signaling peptide domain at the N-terminus, (ii) they are produced as inactive pro-enzymes, and (iii) they share a similar conserved catalytic zinc cleft that serves as the active site for enzymatic activity (84). Substrate specificity is therefore determined by binding sites outside of the catalytic cleft itself, which are also responsible for establishing the correct orientation of the particular substrate. Activation of the MMPs from their proenzyme forms occurs by coordinated cleavage of the zymogen within the extracellular matrix, often by other MMPs, and often with the assistance of a ternary complex formed by tissue inhibitors of matrix metalloproteinases (TIMPs), which may either facilitate proenzyme cleavage or may maintain the inactive form (84). This is indicative of the complexity of the MMP network, and underlies the difficulty in designing targeted therapies that affect only certain enzymatic activities, without blocking the reverse activity.

Endothelial cells are usually kept stationary by the enveloping basement membrane and by mural cells, and sprouting requires degradation of the basement membrane and surrounding ECM in a controlled fashion. Uncontrolled or excessive ECM degradation, as occurs in plasminogen activator inhibitor (PAI) deficiency, prevents adequate matrix support for the branching endothelial tubes (85). MMPs are able to digest most protein components of the ECM, as well as other proteins stored within the ECM, such as chemokines, receptors, and other MMPs (86). They can release pro- and antiangiogenic growth factors incarcerated in the ECM (87), but can also degrade them (88).

In angiogenesis, the gelatinases, MMP-2 and MMP-9, along with TIMP-3, appear to play the dominant role. In cancers, it appears that the infiltrating neutrophils release the MMP-9 that serves as a catalytic stimulator of angiogenesis that is critical for tumor progression (89). VEGF induces production and secretion of MMP-2 from endothelial cells (90), and increases MMP-9 transcription in human RPE cells (91). In turn, MMP-9 feeds back to upregulate VEGF production from the RPE cells (91). Given that sprouting angiogenesis requires disassembly of the surrounding mural cells, it is not surprising to find that VEGF affects the smooth muscle cells as well. VEGF upregulates the expression of MMP-1 and MMP-9 (and to a lesser degree, MMP-3) from smooth muscle cells via VEGFR-1, and also causes smooth muscle cell migration (92). Interestingly, TIMP3 inhibits angiogenesis not only by inhibiting MMPs, but also by directly blocking VEGF binding to VEGFR-2 and thereby inhibiting downstream signaling (93). Independent of VEGF, several other molecules modulate MMP levels, including advanced glycation end products, which upregulate MMP-2 (94), tumor necrosis factor alfa (TNFα), which increases secretion of both MMP-2 and MMP-9 (95), and adenosine monophosphate (AMP)-activated protein kinase, which suppresses MMP-9 (96). MMP-2 and MMP-9, in turn, degrade the antiangiogenic growth factor PEDF in response to hypoxia (88).

Given the barrier role that Bruch's membrane plays in the normal retina, it follows that TIMP-3, a potent inhibitor of angiogenesis, is constitutively present in the ECM component of Bruch's membrane (97). Mice lacking TIMP-3 show increased corneal neovascularization in response to VEGF and more robust choroidal neovascularization in response to laser-induced Bruch's rupture (98). This is consistent with the known pathophysiology and natural history of Sorsby's fundus dystrophy, which is caused by a dominantly inherited mutation of TIMP-3, and is characterized by early-onset macular degeneration and CNV (99).

In contrast, MMP-2 and MMP-9 are positively associated with CNV formation, and are components of the membranes themselves. Consistent with findings in tumor angiogenesis, infiltrating neutrophils appear to be an important source of MMP-9 in CNVMs as well (100), although a recent histopathologic study of an idiopathic membrane that was excised from an infant and was composed entirely of RPE cells and vascular units demonstrated that complete CNV formation can occur even in the absence of any inflammatory cells whatsoever (101). Other histopathologic studies on surgically removed membranes have shown MMP-2 to be localized to vascular endothelial cells and MMP-9 to be localized predominantly near the edges of the CNVMs near Bruch's membrane (102). In fact, plasma levels of MMP-9 are actually elevated systemically in patients with AMD (103).

The difficulty in targeting MMPs in the treatment of neovascular AMD owes to the extreme complexity of the networks, whereby MMPs control not only digestion of ECM and therefore sprouting and migration, but also cleavage of other MMPs themselves. Thus, one will need to target those MMP reactions that lead to sprouting, while not affecting those substrate reactions that curtail angiogenesis. In addition, MMPs generally share a common catalytic zinc cleft that serves as the active site for enzymatic activity (84). This difficulty in achieving the desired specificity and selectivity has led to the failure in clinical trials of many potent MMP inhibitors which target the catalytic domain. Thus, newer generation MMP inhibitors instead target the substrate-specific exosites that are more unique to a given MMP's enzymatic activity on a given target. For example, an inhibitor of MMP-9 was created that selectively blocked its type V collagen-based activity (104). That said, non-selective MMP inhibition with doxycycline was also found to reduce neovascularization and CNV volume in a mouse model in response to laser-induced Bruch's rupture (105,106).

Integrins

Integrins are transmembrane receptor glycoproteins that are the products of 18 α subunits and 8 β subunits and assemble into 24 different $\alpha\beta$ heterodimers (107). The heterodimers have affinities for different ECM components, but a single integrin may bind different ECM components and a single ECM component may bind different integrins. At the simplest level, integrins bind the ECM, and couple it to the actin cytoskeleton inside the cell, thus anchoring the two together (108). The integrins can therefore use ECM proteins and embedded growth factors as a scaffold on which the physical process of migration occurs, which is fundamental to the formation of endothelial cell tubes in the process of angiogenesis. Much more than just a physical attachment, however, integrins have been shown to function as receptors, modulating the intracellular environment to outside signals. Changes in the ECM environment or in growth factors or other extracellular signals can cause intracellular cell responses (so-called "outside-in" signaling), while changes inside the cell, such as integrin interactions with other receptors or with other tyrosine kinases can affect the integrin receptors' affinity for, and attachment to, the ECM (so-called "inside-out" signaling) (109).

The different integrins appear to modulate the affinities of various other receptors for their ligands, based on whether the accompanying integrin is bound to its cognate ECM component, or to the other receptor's cognate ligand. For example, VEGF stimulation of VEGFR-2 causes VEGFR-2 to interact with integrin $\alpha_v\beta_3$, which not only augments the integrin's activity but also promotes VEGFR-2 phosphorylation (110). Conversely, blockade of integrin $\alpha_v\beta_3$ diminishes VEGFR-2 autophosphorylation and PI3K activation, as well as endothelial cell proliferation and migration in response to VEGF-A (111). Integrins $\alpha_v\beta_3$ and $\alpha_5\beta_5$ also modulate FGFR signaling (112–114), and blockade of $\alpha_v\beta_3$ leads to diminished MAPK pathway activation in response to FGF signaling, and therefore leads to a decrease in angiogenesis (115). PDGFR, as well as the PDGF and VEGF-A ligands themselves, also interact with integrin $\alpha_v\beta_3$ (114). Interaction of integrin $\alpha_5\beta_1$ with Tie2 dramatically increases Tie2's affinity for Ang-1, thus leading to

Tie2 phosphorylation at lower Ang-1 concentrations and causes much more prolonged stimulation of Tie2 in response to Ang-1 binding (109). Integrin $\alpha_5\beta_1$ also binds Ang-1 and Ang-2 directly (114).

Lastly, integrins can bind to fragments of proteins that serve as inhibitors of angiogenesis. For example, endostatin (described below) binds to $\alpha_5\beta_1$, and PEX (a noncatalytic fragment of MMP-2) binds to $\alpha_v\beta_3$, and thus functions as a natural antagonist of MMP-2 and therefore of angiogenesis (116). Integrin stimulation also mediates endothelial cell survival in response to binding of various ECM components, by decreasing apoptosis via an NF-κB mediated pathway (117).

In the eye, several integrins play physiological and pathological roles. Integrin $\alpha_v\beta_5$ on the RPE mediates retinal adhesion at the RPE apical microvilli, and is also responsible for diurnal phagocytosis of photoreceptor outer segments (118). Integrin $\alpha_v\beta_5$ as well as $\alpha_v\beta_3$ are found in retinal neovascular tissues from patients with proliferative diabetic retinopathy (119), and integrin $\alpha_5\beta_1$ appears important in both corneal (120) and choroidal (121,122) neovascularization. $\alpha_v\beta_3$ was found in subretinal membranes from patients with AMD (119), and various types of $\alpha_v\beta_3$ antagonists have been effective in reducing angiogenesis in animal models of CNV. An intravenously delivered anti-$\alpha_v\beta_3$ monoclonal antibody inhibited angiogenesis and reduced CNV volume in a laser-induced CNV rat model (123); an intravitreally delivered $\alpha_v\beta_3$-binding peptide antagonist (124) and an intraperitoneally delivered non-peptide antagonist (125) both reduced CNV thickness and leakage in laser-induced CNV models. In addition, a sustained-release intravitreal implant which released a combined antagonist against both $\alpha_v\beta_3$ and $\alpha_v\beta_5$ likewise suppressed laser-induced CNV (126), and an orally bioavailable $\alpha_v\beta_3$ and $a_v\beta_5$ combined antagonist reduced retinal neovascularization in an oxygen-induced retinopathy model (127). Lastly, small-molecule inhibition of integrin $\alpha_5\beta_1$ with JSM6427 delivered either intravitreally (122) or via a subcutaneous pump (121), both inhibited CNV formation in various animal models. The $\alpha_5\beta_1$ inhibitor Volocoxib (Ophthotech) is in a phase I clinical trial (ARVO 2011 Program 1252 Inhibition of $\alpha_5\beta_1$ Integrin in Neovascular AMD - A Phase 1 Study).

Angiostatin and Endostatin

Angiostatin is a 38 kDa peptide that is a naturally occurring internal fragment of plasminogen, which was originally isolated from human Lewis lung carcinoma (128). Endostatin is the 20 kDa C-terminal peptide fragment of collagen XVIII that was originally isolated from murine hemangioendothelioma (129), and subsequently found to also exist in a circulating form in humans (130). Both have been shown to have antiangiogenic, antitumor, and antimetastatic properties (128,129).

Collagen XVIII, as well as its C-terminal fragment representing endostatin, are found ubiquitously in ocular structures in normal, healthy eyes (131). Collagen XVIII fragments of varying sizes that included the C-terminal endostatin fragment were detected in aqueous, vitreous, and in tears (131). There is some evidence that endostatin may be expressed at reduced levels in certain areas in AMD eyes compared to control eyes, including the choriocapillaris, Bruch's membrane, and RPE basal lamina (132,133). In a laser injury model, mice lacking collagen XVIII produced larger and leakier CNVMs. Exogenous endostatin could rescue this increased membranogenesis in these mutant mice, and additional exogenous endostatin could also decrease the size of CNVMs in control mice that produced otherwise normal levels of endostatin (134). Subretinal injection of recombinant viral vectors expressing either endostatin or angiostatin could likewise inhibit laser-induced CNV (135,136). Unfortunately, angiostatin- and endostatin-based therapies have not found success in clinical use thus far.

Placental Growth Factor

Placental growth factor (PlGF) is a VEGF homolog that shares only 42% amino acid identity, yet remarkably similar three-dimensional protein structure (137). Unlike VEGF, PlGF binds only to VEGFR-1 (FLT1), and not to other VEGFRs (138). In addition, *Plgf-/-* (and *Flt1-/-*) mice develop normally, indicating no indispensable role for PlGF in normal developmental vasculogenesis, although adult angiogenesis is impaired (139). It is unclear exactly what role the interactions of PlGF, VEGFR-1 and VEGF play in angiogenesis. On the one hand, VEGFR-1 is only weakly stimulated by VEGF binding, and also exists as an endogenous soluble receptor (140). This has led to the hypothesis that VEGFR-1, either in its membrane-bound or soluble form, may serve as a receptor decoy for VEGF, decreasing VEGF-VEGFR-2 signaling by soaking up the available soluble VEGF (138). In this model, PlGF may potentiate VEGF-mediated signaling by occupying the VEGFR-1 sites, thereby making them inaccessible to VEGF, and thus making more VEGF available to signal via VEGFR-2 (141).

However, other evidence seems to indicate that PlGF plays a more direct role in potentiating VEGF-mediated angiogenesis, rather than just as a VEGF decoy's decoy. PlGF binding to VEGFR-1 results in inter-receptor transphosphorylation of VEGFR-2 by VEGFR-1, potentiating transduction of the VEGFR-2 signal (142). When VEGF and PlGF both bind to VEGFR-1, it results in the phosphorylation of different VEGFR-1 tyrosine residues, and only PlGF binding results in transphosphorylation of VEGFR-2 (142). Likewise, PlGF and VEGF binding to VEGFR-1 leads to activation of different downstream target genes through the VEGFR-1-mediated pathway, irrespective of any effect on VEGFR-2 (142). Lastly, the natural formation of PlGF/VEGF ligand heterodimers facilitates VEGFR-1/VEGFR-2 receptor heterodimerization and angiogenic signaling (142). Therefore, the overall effect of PlGF is to cause VEGFR-1/VEGFR-2 receptor heterodimerization by co-binding of PlGF/VEGF ligand heterodimers and this induces receptor transphosphorylation and potentiation of the VEGF signal in a way not seen in the absence of PlGF (142,143).

In the eye, PlGF is expressed by normal RPE, which also undergoes chemotaxis in response to an exogenous PlGF signal (144). The choroid constitutively produces PlGF, and this is significantly upregulated during the process of CNVM formation in response to laser-induced rupture of Bruch's membrane (145,146). This upregulation of PlGF appears to play an indispensable pathophysiologic role in the process of CNV, as both *Plgf*-null mice, as well as wild-type mice treated with anti-VEGFR-1 antibody, did not produce CNVM in response to laser-induced rupture of Bruch's membrane (145). Similarly, monoclonal antibody directed against PlGF itself likewise inhibited CNVM formation in a dose-dependent manner (146).

The current clinical interest in the role of PlGF blockade in AMD derives from the FDA approval of aflibercept, which is a soluble decoy receptor derived from fusion of the second Ig-like domain of VEGFR-1 with the third Ig-like domain of VEGFR-2 attached to the Fc portion of human IgG1 (147). This engineered fusion protein binds not only VEGF-A, but also VEGF-B and PlGF, with high affinity (148). The VIEW-1 and VIEW-2 clinical trials demonstrated the efficacy of aflibercept in the treatment of neovascular AMD with an apparent increase in durability of action over ranibizumab. However, it is still unclear how much, if any, of this effect derives from anti-PlGF activity. (http://newsroom.regeneron.com/releasedetail.cfm?ReleaseID=629800).

CONCLUSIONS

Numerous molecular pathways are involved in angiogenesis, either by serving as angiogenic or antiangiogenic signals, by facilitating or retarding endothelial migration or tube formation, by desensitizing vessels to regression through the process of vessel maturation, by inducing fibrosis, or by augmenting or diminishing VEGF- or non-VEGF-mediated signals (Fig. 20.1). Therefore, although important, VEGF is far from the entire story in angiogenesis. Targeting multiple pathways in combination with VEGF is the goal of future antiangiogenic therapy. Much of the work in this decade will depend on knowledge about these non-VEGF pathways to maximize patient outcomes.

SUMMARY POINTS

- Although therapies targeting VEGF have dramatically improved patient outcomes, many patients still fail to experience an improvement in visual acuity with anti-VEGF monotherapy.
- Many other cellular pathways mediate or modulate angiogenesis by modulating the processes of:
  ○ angiogenic signaling
  ○ endothelial migration or tube formation
  ○ vessel maturation
  ○ fibrosis
- Each of these mechanisms can be harnessed or blocked to improve antiangiogenic therapeutic effect.
- A combined approach targeting multiple pathways is likely to exploit synergisms and to have a more robust and sustained effect.

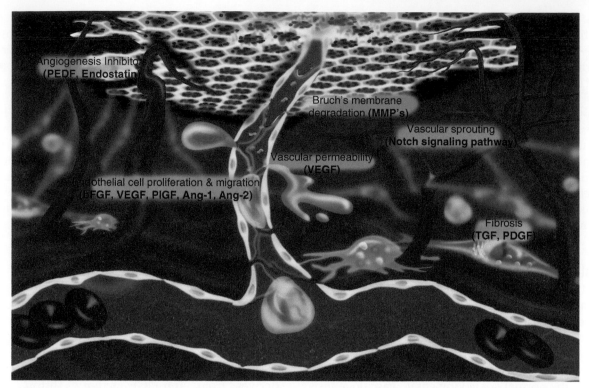

Figure 20.1 Schematic summary of potential treatment targets for neovascular AMD. *Source*: Courtesy of Aristomenis Thanos, MD.

REFERENCES

1. Rosenfeld PJ, Brown DM, Heier JS, et al. Ranibizumab for neovascular age-related macular degeneration. N Engl J Med 2006; 355: 1419–31.

2. Brown DM, Kaiser PK, Michels M, et al. Ranibizumab versus verteporfin for neovascular age-related macular degeneration. N Engl J Med 2006; 355: 1432–44.

3. Singer MA, Awh CC, Sadda S, et al. HORIZON: an open-label extension trial of ranibizumab for choroidal neovascularization secondary to age-related macular degeneration. Ophthalmology 2012; 119: 1175–83.

4. Regillo CD, Brown DM, Abraham P, et al. Randomized, double-masked, sham-controlled trial of ranibizumab for neovascular age-related macular degeneration: PIER Study year 1. Am J Ophthalmol 2008; 145: 239–48.

5. Fung AE, Lalwani GA, Rosenfeld PJ, et al. An optical coherence tomography-guided, variable dosing regimen with intravitreal ranibizumab (Lucentis) for neovascular age-related macular degeneration. Am J Ophthalmol 2007; 143: 566–83.

6. Oubraham H, Cohen SY, Samimi S, et al. Inject and extend dosing versus dosing as needed: a comparative retrospective study of ranibizumab in exudative age-related macular degeneration. Retina 2011; 31: 26–30.

7. Gupta OP, Shienbaum G, Patel AH, et al. A treat and extend regimen using ranibizumab for neovascular age-related macular degeneration clinical and economic impact. Ophthalmology 2010; 117: 2134–40.

8. Knights V, Cook SJ. De-regulated FGF receptors as therapeutic targets in cancer. Pharmacol Ther 2010; 125: 105–17.

9. Beenken A, Mohammadi M. The FGF family: biology, pathophysiology and therapy. Nat Rev Drug Discov 2009; 8: 235–53.

10. Polanska UM, Fernig DG, Kinnunen T. Extracellular interactome of the FGF receptor-ligand system: complexities and the relative simplicity of the worm. Dev Dyn 2009; 238: 277–93.

11. Murakami M, Elfenbein A, Simons M. Non-canonical fibroblast growth factor signalling in angiogenesis. Cardiovasc Res 2008; 78: 223–31.

12. Potente M, Gerhardt H, Carmeliet P. Basic and therapeutic aspects of angiogenesis. Cell 2011; 146: 873–87.

13. Zubilewicz A, Hecquet C, Jeanny JC, et al. Two distinct signalling pathways are involved in FGF2-stimulated proliferation of choriocapillary endothelial cells: a comparative study with VEGF. Oncogene 2001; 20: 1403–13.

14. Browning AC, Dua HS, Amoaku WM. The effects of growth factors on the proliferation and in vitro angiogenesis of human macular inner choroidal endothelial cells. Br J Ophthalmol 2008; 92: 1003–8.

15. Stahl A, Paschek L, Martin G, et al. Combinatory inhibition of VEGF and FGF2 is superior to solitary VEGF inhibition in an in vitro model of RPE-induced angiogenesis. Graefes Arch Clin Exp Ophthalmol 2009; 247: 767–73.

16. Martin G, Schlunck G, Hansen LL, Agostini HT. Differential expression of angioregulatory factors in normal and CNV-derived human retinal pigment epithelium. Graefes Arch Clin Exp Ophthalmol 2004; 242: 321–6.

17. Amin R, Puklin JE, Frank RN. Growth factor localization in choroidal neovascular membranes of age-related macular degeneration. Invest Ophthalmol Vis Sci 1994; 35: 3178–88.

18. Nickel W. Unconventional secretory routes: direct protein export across the plasma membrane of mammalian cells. Traffic 2005; 6: 607–14.

19. Adamis AP, Meklir B, Joyce NC. In situ injury-induced release of basic-fibroblast growth factor from corneal epithelial cells. Am J Pathol 1991; 139: 961–7.

20. Kostyk SK, D'Amore PA, Herman IM, Wagner JA. Optic nerve injury alters basic fibroblast growth factor

localization in the retina and optic tract. J Neurosci 1994; 14(3 Pt 2): 1441–9.

21. Ozaki S, Radeke MJ, Anderson DH. Rapid upregulation of fibroblast growth factor receptor 1 (flg) by rat photoreceptor cells after injury. Invest Ophthalmol Vis Sci 2000; 41: 568–79.

22. Dreyfuss JL, Regatieri CV, Lima MA, et al. A heparin mimetic isolated from a marine shrimp suppresses neovascularization. J Thromb Haemost 2010; 8: 1828–37.

23. Chow LQ, Eckhardt SG. Sunitinib: from rational design to clinical efficacy. J Clin Oncol 2007; 25: 884–96.

24. Becerra SP. Focus on molecules: pigment epithelium-derived factor (PEDF). Exp Eye Res 2006; 82: 739–40.

25. Ogata N, Wada M, Otsuji T, et al. Expression of pigment epithelium-derived factor in normal adult rat eye and experimental choroidal neovascularization. Invest Ophthalmol Vis Sci 2002; 43: 1168–75.

26. Karakousis PC, John SK, Behling KC, et al. Localization of pigment epithelium derived factor (PEDF) in developing and adult human ocular tissues. Mol Vis 2001; 7: 154–63.

27. Dawson DW, Volpert OV, Gillis P, et al. Pigment epithelium-derived factor: a potent inhibitor of angiogenesis. Science 1999; 285: 245–8.

28. Cai J, Jiang WG, Grant MB, Boulton M. Pigment epithelium-derived factor inhibits angiogenesis via regulated intracellular proteolysis of vascular endothelial growth factor receptor 1. J Biol Chem 2006; 281: 3604–13.

29. Ablonczy Z, Prakasam A, Fant J, et al. Pigment epithelium-derived factor maintains retinal pigment epithelium function by inhibiting vascular endothelial growth factor-R2 signaling through gamma-secretase. J Biol Chem 2009; 284: 30177–86.

30. Volpert OV, Zaichuk T, Zhou W, et al. Inducer-stimulated Fas targets activated endothelium for destruction by anti-angiogenic thrombospondin-1 and pigment epithelium-derived factor. Nat Med 2002; 8: 349–57.

31. Matsuoka M, Ogata N, Otsuji T, et al. Expression of pigment epithelium derived factor and vascular endothelial growth factor in choroidal neovascular membranes and polypoidal choroidal vasculopathy. Br J Ophthalmol 2004; 88: 809–15.

32. Ohno-Matsui K, Morita I, Tombran-Tink J, et al. Novel mechanism for age-related macular degeneration: an equilibrium shift between the angiogenesis factors VEGF and PEDF. J Cell Physiol 2001; 189: 323–33.

33. Pons M, Marin-Castano ME. Nicotine increases the VEGF/PEDF ratio in retinal pigment epithelium: a possible mechanism for CNV in passive smokers with AMD. Invest Ophthalmol Vis Sci 2011; 52: 3842–53.

34. Holekamp NM, Bouck N, Volpert O. Pigment epithelium-derived factor is deficient in the vitreous of patients with choroidal neovascularization due to age-related macular degeneration. Am J Ophthalmol 2002; 134: 220–7.

35. Lin JM, Wan L, Tsai YY, et al. Pigment epithelium-derived factor gene Met72Thr polymorphism is associated with increased risk of wet age-related macular degeneration. Am J Ophthalmol 2008; 145: 716–21.

36. Mori K, Gehlbach P, Yamamoto S, et al. AAV-mediated gene transfer of pigment epithelium-derived factor inhibits choroidal neovascularization. Invest Ophthalmol Vis Sci 2002; 43: 1994–2000.

37. Yuan A, Kaiser PK. Emerging therapies for the treatment of neovascular age related macular degeneration. Semin Ophthalmol 2011; 26: 149–55.

38. Patel-Hett S, D'Amore PA. Signal transduction in vasculogenesis and developmental angiogenesis. Int J Dev Biol 2011; 55: 353–63.

39. Dou GR, Wang L, Wang YS, Han H. Notch signaling in ocular vasculature development and diseases. Mol Med 2012; 18: 47–.

40. Garcia A, Kandel JJ. Notch: A key regulator of tumor angiogenesis and metastasis. Histol Histopathol 2012; 27: 151–6.

41. Jakobsson L, Bentley K, Gerhardt H. VEGFRs and Notch: a dynamic collaboration in vascular patterning. Biochem Soc Trans 2009; 37(Pt 6): 1233–6.

42. Liu ZJ, Shirakawa T, Li Y, et al. Regulation of Notch1 and Dll4 by vascular endothelial growth factor in arterial endothelial cells: implications for modulating arteriogenesis and angiogenesis. Mol Cell Biol 2003; 23: 14–25.

43. Phng LK, Gerhardt H. Angiogenesis: a team effort coordinated by notch. Dev Cell 2009; 16: 196–208.

44. Eilken HM, Adams RH. Dynamics of endothelial cell behavior in sprouting angiogenesis. Curr Opin Cell Biol 2010; 22: 617–25.

45. Jakobsson L, Franco CA, Bentley K, et al. Endothelial cells dynamically compete for the tip cell position during angiogenic sprouting. Nat Cell Biol 2010; 12: 943–53.

46. Wang T, Baron M, Trump D. An overview of Notch3 function in vascular smooth muscle cells. Prog Biophys Mol Biol 2008; 96: 499–509.

47. Gridley T. Notch signaling in the vasculature. Curr Top Dev Biol 2010; 92: 277–309.

48. Swift MR, Weinstein BM. Arterial-venous specification during development. Circ Res 2009; 104: 576–88.

49. Dou GR, Wang YC, Hu XB, et al. RBP-J, the transcription factor downstream of Notch receptors, is essential for the maintenance of vascular homeostasis in adult mice. FASEB J 2008; 22: 1606–17.

50. Harrington LS, Sainson RC, Williams CK, et al. Regulation of multiple angiogenic pathways by Dll4 and Notch in human umbilical vein endothelial cells. Microvasc Res 2008; 75: 144–54.

51. Liu Z, Turkoz A, Jackson EN, et al. Notch1 loss of heterozygosity causes vascular tumors and lethal hemorrhage in mice. J Clin Invest 2011; 121: 800–8.

52. Ahmad I, Balasubramanian S, Del Debbio CB, et al. Regulation of ocular angiogenesis by Notch signaling: implications in neovascular age-related macular degeneration. Invest Ophthalmol Vis Sci 2011; 52: 2868–78.

53. Gerhardt H, Golding M, Fruttiger M, et al. VEGF guides angiogenic sprouting utilizing endothelial tip cell filopodia. J Cell Biol 2003; 161: 1163–77.

54. Lindahl P, Johansson BR, Leveen P, Betsholtz C. Pericyte loss and microaneurysm formation in PDGF-B-deficient mice. Science 1997; 277: 242–5.

55. Quaegebeur A, Segura I, Carmeliet P. Pericytes: blood-brain barrier safeguards against neurodegeneration? Neuron 2010; 68: 321–3.

56. Hellstrom M, Kalen M, Lindahl P, Abramsson A, Betsholtz C. Role of PDGF-B and PDGFR-beta in recruitment of vascular smooth muscle cells and pericytes during embryonic blood vessel formation in the mouse. Development 1999; 126: 3047–55.

57. Hou X, Kumar A, Lee C, et al. PDGF-CC blockade inhibits pathological angiogenesis by acting on multiple cellular and molecular targets. Proc Natl Acad Sci USA 2010; 107: 12216–21.

58. Gee MS, Procopio WN, Makonnen S, et al. Tumor vessel development and maturation impose limits on the effectiveness of anti-vascular therapy. Am J Pathol 2003; 162: 183–93.

59. Benjamin LE, Golijanin D, Itin A, Pode D, Keshet E. Selective ablation of immature blood vessels in established human tumors follows vascular endothelial growth factor withdrawal. J Clin Invest 1999; 103: 159–65.

60. Nisancioglu MH, Betsholtz C, Genove G. The absence of pericytes does not increase the sensitivity of tumor vasculature to vascular endothelial growth factor-A blockade. Cancer Res 2010; 70: 5109–15.

61. Jo N, Mailhos C, Ju M, et al. Inhibition of platelet-derived growth factor B signaling enhances the efficacy of anti-vascular endothelial growth factor therapy in multiple models of ocular neovascularization. Am J Pathol 2006; 168: 2036–53.

62. Rossant J, Howard L. Signaling pathways in vascular development. Annu Rev Cell Dev Biol 2002; 18: 541–73.

63. Pardali E, Goumans MJ, ten Dijke P. Signaling by members of the TGF-beta family in vascular morphogenesis and disease. Trends Cell Biol 2010; 20: 556–67.

64. Recalde S, Zarranz-Ventura J, Fernandez-Robredo P, et al. Transforming growth factor-beta inhibition decreases diode laser-induced choroidal neovascularization development in rats: P17 and P144 peptides. Invest Ophthalmol Vis Sci 2011; 52: 7090–7.

65. Nagineni CN, Samuel W, Nagineni S, et al. Transforming growth factor-beta induces expression of vascular endothelial growth factor in human retinal pigment epithelial cells: involvement of mitogen-activated protein kinases. J Cell Physiol 2003; 197: 453–62.

66. Zhang L, Lim SL, Du H, et al. High temperature requirement factor A1 (HTRA1) gene regulates angiogenesis through transforming growth factor-beta family member growth differentiation factor 6. J Biol Chem 2012; 287: 1520–6.

67. Davis S, Aldrich TH, Jones PF, et al. Isolation of angiopoietin-1, a ligand for the TIE2 receptor, by secretion-trap expression cloning. Cell 1996; 87: 1161–9.

68. Maisonpierre PC, Suri C, Jones PF, et al. Angiopoietin-2, a natural antagonist for Tie2 that disrupts in vivo angiogenesis. Science 1997; 277: 55–60.

69. Valenzuela DM, Griffiths JA, Rojas J, et al. Angiopoietins 3 and 4: diverging gene counterparts in mice and humans. Proc Natl Acad Sci USA 1999; 96: 1904–9.

70. Yuan HT, Venkatesha S, Chan B, et al. Activation of the orphan endothelial receptor Tie1 modifies Tie2-mediated intracellular signaling and cell survival. FASEB J 2007; 21: 3171.3183.

71. Makinde T, Agrawal DK. Intra and extravascular transmembrane signalling of angiopoietin-1-Tie2 receptor in health and disease. J Cell Mol Med 2008; 12: 810–28.

72. Witzenbichler B, Maisonpierre PC, Jones P, Yancopoulos GD, Isner JM. Chemotactic properties of angiopoietin-1 and -2, ligands for the endothelial-specific receptor tyrosine kinase Tie2. J Biol Chem 1998; 273: 18514–21.

73. Zhang J, Fukuhara S, Sako K, et al. Angiopoietin-1/Tie2 signal augments basal Notch signal controlling vascular quiescence by inducing delta-like 4 expression through AKT-mediated activation of beta-catenin. J Biol Chem 2011; 286: 8055–66.

74. Hanahan D. Signaling vascular morphogenesis and maintenance. Science 1997; 277: 48–50.

75. Fukuhara S, Sako K, Noda K, et al. Tie2 is tied at the cell-cell contacts and to extracellular matrix by angiopoietin-1. Exp Mol Med 2009; 41: 133–9.

76. Asahara T, Chen D, Takahashi T, et al. Tie2 receptor ligands, angiopoietin-1 and angiopoietin-2, modulate VEGF-induced postnatal neovascularization. Circ Res 1998; 83: 233–40.

77. Hackett SF, Ozaki H, Strauss RW, et al. Angiopoietin 2 expression in the retina: upregulation during physiologic and pathologic neovascularization. J Cell Physiol 2000; 184: 275–84.

78. Otani A, Takagi H, Oh H, et al. Expressions of angiopoietins and Tie2 in human choroidal neovascular membranes. Invest Ophthalmol Vis Sci 1999; 40: 1912–20.

79. Hangai M, Murata T, Miyawaki N, et al. Angiopoietin-1 upregulation by vascular endothelial growth factor in human retinal pigment epithelial cells. Invest Ophthalmol Vis Sci 2001; 42: 1617–25.

80. Nambu H, Nambu R, Oshima Y, et al. Angiopoietin 1 inhibits ocular neovascularization and breakdown of the blood-retinal barrier. Gene Ther 2004; 11: 865–73.

81. Hangai M, Moon YS, Kitaya N, et al. Systemically expressed soluble Tie2 inhibits intraocular neovascularization. Hum Gene Ther 2001; 12: 1311–21.

82. Rennel ES, Regula JT, Harper SJ, et al. A human neutralizing antibody specific to Ang-2 inhibits ocular angiogenesis. Microcirculation 2011; 18: 598–607.

83. Liu J, Lin TH, Cole AG, et al. Identification and characterization of small-molecule inhibitors of Tie2 kinase. FEBS Lett 2008; 582: 785–91.

84. Hadler-Olsen E, Fadnes B, Sylte I, Uhlin-Hansen L, Winberg JO. Regulation of matrix metalloproteinase activity in health and disease. FEBS J 2011; 278: 28–45.

85. Blasi F, Carmeliet P. uPAR: a versatile signalling orchestrator. Nat Rev Mol Cell Biol 2002; 3: 932–43.

86. Butler GS, Overall CM. Updated biological roles for matrix metalloproteinases and new "intracellular" substrates revealed by degradomics. Biochemistry 2009; 48: 10830–45.

87. Arroyo AG, Iruela-Arispe ML. Extracellular matrix, inflammation, and the angiogenic response. Cardiovasc Res 2010; 86: 226–35.

88. Notari L, Miller A, Martinez A, et al. Pigment epithelium-derived factor is a substrate for matrix metalloproteinase type 2 and type 9: implications for downregulation in hypoxia. Invest Ophthalmol Vis Sci 2005; 46: 2736–47.

89. Ardi VC, Kupriyanova TA, Deryugina EI, Quigley JP. Human neutrophils uniquely release TIMP-free MMP-9 to provide a potent catalytic stimulator of angiogenesis. Proc Natl Acad Sci USA 2007; 104: 20262–7.

90. Zucker S, Mirza H, Conner CE, et al. Vascular endothelial growth factor induces tissue factor and matrix metalloproteinase production in endothelial cells: conversion of prothrombin to thrombin results in progelatinase A activation and cell proliferation. Int J Cancer 1998; 75: 780–6.

91. Hollborn M, Stathopoulos C, Steffen A, et al. Positive feedback regulation between MMP-9 and VEGF in human RPE cells. Invest Ophthalmol Vis Sci 2007; 48: 4360–7.

92. Wang H, Keiser JA. Vascular endothelial growth factor upregulates the expression of matrix metalloproteinases in vascular smooth muscle cells: role of flt-1. Circ Res 1998; 83: 832–40.

93. Qi JH, Ebrahem Q, Moore N, et al. A novel function for tissue inhibitor of metalloproteinases-3 (TIMP3): inhibition of angiogenesis by blockage of VEGF binding to VEGF receptor-2. Nat Med 2003; 9: 407–15.

94. Hoffmann S, Friedrichs U, Eichler W, Rosenthal A, Wiedemann P. Advanced glycation end products induce choroidal endothelial cell proliferation, matrix metalloproteinase-2 and VEGF upregulation in vitro. Graefes Arch Clin Exp Ophthalmol 2002; 240: 996–1002.

95. Hoffmann S, He S, Ehren M, et al. MMP-2 and MMP-9 secretion by rpe is stimulated by angiogenic molecules found in choroidal neovascular membranes. Retina 2006; 26: 454–61.

96. Morizane Y, Thanos A, Takeuchi K, et al. AMP-activated protein kinase suppresses matrix metalloproteinase-9 expression in mouse embryonic fibroblasts. J Biol Chem 2011; 286: 16030–8.

97. Fariss RN, Apte SS, Olsen BR, Iwata K, Milam AH. Tissue inhibitor of metalloproteinases-3 is a component of Bruch's membrane of the eye. Am J Pathol 1997; 150: 323–8.

98. Ebrahem Q, Qi JH, Sugimoto M, et al. Increased neovascularization in mice lacking tissue inhibitor of metalloproteinases-3. Invest Ophthalmol Vis Sci 2011; 52: 6117–23.

99. Qi JH, Dai G, Luthert P, et al. S156C mutation in tissue inhibitor of metalloproteinases-3 induces increased angiogenesis. J Biol Chem 2009; 284: 19927–36.

100. Lambert V, Munaut C, Jost M, et al. Matrix metalloproteinase-9 contributes to choroidal neovascularization. Am J Pathol 2002; 161: 1247–53.

101. Daniels AB, Jakobiec FA, Westerfeld CB, et al. Idiopathic subfoveal choroidal neovascular membrane in a 21-month-old child: ultrastructural features and implication for membranogenesis. J AAPOS 2010; 14: 244–50.

102. Steen B, Sejersen S, Berglin L, Seregard S, Kvanta A. Matrix metalloproteinases and metalloproteinase inhibitors in choroidal neovascular membranes. Invest Ophthalmol Vis Sci 1998; 39: 2194–200.

103. Chau KY, Sivaprasad S, Patel N, et al. Plasma levels of matrix metalloproteinase-2 and -9 (MMP-2 and MMP-9) in age-related macular degeneration. Eye (Lond) 2007; 21: 1511–15.

104. Lauer-Fields JL, Whitehead JK, Li S, et al. Selective modulation of matrix metalloproteinase 9 (MMP-9) functions via exosite inhibition. J Biol Chem 2008; 283: 20087–95.

105. Samtani S, Amaral J, Campos MM, Fariss RN, Becerra SP. Doxycycline-mediated inhibition of choroidal neovascularization. Invest Ophthalmol Vis Sci 2009; 50: 5098–106.

106. Cox CA, Amaral J, Salloum R, et al. Doxycycline's effect on ocular angiogenesis: an in vivo analysis. Ophthalmology 2010; 117: 1782–91.

107. Bussolino F, Caccavari F, Valdembri D, Serini G. Angiogenesis: a balancing act between integrin activation and inhibition? Eur Cytokine Netw 2009; 20: 191–6.

108. Joseph-Silverstein J, Silverstein RL. Cell adhesion molecules: an overview. Cancer Invest 1998; 16: 176–82.

109. Serini G, Napione L, Arese M, Bussolino F. Besides adhesion: new perspectives of integrin functions in angiogenesis. Cardiovasc Res 2008; 78: 213–22.

110. Somanath PR, Malinin NL, Byzova TV. Cooperation between integrin alphavbeta3 and VEGFR2 in angiogenesis. Angiogenesis 2009; 12: 177–85.

111. Soldi R, Mitola S, Strasly M, et al. Role of alphavbeta3 integrin in the activation of vascular endothelial growth factor receptor-2. EMBO J 1999; 18: 882–92.

112. Brooks PC, Clark RA, Cheresh DA. Requirement of vascular integrin alpha v beta 3 for angiogenesis. Science 1994; 264: 569–71.

113. Friedlander M, Brooks PC, Shaffer RW, et al. Definition of two angiogenic pathways by distinct alpha v integrins. Science 1995; 270: 1500–2.

114. Somanath PR, Ciocea A, Byzova TV. Integrin and growth factor receptor alliance in angiogenesis. Cell Biochem Biophys 2009; 53: 53–64.

115. Eliceiri BP, Klemke R, Stromblad S, Cheresh DA. Integrin alphavbeta3 requirement for sustained mitogen-activated protein kinase activity during angiogenesis. J Cell Biol 1998; 140: 1255–63.

116. Brooks PC, Silletti S, von Schalscha TL, Friedlander M, Cheresh DA. Disruption of angiogenesis by PEX, a noncatalytic metalloproteinase fragment with integrin binding activity. Cell 1998; 92: 391–400.

117. Scatena M, Almeida M, Chaisson ML, et al. NF-kappaB mediates alphavbeta3 integrin-induced endothelial cell survival. J Cell Biol 1998; 141: 1083–93.

118. Nandrot EF, Anand M, Almeida D, et al. Essential role for MFG-E8 as ligand for alphavbeta5 integrin in diurnal retinal phagocytosis. Proc Natl Acad Sci USA 2007; 104: 12005–10.

119. Friedlander M, Theesfeld CL, Sugita M, et al. Involvement of integrins alpha v beta 3 and alpha v beta 5 in ocular neovascular diseases. Proc Natl Acad Sci USA 1996; 93: 9764–9.

120. Muether PS, Dell S, Kociok N, et al. The role of integrin alpha5beta1 in the regulation of corneal neovascularization. Exp Eye Res 2007; 85: 356–65.

121. Umeda N, Kachi S, Akiyama H, et al. Suppression and regression of choroidal neovascularization by systemic administration of an alpha5beta1 integrin antagonist. Mol Pharmacol 2006; 69: 1820–8.

122. Zahn G, Vossmeyer D, Stragies R, et al. Preclinical evaluation of the novel small-molecule integrin alpha5beta1 inhibitor JSM6427 in monkey and rabbit models of choroidal neovascularization. Arch Ophthalmol 2009; 127: 1329–35.

123. Kamizuru H, Kimura H, Yasukawa T, et al. Monoclonal antibody-mediated drug targeting to choroidal neovascularization in the rat. Invest Ophthalmol Vis Sci 2001; 42: 2664–72.

124. Yasukawa T, Hoffmann S, Eichler W, et al. Inhibition of experimental choroidal neovascularization in rats by an alpha(v)-integrin antagonist. Curr Eye Res 2004; 28: 359–66.

125. Honda S, Nagai T, Negi A. Anti-angiogenic effects of non-peptide integrin alphavbeta3 specific antagonist on laser-induced choroidal neovascularization in mice. Graefes Arch Clin Exp Ophthalmol 2009; 247: 515–22.

126. Fu Y, Ponce ML, Thill M, et al. Angiogenesis inhibition and choroidal neovascularization suppression by sustained delivery of an integrin antagonist, EMD478761. Invest Ophthalmol Vis Sci 2007; 48: 5184–90.

127. Santulli RJ, Kinney WA, Ghosh S, et al. Studies with an orally bioavailable alpha V integrin antagonist in animal models of ocular vasculopathy: retinal neovascularization in mice and retinal vascular permeability in diabetic rats. J Pharmacol Exp Ther 2008; 324: 894–901.

128. O'Reilly MS, Holmgren L, Shing Y, et al. Angiostatin: a novel angiogenesis inhibitor that mediates the suppression of metastases by a Lewis lung carcinoma. Cell 1994; 79: 315–28.

129. O'Reilly MS, Boehm T, Shing Y, et al. Endostatin: an endogenous inhibitor of angiogenesis and tumor growth. Cell 1997; 88: 277–85.

130. Standker L, Schrader M, Kanse SM, et al. Isolation and characterization of the circulating form of human endostatin. FEBS Lett 1997; 420: 129–33.

131. Maatta M, Heljasvaara R, Pihlajaniemi T, Uusitalo M. Collagen XVIII/endostatin shows a ubiquitous distribution in human ocular tissues and endostatin-containing fragments accumulate in ocular fluid samples. Graefes Arch Clin Exp Ophthalmol 2007; 245: 74–81.

132. Bhutto IA, Kim SY, McLeod DS, et al. Localization of collagen XVIII and the endostatin portion of collagen XVIII in aged human control eyes and eyes with age-related macular degeneration. Invest Ophthalmol Vis Sci 2004; 45: 1544–52.

133. Bhutto IA, Uno K, Merges C, et al. Reduction of endogenous angiogenesis inhibitors in Bruch's membrane of the submacular region in eyes with age-related macular degeneration. Arch Ophthalmol 2008; 126: 670–8.

134. Marneros AG, She H, Zambarakji H, et al. Endogenous endostatin inhibits choroidal neovascularization. FASEB J 2007; 21: 3809–18.

135. Lai CC, Wu WC, Chen SL, et al. Suppression of choroidal neovascularization by adeno-associated virus vector expressing angiostatin. Invest Ophthalmol Vis Sci 2001; 42: 2401–7.

136. Balaggan KS, Binley K, Esapa M, et al. EIAV vector-mediated delivery of endostatin or angiostatin inhibits angiogenesis and vascular hyperpermeability in experimental CNV. Gene Ther 2006; 13: 1153–65.

137. Iyer S, Leonidas DD, Swaminathan GJ, et al. The crystal structure of human placenta growth factor-1 (PlGF-1), an angiogenic protein, at 2.0 A resolution. J Biol Chem 2001; 276: 12153–61.

138. Park JE, Chen HH, Winer J, Houck KA, Ferrara N. Placenta growth factor. Potentiation of vascular endothelial growth factor bioactivity, in vitro and in vivo, and high affinity binding to Flt-1 but not to Flk-1/KDR. J Biol Chem 1994; 269: 25646–54.

139. Carmeliet P, Moons L, Luttun A, et al. Synergism between vascular endothelial growth factor and placental growth factor contributes to angiogenesis and plasma extravasation in pathological conditions. Nat Med 2001; 7: 575–83.

140. Kendall RL, Thomas KA. Inhibition of vascular endothelial cell growth factor activity by an endogenously encoded soluble receptor. Proc Natl Acad Sci USA 1993; 90: 10705–9.

141. Ferrara N, Gerber HP, LeCouter J. The biology of VEGF and its receptors. Nat Med 2003; 9: 669–76.

142. Autiero M, Waltenberger J, Communi D, et al. Role of PlGF in the intra- and intermolecular cross talk between the VEGF receptors Flt1 and Flk1. Nat Med 2003; 9: 936–43.

143. Tjwa M, Luttun A, Autiero M, Carmeliet PVEGF. and PlGF: two pleiotropic growth factors with distinct roles in development and homeostasis. Cell Tissue Res 2003; 314: 5–14.

144. Hollborn M, Tenckhoff S, Seifert M, et al. Human retinal epithelium produces and responds to placenta growth factor. Graefes Arch Clin Exp Ophthalmol 2006; 244: 732–41.

145. Rakic JM, Lambert V, Devy L, et al. Placental growth factor, a member of the VEGF family, contributes to the development of choroidal neovascularization. Invest Ophthalmol Vis Sci 2003; 44: 3186–93.

146. Van de Veire S, Stalmans I, Heindryckx F, et al. Further pharmacological and genetic evidence for the efficacy of PlGF inhibition in cancer and eye disease. Cell 2010; 141: 178–90.

147. Holash J, Davis S, Papadopoulos N, et al. VEGF-Trap: a VEGF blocker with potent antitumor effects. Proc Natl Acad Sci USA 2002; 99: 11393–8.

148. Papadopoulos N, Martin J, Ruan Q, et al. Binding and neutralization of vascular endothelial growth factor (VEGF) and related ligands by VEGF Trap, ranibizumab and bevacizumab. Angiogenesis 2012; 15: 171–85.

21

Radiation therapy for age-related macular degeneration

Madhavi Kurli, Paul T. Finger, and Pravin U. Dugel

INTRODUCTION

Neovascular age-related macular degeneration (AMD) is the leading cause of severe, irreversible blindness in the western world. Typically, patients with neovascular AMD are older than 50 years and white, although other races and ages may be affected.

The characteristic feature of neovascular AMD is the development of a subfoveal choroidal neovascular membrane (CNV). When CNV lesions leak or rupture, components (serum, fats, and blood cells) extravasate into the surrounding choroid and retina. This leads to retinal edema, inflammation, and subsequent scarring with damage to the photoreceptor layer (1).

Multiple treatments have been tried over the past few years with variable results. The advent of anti-angiogenic (anti-VEGF) treatment has been shown to produce a significant visual gain in a third of patients (2,3). However, visual results are still limited with continued retinal pigment epithelial degeneration and subsequent neurosensory retinal atrophy. Also, the majority of patients require frequent intravitreal injections and follow-up visits, posing challenges to both patients and their caregivers. Newer treatments including radiation therapy have been investigated as an alternative or adjunct to anti-VEGF agents in the treatment of neovascular AMD.

RADIATION AND ANGIOGENESIS
Radio Biology

Radiation is known to induce acute vasculitis followed by a slowly progressive vascular closure that can take years to develop (4–6). Radiation of a macula containing classic or occult CNV could affect angiogenesis either directly (by destroying neovascular endothelial cells and cytokine-producing macrophages) or indirectly (affecting regulatory genes within cells that produce endothelial growth-regulating cytokines). Commonly employed to prevent aberrant scar formation, low doses have been used to inhibit formation of scars such as cutaneous keloids and later, to prevent arterial stenosis. The experience of Hart et al. suggests that radiotherapy may inhibit the scar formation associated with end-stage neovascular macular degeneration (7). This could occur because the development of neovascular AMD is considered to be similar to a proliferative wound healing process. Radiation causes irreparable damage to DNA and protein synthesis thereby preventing further replication and protein synthesis. This effect is selective and proliferative cells discontinue the cell division cycle while nondividing cells repair the damage to the DNA (8).

Synergistic Effect of Radiation Therapy and Anti-VEGF

Radiation and anti-VEGF agents target the neovascular disease in different ways. Radiation produces a delayed response that has a longer duration of action while anti-VEGF therapy produces a rapid response and has a shorter duration of action. Anti-VEGF inhibits growth factors in the local lesion while radiation disarms the local inflammatory cellular response and produces apoptosis of the vascular endothelium. These effects have the potential to produce a faster and complete recovery as seen in the treatment of colon cancer (9,10). The synergistic effect of radiation and anti-VEGF treatment may prove to be efficacious in the treatment of the neovascular process in wet AMD; this combined treatment is currently being investigated in ongoing clinical trials.

METHODS OF DELIVERY

Radiation can be delivered to tissues via two different methods:

Brachytherapy (*brachy* in Greek means short-distance) uses a source, usually a radionuclide (an isotope that produces ionizing radiation as it decays and emits energy), close to the target. This radioactive source is typically delivered directly to the lesion via a surgical procedure.

Teletherapy, or external beam radiotherapy, uses an isotope or an electronically produced ionizing radiation source that is external and is projected as a beam at a target within the body tissue.

USE OF RADIATION THERAPY FOR AMD IN THE PAST

Multiple phase I clinical studies have investigated a range of radiation doses for treatment of neovascular AMD in the past (11–20). Most centers initially used external beam irradiation because it was readily available, noninvasive, and inexpensive. A few centers investigated temporary surgical implantation of radioactive materials for the treatment of neovascular AMD. Finger et al. reported results of palladium-103 (103Pd) ophthalmic plaque radiotherapy for neovascular AMD, while Immonen and Freire studied the use of strontium-90 (90Sr) applicators and Berta et al. studied ruthenium-106 (106Ru) for the treatment of neovascular AMD. Although none of these groups performed a prospective, randomized clinical trial to prove whether radiation effectively treats macular degeneration, the phase I results were encouraging (14–17).

The overwhelming majority of phase-I clinical studies employing radiation to treat CNV in the past have used 4–6 MV external beam radiotherapy (EBRT) (11,12). Advantages included the ability to noninvasively radiate one or both eyes as well as radiographic localization of the targeted macular volume. Unfortunately, EBRT required a relatively large number of fractions (days) to deliver the dose (e.g., 200 cGy over 3–10 working days). Further, unlike brachytherapy the EBRT-dose to target volume (macula) was fairly uniform. Lastly, EBRT photons typically continue past the eye, resulting in unnecessary irradiation of the sinuses and the brain.

Proton Beam

Proton beam therapy (charged-particle external irradiation) is another form of EBRT, but is more focused. Like photon-based EBRT, proton therapy is typically nonsurgical. However, protons are delivered at a high-dose rate given over fewer (e.g., one to three) days (18). Like photon-based EBRT, proton beam therapy can be used unilaterally or bilaterally. However, high-dose-rate radiation therapy is known to cause more long-term side effects.

Both photon and proton-based EBRT can be thought of as a cylinder or column of radiation that courses from the front to the back of the eye. Therefore, the accuracy of the macular dose is affected by eye movements. Although a number of proton facilities are under construction, they are currently not widely available in North America.

Implant Brachytherapy

Implant radiotherapy or brachytherapy involves placing a radiation source directly beneath the macula. Palladium-103 (103Pd) ophthalmic plaques, ruthenium-106 (106Ru), and strontium-90 (90Sr) applicators have been employed. Implant brachytherapy delivers a relatively high dose within the targeted volume (macula) over a relatively short duration (minutes to 36 hours). Implant radiation therapy is a monocular treatment that delivers almost no radiation to the fellow eye, sinuses, or brain. Although the involved macula received a larger dose than with photon-based EBRT, most normal ocular structures of the treated eye received less irradiation with implant radiotherapy.

Although there was a trend toward progressive visual loss at two years with these treatment methods, some authors noted a resolution of the neovascular component of the AMD and subsequent atrophy (11–20). In general, the visual outcomes from these studies were variable and do not compare favorably with the visual stabilization or improvement obtained with anti-VEGF treatment.

EPIMACULAR BRACHYTHERAPY

In epimacular brachytherapy, beta radiation from a strontium-90/yttrium-90 source is placed close to the macula. The dose of beta radiation decreases with increasing distance thereby reducing radiation exposure of adjacent normal tissue.

In epimacular brachytherapy, the beta radiation is delivered to the CNV lesion after a pars plana vitrectomy. The radiation delivery probe is then positioned over the CNV lesion so that the maximum radiation dose is delivered to the area with the greatest disease activity as determined by a preoperative fluorescein angiogram. The probe is held for four minutes over the lesion and then removed. However, the potential risks include radiation retinopathy, optic neuropathy and cataract; the dose to adjacent structures is reported to be below the safety threshold for these tissues (21–26).

In the Neovista-sponsored epimacular brachytherapy clinical trials, patients received anti-VEGF treatment at the time of surgery, one month later and thereafter based on disease activity. This combination of vitrectomy, radiation, and anti-VEGF therapy was proposed to treat the CNV lesions in AMD. Vitrectomy is said to increase oxygenation of the inner retinal layers and thus decrease free-radical formation which in turn prevents further CNV (27–31). This in combination with the anti-angiogenic effect of radiation and anti-VEGF treatment was postulated to be an effective treatment of neovascular AMD.

Epimacular Brachytherapy Trials
Preliminary Studies

NVI-68 was a nonrandomized multicenter feasibility study. Thirty-four treatment-naïve patients were enrolled. Patients received 24 Gy (26 patients) or 15 Gy (8 patients) of beta radiation. After 12 months, a significant difference in visual outcome was noted and there were no radiation-related complications. In the 24 Gy group, a mean gain of 10.3 letters (using the ETDRS chart) was noted while the 15 Gy group had a loss of –1.0 letters (32).

NV-111 was a prospective, nonrandomized, multicenter study with 34 treatment-naïve patients. Patients received 24 Gy of beta-radiation and two injections of anti-VEGF, initially at the time of surgery and another injection one month later. Further injections were given based on disease activity. At the end of 12 months, there was a mean gain of 8.9 letters with 91% maintaining vision and 68% showing stable or improved vision. Almost 75% received no further anti-VEGF treatment during that year. This was in contrast to patients receiving ranibizumab monotherapy who were anticipated to receive eight injections during this time. No radiation-related side effects were noted.

These early feasibility trials demonstrated the preliminary safety and efficacy of epimacular brachytherapy and led to the larger clinical trials.

MERITAGE Study

The Macular Epiretinal Brachytherapy in Treated Age-Related Macular Degeneration (MERITAGE) study was conducted in two centers in the Unites States, one center in the United Kingdom, and two centers in Israel. The study was designed to examine NeoVista's epimacular brachytherapy procedure when used in patients who require chronic therapy with anti-VEGF agents on an ongoing basis to control neovascular age-related macular degeneration. The study enrolled patients who had as many as 38 prior injections of anti-VEGF therapy before receiving epimacular brachytherapy.

The study population (53 patients) had a trend toward losing vision, even with regular anti-VEGF therapy in the year prior to enrollment. Prior to entry into the study, all patients were required to have received a loading dose of three monthly anti-VEGF injections and then a minimum of five additional injections in the 12 months preceding enrollment or three injections in the six months preceding enrollment. This ensured that the full benefit of anti-VEGF therapy was realized prior to entry into the study.

Study results suggest that a single procedure of epimacular brachytherapy can stabilize visual acuity in a majority of this patient population (79%) while decreasing the number of anti-VEGF injections required. Most importantly, 47% of patients enrolled in the study experienced some improvement in their visual acuity while 10% of patients gained 15 or more letters of visual acuity at 12 months. This improvement is significant in patients who had been receiving chronic anti-VEGF treatment with no vision improvement in the year prior to enrollment.

The study results also pointed to a favorable trend with respect to a reduced number of anti-VEGF injections following delivery of epimacular brachytherapy (mean of 3.9) versus the period of time leading up to epimacular brachytherapy intervention (mean of 12.3). In addition, 25% of patients remained injection-free at 12 months following the epimacular brachytherapy procedure.

CABERNET Study
The CNV secondary to AMD treated with Beta RadiatioN Epiretinal Therapy (CABERNET) is a phase 3, multicenter, prospective, randomized, noninferiority-design study that included 457 treatment-naïve patients, who were divided into two arms. Patients in the treatment arm (n = 302) underwent strontium-90 beta radiation with epimacular brachytherapy (NeoVista's Epi-Rad 90™ device) and two mandatory ranibizumab (Lucentis, Genentech) injections. Patients in the control arm (n = 155) received ranibizumab injections following a modified PIER protocol, which included three initial monthly injections followed by injections once every three months. In the CABERNET study, patients were seen on a monthly basis, and rescue therapy was permitted, as per the investigators' discretion.

The primary end point of CABERNET was visual acuity, specifically, the percentage of patients losing fewer than 15 letters of vision. In patients treated with epimacular brachytherapy, 77% of patients lost fewer than 15 letters of vision. Noninferiority was not met in this study.

They also found that injections were required at the two-year mark; mean visual acuity change was a 2.5 letter loss. Patients treated with ranibizumab required 11 injections and achieved a mean 4.4 letter gain.

In an unplanned subgroup analysis post study that included patients with lesions of all sizes and both classic and occult membranes, the investigators identified 44% of patients in the epimacular brachytherapy group who required no rescue injections through the first 12 months and one rescue injection through the second 12 months, with a mean 3.3 letter gain. No baseline predictive factors were identified in these patients. In a similar analysis, the investigators identified 25% of patients in the epimacular brachytherapy arm who required no rescue injections throughout the two-year course of the study, with a mean gain of 5.7 letters.

Cataract formation occurred in 48% of patients in the epimacular brachytherapy arm, which was likely due to the vitrectomy procedures.

At the two-year mark, there were ten patients with suspected radiation-based retinopathy that was nonproliferative and nonprogressive throughout the two-year course of the study.

The CABERNET demonstrated an acceptable safety profile for epimacular brachytherapy at the two-year mark and identified a subgroup of patients who tended to respond well to the treatment and required fewer rescue injections. However, the CABERNET study did not achieve its primary end point with a 10% noninferiority margin, and it is not yet known whether the subgroup of patients who benefited from the device can be reliably and consistently identified in clinical practice.

MERLOT Study
MERLOT (Macular EpiRetinal brachytherapy versus Lucentis® Only Treatment) is an ongoing, investigator-initiated, multicenter (U. K. based) randomized controlled trial in patients who have received anti-VEGF treatment. MERLOT has enrolled patients in 16 National Health Service (NHS) hospitals in the United Kingdom (n = 363). Epimacular brachytherapy treatment (Neovista's VIDION® ANV® system) with as-required ranibizumab injections is compared with ranibizumab monotherapy in this trial.

STEREOTACTIC RADIOSURGERY
External beam radiotherapy has been revisited using stereotactic radiosurgery. The IRay system (Oraya Therapeutics, Newark, California, USA) includes a low-voltage x-ray source, an eye tracking system, and a robotically controlled in-office delivery system. The radiation dose is delivered via three x-ray beams that pass into the eye through different locations on the sclera (avoiding the lens). It precisely targets the radiation on the CNV lesion and minimizes the radiation exposure of adjacent tissues. The system uses a low-voltage X-ray source that does not require radiation shielding like the previously used linear accelerators thus eliminating expensive safety precautions.

A robotically controlled radiation source is used to deliver the beam and is connected to the patient using a contact lens and a suction cup. The low-voltage x-ray based system does not require room shielding and could be performed as an office procedure. The patient is secured in place with a head restraint that has a lead backing. A self-retaining lid retractor is used and the eye is secured in position with a vacuum-coupled contact lens interface with suction. The system has eye-tracking abilities (I-Guide) and stabilizes the eye during treatment. Three separate beams (8 Gy each) are then delivered through the sclera in the region of the inferior pars plana (5, 6, and 7 o'clock) to target the CNV lesion in the fovea. The exposure of the lens and optic nerve is reduced by the dispersing scleral entry dose (33,34).

Clinical Trials
CLH001
This phase I trial is a single-center, uncontrolled, pilot study to evaluate the safety and tolerability of the IRay stereotactic radiosurgery system in patients with CNV secondary to AMD. The study aims to determine safety, preliminary efficacy, and dose evaluation of the stereotactic radiosurgery system. The study includes two cohorts: those without previous treatment and those previously treated with anti-VEGF therapy requiring additional treatment due to persistent or recurring disease activity. The study investigated two radiation doses (16 and 24 Gy) and different induction regimens. Induction involved anti-VEGF treatment at baseline and at one month with radiosurgery in between or radiotherapy alone at baseline. Monthly re-treatment with additional anti-VEGF drug was performed if needed.

The initial results with up to 12 months' follow-up showed that in the majority of patients, the visual acuity had stabilized or improved; mean visual acuity gain was 8–10 ETDRS letters. The rate of anti-VEGF re-treatment injections (following the two mandatory "baseline" doses) was 0.9 per patient over 10 months, and approximately 56% of patients needed no additional anti-VEGF injections, while still demonstrating visual acuity preservation and gain (35).

There were no device-related serious adverse events and no evidence of radiation-related abnormalities. Some superficial keratopathy was noted and was attributed mostly to placement of the I-Guide and required no intervention by the physician.

The results of this feasibility study, while meant to evaluate primarily the safety and tolerability of the IRay therapy, demonstrated a number of encouraging visual outcomes, including substantial preservation and gain of vision in both the treatment-naïve and previously treated cohorts, as well as low numbers of required anti-VEGF re-treatment injections.

CLH002 Study (INTREPID)
CLH002 is a commercial, randomized controlled feasibility study that evaluates the safety and effectiveness of stereotactic radiosurgery in patients who have been previously treated with anti-VEGF therapy. The patients are randomized to groups treated with 16 Gy, 24 Gy, or sham stereotactic radiosurgery with as-required ranibizumab in all patients. This European trial is ongoing and has completed recruitment.

CONCLUSION
The management of neovascular AMD remains a challenge across the globe. The advent of anti-VEGF treatment has provided an important and invaluable step forward in the management of this sight-threatening disease. However, regular intravitreal injections and the need for frequent follow-up impose a considerable burden on patients besides the risk of endophthalmitis with repeated injections.

Epimacular brachytherapy and stereotactic radiosurgery have the potential to provide stabilization or improvement in vision while reducing frequent injections and follow-up visits in patients with neovascular AMD. However, the results of the larger clinical trials are awaited to assess the role of radiation treatment therapy possibly as an adjunct to anti-VEGF treatment in patients with CNV secondary to AMD.

SUMMARY POINTS

- Radiation may affect angiogenesis either directly (by destroying neovascular endothelial cells and cytokine-producing macrophages) or indirectly (affecting regulatory genes within cells that produce endothelial growth-regulating cytokines)
- Radiation disarms the local inflammatory cellular response and produces apoptosis of the vascular endothelium
- Epimacular brachytherapy and stereotactic radiosurgery may prove to be valuable adjuncts to anti-VEGF therapy for neovascular AMD.
- Radiation therapy given in conjunction with anti-VEGF agents may reduce the number of intravitreal injections required.
- The risk of radiation-related adverse effects appears to be minimal with these radiation treatments.
- Further trials will reveal the role of radiation therapy in the management of neovascular AMD.

REFERENCES

1. Ferris FL 111, Fine SL, Hyman L. Age-related macular degeneration and blindness due to neovascular maculopathy. Arch Ophthalnol 1984; 102: 1640–2.
2. Rosenfeld PJ, Brown DM, Heier JS, et al. Ranibizumab for neovascular age-related macular degeneration. N Engl J Med 2006; 355: 1419–31.
3. Brown DM, Kaiser PK, Michels M, et al. Ranibizumab versus verteporfin for neovascular age-related macular degeneration. N Engl J Med 2006; 255: 1432–44.
4. Chakravarthy U, Biggart JH, Gardiner TA, et al. Focal irradiation of perforating eye injuries. Curr Eye Res 1989; 8: 1241–50.
5. Chakravarthy U, Gardiner TA, Archer DB, et al. A light microscopic and auto radiographic study of non-irradiated and irradiated ocular wounds. Curr Eye Res 1989; 8: 337–48.
6. Flickinger JC, Pollock BE, Kondziolka D, Lunsford LD. A dose–response analysis of arteriovenous malformation

obliteration after radiosurgery. Int J Radiat Oncol Biol Phys 1996; 36: 873–9.

7. Hart PM, Archer DP, Chakravarthy U. Asymmetry of disciform scarring in bilateral disease when one eye is treated with radiotherapy. Br J Ophthalmol 1995; 79: 562–8.

8. Kirwan JF, Constable PH, Murdoch IE, et al. Beta irradiation: new uses for an old treatment: a review. Eye 2003; 17: 207–15.

9. Willett CG, Boucher Y, di Tomaso E, et al. Direct evidence that the VEGF-specific antibody bevacizumab has antivascular effects in human rectal cancer. Nat Med 2004: 10. 145.7.

10. Senan S, Smit EF. Design of clinical trials of radiation combined with antiangiogenic therapy. Oncologist 2007; 12: 465–77.

11. Chakravarthy U, Houston RF, Archer DB. Treatment of age-related subfoveal neovascular membranes by teletherapy: a pilot study. Br J Ophthalmol 1993; 77: 265–73.

12. Bergink GJ, Deutman AF, van der Briek JF, et al. Radiation therapy for subfoveal choroidal neovascular membranes in age-related macular degeneration: a pilot study. Graefes Arch Clin Exp Ophthalmol 1994; 232: 591–8.

13. Berta A, Vezendi L, Vamosi P. Irradiation of macular subretinal neovascularization using ruthenium applicators. Szemeset (Hung J Ophthalmol) 1995; 132: 67–75.

14. Finger PT, Berson A, Sherr DA, et al. Radiation therapy for subretinal neovascularization. Ophthalmology 1996; 103: 878–9.

15. Finger PT, Gelman YP, Berson AM, et al. Palladium-103 plaque radiation therapy for macular degeneration: results of a 7-year study. Br J Ophthalmol 2003; 87: 1497–503.

16. Berson AM, Finger PT, Sherr DL, et al. Radiotherapy for age-related macular degeneration: preliminary results of a potentially new treatment. Int J Radiat Oncol Biol Phys 1996; 36: 861–5.

17. Freire J, Longton WA, Miyamoto CT, et al. External radiotherapy in macular degeneration: technique and preliminary subjective response. Int J Radiat Oncol Biol Phys 1996; 36: 857–60.

18. Yonemoto LT, Slater JD, Friedrichsen EJ, et al. Phase I/II study of proton beam irradiation for the treatment of subfoveal choroidal neovascularization in age-related macular degeneration: treatment, techniques and preliminary results. Int J Radiat Oncol Biol Phys 1996; 36: 867–71.

19. Jaakkola A, Heikkonen J, Tommila P, et al. Strontium plaque irradiation of subfoveal neovascular membranes in age-related macular degeneration. Graefes Arch Clin Exp Ophthalmol 1998; 236: 24–30.

20. Sralmans P, Leys A, Limbergen E. External beam radiotherapy (20_Gy, 2_Gy fractions) fails to control the growth of choroidal neovascularization in age-related macular degeneration: a review of 11 cases. Retina 1997; 17: 491–2.

21. Avila MP, Farah ME, Santos A, et al. Twelve-month short-term safety and visual acuity results from a multi-centre prospective study of epiretinal strontium-90 brachytherapy with bevacizumab for the treatment of subfoveal choroidal neovascularization secondary to age-related macular degeneration. Br J Ophthalmol 2009; 93: 305–9.

22. Parsons JT, Bova FJ, Fitzgerald CR, et al. Radiation retinopathy after external-beam irradiation: analysis of time-dose factors. Int J Radiat Oncol Biol Phys 1994; 30: 765–73.

23. Boozalis GT, Schachat AP, Green WR. Subretinal neovascularization from the retina in radiation retinopathy. Retina 1987; 7: 156–61.

24. Gordon KB, Char DH, Sagerman RH. Late effects of radiation on the eye and ocular adnexa. Int J Radiat Oncol Biol Phys 1995; 31: 1123–39.

25. Hanlon J, Lee C, Chell E, et al. Kilovoltage stereotactic radiosurgery for age-related macular degeneration: assessment of optic nerve dose and patient-effective dose. Med Phys 2009; 36: 3671–81.

26. Finger PT, Berson A, Ng T, et al. Ophthalmic plaque brachytherapy for age-related macular degeneration associated with subretinal neovascularization. Am J Ophthalmol 1999; 127: 170–7.

27. Stefansson E, Landers MB 3rd, Wolbarsht ML. Increased retinal oxygen supply following pan-retinal photocoagulation and vitrectomy and lensectomy. Trans Am Ophthalmol Soc 1981; 79: 307–34.

28. Jampol LM. Oxygen therapy and intraocular oxygenation. Trans Am Ophthalmol Soc 1987; 85: 407–37.

29. Hashimoto E, Hirakata A, Hotta K, et al. Unusual macular retinal detachment associated with vitreomacular traction syndrome. Br J Ophthalmol 1998; 82: 326.

30. Nordsmark M, Overgaard M, Overgaard J. Pretreatment oxygenation predicts radiation response in advanced squamous cell carcinoma of head and neck. Radiother Oncol 1996; 41: 31–9.

31. Brizel DM, Scully SP, Harrelson JM, et al. Tumor oxygenation predicts for the likelihood of distant metastases in human soft tissue sarcoma. Cancer Res 1996; 56: 941–3.

32. Avila MP, Farah ME, Santos A, et al. Twelve-month safety and visual acuity results from a feasibility study of intraocular, epiretinal radiation therapy for the treatment of subfoveal CNV secondary to AMD. Retina 2009; 29: 157–69.

33. Moshfeghi DM, Kaiser PK, Gertner M. Stereotactic low-voltage x-ray irradiation for age-related macular degeneration. Br J Ophthalmol 2010; 95: 185–8.

34. Lee C, Chell E, Gertner M, et al. Dosimetry characterization of a multibeam radiotherapy treatment for age-related macular degeneration. Med Phys 2008; 35: 5151–60.

35. Canton VM, Quiroz-Mercado H, Velez-Montoya R, et al. 24-Gy low-voltage x-ray irradiation with ranibizumab therapy for neovascular AMD: 6-month safety and functional outcomes. Ophthalmic Surg Lasers Imaging 2012; 43: 20–4.

22

Combination therapy for age-related macular degeneration

Darin R. Goldman, Chirag P. Shah, and Jeffrey S. Heier

INTRODUCTION

Advances in diagnostic imaging and pharmacotherapy have dramatically altered our ability to treat neovascular age-related macular degeneration (AMD). Clinical experience coupled with ongoing research has allowed our understanding of this process to evolve rapidly. Neovascular, or wet AMD, with development of choroidal neovascularization (CNV) accounts for a significant amount of vision loss, especially throughout the developed world. Prior to the advent of anti-vascular endothelial growth factor (VEGF) therapy, advanced AMD (including neovascular disease and geographic atrophy) accounted for the most common cause of blindness in people older than 50 years in the United States and many other developed nations (1–3). In the United States, the prevalence of vision loss from advanced AMD was estimated at 1.75 million in 2004, which was predicted to increase to 2.95 million by 2020 (4). More recent predictions suggest that the prevalence of legal blindness from neovascular AMD may be reduced by 70–74% with the advent of anti-VEGF therapy (5).

Treatment options for wet AMD have evolved rapidly over the past three decades. This process began in the late 1980s with the advent of thermal laser photocoagulation (6,7), which offered the first therapeutic treatment modality for wet AMD. Thermal laser was made nearly obsolete by the advent of nonthermal laser, which followed in the late 1990s with the development of verteporfin photodynamic therapy (PDT) (8–11). Both thermal laser and PDT represented therapeutic advances by slowing down the rate of visual loss, but neither led to overall improvements in vision.

The advent of the first anti-VEGF agent for the treatment of neovascular AMD, pegaptanib, which was approved by the FDA for treatment of neovascular AMD in 2004 (12,13), led to a shift in therapeutic strategy that would open the door to modern wet AMD treatment. The therapeutic effect of pegaptanib was similar to prior laser therapies by stabilizing disease without significant improvement in vision. Shortly following pegaptanib's approval, the FDA approved ranibizumab in 2006 after efficacy was proven in the Minimally Classic/Occult Trial of the Anti-VEGF Antibody Ranibizumab in the Treatment of Neovascular Age-Related Macular Degeneration (MARINA) and Anti-VEGF Antibody for the Treatment of Predominantly Classic Choroidal Neovascularization in Age-related Macular Degeneration (ANCHOR) trials (14,15).

The arrival of ranibizumab for the treatment of neovascular AMD was revolutionary as it provided the first therapeutic agent that could improve vision in a significant proportion of patients. Ranibizumab was directly compared with PDT in the ANCHOR trial and found to have a greater clinical benefit (15).

The intravitreal use of bevacizumab has gained widespread acceptance along with ranibizumab for the treatment of wet AMD. Both ranibizumab and bevacizumab were compared head to head in the Comparison of Age-related Macular Degeneration Treatments Trials (CATT), which showed similar efficacy at one year (16). The current standard care for neovascular AMD with bevacizumab or ranibizumab monotherapy requires regular, indefinite follow-up intervals as frequent as every four weeks to maintain maximal efficacy. Such frequent follow-up can be a significant time commitment for patients and their families who accompany them to office visits, while also increasing health care costs. Additionally, frequent repeated intravitreal injections carry an increased risk to the patient for a serious adverse event such as endophthalmitis. Even with the impressive efficacy of anti-VEGF therapy compared with older modalities, there remains a portion of patients (10%) who lose vision despite two years of monthly monotherapy with ranibizumab (14). For patients with neovascular AMD, researchers have developed various strategies to address the frequency of injections and to try to improve efficacy. One of these strategies employs the combination of different treatment modalities in addition to an anti-VEGF agent. This strategy is referred to as "combination therapy." Most patients with neovascular AMD exhibit a profound anatomical response to anti-VEGF therapy with resolution of intraretinal and subretinal fluid. Some patients, however, retain persistent fluid despite regular, monthly anti-VEGF therapy. This population of patients may have the potential to gain even more vision by therapeutically extinguishing their residual fluid. Combination therapy may also be of potential benefit in this population of patients, who are referred to as suboptimal responders. This chapter focuses on the efficacy and utility of the three most common modalities currently used in combination therapy for neovascular AMD including anti-VEGF agents, PDT, and corticosteroids. These agents are used in either double or triple combinations to target inflammation, CNV formation, and VEGF load.

PATHOPHYSIOLOGY OF CNV FORMATION AND THE RATIONALE FOR COMBINATION THERAPY

The rationale for combination therapy comes from our understanding of the underlying pathophysiology of neovascular AMD, whose hallmark feature is CNV formation. Neovascular AMD is a multifactorial process undermined by aberrant growth factor signaling (17,18). The pathogenic process is thought to be initiated by oxidative stress (19), which subsequently causes retinal pigment epithelium (RPE) dysfunction, followed by a cascade of active inflammation mediated by vasculogenic and angiogenic factors, CNV formation with hemorrhage and exudation, and disciform scarring (20). There is a potential role for intervention at each pathogenic stage of neovascular AMD with the goal of mitigating both CNV formation and disciform scarring, which have the greatest effects on visual acuity.

Within the cascade of neovascular AMD pathophysiology, CNV formation usually causes the first visual symptoms owing to associated serous and hemorrhagic detachments of the RPE with exudation of fluid and lipid into and below the retina. Histopathologically, CNV is composed of cellular and extracellular components (21). Spaide has proposed that CNV formation and maintenance are due to two main components, both vascular and extravascular (22). The vascular component includes endothelial cells, endothelial precursors, and pericytes, whose organization into functional vasculature is mediated by growth factors such as VEGF and platelet-derived growth factor (PDGF) (23). VEGF, in particular, plays a critical role in physiologic and pathologic vascular permeability and angiogenesis (24). Aberrant signaling by VEGF and other growth factors can lead to the formation and potentiation of CNV. The extravascular component of CNV formation consists of inflammatory cells and other extracellular matrix components such as glial cells and fibroblasts, contributing a significant portion by volume to the composition of CNV. Irregular cytokine and inflammatory signaling can result in faulty extracellular matrix construction and flawed support structures that can also potentiate CNV formation. Both the vascular and extravascular components of CNV can produce angiogenic factors and potentiate CNV formation with some degree of redundancy, thereby providing targets for various directed therapies.

By simultaneously targeting multiple different pathogenic factors in neovascular AMD development and progression, it may be possible to improve upon the efficacy of monotherapy by improving visual acuity outcomes, lengthening treatment-free intervals, and decreased re-treatment rates. The most common combination therapy strategies in clinical practice utilize anti-VEGF agents, PDT, and corticosteroids. As we better understand the pathophysiology of CNV formation and progression, additional therapeutic targets may be revealed. Currently, clinical trials are ongoing investigating various new targets for neovascular AMD treatment including integrin α5β1, complement factor 5, PDGF, tyrosine kinase, and tumor necrosis factor (25,26).

MONOTHERAPEUTIC AGENTS CURRENTLY USED IN COMBINATION FOR THE TREATMENT OF NEOVASCULAR AMD

Photodynamic Therapy: Targeting Vasculogenesis

PDT with verteporfin directly targets the vascular component of CNV, causing localized thrombosis and occlusion within CNV endothelium, while minimizing collateral damage to nearby neural retina and Bruch's membrane (27,28). PDT utilizes Visudyne® (QLT Ophthalmics, Vancouver BC and Novartis AG, Basel, Switzerland), which is a light-activated pharmacologic agent that requires intravenous administration of verteporfin followed by activation with 689 nm nonthermal infrared laser (29). Photoactivation of verteporfin causes localized endothelial cytoskeletal damage with resultant vessel occlusion. The degree of photoactivation is controlled by the total dose of light delivered. The manufacturer recommends 50 J/cm^2 at an intensity of 600 mW/cm, administered over 83 seconds, which is referred to as standard- or full-fluence PDT. PDT is indicated as monotherapy for the treatment of predominantly classic CNV due to neovascular AMD based on the Treatment of AMD with Photodynamic Therapy (TAP) study (8,30). PDT is also indicated for the treatment of smaller occult and minimally classic CNV based on the Verteporfin in Photodynamic Therapy (VIP) (9) and Verteporfin in Minimally Classic CNV due to AMD (VIM) studies (10). As monotherapy, PDT has demonstrated efficacy against CNV but this has been limited by CNV recurrence (31). In typical neovascular AMD, PDT monotherapy has been supplanted by anti-VEGF therapy because of more robust visual acuity outcomes with the latter. Additional factors limiting the use of PDT as monotherapy are its selective efficacy in certain types of CNV (i.e., classic) and failure to improve vision in most patients. Full-fluence PDT has been associated with transient choroidal ischemia and there are also reports of permanent ischemia, which may be more likely in purely occult or minimally classic lesions (32). Transient ischemia immediately following PDT can cause release of proangiogenic and pro-inflammatory factors such as VEGF within choroidal endothelial cells, which is associated with some degree of collateral damage to the nearby choriocapillaris and RPE (31). Reduced- or half-fluence (25 J/cm^2) PDT may minimize the associated choroidal hypoperfusion that accompanies full-fluence PDT and therefore minimize the adverse effects to the surrounding physiologic choroid (33). The combination of anti-inflammatory agents with PDT may blunt some of the adverse effects that are inherent with PDT and prevent CNV recurrence. Further details on the PDT clinical trials results are available in chapter 23, "PDT for Neovascular AMD."

Anti-VEGF: Targeting Angiogenesis

VEGF plays a critical role in the mediation of both physiologic and pathologic neovascularization with the eye (34,35). Normal VEGF secretion occurs from a variety of cell types within the eye. In patients with neovascular AMD, high levels of VEGF are found in CNV (36), RPE

(37), surrounding extracellular tissue, and vitreous (38,39). Hypoxia is known to be one of the predominant cues for secretion of VEGF, which occurs abnormally following oxidative damage to RPE cells, pericytes, and endothelial cells (40). VEGF receptors are present on various inflammatory cell membranes such as neutrophils (41), which are involved as effectors of local inflammation and pathologic angiogenesis. Treatment with anti-VEGF therapy has been shown to significantly reduce the levels of VEGF in eyes with neovascular AMD (39). Anti-VEGF therapy is thought to directly target the angiogenic component of CNV formation.

Clinically, there is ample evidence to support the role of anti-VEGF therapy in the treatment of neovascular AMD and its use as monotherapy is the current gold standard. Current anti-VEGF therapy consists predominantly of monotherapy with either bevacizumab or ranibizumab, though another anti-VEGF agent, aflibercept, was FDA approved (42) for the treatment of neovascular AMD. Ranibizumab is a recombinant, humanized monoclonal antibody Fab that blocks all forms of VEGF-A. Ranibizumab gained FDA approval for the treatment of all subtypes of CNV caused by neovascular AMD following the MARINA (14) and ANCHOR (15) trials, which showed a significant improvement in mean visual acuity in eyes treated with monthly ranibizumab over two years. Ranibizumab is typically administered as a single intravitreal injection of 0.5 mg in a volume of 0.5 mL. Bevacizumab is a humanized monoclonal antibody that blocks all forms of VEGF-A. Bevacizumab is FDA approved for certain metastatic neoplasms and is currently used off-label for the treatment of neovascular AMD. The CATT trial provides evidence supporting similar clinical efficacy of bevacizumab to ranibizumab as monotherapy for neovascular AMD at one year (16). Bevacizumab is typically administered as a single intravitreal injection of 1.25 mg in a volume of 0.5 mL. Current anti-VEGF treatment requires regular monthly treatment for optimal efficacy without a clearly defined end point of treatment.

Anti-Inflammatory Agents: Targeting Inflammation

The use of corticosteroids for neovascular AMD is based on the association of inflammation as an integral part of the underlying pathophysiology of AMD. Inflammatory mechanisms have been directly linked to drusen formation whereby primary RPE pathology is aggravated by local inflammation and complement activation (43). Inflammatory cells have also been identified histologically in excised CNVs (44). There are various other anatomical, molecular, and pathological links implicating inflammation in the pathogenesis of AMD (17). Corticosteroids may reduce VEGF expression (45) and have been shown to reduce the incidence of laser-induced CNV in primates (46). Certain steroids have been shown to be antiangiogenic (47) but their role in the treatment of neovascular AMD is thought to be mediated predominantly via their anti-inflammatory properties such as antifibrosis and antipermeability (48). Intravitreal corticosteroids have shown a lack of clinical efficacy in a large prospective trial, though there was a positive anatomical

effect on CNV lesion size (49). Intravitreal steroids also exhibit a significant complication profile including glaucoma and cataract formation, which become more prevalent with re-treatments. Given these shortcomings, corticosteroids have limited clinical utility as monotherapy in neovascular AMD. Nonetheless, there has been a renewed interest in combining intravitreal corticosteroids with other monotherapies for neovascular AMD in the hopes of achieving a synergistic effect (23). The use of intravitreal corticosteroids in combination with anti-VEGF agents and/or PDT for neovascular AMD is the subject of numerous clinical studies. The most common intravitreal corticosteroids that are currently used (their use is off-label) in combination with other agents for neovascular AMD are triamcinolone acetonide (dose ranging from 4 to 25 mg) and dexamethasone (dose ranging from 200 to 800 µg). After intravitreal injection in humans, triamcinolone has been found to have a mean half-life of 15.6 days and would be expected to last approximately three months in a nonvitrectomized eye (50). The half-life of dexamethasone was found to be 3.45 days after intravitreal injection in rabbits (51). Dexamethasone is five times more potent than triamcinolone. Given the longer half-life of triamcinolone, it is associated with a higher incidence of intraocular pressure spikes and cataract formation compared with dexamethasone when injected intravitreally.

CURRENT COMBINATION THERAPY REGIMENS FOR NEOVASCULAR AMD
PDT and Triamcinolone

There are numerous studies investigating the efficacy of PDT combined with intravitreal triamcinolone acetonide (IVTA) for the treatment of neovascular AMD (52–65). See Table 22.1 for a detailed summary of all studies. There was an additional study investigating PDT combined with sub-Tenon's triamcinolone acetonide (66). Based on the underlying mechanism of action of both PDT and IVTA, there is reason to believe that combination therapy with the two agents may be better than PDT monotherapy.

Maberly et al. conducted the only prospective, randomized, double-blind, sham-controlled multicenter trial investigating the combination therapy of PDT and IVTA for neovascular AMD (64). They used full-fluence PDT in all 100 eyes, 4 mg IVTA in 50 eyes, and sham intraocular injection in 50 eyes. They included eyes with subfoveal, predominantly classic CNV only. They found no significant difference in final visual acuity at one year between groups. The trend toward visual benefit with combination therapy may have been lost at month 12 due to cataract formation. Eyes receiving IVTA required significantly less re-treatments during the study period (1.28 vs. 1.94).

Arias et al. examined full-fluence PDT in 61 eyes with predominantly classic subfoveal CNV immediately followed by 11 mg of IVTA in 31 of these eyes (55). At 12 months, they found that visual acuity was better, lesion size and foveal thickness were reduced, and re-treatment rates were lower in the combination group compared with the PDT monotherapy group. The re-treatment rate

Table 22.1 Combination Therapy with PDT and Intravitreal Triamcinolone for Neovascular AMD

Reference (year of publication)	No. of eyes, follow-up duration	Study design	CNV type	Treatment protocol	Outcome measures
Randomized Controlled Trials					
Maberley et al. (64) (2009)	n = 100, 12 mos	Prospective, randomized, double-blind, sham-controlled, multicenter	Subfoveal CNV, predominantly classic	Full-fluence PDT in all eyes; 4 mg intravitreal triamcinolone in 50 eyes and sham intraocular injection in 50 eyes	No significant difference in final visual acuity at 1 yr between groups. Eyes receiving intravitreal triamcinolone required significantly less re-treatments during the study period (1.28 vs. 1.94). The trend toward visual benefit with combination therapy may have been lost at month 12 due to cataract formation.
Prospective, comparative					
Piermarocchi et al. (62) (2008)	n = 84, 24 mos	Prospective, randomized	Subfoveal CNV, all subtypes	Full-fluence PDT followed within 7–15 days by 4 mg intravitreal triamcinolone in 43 eyes	Mean visual acuity increased at 1 mo but then decreased at each subsequent follow-up interval (3, 6, 12, and 24 mos) in both groups. The re-treatment rate was significantly lower in the combination therapy group. Choroidal hypo- and nonperfusion on ICGA were greater with combined therapy.
Chadhaury et al. (61) (2007)	n = 30, 12 mos	Prospective, randomized	Subfoveal CNV, occult and minimally classic only, included RAP	Full-fluence PDT in all eyes followed 30 min later by 12 mg intravitreal triamcinolone in 15 eyes	Mean visual acuity remained stable in the combination group but declined in the PDT-only group. The re-treatment rate was significantly higher in the PDT-only group (2.6 vs.0.13) over the study period. Cataract progression occurred in 57% of phakic eyes in the combination group. Topical glaucoma therapy was required in 40% of eyes in the combination group.
Chan et al. (58) (2006)	n = 48, 12 mos	Prospective, nonrandomized, comparative	Subfoveal CNV, predominantly classic or occult	Full-fluence PDT in all eyes followed 5 min later by 4 mg intravitreal triamcinolone in 24 eyes	Eyes in the combination group had less vision loss compared with the PDT monotherapy group at 1 yr. The combination group required less frequent treatments (1.5 vs.1.96 treatments). In the combination group, 33% required initiation of glaucoma drops, 26% of phakic eyes developed progressive cataract, with 16% requiring cataract surgery.
Arias et al. (55) (2006)	n = 61 12 mos	Prospective, randomized, comparative	Subfoveal CNV, predominantly classic	Full-fluence PDT in all eyes immediately followed by 11 mg intravitreal triamcinolone in 31 eyes	Visual acuity was better, lesion size and foveal thickness were reduced, and re-treatment rates were lower in the combination group compared with the PDT-only group. The re-treatment rate was 1.8 in the combination group and 2.9 in the PDT-only group. Glaucoma occurred in 26% of eyes and cataract progression in 32% of phakic patients.
Prospective, noncomparative					
Augustin et al. (57) (2006)	n = 41, 24 mos	Prospective, noncomparative	Occult CNV only	Full-fluence PDT and 25 mg intravitreal triamcinolone 16 hrs after PDT in all eyes	Mean number of treatments was 1.8. A significant improvement in visual acuity was found in the majority of eyes and was maintained at 2 years of follow-up (mean 20/133 baseline vs.20/81 at 2 yrs); 26% of eyes required cataract surgery within 15 mos of the first treatment; 22% of eyes required management of glaucoma (7 eyes managed topically and 2 required systemic carbonic anhydrase inhibitors).

(Continued)

Table 22.1 Combination Therapy with PDT and Intravitreal Triamcinolone for Neovascular AMD (*Continued*)

Reference (year of publication)	No. of eyes, follow-up duration	Study design	CNV Type	Treatment protocol	Outcome measures
Augustin et al. (56) (2006)	n = 184 Median = 9.7 mos	Prospective, noncomparative	Subfoveal, juxtafoveal, and extrafoveal CNV, all subtypes	Full-fluence PDT and 25 mg intravitreal triamcinolone 16 hrs after PDT in all eyes	Mean number of treatments was 1.21. A significant improvement in visual acuity was found in most of the eyes (mean LogMAR visual acuity 0.83 baseline vs.0.71 last follow-up); 25% of eyes required glaucoma therapy (44 eyes treated medically and 2 eyes required surgical management); 48% of phakic eyes experienced cataract progression.
Smaller retrospective and prospective, noncomparative					
Lie et al. (65) (2010)	n = 40 3 mos	Retrospective, noncomparative	subfoveal CNV, all subtypes	Full-fluence PDT and 4 mg intravitreal triamcinolone within 1 hr of PDT in all eyes	Mean visual acuity improved from baseline (0.74 LogMAR) to 3 mo follow-up (0.69 LogMAR). Mean central retinal thickness increased from baseline 334 μm to 439 μm on day 1, subsequently decreasing to 255 μm by mo 3. The mean size of leakage are on FA did not change during the study period; 38% of eyes required re-treatment at mo 3.
Singh et al. (63) (2008)	n = 23 6 mos	Retrospective, noncomparative	Subfoveal CNV	Varying-fluence PDT (50, 40, and 25 J/cm2) immediately followed by 4 mg intravitreal triamcinolone in all eyes	Dose–response trend toward better visual outcomes and fewer treatments in the reduced fluence PDT group combined with intravitreal triamcinolone.
Nicolo et al. (60) (2006)	n = 11, 12 mos	Prospective, noncomparative	Subfoveal CNV, occult only	Full-fluence PDT and 25 mg intravitreal triamcinolone 1 mo after PDT in all eyes	Mean visual acuity improved from baseline at 1, 3 and 6 mos but not at 12 mos. No re-treatments were given during the entire study period. Fluorescein leakage and retinal thickness were significantly reduced during the study period. Prophylactic ophthalmic glaucoma medications were utilized in all patients, progression of cataract was observed in one patient.
Ergun et al. (59) (2006)	n = 60 Median = 15 mos	Retrospective, noncomparative	Subfoveal CNV, all subtypes	Full-fluence PDT followed by 4 mg intravitreal triamcinolone in all eyes	Mean visual acuity remained stable or improved in 43% of eyes at 12 mos. Mean number of treatments over 12 mos was 1.45.
Spaide et al. (54) (2005) (Ophthalmology)	n = 26 12 mos	Prospective, noncomparative	Subfoveal CNV, all subtypes	Full-fluence PDT followed by 4 mg intravitreal triamcinolone in all eyes	Re-treatment rate was 1.2. Treatment-naive eyes had better visual acuity outcomes than eyes previously treated with PDT; 38.5% of eyes required topical glaucoma therapy.
Spaide et al. (53) (2005) (Retina)	n = 15 , 12 mos	Prospective, non-comparative	Extrafoveal and juxtafoveal CNV	Full-fluence PDT followed by 4 mg intravitreal triamcinolone in all eyes	Mean number of treatments was 1.9. A significant improvement in visual acuity occurred at 3, 6, and 9 mos, but not at 12 mos; 20% of eyes required topical glaucoma therapy.
Rechtman et al. (52) (2004)	n = 14 , median = 18 mos	Retrospective, noncomparative	Subfoveal CNV, all subtypes	Full-fluence PDT followed by 4 mg intravitreal triamcinolone within 6 in all eyes	Mean visual acuity remained stable or improved in 57% of eyes. Mean number of PDT treatments during the first year was 2.57. Intraocular pressure elevation was noted in 28.5% of eyes and cataract progression in 50% of phakic eyes.

Abbreviations: CNV, choroidal neovascularization; mo/s, month/s; RAP, retinal angiomatous proliferation P.

was 1.8 in the combination group and 2.9 in the PDT-only group. Glaucoma occurred in 26% of eyes and cataract progression occurred in 32% of phakic patients.

Chan et al. investigated full-fluence PDT in 48 eyes followed five minutes later by 4 mg IVTA in 24 eyes (58). They found that eyes in the combination group had less vision loss compared to the PDT monotherapy group at one year. The combination group required less treatment (1.5 vs. 1.96 treatments). In the combination group, 33% required initiation of glaucoma drops, 26% of phakic eyes developed progressive cataract, with 16% requiring cataract surgery.

Chadhaury et al. examined full-fluence PDT in 30 eyes followed 30 minutes later by 12 mg IVTA in 15 eyes (61). They looked at occult and minimally classic CNV only and also included retinal angiomatous proliferation (RAP) lesions. Mean visual acuity remained stable in the combination group but declined in the PDT-only group. The re-treatment rate was significantly higher in the PDT-only group (2.6 vs. 0.13) over the 12-month study period. Cataract progression occurred in 57% of phakic eyes in the combination group and topical glaucoma therapy was required in 40% of eyes in the combination group.

Piermarocchi et al. investigated full-fluence PDT in 84 eyes with all subtypes of CNV followed within 7–15 days by 4 mg IVTA in 43 eyes (62). They found that mean visual acuity increased at one month but then decreased at each subsequent follow-up interval (3, 6, 12, and 24 months) in both groups. The re-treatment rate was significantly lower in the combination therapy group. In the combination therapy group, they found atrophic macular changes in the central choroid and retina as evidenced by choroidal hypo- and nonperfusion on ICGA (defined as closure of 1 or more major or midsize choroidal vessels within the treated area) and reduced or absent macular fundus autofluorescence. This series is the largest prospective, randomized, comparative study with the longest follow-up of combination therapy with PDT and IVTA. The authors suggest a concern that IVTA is responsible for the atrophic changes and poor visual outcomes at 24 months due to an anti-VEGF effect, which they feel limits the ability of the choroidal vasculature to restore normal blood flow within the treated area following PDT. This conclusion may not be accurate and consideration should also be given to the full-fluence PDT dosing, which may have had a direct ischemic effect.

Augustin et al. conducted a large prospective, non-comparative series of full-fluence PDT and 25 mg IVTA 16 hours after PDT in 184 eyes with subfoveal, juxtafoveal, and extrafoveal CNV of all subtypes (56) and in 41 eyes with occult CNV only (57). The mean number of treatments was 1.21 and 1.8, respectively. A significant improvement in visual acuity was found in the majority of eyes in both studies, but a significant proportion of eyes also required glaucoma therapy or experienced cataract progression.

There are a number of smaller noncomparative, prospective, and retrospective studies that examine full-fluence PDT in combination with a varied dose of IVTA given at a variable time following initial PDT (52–54,59,60,63,65). These studies included eyes with a mixture of all CNV subtypes. Intraocular pressure elevation and cataract progression were common. One of these studies used varying-fluence PDT and found a dose–response trend toward better visual outcomes and fewer treatments in the reduced-fluence (25 J/cm²) PDT combination group (63). Their results support the idea that reduced-fluence PDT minimizes choroidal hypoperfusion, which in turn may be associated with less collateral damage to surrounding normal choroidal tissue, a finding that warrants further investigation.

Van de Moere et al. investigated full-fluence PDT in 117 eyes with classic subfoveal CNV followed by 40 mg sub-Tenon's triamcinolone acetonide in 38 eyes (66). There was significantly less lesion growth at three and six months in the combination group. Visual acuity outcomes were similar between groups. Fewer PDT re-treatments were required in the combination group (2.03 vs. 2.47).

In summary, the studies investigating the efficacy of PDT combined with IVTA show efficacy that may be superior to PDT alone but is definitely inferior to intravitreal anti-VEGF monotherapy. The number of re-treatments with PDT that are required tend to be less when PDT is combined with IVTA rather than used as monotherapy. There is a significant risk of glaucoma development and cataract progression or development with IVTA. There may be an association of increased and persistent choroidal hypoperfusion within the PDT spot area when full-fluence PDT is accompanied by IVTA, (62), but this may be abated by using reduced-fluence PDT (63).

PDT and Anti-VEGF Agents

There are various studies investigating the efficacy of PDT combined with intravitreal bevacizumab (67–79) or ranibizumab (Tables 22.2 and 22.3) (80–87).

PDT and Intravitreal Bevacizumab

PDT combined with intravitreal bevacizumab has been the subject of more than 10 published, peer-reviewed, studies since 2006 (Table 22.2). Most studies used a standard dose of 1.25 mg/0.05 mL of bevacizumab for the intravitreal injection.

There have been two randomized, controlled trials studying PDT and bevacizumab (69,79). The study by Lazic et al. is the largest to date, but has limited follow-up (69). They included three parallel groups of PDT monotherapy (n = 55), intravitreal monotherapy (n = 55), and combination PDT with intravitreal bevacizumab (n = 55). They found that visual acuity improvement and central foveal thickness reduction occurred after one month in all groups but was more significant in the combination group. This effect was maintained at three months in the combination and bevacizumab monotherapy groups only, being more significant in the combination group. Patients may have been undertreated with bevacizumab, which could have biased their results in favor of combination therapy. Potter et al. investigated intravitreal bevacizumab in 36 eyes 2 hours following variably reduced-fluence PDT in 24 eyes (12 eyes with 25 J/cm² and 12 eyes with 12 J/cm²) (79). This study was the first prospective, randomized, double-masked, controlled clinical trial designed to determine

Table 22.2 Combination Therapy with Photodynamic Therapy (PDT) and Intravitreal Bevacizumab for Neovascular Age-Related Macular Degeneration

Reference (year of publication)	No. of eyes & follow-up duration	Study design	CNV type	Treatment protocol	Outcome measures
Randomized controlled trials					
Potter et al. (79) (2010)	n = 36 6 mos	Prospective, randomized, double-masked, controlled	Subfoveal CNV	Intravitreal bevacizumab in all eyes 2 hrs following variably reduced-fluence PDT in 24 eyes (12 with 25 J/cm2 and 12 with 12 J/cm2)	Patients required a mean of 2.5–2.8 treatments with beva-cizumab in the combination group and 5.1 in the monotherapy group. Mean overall visual acuity improved. Each group had a significant decrease in central retinal thickness.
Lazic et al. (69) (2007)	n = 165 3 mos	Prospective, randomized, controlled	Subfoveal CNV, minimally classic or occult	3 parallel groups, evenly divided: bevacizumab and full-fluence PDT monotherapies and their combination, no re-treatment allowed	Visual acuity improvement and central foveal thickness reduction occurred after one mo in all groups, which was more significant in the combination group compared with either monotherapy group. This was maintained till three mos in the combination and bevacizumab monotherapy group only. Combination treatment resulted in 2.2 lines of visual improvement versus 0.8 lines in eyes treated with bevacizumab alone.
Large prospective and retrospective, comparative					
Costagliola et al. (76) (2010)	n = 85, 12 mos	Prospective, randomized	Subfoveal CNV, classic or predominantly classic	Intravitreal bevacizumab in all eyes followed by half-fluence PDT within 2 wks in 40 eyes	There was no difference between groups in visual acuity outcomes. Eyes in the combination group received statistically significant less re-treatments with bevacizumab (2.8–3.2 vs.1.4–2.2).
Rudnisky et al. (77) (2010)	n = 375 mean = 13.5 mos	Retrospective, comparative	Subfoveal CNV, all subtypes	Intravitreal bevacizumab in all eyes following half-fluence PDT in 236 eyes on the same day	There was no difference between groups in visual acuity outcome or the number of bevacizumab injections.
Large retrospective, noncomparative					
Wan et al. (78) (2010)	n = 174 mean = 10 mos	Retrospective, noncomparative	Subfoveal CNV	Intravitreal bevacizumab 30 min following half-fluence PDT in all eyes	The mean visual acuity showed statistically significant improvement over the first 6 mos of follow-up. Subgroup analysis revealed that patients who were treatment naive had significantly better outcomes compared with patients who had received previous treatment. The mean number of treatments with bevacizumab was 3.0 and with PDT was 1.4
Kaiser et al. (73) (2009)	n = 1073 mean = 15 mos	Retrospective, noncomparative	Subfoveal CNV, all subtypes	Varied	Patients received a mean of 0.6 additional PDT re-treatments and 2.0 bevacizumab re-treatments over 15 mos; 82% of patients followed for 12 mos had stable or improved visual acuity. Patients who were treatment-naïve had better visual acuity outcomes compared with patients who had been previously treated.

(Continued)

Table 22.2 Combination Therapy with Photodynamic Therapy (PDT) and Intravitreal Bevacizumab for Neovascular Age-Related Macular Degeneration (*Continued*)

Reference (year of publication)	No. of eyes & follow-up duration	Study design	CNV type	Treatment protocol	Outcome measures
Smaller retrospective and prospective, noncomparative					
Navea et al. (75) (2009)	n = 63 12 mos	Prospective, noncomparative	Subfoveal CNV	Intravitreal bevacizumab following full-fluence PDT in all eyes	Mean visual acuity improved. Mean number of PDT treatments was 1.46. Mean number of bevacizumab injections was 2.0.
Liu et al. (74) (2009)	n = 15, 6 mos	Prospective, noncomparative	Subfoveal CNV, all subtypes	Intravitreal bevacizumab 3 days following full-fluence PDT in all eyes	Macular function was evaluated with multifocal electroretinography. There was an increase from baseline in mean retinal response amplitudes at 1, 3, and 6 mos after combination therapy.
Ladewig et al. (70) (2008)	n = 30 3 mos	Prospective, noncomparative	Subfoveal CNV, all subtypes	Intravitreal bevacizumab following full-fluence PDT in all eyes on the same day	Short-term results showed stabilization of visual acuity and decrease in central retinal thickness.
Smith et al. (71) (2008)	n = 40, mean = 9.5 mos	Retrospective, noncomparative	Juxtafoveal and subfoveal CNV, predominantly classic or occult	Intravitreal bevacizumab within 2 wks following full-fluence PDT in all eyes	Mean visual acuity stabilized or improved in 83% of eyes. Only 33% of eyes required re-treatment during the study period.
Costa et al. (68) (2007)	n = 11, 6 mos	Prospective, noncomparative	CNV progression following PDT	Intravitreal bevacizumab (1.5 mg) one wk following PDT (fluence not specified) in all eyes	A improvement in mean visual acuity was found at all study time points (1 and 2 weeks, 3 and 6 mos).
Dhalla et al. (67) (2006)	n = 24, 7 mos	Retrospective, noncomparative	Juxtafoveal and subfoveal CNV	Intravitreal bevacizumab and PDT within 2 wks in all eyes	Mean visual acuity stabilized or improved in 83% of eyes. A single combined re-treatment was required in 63% of eyes.

Abbreviations: CNV, choroidal neovascular membrane; mo/s, month/s; PDT, photodynamic therapy.

Table 22.3   Combination Therapy with Photodynamic Therapy (PDT) and Intravitreal Ranibizumab for Neovascular Age-Related Macular Degeneration

Reference (year of publication)	No. of eyes & follow-up duration	Study design	CNV type	Treatment protocol	Outcome measures
Randomized controlled trials					
DENALI, unpublished (89) 2010	n = 321, 12 mos, terminated early	Prospective, randomized, double-masked, multicenter	Subfoveal CNV, subtypes not specified	Intravitreal ranibizumab in all eyes, standard-fluence and half-fluence combination groups	Did not show noninferior visual acuity gains between either PDT combination group (5.3[reduced fluence] and 4.4[standard fluence] mean letters gained) and ranibizumab monotherapy (8.1 mean letters gained). Patients in the combination groups required an average of 2.2 (standard fluence) or 2.8 (reduced fluence) additional ranibizumab injections after the mandatory 3 loading doses, compared with an average of 7.6 additional injections in the ranibizumab moly monotherapy group.
MONT BLANC, unpublished (88) 2009	n = 255 12 mos, terminated early	Prospective, randomized, double-masked, multicenter	Subfoveal CNV, subtypes not specified	Intravitreal ranibizumab in all eyes following standard-fluence PDT or placebo	A mean VA improvement in the combination group that was noninferior to the ranibizumab monotherapy group (2.5 vs.4.4 letters) was found. The percentage of patients achieving a 3 mo treatment-free interval was not statistically significant between the two groups. A treatment-free interval of at least 4 mos was achieved in 85% of patients in the combination arm and 72% in the ranibizumab monotherapy arm. Time to first re-treatment was longer in the combination group (median 6 mos vs.5 mos).
Antoszyk et al. FOCUS (81) (2008)	n = 138, 24 mos	Prospective, randomized, single-masked, controlled	Subfoveal, predominantly classic (but reading center determined presence of minimally classic and occult lesion)	see below	In the combination group, 88% of the patients lost fewer than 15 letters compared with 75% of the eyes treated with PDT alone. In the combination group, 25% gained 15 letters or more compared to 7% in the eyes treated with PDT alone. The combination group had a mean change in visual acuity of 12.4 letters compared with the PDT-alone group. A significantly greater proportion of the PDT-alone group than the combination group received additional PDT treatments after day zero (93% vs.29%; mean numberof PDT treatments 3.0 vs.0.4).
Heier et al. FOCUS (80) (2006)	n = 162, 12 mos	Prospective, randomized, single-masked, controlled	Subfoveal, predominantly classic (but reading center determined presence of minimally classic and occult lesion)	Intravitreal ranibizumab (n = 106) or sham (n = 56) one week following full fluence PDT in all eyes	In the combination group, 91% of the patients lost fewer than 15 letters compared with 68% of the eyes treated with PDT alone. In the combination group, 24% gained 15 letters or more compared to 5% in the eyes treated with PDT alone. The mean number of injections was 10.9 in the ranibizumab group and 10.4 in the sham group. A marked difference in the proportion of study eyes requiring repeated PDT was evident by 3 mos (80% of the PDT monotherapy study eyes vs.16% of the combination study eyes) and was also observed at each subsequent 3-mo interval.
Prospective, comparative					
Bashshur et al. (83) (2011)	n = 40 12 mos	Prospective, comparative	Subfoveal CNV, all subtypes	Intravitreal ranibizumab in all eyes following full-fluence PDT in 13 eyes	There was a significantly greater mean visual acuity improvement for the monotherapy group. The time until ranibizumab re-treatment was longer and the number of ranibizumab injections was less in the combination group.

(Continued)

Table 22.3 Combination Therapy with Photodynamic Therapy (PDT) and Intravitreal Ranibizumab for Neovascular Age-Related Macular Degeneration (*Continued*)

Reference (year of publication)	No. of eyes & follow-up duration	Study design	CNV type	Treatment protocol	Outcome measures
Smaller retrospective and prospective, non-comparative					
Nakamura et al. (87) (2012)	n = 38 mean = 14 mos	Retrospective, non-comparative	Not specified	Intravitreal ranibizumab followed by full fluence PDT within one week in all eyes	The mean visual acuity and central macular thickness improved at 12 mos. The mean number of treatments was 1.1 for PDT and 2.9 for ranibizumab.
Wolf-Schnurrbusch et al. (86) (2011)	n = 15 12 mos	Prospective, non-comparative	Subfoveal CNV, predominantly classic or occult	Intravitreal ranibizumab following full fluence PDT in all eyes	Mean visual acuity improved by 10.9 letters. Mean central retinal thickness decreased by 85 μm.
Mataix et al. (84) (2010)	n = 53 12 mos	Prospective, non-comparative	Juxtafoveal and subfoveal CNV	Intravitreal ranibizumab 2–3 days following full fluence PDT in all eyes	Mean visual acuity stabilized or improved in 79% of eyes. Re-treatment was required in 60% of eyes. The mean number of treatments was 1.22 for PDT and 2.37 for ranibizumab.
Spielberg et al. (85) (2010)	n = 25 24 mos	Prospective, non-comparative	Subfoveal CNV, all subtypes including retinal angiomatous proliferative lesions	Intravitreal ranibizumab following one-time half fluence PDT in all eyes	The mean visual acuity improved by 7.2 letters and the mean central macular thickness decreased by 146 μm. Eighty-four percent of patients had stable or improved vision at mo 24. An average of 5.1 injections were administered during the first 12 mos, and 7.1 injections over 24 mos.
Kumar et al. (82) (2008)	n = 17 6 mos	Prospective, non-comparative	Subfoveal CNV, all subtypes	Intravitreal ranibizumab following full-fluence PDT in all eyes on the same day	Mean visual acuity stabilized in 82% of eyes. Re-treatment was required in only 12% of eyes.

Abbreviations: CNV, choroidal neovascular membrane; mo/s, month/s; PDT, photodynamic therapy.

whether the number of bevacizumab treatments can be decreased when combined with reduced-fluence PDT compared with bevacizumab alone. They found that the patients required a mean of 2.5–2.8 treatments with bevacizumab in the combination group and 5.1 in the monotherapy group after six months. Mean visual acuity improved in all groups. Each group had a significant decrease in central retinal thickness from baseline to month 6. Based on their results, they postulated that the combination of PDT and bevacizumab led to a quicker and more robust treatment effect compared with monotherapy with bevacizumab. Using a reduced fluence of 12 J/cm² did not appear to decrease the efficacy of PDT but may have decreased potential adverse effects.

Costagliola et al. conducted a large prospective investigation of intravitreal bevacizumab in 85 eyes followed by half-fluence PDT within two weeks in 40 eyes in a prospective, randomized fashion (76). They found no difference between groups in visual acuity outcomes. Eyes in the combination group received statistically significant less re-treatments with bevacizumab (2.8–3.2 vs. 1.4–2.2).

There was a large, comparative, retrospective series, conducted by Rudnisky et al. (78). They investigated intravitreal bevacizumab in 375 eyes following half-fluence PDT in 236 eyes on the same day. Their conclusions did not support any benefit from the combination of PDT with bevacizumab. Though both treatment groups appreciated a mean improvement of 1 line in visual acuity at one year, there was no difference between groups in visual acuity outcome or the number of bevacizumab injections. This study has findings which are in contrast to the results of a large prospective, comparative series with a short follow-up by Lazic et al. which will be discussed in the following text. The study by Rudnisky is retrospective with variable follow-up but suggests the short-term positive results seen by Lazic et al. may be temporary.

Two other large, noncomparative, retrospective investigations have been performed (73,78). Kaiser et al. conducted the largest series on combination intravitreal bevacizumab and PDT to date, which included a variable follow-up interval (mean of 15 months) (73). They investigated a variable treatment regimen of combination therapy in 1073 eyes. At the initial treatment, 14% of patients received reduced-fluence PDT and 6% received triple therapy (PDT and bevacizumab with either intravitreal dexamethasone or triamcinolone). The remaining patients presumably were treated with full-fluence PDT, though this was not explicitly specified. After the initial combination treatment at baseline, patients received a mean of 0.6 additional PDT re-treatments and 2.0 bevacizumab re-treatments. Eighty-two percent of patients followed for 12 months had stable or improved visual acuity. A subgroup analysis at 12 months revealed that patients who were treatment-naïve had better visual acuity outcomes compared with patients who had been previously treated. Visual acuity outcomes were analyzed by a subtype of CNV, which showed that patients with occult CNV were the largest gainers, followed by predominantly classic CNV, then minimally classic CNV, though these results were not statistically significant. Wan et al. investigated the effect of intravitreal bevacizumab 30 minutes following half-fluence PDT in 174 eyes (78). They found that mean best-corrected visual acuity improved significantly over the first six months of follow-up. A subgroup analysis revealed that patients who were treatment-naïve had significantly better outcomes than those who had received prior treatment. The mean number of treatments with bevacizumab was 3.0 and the mean number of treatments with PDT was 1.4.

There have been six smaller noncomparative retrospective and prospective studies of combination therapy with PDT and bevacizumab (67,68,70,71,74,75). These studies as a group found that visual acuity improved or stabilized in the majority of eyes. The study by Liu et al. evaluated multifocal electroretinography and found an increase from baseline in mean retinal response amplitudes one, three, and six months after combination therapy (74). They believed their results showed evidence that bevacizumab could offset the decreased retinal function that was associated with the immediate interval following PDT when used as monotherapy. This conclusion warrants further investigation in a larger study. One of these noncomparative studies that included 63 eyes required a mean number of PDT treatments of 1.46 and a mean number of bevacizumab injections of 2.0 over 12 months (75).

In summary, there are a number of studies investigating the combination of PDT and bevacizumab for neovascular AMD, many with varying study design. There are no long-term prospective randomized, controlled trials. Most studies suggest that this combination allows for less re-treatments with bevacizumab while maintaining good visual acuity results, though these findings are not supported by one of the larger series (77). Reduced-fluence PDT may have similar efficacy to full-fluence PDT, but with less potential for adverse effects, when used in combination with bevacizumab (79). Bevacizumab used in combination with PDT may be protective of the adverse effects on the retina that are noted in the short term following full-fluence PDT (74).

PDT and Intravitreal Ranibizumab

PDT combined with intravitreal ranibizumab (Table 22.3) has been the subject of significant interest since the 12-month results of the FOCUS (RhuFab V2 Ocular Treatment Combining the Use of Visudyne® to Evaluate Safety) trial were published in 2006 (80). This study by Heier et al. was a prospective, randomized, single-masked, controlled trial investigating intravitreal ranibizumab (n = 106) or sham (n = 56) one week following full-fluence PDT in 162 eyes. In the combination group, they found that 91% of the patients lost fewer than 15 letters compared with 68% of the eyes treated with PDT alone. In the combination group, 24% gained 15 letters or more compared with 5% in the eyes treated with PDT alone. The mean number of injections was 10.9 in the ranibizumab group and 10.4 in the sham group. A marked difference in the proportion of study eyes requiring repeat PDT was evident by three months (80% of the PDT monotherapy study eyes vs. 16% of the combination study eyes) and was also observed at each subsequent three-month interval. The addition of ranibizumab reduced the frequency of PDT from 3.4 treatments to 1.3. Twenty-four month results of the FOCUS trial revealed similar findings (81). The difference between the ranibizumab combination group and the PDT monotherapy group in mean change from baseline visual acuity was 12.4 letters, in favor of the combination group.

Since the FOCUS trial, there have been a number of completed randomized clinical trials directly comparing combination ranibizumab and PDT to ranibizumab monotherapy for neovascular AMD (DENALI in North America and MONT BLANC in Europe) and also macular polypoidal choroidal vasculopathy (EVEREST in Asia). The MONT BLANC trial used standard-fluence PDT exclusively, whereas the DENALI trial included standard-fluence and reduced-fluence PDT groups. Together, these studies are referred to as the SUMMIT clinical trial program, which was sponsored by Novartis.

MONT BLANC was designed as a 24-month, randomized, double-masked, multicenter trial but was terminated early at 12 months. The 12-month results have not been published in the peer-reviewed literature but are available on the study sponsor's website (88). They enrolled 255 patients. Patients were randomized evenly at baseline to standard-fluence PDT or placebo and subsequently were treated at intervals of at least three months. Intravitreal ranibizumab was administered at baseline, month 1, and month 2 in all patients followed by as-needed dosing. The 12-month results showed a mean VA improvement in the combination group that was noninferior to the ranibizumab monotherapy group (2.5 vs. 4.4 letters). The percentage of patients achieving a three-month treatment-free interval was not statistically significant between the two groups. A treatment-free interval of at least four months was achieved in 85% of patients in the combination arm and 72% in the ranibizumab monotherapy arm. Time to first re-treatment was longer in the combination group (median six months vs. five months). Two-year results from this study would certainly be helpful to determine any true treatment effect with combination therapy. It is unclear why the study sponsor chose not to complete the full 24 months as planned at the onset of the study design, but can only be assumed due to anticipation of negative results.

DENALI was designed as a 24-month, randomized, double-masked, multicenter trial for patients with subfoveal neovascular AMD, but was also terminated early at 12 months due to negative results at 12 months. Results have not been published in the peer-reviewed literature but the 12-month results are available on the study sponsor's website (89). The study enrolled 321 patients into three groups who received either same-day ranibizumab plus standard-fluence PDT, same-day ranibizumab plus reduced-fluence PDT, or ranibizumab monotherapy. In the first two treatment groups, ranibizumab was given at baseline, month 1, month 2, and then as needed. In the third group, ranibizumab was given monthly for the first year. The 12-month results of the DENALI trial were not able to show noninferior visual acuity gains between either PDT combination group [5.3 (reduced-fluence) and

4.4 (standard-fluence) mean letters gained] and ranibizumab monotherapy (8.1 mean letters gained). Patients in the combination groups required an average of 2.2 (standard fluence) or 2.8 (reduced-fluence) additional ranibizumab injections after the mandatory three loading doses, compared with an average of 7.6 additional injections in the ranibizumab monthly monotherapy group.

Bashshur et al. conducted a prospective, comparative investigation of intravitreal ranibizumab in 40 eyes following full-fluence PDT in 13 eyes (83). There was a significantly greater mean visual acuity improvement for the monotherapy group. The time until ranibizumab re-treatment was longer and the number of ranibizumab injections was less in the combination group.

A number of subsequent smaller noncomparative prospective and retrospective investigations have been performed (82,84–87). Mean visual acuity improved or stabilized in 79–84% of eyes while treatments with PDT and ranibizumab over one year ranged from 1.1 to 1.22 and 2.37 to 5.1 respectively in these varying studies. One study suggested that the treatment of neovascular AMD with initial one-time, reduced-fluence PDT in conjunction with an as-needed ranibizumab dosing regimen yielded visual acuity and anatomical results comparable to monthly ranibizumab monotherapy (85), a finding that has not been clearly validated in randomized controlled trials (80,81,88,89).

EVEREST was designed as a six-month randomized, double-masked, multicenter trial for patients with macular polypoidal choroidal vasculopathy (PCV). The six-month results were published on the study sponsor's website in 2009 (90). A total of 61 patients were enrolled into three groups including PDT and ranibizumab combination (n = 19), PDT monotherapy (n = 21), and ranibizumab monotherapy (n = 21). Standard-fluence PDT was used in all PDT arms. Patients were treated as needed, starting at month 3. At six months, complete polyp regression was achieved in 77.8% of eyes in the combination group, 71.4% of eyes in the PDT monotherapy group, and 28.6% of eyes in the ranibizumab monotherapy group. Mean VA improved from baseline in all groups, but the difference was not statistically significant.

In summary, there have been many studies of various design investigating combination PDT and ranibizumab, including randomized, controlled trials. Follow-up is limited. Smaller, noncontrolled trials show an improvement in visual acuity and a decrease in central macular thickness with combination PDT and ranibizumab. They also suggest less frequent re-treatment with ranibizumab may be possible, while maintaining adequate visual acuity outcomes. Visual acuity outcomes have varied between studies. Of note, one study showed a significantly greater mean visual acuity improvement for ranibizumab monotherapy compared with full-fluence PDT combination therapy (83). Larger, randomized, controlled, multicenter trials have been undertaken but their results have not been published in the peer-reviewed literature. The MONT BLANC study showed visual acuity outcomes that were noninferior at 12 months between combination therapy with PDT and ranibizumab compared with ranibizumab monotherapy (88). The DENALI study, in contrast to MONT BLANC, was unable to show noninferiority of both full-fluence and half-fluence PDT combination therapy versus ranibizumab monotherapy at 12 months (89). However, re-treatments with ranibizumab were significantly less frequent in the combination groups. Both of these studies were cut short from 24 months to 12 months and results have not been published in peer-reviewed journals.

Triple Therapy with PDT, Anti-VEGF, and Corticosteroid

Triple therapy with PDT, an anti-VEGF agent (bevacizumab or ranibizumab) and a corticosteroid (triamcinolone or dexamethasone) have been studied in various combinations (Table 22.4) (91–99).

Two randomized, single-masked, multicenter trials were completed in 2009, comparing reduced-fluence PDT, ranibizumab, and dexamethasone triple therapy with ranibizumab monotherapy (RADICAL and PDEX) (100,101). The purpose of the RADICAL (Reduced Fluence Visudyne-Anti-VEGF-Dexamethasone In Combination for AMD Lesions) trial was to determine whether PDT combined with ranibizumab and/or dexamethasone reduces re-treatment rates compared with ranibizumab monotherapy. A total of 162 patients were enrolled into four treatment groups. The preliminary 12-month results showed that statistically significantly fewer re-treatments were required in the combination therapy groups compared with ranibizumab monotherapy (3 vs. 5.4). Mean visual acuity improved in all groups but there were no statistically significant differences found between groups. The second trial, PDT Plus IVD and Intravitreal Ranibizumab Versus Lucentis Monotherapy to Treat Age-Related Macular Degeneration (PDEX), was designed to examine whether PDT combined with ranibizumab and dexamethasone had better visual acuity outcomes compared with ranibizumab monotherapy after one year. They enrolled 60 patients. The results of this study have not been released yet.

Two large retrospective, comparative studies have been conducted (96,97). Hatta et al. studied 92 eyes treated with PDT alone, 90 eyes treated with sub-Tenon's injection of triamcinolone followed by PDT one week later, and 60 eyes treated with intravitreal bevacizumab followed by PDT one week later (97). Full-fluence PDT was used in the PDT groups. The aim of this study was to determine the incidence of transient choroidal hypofluorescence by indocyanine green angiography after PDT alone or after PDT combined with sub-Tenon's triamcinolone or intravitreal bevacizumab. The combined use of sub-Tenon's triamcinolone or intravitreal bevacizumab with PDT significantly prolonged the time of choroidal hypofluorescence on ICGA compared with the PDT monotherapy group. Fewer PDT re-treatments were required in the combination groups. The prolongation of choroidal hypofluorescence in the combination groups may have contributed to the reduction in the number of re-treatments. No adverse events were reported. Forte et al. investigated the effect of intravitreal ranibizumab or bevacizumab in monotherapy (n = 40) or in combination with PDT followed by 400 μg intravitreal dexamethasone

within 16 hours (n = 61) (96). All eyes were treatment naïve. There were fewer treatments required (1.92 vs. 3.12) and a longer treatment-free interval (3.6 vs. 5.4 months) after initial treatment in the triple therapy group compared with monotherapy. A significant improvement in visual acuity and foveal thickness was achieved in both groups. No adverse events were reported.

Augustin et al. conducted a large prospective, noncomparative investigation of reduced-fluence PDT (42 J/cm^2) followed within a mean of 16 hours by retrobulbar anesthesia and 800 μg dexamethasone and 1.5 mg bevacizumab administered via a 25-gauge vitrector incision in an operating room setting in 104 eyes (92). There was a mean increase in visual acuity of 1.8 lines and a mean decrease in retinal thickness of 182 μm over a mean follow-up of 10 months. Seventeen percent of eyes received an additional injection of bevacizumab (mean of 15 weeks after triple therapy). An additional cycle of PDT was required in five eyes due to recurrent angiographic CNV activity. There were no adverse events reported. Based on their results, they felt that a similar benefit may be gained from one triple therapy cycle compared with up to three anti-VEGF monotherapy courses, with sustained benefit from the triple therapy. They felt that delaying 16 hours before administering dexamethasone reduces the risk of an overactivated PDT-mediated inflammatory cascade. Their treatment procedure was invasive and would need to be adapted to an office-based procedure to offer utility to most patients.

There have been a number of smaller noncomparative prospective and retrospective series investigating various triple therapy regimens (91,93–95,98,99). These studies used both triamcinolone and dexamethasone as the steroid. They showed variable visual acuity outcomes with a general trend of a reduction in re-treatment over one year. Adverse events intraocular pressure rise and cataract formation in a minority of patients.

In summary, triple therapy with PDT, an anti-VEGF agent, and intravitreal corticosteroid for neovascular AMD can be administered in a variety of different dosing and timing schemes. An approach utilizing PDT at baseline followed by delayed anti-VEGF and corticosteroid has been advocated to maximize the therapeutic effect of PDT while also subduing the associated inflammatory and pro-VEGF reaction that follows in the immediate period after PDT (91,92,96). From a theoretical standpoint, this approach addresses the damaging components of the angiogenic and inflammatory processes in neovascular AMD. Administration of all three agents in a single, office-based session offers the most practical approach. Such a single-session approach has been shown to be feasible and safe (93,94). Other variations have also been studied, including initial anti-VEGF at baseline followed by later treatment of corticosteroid and PDT (98), quadruple therapy with minocycline (99), and initial PDT and corticosteroid followed by later anti-VEGF (95). Another proposed triple therapy regimen that is commonly used in practice, which has not been studied, combines initial PDT with an anti-VEGF agent at baseline. Intravitreal corticosteroid can then be administered at a later interval depending on the presence of persistent or increased

Table 22.4 Triple Therapy with PDT, Intravitreal Anti-VEGF, and Intravitreal or Sub-Tenon's Steroid for Neovascular Age-Related Macular Degeneration

Reference (year of publication)	No. of eyes and follow-up duration	Study design	CNV type	Treatment protocol	Outcome measures and findings
Randomized controlled trials					
RADICAL unpublished (100) 2009	n = 162 and 24 mos	Prospective, random-ized, single-masked, multicenter	Subfoveal CNV	Reduced-fluence PDT, ranibizumab, and dexamethasone triple therapy compared with ranibizumab monotherapy	12 mo results: statistically significantly fewer re-treatments were required in the combination therapy groups compared with ranibizumab monotherapy (3 vs.5.4). Mean visual acuity improved in all groups and there were no statistically significant differences found between groups.
PDEX unpublished (101) 2009	n = 60 12 mos	Prospective, random-ized, single-masked, multicenter	Not specified	reduced fluence PDT, ranibizumab, and dexamethasone triple therapy compared to ranibizumab monotherapy	Results not released
Retrospective, comparative					
Forte et al. (96) (2010)	n = 101 mean = 14.1 to 16.3	Retrospective, comparative	Subfoveal CNV, all subtypes	intravitreal anti-VEGF (ranibizumab or bevacizumab) in monotherapy (40 eyes) or in combination with 400 μg intravitreal dexamethasone within 16 hrs following full fluence PDT (61 eyes)	All eyes were treatment naïve. There were fewer treat-ments required (1.92 vs.3.12) and a longer treatment-free interval (5.4 vs.3.6 mos) after initial treatment in the triple therapy group. A significant improvement in visual acuity and foveal thickeness was present in both groups. No adverse events were noted.
Hatta et al. (97) (2010)	n = 242 3 mos	Retrospective, comparative	Subfoveal CNV, caused by either AMD or PCV	Ninety-two eyes underwent PDT alone, 90 eyes underwent PDT with sub-Tenon's injection of triamcinolone one week prior, and 60 eyes underwent PDT with intravitreal bevacizumab one week prior. Full fluence PDT was used.	The combined use of sub-Tenon's triamcinolone or intravitreal bevacizumab with PDT significantly prolonged the time of choroidal hypofluorescence on ICGA compared with the PDT monotherapy group. Less PDT re-treatments were required in the combination groups. The prolongation of choroidal hypofluorescence in the combination groups may have contributed to the reduction of re-treatments. No adverse events were reported
Prospective, non-comparative					
Augustin et al. (92) (2007)	n = 104 mean = 10 mos	Prospective, non-comparative	Subfoveal CNV, all subtypes	Reduced fluence PDT (42 J/cm2) followed within a mean of 16 hours by retrobulbar anesthesia and 800 μg dexamethasone and 1.5 mg bevacizumab administered via a 25-gauge vitrector incision.	There was a mean increase in visual acuity of 1.8 lines and a mean decrease in retinal thickness of 182 μm. Seventeen percent of eyes received an additional injection of bevacizumab (mean of 15 wks after triple therapy). There were no adverse events.
Smaller retrospective and prospective, noncomparative					
Kovacs et al. (98) (2011)	n = 31 3–12 mos	Retrospective, noncomparative	Not specified	Intravitreal bevacizumab was given, immediately followed by 40 mg sub-Tenon's triamcinolone. Half-fluence PDT was then administered at a later time in all eyes.	Visual acuity improved from baseline (not statistically significant) and retinal thickness decreased. Re-treatments were required in 61% of eyes (11 of 18) that reached 1 year of follow-up. No significant differences in treatment naïve vs.previously treated eyes were found. An increase in intraocular pressure occurred in 9.7% of eyes.

(Continued)

Table 22.4 Triple Therapy with PDT, Intravitreal Anti-VEGF, and Intravitreal or Sub-Tenon's Steroid for Neovascular Age-Related Macular Degeneration (*Continued*)

Reference (year of publication)	No. of eyes and follow-up duration	Study design	CNV type	Treatment protocol	Outcome measures and findings
Sivaprasad et al. (99) (2011)	n = 18, 12 mos	Prospective, noncomparative	Subfoveal CNV, all subtypes	Quadruple therapy: Half-fluence PDT followed by intravitreal ranbizumab (0.3 mg) and 200 µg dexamethasone in one injection at baseline in all eyes. Oral minocycline 100 mg was begun the following day and continued for 3 mos.	There was a mean decrease in visual acuity of 5 letters. The mean reduction of central retinal thickenss was 66 µm. The mean total number of ranibizumab injections was 3.4. The mean time from baseline to re-treatment was 2.6 mos. No eyes experienced a raise in intraocular pressure or cataract progression.
Ehmann et al. (95) (2010)	n = 32, 12 mos	Retrospective, noncomparative	Subfoveal and juxtafoveal CNV	Half fluence PDT followed immediately by 800 µg of intravitreal dexamethasone in all eyes. Intravitreal bevacizumab was injected at 1 and 7 wks after initial treatment in all eyes.	Mean visual acuity improved and mean foveal thickness decreased. Ninety-four percent of eyes lost fewer than 3 lines. The mean number of treatment cycles was 1.4 and the mean number of bevacizumab injections was 2.8. No rise in intraocular pressure or other adverse events was noted.
Yip et al. (94) (2009)	n = 36 mean = 14.7 mos	Prospective, noncomparative	Subfoveal CNV, all subtypes, 58% treatment-naïve	Single session triple therapy: full fluence PDT followed within 1 hr by intravitreal bevacizumab and 4 mg intravitreal triamcinolone.	At 6 mos, 67% of eyes showed an improvement or stabilization of visual acuity. Complete resolution of angiographic evidence of CNV occurred after a single session of triple therapy in 78% of eyes. Increased intraocular pressure occurred in 6% of eyes and cataract requiring surgery occurred in 8% of eyes.
Bakri et al. (93) (2009)	n = 31, mean = 13.7 mos	Retrospective, noncomparative	Subfoveal CNV, all subtypes	Single session triple therapy: half fluence PDT followed by intravitreal bevacizumab and 200 µg dexamethasone.	Same-day triple therapy maintained visual acuity and decreased macular thickness in patients with and without previous anti-VEGF therapy. Visual acuity outcomes confounded by variable followup.
Ahmadieh et al. (91) (2007)	n = 17 mean = 12.6 mos	Prospective, noncomparative	Subfoveal CNV, all subtypes	Full-fluence PDT followed by intravitreal bevacizumab and 2 mg intravitreal triamcinolone 48 hours later in all eyes.	Mean visual acuity improved and mean central macular thickness decreased at 6 mos. The mean interval between initial triple therapy and subsequent re-treatment with bevacizumab was 5 mos (required in 59% of eyes). No adverse events were reported. Bevacizumab and triamcinolone were injected 48 hrs after PDT to reduce the risk of light toxicity and to counteract the adverse effects of PDT-induced release of VEGF per the authors.

Abbreviations: CNV, choroidal neovascular membrane; ICGA, indocyanine green angiography; mo/s, month/s; PDT, photodynamic therapy.

subretinal fluid. This method may alleviate the risks of intraocular steroid therapy in patients who respond well to double combination therapy. The various published studies suggest that combination triple therapy can allow for less re-treatment and a longer treatment-free interval, while maintaining visual acuity outcomes in patients with neovascular AMD. The RADICAL study, which is the only prospective, randomized, multicenter study with reported results, supports the findings of smaller studies. This study showed a reduction in re-treatment and equal visual acuity outcomes with combination therapy compared with ranibizumab monotherapy at one year, but two-year results were not reported.

SUBGROUP OF SUBOPTIMAL RESPONDERS

In addition to aspiring for improved efficacy and a longer treatment-free interval with combination therapy for neovascular AMD, there is a subgroup of patients who could achieve better results. Despite excellent anatomical results in the majority of neovascular AMD patients who are treated with anti-VEGF therapy, there remains a significant proportion of patients who retain residual fluid despite aggressive therapy. This subgroup of patients are referred to as suboptimal responders and make up an ill-defined cohort of neovascular AMD patients that are not well studied. When imaged with indocyanine green angiography, suboptimal responders disproportionately show evidence of retinal angiomatous proliferation and polypoidal choroidal vasculopathy compared with neovascular AMD patients who respond well to anti-VEGF monotherapy. These suboptimal responders warrant further study, as evidence suggests better PCV lesion regression using combination therapy with anti-VEGF and PDT compared with anti-VEGF monotherapy (90). Triple combination therapy with the addition of corticosteroid may offer additional benefits and has not been adequately studied to date.

SUMMARY

Treatment for neovascular AMD has evolved rapidly and will likely continue to do so in the foreseeable future. Current standard of care for neovascular AMD with anti-VEGF monotherapy provides visual acuity efficacy not possible prior to FDA approval of ranibizumab in 2006. But, with anti-VEGF monotherapy comes a requirement for frequent re-treatment with no defined endpoint. Additionally, anti-VEGF therapy targets only one facet of a complex multifactorial pathophysiology, which results in vision loss from CNV formation and scarring. The evidence shows ranibizumab monotherapy has greater efficacy than combination therapy with PDT for neovascular AMD. Some evidence from randomized controlled trials suggest that the double combination (intravitreal anti-VEGF agent combined with intravitreal triamcinolone) therapy is inferior to ranibizumab monotherapy (89) and the triple combination (PDT, intravitreal anti-VEGF, and intravitreal dexamethasone) therapy may offer equivalent efficacy to ranibizumab monotherapy while reducing the re-treatment rate (100). Additionally, a randomized controlled trial has shown promise for combination therapy in the treatment of macular PCV (90), which may make up a

portion of suboptimal AMD responders. Though current combination therapy strategies do not offer an improvement in efficacy over monotherapy with anti-VEGF for neovascular AMD, future combination strategies may still be able to achieve this end point. In current practice, anti-VEGF monotherapy remains first line for neovascular AMD but combination therapy should be considered for patients who do not respond to standard anti-VEGF monotherapy.

SUMMARY POINTS

- Neovascular AMD has a complex disease pathophysiology with multiple potential targets for pharmacotherapy, including mediators of vasculogenesis, angiogenesis, and inflammation.
- Monotherapy with anti-VEGF agents offer tremendous efficacy in many patients with neovascular AMD but targets only the vasculogenic component, leaving a small proportion of patients who respond suboptimally.
- A combination strategy targeting different steps within the pathologic cascade in AMD, which results in CNV formation and progression, theoretically may offer improved efficacy over monotherapy with anti-VEGF, but this has not been proven in any randomized controlled trials to date.
- Combination therapy in neovascular AMD most commonly includes treatment with a PDT, an anti-VEGF agent, and/or a corticosteroid.

REFERENCES

1. Congdon N, O'Colmain B, Klaver CC, et al. Causes and prevalence of visual impairment among adults in the United States. Arch Ophthalmol 2004; 122: 477–85.
2. Pascolini D, Mariotti SP, Pokharel GP, et al. 2002 global update of available data on visual impairment: a compilation of population-based prevalence studies. Ophthalmic Epidemiol 2004; 11: 67–115.
3. Jager RD, Mieler WF, Miller JW. Age-related macular degeneration. N Engl J Med 2008; 358: 2606–17.
4. Friedman DS, O'Colmain BJ, Munoz B, et al. Prevalence of age-related macular degeneration in the United States. Arch Ophthalmol 2004; 122: 564–72.
5. Bressler NM, Doan QV, Varma R, et al. Estimated cases of legal blindness and visual impairment avoided using ranibizumab for choroidal neovascularization: non-Hispanic white population in the United States with age-related macular degeneration. Arch Ophthalmol 2011; 129: 709–17.
6. Argon laser photocoagulation for senile macular degeneration. Results of a randomized clinical trial. Arch Ophthalmol 1982; 100: 912–18.
7. Macular Photocoagulation Study Group. Argon laser photocoagulation for neovascular maculopathy. Five-year results from randomized clinical trials. Arch Ophthalmol 1991; 109: 1109–14.
8. Bressler NM. Photodynamic therapy of subfoveal choroidal neovascularization in age-related macular degeneration with verteporfin: two-year results of 2

randomized clinical trials-tap report 2. Arch Ophthalmol 2001; 119: 198–207.

9. Verteporfin In Photodynamic Therapy Study Group. Verteporfin therapy of subfoveal choroidal neovascularization in age-related macular degeneration: two-year results of a randomized clinical trial including lesions with occult with no classic choroidal neovascularization–verteporfin in photodynamic therapy report 2. Am J Ophthalmol 2001; 131: 541–60.

10. Azab M, Boyer DS, Bressler NM, et al. Verteporfin therapy of subfoveal minimally classic choroidal neovascularization in age-related macular degeneration: 2-year results of a randomized clinical trial. Arch Ophthalmol 2005; 123: 448–57.

11. Cruess AF, Zlateva G, Pleil AM, Wirostko B. Photodynamic therapy with verteporfin in age-related macular degeneration: a systematic review of efficacy, safety, treatment modifications and pharmacoeconomic properties. Acta Ophthalmol 2009; 87: 118–32.

12. Gragoudas ES, Adamis AP, Cunningham ET Jr, Feinsod M, Guyer DR. Pegaptanib for neovascular age-related macular degeneration. N Engl J Med 2004; 351: 2805–16.

13. Chakravarthy U, Adamis AP, Cunningham ET Jr, et al. Year 2 efficacy results of 2 randomized controlled clinical trials of pegaptanib for neovascular age-related macular degeneration. Ophthalmology 2006; 113: 1508 e1–25.

14. Rosenfeld PJ, Brown DM, Heier JS, et al. Ranibizumab for neovascular age-related macular degeneration. N Engl J Med 2006; 355: 1419–31.

15. Brown DM, Michels M, Kaiser PK, et al. Ranibizumab versus verteporfin photodynamic therapy for neovascular age-related macular degeneration: Two-year results of the ANCHOR study. Ophthalmology 2009; 116: 57–65 e5.

16. Martin DF, Maguire MG, Ying GS, et al. Ranibizumab and bevacizumab for neovascular age-related macular degeneration. N Engl J Med 2011; 364: 1897–908.

17. Zarbin MA. Current concepts in the pathogenesis of age-related macular degeneration. Arch Ophthalmol 2004; 122: 598–614.

18. Schlingemann RO. Role of growth factors and the wound healing response in age-related macular degeneration. Graefes Arch Clin Exp Ophthalmol 2004; 242: 91–101.

19. Kannan R, Zhang N, Sreekumar PG, et al. Stimulation of apical and basolateral VEGF-A and VEGF-C secretion by oxidative stress in polarized retinal pigment epithelial cells. Mol Vis 2006; 12: 1649–59.

20. Ambati J, Ambati BK, Yoo SH, Ianchulev S, Adamis AP. Age-related macular degeneration: etiology, pathogenesis, and therapeutic strategies. Surv Ophthalmol 2003; 48: 257–93.

21. Grossniklaus HE, Martinez JA, Brown VB, et al. Immunohistochemical and histochemical properties of surgically excised subretinal neovascular membranes in age-related macular degeneration. Am J Ophthalmol 1992; 114: 464–72.

22. Spaide RF. Rationale for combination therapies for choroidal neovascularization. Am J Ophthalmol 2006; 141: 149–56.

23. Spaide RF. Rationale for combination therapy in age-related macular degeneration. Retina 2009; 29(6 Suppl): S5–7.

24. Campochiaro PA. Ocular neovascularisation and excessive vascular permeability. Expert Opin Biol Ther 2004; 4: 1395–402.

25. Patel S. Combination therapy for age-related macular degeneration. Retina 2009; 29(6 Suppl): S45–8.

26. Bradley J, Ju M, Robinson GS. Combination therapy for the treatment of ocular neovascularization. Angiogenesis 2007; 10: 141–8.

27. Schmidt-Erfurth U, Hasan T, Gragoudas E, et al. Vascular targeting in photodynamic occlusion of subretinal vessels. Ophthalmology 1994; 101: 1953–61.

28. Schmidt-Erfurth U, Laqua H, Schlotzer-Schrehard U, Viestenz A, Naumann GO. Histopathological changes following photodynamic therapy in human eyes. Arch Ophthalmol 2002; 120: 835–44.

29. Visudyne package insert. East Hanover, NJ: Novartis Pharmaceuticals, 2007.

30. Kaiser PK. Verteporfin therapy of subfoveal choroidal neovascularization in age-related macular degeneration: 5-year results of two randomized clinical trials with an open-label extension: TAP report no. 8. Graefes Arch Clin Exp Ophthalmol 2006; 244: 1132–42.

31. Schmidt-Erfurth U, Schlotzer-Schrehard U, Cursiefen C, et al. Influence of photodynamic therapy on expression of vascular endothelial growth factor (VEGF), VEGF receptor 3, and pigment epithelium-derived factor. Invest Ophthalmol Vis Sci 2003; 44: 4473–80.

32. Klais CM, Ober MD, Freund KB, et al. Choroidal infarction following photodynamic therapy with verteporfin. Arch Ophthalmol 2005; 123: 1149–53.

33. Michels S, Hansmann F, Geitzenauer W, Schmidt-Erfurth U. Influence of treatment parameters on selectivity of verteporfin therapy. Invest Ophthalmol Vis Sci 2006; 47: 371–6.

34. Adamis AP, Shima DT. The role of vascular endothelial growth factor in ocular health and disease. Retina 2005; 25: 111–18.

35. Ferrara N. Vascular endothelial growth factor: basic science and clinical progress. Endocr Rev 2004; 25: 581–611.

36. Kvanta A, Algvere PV, Berglin L, Seregard S. Subfoveal fibrovascular membranes in age-related macular degeneration express vascular endothelial growth factor. Invest Ophthalmol Vis Sci 1996; 37: 1929–34.

37. Kliffen M, Sharma HS, Mooy CM, Kerkvliet S, de Jong PT. Increased expression of angiogenic growth factors in age-related maculopathy. Br J Ophthalmol 1997; 81: 154–62.

38. Wells JA, Murthy R, Chibber R, et al. Levels of vascular endothelial growth factor are elevated in the vitreous of patients with subretinal neovascularisation. Br J Ophthalmol 1996; 80: 363–6.

39. Funk M, Karl D, Georgopoulos M, et al. Neovascular age-related macular degeneration: intraocular cytokines and growth factors and the influence of therapy with ranibizumab. Ophthalmology 2009; 116: 2393–9.

40. Aiello LP, Northrup JM, Keyt BA, Takagi H, Iwamoto MA. Hypoxic regulation of vascular endothelial growth factor in retinal cells. Arch Ophthalmol 1995; 113: 1538–44.

41. Gaudry M, Bregerie O, Andrieu V, et al. Intracellular pool of vascular endothelial growth factor in human neutrophils. Blood 1997; 90: 4153–61.

42. Regeneron Announces FDA Approval of EYLEA™ (aflibercept) Injection for the Treatment of Wet Age-Related Macular Degeneration. [Available from: http://www.multivu.com/mnr/51268-eylea-aflibercept-wet-age-related-macular-degeneration-AMD-FDA-approval/] (January 22, 2012).

43. Johnson LV, Leitner WP, Staples MK, Anderson DH. Complement activation and inflammatory processes in Drusen formation and age related macular degeneration. Exp Eye Res 2001; 73: 887–96.

44. Seregard S, Algvere PV, Berglin L. Immunohistochemical characterization of surgically removed subfoveal fibrovascular membranes. Graefes Arch Clin Exp Ophthalmol 1994; 232: 325–9.

45. Nauck M, Karakiulakis G, Perruchoud AP, Papakonstantinou E, Roth M. Corticosteroids inhibit the expression of the vascular endothelial growth factor gene in human vascular smooth muscle cells. Eur J Pharmacol 1998; 341: 309–15.

46. Ishibashi T, Miki K, Sorgente N, Patterson R, Ryan SJ. Effects of intravitreal administration of steroids on experimental subretinal neovascularization in the subhuman primate. Arch Ophthalmol 1985; 103: 708–11.

47. Folkman J, Ingber DE. Angiostatic steroids. Method of discovery and mechanism of action. Ann Surg 1987; 206: 374–83.

48. Kaiser PK. Steroids for choroidal neovascularization. Am J Ophthalmol 2005; 139: 533–5.

49. Gillies MC, Simpson JM, Luo W, et al. A randomized clinical trial of a single dose of intravitreal triamcinolone acetonide for neovascular age-related macular degeneration: one-year results. Arch Ophthalmol 2003; 121: 667–73.

50. Beer PM, Bakri SJ, Singh RJ, et al. Intraocular concentration and pharmacokinetics of triamcinolone acetonide after a single intravitreal injection. Ophthalmology 2003; 110: 681–6.

51. Kwak HW, D'Amico DJ. Evaluation of the retinal toxicity and pharmacokinetics of dexamethasone after intravitreal injection. Arch Ophthalmol 1992; 110: 259–66.

52. Rechtman E, Danis RP, Pratt LM, Harris A. Intravitreal triamcinolone with photodynamic therapy for subfoveal choroidal neovascularisation in age related macular degeneration. Br J Ophthalmol 2004; 88: 344–7.

53. Spaide RF, Sorenson J, Maranan L. Combined photodynamic therapy and intravitreal triamcinolone for nonsubfoveal choroidal neovascularization. Retina 2005; 25: 685–90.

54. Spaide RF, Sorenson J, Maranan L. Photodynamic therapy with verteporfin combined with intravitreal injection of triamcinolone acetonide for choroidal neovascularization. Ophthalmology 2005; 112: 301–4.

55. Arias L, Garcia-Arumi J, Ramon JM, et al. Photodynamic therapy with intravitreal triamcinolone in predominantly classic choroidal neovascularization: one-year results of a randomized study. Ophthalmology 2006; 113: 2243–50.

56. Augustin AJ, Schmidt-Erfurth U. Verteporfin therapy combined with intravitreal triamcinolone in all types of choroidal neovascularization due to age-related macular degeneration. Ophthalmology 2006; 113: 14–22.

57. Augustin AJ, Schmidt-Erfurth U. Verteporfin and intravitreal triamcinolone acetonide combination therapy for occult choroidal neovascularization in age-related macular degeneration. Am J Ophthalmol 2006; 141: 638–45.

58. Chan WM, Lai TY, Wong AL, et al. Combined photodynamic therapy and intravitreal triamcinolone injection for the treatment of subfoveal choroidal neovascularisation in age related macular degeneration: a comparative study. Br J Ophthalmol 2006; 90: 337–41.

59. Ergun E, Maar N, Ansari-Shahrezaei S, et al. Photodynamic therapy with verteporfin and intravitreal triamcinolone acetonide in the treatment of neovascular age-related macular degeneration. Am J Ophthalmol 2006; 142: 10–16.

60. Nicolo M, Ghiglione D, Lai S, et al. Occult with no classic choroidal neovascularization secondary to age-related macular degeneration treated by intravitreal triamcinolone and photodynamic therapy with verteporfin. Retina 2006; 26: 58–64.

61. Chaudhary V, Mao A, Hooper PL, Sheidow TG. Triamcinolone acetonide as adjunctive treatment to verteporfin in neovascular age-related macular degeneration: a prospective randomized trial. Ophthalmology 2007; 114: 2183–9.

62. Piermarocchi S, Sartore M, Lo Giudice G, et al. Combination of photodynamic therapy and intraocular triamcinolone for exudative age-related macular degeneration and long-term chorioretinal macular atrophy. Arch Ophthalmol 2008; 126: 1367–74.

63. Singh CN, Saperstein DA. Combination treatment with reduced-fluence photodynamic therapy and intravitreal injection of triamcinolone for subfoveal choroidal neovascularization in macular degeneration. Retina 2008; 28: 789–93.

64. Maberley D. Photodynamic therapy and intravitreal triamcinolone for neovascular age-related macular degeneration: a randomized clinical trial. Ophthalmology 2009; 116: 2149–57, e1.

65. Lie S, Aue A, Sacu S, et al. Time-course and characteristic morphology of retinal changes following combination of verteporfin therapy and intravitreal triamcinolone in neovascular age-related macular degeneration. Acta Ophthalmol 2008; 88: 212–17.

66. Van de Moere A, Sandhu SS, Kak R, Mitchell KW, Talks SJ. Effect of posterior juxtascleral triamcinolone acetonide on choroidal neovascular growth after photodynamic therapy with verteporfin. Ophthalmology 2005; 112: 1896–903.

67. Dhalla MS, Shah GK, Blinder KJ, et al. Combined photodynamic therapy with verteporfin and intravitreal bevacizumab for choroidal neovascularization in age-related macular degeneration. Retina 2006; 26: 988–93.

68. Costa RA, Jorge R, Calucci D, et al. Intravitreal bevacizumab (Avastin) in combination with verteporfin photodynamic therapy for choroidal neovascularization associated with age-related macular degeneration (IBeVe Study). Graefes Arch Clin Exp Ophthalmol 2007; 245: 1273–80.

69. Lazic R, Gabric N. Verteporfin therapy and intravitreal bevacizumab combined and alone in choroidal neovascularization due to age-related macular degeneration. Ophthalmology 2007; 114: 1179–85.

70. Ladewig MS, Karl SE, Hamelmann V, et al. Combined intravitreal bevacizumab and photodynamic therapy for neovascular age-related macular degeneration. Graefes Arch Clin Exp Ophthalmol 2008; 246: 17–25.

71. Smith BT, Dhalla MS, Shah GK, et al. Intravitreal injection of bevacizumab combined with verteporfin photodynamic therapy for choroidal neovascularization in age-related macular degeneration. Retina 2008; 28: 675–81.

72. Weigert G, Michels S, Sacu S, et al. Intravitreal bevacizumab (Avastin) therapy versus photodynamic therapy plus intravitreal triamcinolone for neovascular age-related macular degeneration: 6-month results of a prospective, randomised, controlled clinical study. Br J Ophthalmol 2008; 92: 356–60.

73. Kaiser PK, Boyer DS, Garcia R, et al. Verteporfin photodynamic therapy combined with intravitreal bevacizumab for neovascular age-related macular degeneration. Ophthalmology 2009; 116: 747–55; 55 e1.

74. Liu Y, Wen F, Li J, Zuo C, Li M. Transitions of multifocal electroretinography in patients with age-related macular degeneration after combination therapy with

photodynamic therapy and intravitreal bevacizumab. Doc Ophthalmol 2009; 119: 163–9.

75. Navea A, Mataix J, Desco MC, Garcia-Pous M, Palacios E. One-year follow-up of combined customized therapy. Photodynamic therapy and bevacizumab for exudative age-related macular degeneration. Retina 2009; 29: 13–19.

76. Costagliola C, Romano MR, Rinaldi M, et al. Low fluence rate photodynamic therapy combined with intravitreal bevacizumab for neovascular age-related macular degeneration. Br J Ophthalmol 2009; 94: 180–4.

77. Rudnisky CJ, Liu C, Ng M, Weis E, Tennant MT. Intravitreal bevacizumab alone versus combined verteporfin photodynamic therapy and intravitreal bevacizumab for choroidal neovascularization in age-related macular degeneration: visual acuity after 1 year of follow-up. Retina 2010; 30: 548–54.

78. Wan MJ, Hooper PL, Sheidow TG. Combination therapy in exudative age-related macular degeneration: visual outcomes following combined treatment with photodynamic therapy and intravitreal bevacizumab. Can J Ophthalmol 2010; 45: 375–80.

79. Potter MJ, Claudio CC, Szabo SM. A randomised trial of bevacizumab and reduced light dose photodynamic therapy in age-related macular degeneration: the VIA study. Br J Ophthalmol 2009; 94: 174–9.

80. Heier JS, Boyer DS, Ciulla TA, et al. Ranibizumab combined with verteporfin photodynamic therapy in neovascular age-related macular degeneration: year 1 results of the FOCUS Study. Arch Ophthalmol 2006; 124: 1532–42.

81. Antoszyk AN, Tuomi L, Chung CY, Singh A. Ranibizumab combined with verteporfin photodynamic therapy in neovascular age-related macular degeneration (FOCUS): year 2 results. Am J Ophthalmol 2008; 145: 862–74.

82. Kumar A, Gopalakrishnan K, Sinha S. Combination photodynamic therapy and intravitreal ranibizumab in neovascular age-related macular degeneration in a North Indian population: a pilot study. Retina 2008; 28: 1296–301.

83. Bashshur ZF, Schakal AR, El-Mollayess GM, et al. Ranibizumab monotherapy versus single-session verteporfin photodynamic therapy combined with as-needed ranibizumab treatment for the management of neovascular age-related macular degeneration. Retina 2010; 31: 636–44.

84. Mataix J, Palacios E, Carmen DM, Garcia-Pous M, Navea A. Combined ranibizumab and photodynamic therapy to treat exudative age-related macular degeneration: an option for improving treatment efficiency. Retina 2010; 30: 1190–6.

85. Spielberg L, Leys A. Treatment of neovascular age-related macular degeneration with a variable ranibizumab dosing regimen and one-time reduced-fluence photodynamic therapy: the TORPEDO trial at 2 years. Graefes Arch Clin Exp Ophthalmol 2010; 248: 943–56.

86. Wolf-Schnurrbusch UE, Brinkmann CK, Berger L, Wolf S. Effects of combination therapy with verteporfin photodynamic therapy and ranibizumab in patients with age-related macular degeneration. Acta Ophthalmol 2009; 89: 585–90.

87. Nakamura T, Miyakoshi A, Fujita K, et al. One-year results of photodynamic therapy combined with intravitreal ranibizumab for exudative age-related macular degeneration. J Ophthalmol 2012; 2012: 154659.

88. QLT announces 12-month results from Novartis sponsored MONT BLANC study evaluating standard-fluence Visudyne® combination therapy. 2009. [Available from: http://www.qltinc.com/newsCenter/2009/090615.htm] (January 26, 2012).

89. 12-month results from DENALI study evaluation verteporfin PDT (Visudyne®) combination therapy. 2010. [Available from: http://www.qltinc.com/newsCenter/2010/100615.htm] (January 29, 2012).

90. Koh A, Lee WK, Chen LJ, et al. EVEREST STUDY: Efficacy and safety of verteporfin photodynamic therapy in combination with ranibizumab or alone versus ranibizumab monotherapy in patients with. symptomatic macular polypoidal choroidal vasculopathy. Retina 2012. [Epub ahead of print].

91. Ahmadieh H, Taei R, Soheilian M, et al. Single-session photodynamic therapy combined with intravitreal bevacizumab and triamcinolone for neovascular age-related macular degeneration. BMC Ophthalmol 2007; 7: 10.

92. Augustin AJ, Puls S, Offermann I. Triple therapy for choroidal neovascularization due to age-related macular degeneration: verteporfin PDT, bevacizumab, and dexamethasone. Retina 2007; 27: 133–40.

93. Bakri SJ, Couch SM, McCannel CA, Edwards AO. Same-day triple therapy with photodynamic therapy, intravitreal dexamethasone, and bevacizumab in wet age-related macular degeneration. Retina 2009; 29: 573–8.

94. Yip PP, Woo CF, Tang HH, Ho CK. Triple therapy for neovascular age-related macular degeneration using single-session photodynamic therapy combined with intravitreal bevacizumab and triamcinolone. Br Ophthalmol 2009; 93: 754–8.

95. Ehmann D, Garcia R. Triple therapy for neovascular age-related macular degeneration (verteporfin photodynamic therapy, intravitreal dexamethasone, and intravitreal bevacizumab). Can J Ophthalmol 2010; 45: 36–40.

96. Forte R, Bonavolonta P, Benayoun Y, Adenis JP, Robert PY. Intravitreal ranibizumab and bevacizumab in combination with full-fluence verteporfin therapy and dexamethasone for exudative age-related macular degeneration. Ophthalmic Res 2010; 45: 129–34.

97. Hatta Y, Ishikawa K, Nishihara H, et al. Effect of photodynamic therapy alone or combined with posterior sub-tenon triamcinolone acetonide or intravitreal bevacizumab on choroidal hypofluorescence by indocyanine green angiography. Retina 2009; 30: 495–502.

98. Kovacs KD, Quirk MT, Kinoshita T, et al. A retrospective analysis of triple combination therapy with intravitreal bevacizumab, posterior sub-Tenon's triamcinolone acetonide, and low-fluence verteporfin photodynamic therapy in patients with neovascular age-related macular degeneration. Retina 2011; 31: 446–52.

99. Sivaprasad S, Patra S, DaCosta J, et al. A pilot study on the combination treatment of reduced-fluence photodynamic therapy, intravitreal ranibizumab, intravitreal dexamethasone and oral minocycline for neovascular age-related macular degeneration. Ophthalmologica 2011; 225: 200–6.

100. QLT announces positive results from the evaluation of Visudyne® combination therapy. 2009. [Available from: http://www.qltinc.com/newsCenter/2009/090602.htm] (January 29, 2012).

101. Triple Therapy - PDT Plus IVD and Intravitreal Ranibizumab Versus Lucentis Monotherapy to Treat Age-Related Macular Degeneration (PDEX). 2009. [Available from: http://www.clinicaltrials.gov/ct2/show/NCT00390208?term=NCT00390208&rank=1] (January 29, 2012).

23

Photodynamic therapy for neovascular age-related macular degeneration

Kelly M. Bui and Yannek I. Leiderman

Photodynamic therapy (PDT) entails the administration of a photosensitizer with its subsequent accumulation in the target tissue and then activation by monochromatic light corresponding to the sensitizer's absorption profile (1). Cytotoxic singlet oxygen and free radicals are produced causing irreversible cellular damage. PDT has traditionally been used in the treatment of cancer (2), but the potential for selective destruction of diseased vessels, while sparing normal overlying tissues, coupled with promising clinical efficacy, resulted in its use for the treatment of age-related macular degeneration (AMD), particularly subfoveal choroidal neovascularization (CNV). PDT's relative selectivity for CNV is achieved both through photosensitizer retention in choroidal neovascular membranes and through targeted light application. This chapter will provide an overview of the photochemistry of PDT and the clinical trials that have established its clinical effectiveness in the treatment of neovascular AMD.

VASCULAR TARGETING

PDT causes direct cellular injury in addition to microvascular damage and nonperfusion within illuminated tissue. Uptake is due to the increased expression of low-density lipoprotein receptors on tumor cells and neovascular endothelium. Porphyrin photosensitization in mammals was studied beginning in 1910 when Hausmann investigated the effects of hematoporphyrin and light in mice (3). The results established the phototoxic capability of porphyrins, and Hausmann concluded that peripheral vasculature was targeted by PDT. In 1963, Castellani and colleagues demonstrated microvasculature to be a crucial target (4). Vascular occlusion following PDT is marked by the release of vasoactive molecules, vasoconstriction, blood cell aggregation, endothelial cell damage, blood flow stasis, and hemorrhage. The response is dependent on the sensitizer type, concentration, and the time interval between administration and treatment. Benzoporphyrin derivative monoacid ring A (BPD-MA)-induced PDT resulted in selective destruction of tumor microvasculature in a chondrosarcoma rodent model when compared with the surrounding normal microvasculature (5).

LIGHT APPLICATION

The light used for ophthalmic application is monochromatic laser light matched to the sensitizer's infrared absorbance profile. Infrared light confers greater transmission through both blood and tissue than light at shorter wavelengths thereby enabling the treatment of pigmented or hemorrhagic lesions. The energy at which light is delivered is a product of the radiant power [expressed in milliwatts per square centimeter (mW/cm^2)] and the time of illumination. The radiant energy, often termed fluence, is expressed as joules per square centimeter (J/cm^2). Therefore, to deliver a fluence of $50 J/cm^2$ at a power density of $600 mW/cm^2$, an illumination time of 83 seconds is required.

Upon illumination, photons interact with the ground singlet state sensitizer causing it to undergo an electronic transition to an activated short-lived excited singlet state. Singlet oxygen is highly electrophilic, oxidizing biological substrates and initiating a cascade of radical-generating reactions that damage cellular components. Singlet oxygen possesses a reactive path length of less than $0.02 \mu m$ so that any effect has limited potency (2). The photochemical processes involved are complex and are different for each sensitizer and are subject to the microenvironment.

PHOTOSENSITIZERS

BPD-MA (verteporfin, Visudyne™) consists of equal amounts of two regioisomers that differ in the location of the carboxylic acid and methyl ester moieties on the lower pyrrole rings of the chlorin macrocycle. BPD-MA, due to its hydrophobicity, is formulated with liposomes.

PDT studies undertaken using experimentally induced CNV in primates resulted in the closure of the neovascular membranes and choriocapillaris, but not the retinal vasculature. Liposomal BPD-MA was infused at a dose of 0.375 mg/kg for 10–32 minutes and illumination with infrared light at a fluence of $150 J/cm^2$ (689–692 nm laser light at $600 mW/cm^2$) occurred 30–55 minutes following the start of the infusion (6). When the same treatment parameters were performed on normal primate eyes, some retinal pigment epithelium (RPE) damage and choriocapillaris closure occurred locally with little damage in contiguous tissues. BPD-MA localization in the choroid and RPE was confirmed using fluorescence microscopy in rabbits. No BPD-MA was detected within the choroid or photoreceptors at two hours; however, a small trace was detected in the RPE at 24 hours (7). A similar pharmacokinetic pattern was observed in monkeys using in-vivo fluorescence imaging (8).

The long-term effects on the retina and choroid were evaluated in cynomolgus monkeys (9). CNV closure also resulted in the closure of the choriocapillaris with damage occurring in RPE cells. However, these areas appeared to regenerate somewhat in the four to seven-week study period. Of the 28 CNV lesions observed for four weeks, 72% remained closed. However, lesion re-treatment was necessary to sustain vascular closure.

Other photosensitizer agents including tin ethyl etiopurpurin (Purlytin™, SnET2), Optrin™, lutetium texaphyrin (Lu-Tex), mono-L-aspartyl chlorin e6 (NPe6 or MACE), chloroaluminum sulfonated phthalocyanine (AlPcS4), and ATX-S10 have been explored for the treatment of neovascular AMD and other retinal conditions (10–22); however, they have not been used in clinical practice. Verteporfin PDT has emerged as the dominant therapeutic option for neovascular AMD.

Laboratory and preclinical investigations have shown that PDT with verteporfin is superior to thermal laser photocoagulation for subfoveal CNV. Using experimental CNV models, the neovascularization and normal choriocapillaris can be closed while preserving the outer and inner retina. In contrast, treatment of neovascularization beneath the RPE and sensory retina with laser photocoagulation induces thermal conductance to the retina resulting in acute necrosis of all layers of the retina.

CLINICAL STUDIES

The safety and efficacy of verteporfin (BPD-MA, Visudyne™) for AMD were established in phase I, II, and III clinical trials in 1999 (23–25). Phase I and phase II studies proved that a single treatment of verteporfin PDT could occlude CNV vessels for one to four weeks following administration, as measured by fluorescein angiography (24). The maximal tolerated dose, defined by retinal closure, was 150 J/cm². The minimal light dose required to achieve the closure of the vessels was 25 J/cm².

Monotherapy

TAP Trial – Verteporfin in Predominantly Classic CNV
The preliminary results of the Treatment of Age-Related Macular Degeneration with Photodynamic Therapy (TAP) study were published in 1999 (23). Two concurrent, multicenter, double-masked, placebo-controlled, randomized trials were conducted in Europe and North America. Six-hundred-and-nine patients with subfoveal CNV, exhibiting at least some classic-type CNV features by fluorescein angiography, lesion size 5400 µm or less (9 DA), and visual acuity of 20/40 to 20/200 were enrolled. Four-hundred-and-two patients were randomized to the verteporfin group and 207 were randomized to the placebo group. Verteporfin or placebo (5% dextrose in water) was injected, followed 15 minutes later by diode laser application (689 nm) via a slit-lamp delivery system that yielded a fluence dose of 50 J/cm². Patients were examined every three months until the 24-month study completion period. If there was evidence of residual or new leakage on fluorescein angiography (FA), patients could undergo re-treatment with PDT at the discretion of the treating physician. The primary outcome of interest was the percentage of eyes that lost fewer than 15 letters. In the treatment group, 246 of

402 eyes (61%) lost fewer than 15 letters of visual acuity from baseline, compared with 96 of 207 placebo eyes (47%), a difference that was statistically significant (23). Similar results was found at 24 months (26). Subgroup analysis demonstrated the greatest benefit in eyes with predominantly classic CNV (defined as classic CNV comprising 50% or more of the total CNV lesion), and no treatment benefit was seen in eyes with minimally classic CNV (defined as classic CNV comprising less than 50% of the total CNV lesion). There was a trend toward benefit in the occult CNV group but the group was small (54 patients) and did not meet the eligibility criteria for these two trials. No significant lasting adverse effects were reported. The average number of PDT treatments was 3.4 by 12 months and 5.6 by 24 months (23,26). The treatment effect for PDT of predominantly classic subfoveal CNV persisted up to 24 months (26). Additionally, the subgroup analysis revealed that patients with predominantly classic CNV who were treated with PDT were more likely to have visual acuity greater than 20/200 at the 24-month follow-up (27).

An open-label extension of the TAP study for an additional three years was performed (28). At month 60, 35% of patients had lost 3 lines or more of visual acuity. The mean change in visual acuity from baseline was similar to results from month 12 and month 24, which was a loss of 1.5 lines of visual acuity at month 48 and month 60. On an average, patients received two PDT treatments during the three-year extension period.

VIP Trial: Verteporfin in Occult CNV
The Verteporfin in Photodynamic Therapy (VIP) study group conducted two concurrent trials in Europe and North America assessing PDT with verteporfin in patients with CNV from pathologic myopia, and AMD related occult CNV and classic CNV. The results of the AMD cohort were the first to establish the clinical efficacy of verteporfin in occult CNV (29). Three-hundred-and-thirty-nine patients with occult CNV lesions no greater than 5400 µm and visual acuity 20/100 or better with recent hemorrhage or disease progression, or classic CNV lesions no greater than 5400 µm and visual acuity of at least 20/40, were enrolled. There were 225 patients in the treatment group and 114 in the placebo group. Patients received either standard fluence PDT (50 J/cm²) with verteporfin or sham PDT. Patients were examined every three months and re-treatment given if there was evidence of leakage on FA. The primary outcome of interest was the proportion of eyes that lost at least 15 letters.

Treatment benefit was found at month 24, though not month 12, with 54% of the verteporfin-treated group compared with 67% of the placebo group losing at least 15 letters. Thirty percent of the verteporfin-treated group compared with 47% in placebo group lost at least 30 letters. The PDT group exhibited superior visual acuity, contrast sensitivity, final lesion size, and rate of progression to classic CNV at month 24. Subgroup analyses revealed a similar treatment benefit for occult CNV lesions (55% verteporfin-treated compared with 68% placebo-treated lost at least 15 letters). Patients with smaller CNV lesions (≤4 DA) or worse vision (≤20/50) at presentation had a greater treatment benefit. Patients in the treatment group received an average of 3.1 treatments in the first 12 months, and a total of 4.9 treatments at 24 months.

Safety Profile

A meta-analysis of the two-year safety results of the TAP and VIP trial was performed (30). There were 627 patients in the verteporfin group and 321 patients in the placebo group, and patients on an average received 5.4 courses of PDT. The percentage of patients who reported at least one adverse event, regardless of the relationship to treatment, was 92.3% in the verteporfin group compared with 89.1% in the placebo group. Significant differences in ocular adverse events between the two groups were seen only in the VIP trial and included reduction in visual acuity, especially acute severe decrease in vision, and visual field deficit, both of which occurred more often in the verteporfin group. Blepharitis occurred more commonly in the verteporfin group, whereas subretinal hemorrhage occurred more often in the placebo group. Other commonly reported ocular adverse events, with similar rates between the two groups, included cataract formation, conjunctival injection, dry eyes, and ocular itching. Systemic adverse events that occurred more commonly in the verteporfin group included injection site reaction, infusion-related back pain, photosensitivity reaction, constipation, and sleep disorder. Other commonly reported systemic adverse reactions included allergic reaction, asthenia, chest pain, flu syndrome, hypertension (HTN), nausea, anemia, arthralgia, and respiratory symptoms.

VIO Trial: Verteporfin in Occult CNV

The Visudyne In Occult CNV (VIO) study in 2009 attempted to replicate the results of the VIP trial (31). This was a multicenter, double-masked, placebo-controlled, randomized clinical trial conducted at 43 centers in the US and Canada. The study population consisted of 364 patients with subfoveal occult CNV, lesion size ≤6 DA, visual acuity between 20/40 to 20/200, and evidence of progression of CNV within three months prior to enrollment. Patients in the treatment group (n = 244) received standard fluence PDT with verteporfin and the placebo group (n = 120) received sham PDT. Patients in the verteporfin group received an average of 2.9 treatments at 12 month, and a total of 4.2 treatments at 24 months.

There was no statistically significant difference between the treatment and placebo groups in the percentage of patients with vision loss of at least 15 letters (primary outcome) or at least 30 letters (secondary outcome) at 12 or 24 months. At 2 years, the treatment group was more likely to avoid legal blindness (VA ≤ 20/200), and have stable (<5 letters lost or gained) or improved vision (≥ 5 letters gained) compared with the placebo group.

VIM Trial: Verteporfin in Minimally Classic CNV

The Visudyne In Minimally Classic CNV (VIM) study (32) evaluated the efficacy of verteporfin therapy for minimally classic CNV (for which treatment had not been demonstrated to be beneficial in the TAP and VIP trials), and compared a reduced fluence (RF) PDT (25 J/cm^2) to standard fluence (SF) PDT (50 J/cm^2). RF PDT is thought to enhance selectivity for neovascular lesions and reduce surrounding inflammation. One-hundred-and-seventeen patients with subfoveal CNV with a classic CNV component occupying less than 50% of the total CNV lesion, visual acuity of ≥20/250 and lesion size ≤4 DA or visual acuity of 20/50 to 20/250 and lesion size between 4 and 6 DA were enrolled from 19 clinical centers in North America and Europe.

At 12 months, 47% in the placebo group, 14% in the RF group, and 28% in the SF group had lost at least 15 letters. At 24 months, 62% in the placebo group, 26% in the RF group, and 53% in the SF group had lost at least 15 letters. Statistical significance in favor of treatment with verteporfin was maintained when the RF and SF groups were pooled. The mean changes in visual acuity from baseline to 24 months were -2 letters in the RF group, -16 letters in the SF group, and -21 letters in the placebo group. At month 24, progression to predominantly classic CNV was more prevalent in the placebo group (28%) compared with the RF (5%) and SF (3%) groups. Notably, when subanalyses were performed to look at CNV lesions <4 DA compared with lesions between 4 and 6 DA, similar treatment benefits were found. In addition, when visual outcomes of the two fluence groups were compared, there was a statistically significant difference favoring the RF group at month 12; however, this difference abated by month 24. Adverse events were similar in the pooled verteporfin groups compared with the control group.

ANCHOR: Verteporfin Vs. Ranibizumab for Predominantly Classic CNV

Anti-vascular endothelial growth factor (anti-VEGF) therapy has become the most widely used treatment modality for neovascular AMD in the developed world, after multiple clinical trials emerged in 2000 supporting its efficacy. The ANCHOR study (33,34) (ANti-VEGF antibody for the treatment of predominantly classic CHORoidal neovascularization in AMD) compared the efficacy of ranibizumab, a recombinant monoclonal antibody that binds VEGF-A, to PDT with verteporfin. This was a multicenter, double blind, randomized trial conducted in the United States, Germany, and Australia. Four-hundred-and-twenty-three patients with subfoveal CNV, lesion size 5400 μm or less, visual acuity 20/40 to 20/320, with no evidence of damage to the fovea, and no previous treatments with PDT or anti-VEGF therapy, were enrolled. Patients were assigned to one of three groups: 0.3 mg or 0.5 mg ranibizumab with sham PDT, or SF PDT with sham intravitreal injection. Ranibizumab or sham injections were performed monthly. The mean numbers of injections were 11.1 and 19.2 in the verteporfin group, 11.0 and 21.5 in the 0.3 mg group, and 11.2 and 21.3 in the 0.5 mg group, at 12 months and 24 months, respectively. PDT (active or sham) was administered 2.8 times and 3.8 times in the verteporfin group, 1.7 times and 2.2 times in the 0.3 mg group, and 1.7 and 1.9 times in the 0.5 mg group, at 12 and 24 months respectively.

At 12 months, 94.3% of the 0.3 mg ranibizumab group and 96.4% of the 0.5 mg ranibizumab group compared with 64.3% in the verteporfin group had lost fewer than 15 letters. At 24 months, 90% of 0.3 mg group, 89.9% of 0.5 mg group, and 65.7% of the verteporfin group had lost fewer than 15 letters. The proportion of patients with severe vision loss (30 letters or more) was low in the ranibizumab groups: 1.4% in the 0.3 mg group and 0% in the 0.5 mg group, compared with 16.1% in the verteporfin group at 24 months.

Visual gains were apparent in the ranibizumab groups: 35.7% in the 0.3 mg group and 40.3% in the 0.5 mg group, compared with 5.6% in the verteporfin group, gained 15 or more letters at 12 months. Similar results were found at 24 months. On an average, the 0.3 mg group gained 8.5 letters, the 0.5 mg group gained 11.3 letters and the verteporfin group lost 9.5 letters at 12 months. At 24 months, there was a gain of 8.1 letters in the 0.3 mg and 10.7 letters in the 0.5 mg ranibizumab groups, and a loss of 9.8 letters in the verteporfin group. Angiographic outcomes were also superior in the ranibizumab groups with minimal change in CNV lesion size at 24 months (small increase of 0.33 DA in the 0.3 mg group and 0.27 DA in the 0.5 mg group) compared with an increase of 1.60 DA in the verteporfin group.

There was no statistically significant difference in serious adverse events, ocular or non-ocular, between the pooled ranibizumab groups and the verteporfin group. The rate of presumed endophthalmitis was 1.1% in the ranibizumab groups (0.05% per injection), whereas none occurred in the verteporfin group. Vitreous hemorrhage occurred in 0.7% of the ranibizumab groups compared with 0% in the verteporfin group. Rhegmatogenous retinal detachment occurred in 0.7% of both the pooled ranibizumab and verteporfin groups. Transient increases in intraocular pressure were common in the ranibizumab groups. Although no treatment-associated lens trauma occurred, there was a trend toward a higher rate of cataract formation in the ranibizumab groups compared with the verteporfin group (16.8% in the 0.3 mg group, 20% in the 0.5 mg group, 10.5% in the verteporfin group).

Systemic adverse events including the rate of arterial thromboembolic events were similar in all groups, 4.4% in the 0.3 mg and 5% in the 0.5 mg ranibizumab groups, and 4.2% in the verteporfin group. No fatal myocardial infarctions (MI) or cerebral vascular accidents (CVAs) occurred during the study period. The rates of nonfatal stroke were 2.2%, 0%, and 1.4% in the 0.3 mg, 0.5 mg, and verteporfin groups, respectively. There was a trend toward an increase in non-ocular hemorrhage (gastrointestinal and subdural hematoma) in the ranibizumab groups (8.8% in the 0.3 mg group and 9.3% in the 0.5 mg group) compared with the verteporfin group (4.9%).

Several strategies have been proposed to optimize the effectiveness of PDT, including altering the time to application of nonthermal laser for occult CNV lesions and reducing the re-treatment interval for predominantly classic CNV (to 2-month from 3-month treatment intervals); both strategies have been evaluated in randomized clinical trials with no statistically significant differences among treatment groups (35–37).

Combination Therapy

Following the emergence of anti-VEGF therapy for AMD and the proven benefits for the subsets of patients described above, the use of PDT monotherapy waned. Subsequently, there has been a growing body of clinical investigation of PDT as part of a strategy of combination therapy—the use of two or more treatment modalities including various combinations of anti-VEGF agents, corticosteroids, and PDT. The rationale for combination therapy is the theoretical advantage of increasing the number of targets addressed in the pathobiology of neovascular AMD: occluding choroidal neovascular vessels via PDT, binding intraocular VEGF, and harnessing the pleomorphic benefits of intraocular steroid.

PDT and Corticosteroid

Arias and colleagues from Spain conducted a prospective, randomized, controlled trial directly comparing PDT monotherapy with PDT plus intravitreal triamcinolone (IVTA) combination therapy in patients with subfoveal predominantly classic CNV, lesion size <5400 μm, visual acuity 20/40 to 20/400, and no prior PDT treatment (38). Thirty-one patients were enrolled to the SF PDT plus 11 mg IVTA combination group, and 30 patients were enrolled to the SF PDT with sham injection group. All patients were examined every 3 months for 12 months, and re-treatment with either PDT alone or PDT plus IVTA was provided on an as-needed basis. Results at 12 months showed a statistically significant difference in visual outcome in favor of the combination group: the proportion of patients that lost fewer than 15 letters at 12 months was 74% in the combination group compared with 61% in the monotherapy group. Patients in the combination group had a reduction in the total size of CNV lesions and in foveal thickness compared with the monotherapy group. The re-treatment rate was 1.8 in the combination therapy group compared with 2.9 in the PDT monotherapy group.

However, a subsequent study with a larger sample size and longer duration of follow-up (planned for 24 months) failed to show a similar visual benefit (39). In a multicenter, double-blind, randomized trial in Canada, patients with predominantly classic subfoveal CNV less than 5400 μm in size and VA ≥20/320, were randomized to receive either SF PDT plus 4 mg IVTA (n = 50) or monotherapy with SF PDT (n = 50). Results at 12 months showed that there was no statistically significant difference between the two groups in mean change in visual acuity from baseline or proportion of patients who had lost fewer than 15 letters. There were fewer subsequent treatments administered in the combination group

(1.28 per patient) compared with the monotherapy group (1.94 per patient). Results from the second year of this study are pending. Adverse events included increased intraocular pressure (IOP), which occurred more often in the combination group up to month 9 (the two groups had similar rates of increased IOP at month 12). Cataract progression was more rapid in the combination group, and was thought to contribute to the observed lack of significant difference in visual acuities between the two treatment groups. However, a subgroup analysis of pseudophakic patients still failed to demonstrate a difference in vision between the two treatment groups.

PDT and Anti-VEGF
Several prospective pilot studies of combination therapy with PDT and anti-VEGF agents suggested benefits in both vision and reduction in the total number of treatments (40–42). The PROTECT study in 2008 established the safety of administering PDT with verteporfin and intravitreal ranibizumab on the same day (43). This was a multicenter, open-label, prospective study of 32 patients who received concomitant SF PDT with verteporfin and 0.5 mg intravitreal ranibizumab. This trial showed that the simultaneous administration of verteporfin and ranibizumab was not associated with serious adverse events and resulted in mean improvements in visual acuity of 6.9 letters and 2.4 letters after four and nine months of follow-up, respectively. Large, multicenter, randomized controlled trials evaluating the combination of ranibizumab and PDT with verteporfin soon followed, and included the DENALI trials in the United States and Canada and the MONT BLANC trial in Europe. In addition, the EVEREST trial specifically assessed PDT and anti-VEGF combination therapy in polypoidal choroidal vasculopathy (PCV).

MONT BLANC: Ranibizumab Monotherapy Vs. Combination Therapy with Ranibizumab Plus SF PDT
Two-hundred-and-fifty-five patients were enrolled in this multicenter, double blind, randomized trial comparing ranibizumab monotherapy (n = 133) with ranibizumab plus SF PDT (n = 122) combination therapy (44). In both groups patients received three initial consecutive monthly injections of ranibizumab and one initial PDT treatment, followed by ranibizumab and PDT administered on an as-needed basis over 30-day and 90-day intervals, respectively. Re-treatment criteria were based on CNV leakage on FA, an increase in central retinal thickness ≥100 µm, the presence of subretinal fluid as assessed optical coherence topography (OCT), worsening in visual acuity by more than 5 letters, or presence of new subretinal hemorrhage on fundoscopic examination. Noninferiority of combination therapy in mean change in visual acuity and proportion of patients with treatment-free interval of at least three months were the two main outcomes of interest.

The mean change in visual acuity was a gain of 4.4 letters in the monotherapy group compared with 2.5 letters in the combination group, a noninferior result based on a pre-defined noninferiority margin of 7 letters (p = 0.0048). The percentage of patients who had a ranibizumab treatment-free interval of at least 3 months was similar in both groups, 95.8% in the combination group compared with 92.2% in the monotherapy group. Thus, although the visual results with combination therapy were noninferior to ranibizumab monotherapy, no significant decrease in treatment burden was found at one year.

Post-hoc analyses showed that 85% of patients in the combination group compared with 72% in the monotherapy group had a treatment-free interval of at least 4 months (45). Median time to re-treatment was extended by one month in the combination group (at month 6) compared with the monotherapy group (at month 5). The percentage of patients with residual fluorescein leakage at month 12 was 28.9% in the combination group and 25.2% in the monotherapy group. Both groups had a reduction in the total area of leakage (-5.3 mm² in the combination group, -6.1 mm² in the monotherapy group) and central retinal thickness (-115.3 µm in the combination group, -124.6 µm in the monotherapy group) at month 12 (46). On average, the combination group received 4.8 ranibizumab injections and 1.7 PDT treatments compared with 5.1 ranibizumab injections and 1.9 sham PDT in the monotherapy group.

The rates of adverse events were comparable between the two groups. There was no incidence of endophthalmitis or uveitis in either group. RPE tears occurred in five patients in the combination group and three patients in the monotherapy group. Systemic adverse effects were rare and similar to those reported in previous studies and included few cases of HTN, CVA, angina pectoris, MI, transient ischemic attack (TIA), gastrointestinal hemorrhage, and periorbital hematoma.

DENALI: Monotherapy Vs. Combination Therapy with Ranibizumab Plus SF or RF PDT
Three-hundred-and-twenty-one patients were enrolled in this multicenter, double blind, randomized trial comparing 0.5 mg ranibizumab monotherapy (n = 112) with a combination therapy of SF PDT plus ranibizumab (n = 104) and RF PDT plus ranibizumab (n = 105) (47,48). Patients in the combination groups received three consecutive monthly ranibizumab injections initially, and one initial treatment of SF or RF PDT based on randomization. Subsequent treatments with ranibizumab and PDT were administered as needed, at 30-day and 90-day intervals respectively, based on re-treatment criteria similar to the MONT BLANC trial. Patients in the ranibizumab monotherapy group received monthly treatments for 12 months and then as needed thereafter. The purpose of this study was to demonstrate noninferiority (visual acuity, 7 letter margin) of combination therapy with PDT plus ranibizumab to monotherapy with ranibizumab, and to evaluate the treatment-free interval in each group.

At 12 months, the mean change in visual acuity was a gain of 5.3 letters, 4.4 letters, and 8.1 letters in the SF combination group, the RF combination group, and the ranibizumab monotherapy group, respectively.

Noninferiority of either combination therapy compared with monotherapy was not demonstrated (SF combination vs. monotherapy p = 0.0666; RF combination *vs.* monotherapy p = 0.1178). The percentage of patients with a treatment-free interval of at least 3 months was higher in the SF group (92.6%) compared with the RF group (83.5%); the ranibizumab monotherapy group was not included in analyses because all patients received monthly ranibizumab for 12 months according to protocol. The SF group required an additional 2.2 ranibizumab injections and the RF group required 2.8 additional ranibizumab injections after the mandated three consecutive injections. Patients in all groups had similar reductions in the area of leakage by FA at 12 months (-3.2 mm^2 in SF and RF groups, and -3.8 mm^2 in the monotherapy group). There was a greater reduction in retinal thickness by OCT in the monotherapy group (-172 μm) compared with both combination groups (-151.7 μm in the SF group and -140.9 μm in the RF group).

Overall, the rates of serious adverse events were 30.8%, 27.4%, and 36.9% in the SF, RF, and monotherapy groups, respectively. Rates of acute MI (0% in SF, 0.9% RF, 0.9% monotherapy) and CVA (0.96% in SF, 0.94% in RF, 0.90% in monotherapy) were very low. There were three patients (2.7%) in the monotherapy group who had a TIA compared with one in the RF and none in the SF group. There were six patients in the monotherapy group (5.4%) who had congestive heart failure compared with two in each of the combination groups. The rate of nonserious reduction in visual acuity was higher in the SF group (9.6%) compared with the RF group (8.5%) and monotherapy group (4.5%). The rate of more serious reduction in visual acuity was also higher in the SF group (3.9%) compared with the RF (0.94%) and the monotherapy groups (2.7%). A serious retinal hemorrhage occurred only in one patient in the monotherapy group, whereas nonserious retinal hemorrhage occurred in approximately 7% of patients in each of the combination treatment groups. Cataract developed in 6% of patients in each of the treatment groups. The rate of endophthalmitis was 0.96% in the SF group, 0% in the RF group, and 1.8% in the monotherapy group.

EVEREST: Verteporfin Monotherapy Vs. Ranibizumab Monotherapy Vs. Combination Therapy with Verteporfin plus Ranibizumab in Polypoidal Choroidal Vasculopathy

This multicenter, double masked, randomized controlled trial was conducted in Asia to compare the efficacy of verteporfin monotherapy, ranibizumab monotherapy, and combination therapy with both agents in PCV (49–51). Sixty-one patients were randomized to one of three groups: Verteporfin monotherapy (n = 21), ranibizumab monotherapy (n = 21), and verteporfin plus ranibizumab combination therapy (n = 19). Inclusion criteria were BCVA between 20/40 and 20/320 and lesion size ≤5400 μm. All patients received one initial SF PDT with verteporfin or sham PDT if in the ranibizumab monotherapy group and three consecutive

monthly injections with 0.5 mg ranibizumab or sham injection if in the PDT monotherapy group. At month 3, patients received ranibizumab or sham injection and verteporfin or sham PDT based on randomization on an as-needed basis over 30-day and 90-day treatment intervals, respectively, based on re-treatment criteria of polyp progression on ICG, leakage on FA, and reduction in visual acuity of ≥5 letters.

At month 6, complete polyp regression was achieved in 71.8% of patients in the verteporfin monotherapy group and 77.8% in the combination therapy group, compared with 28.6% in the ranibizumab monotherapy group (p < 0.01). On average, patients in all groups gained vision at month 6, with the greatest gain in the combination group (+10.9 letters in combination group, +9.2 letters in the ranibizumab monotherapy group, and +7.5 letters in the Verteporfin monotherapy group). All groups had a reduction in central retinal thickness on OCT, with the greatest mean reduction seen in the combination therapy group (-145.6 μm in the combination group, -98.1 μm in the verteporfin monotherapy group, and -65.7 μm in the ranibizumab monotherapy group). The rates of serious adverse events were low across all groups (5.3% in the combination group, 4.8% in the verteporfin monotherapy group, and 9.5% in the ranibizumab monotherapy group). These results were significant in that verteporfin monotherapy and combination therapy were shown to result in significantly higher rates of polyp regression than anti-VEGF monotherapy.

RADICAL: Verteporfin plus Ranibizumab plus Dexamethasone Vs. Verteporfin plus Ranibizumab Vs. Ranibizumab Monotherapy

In this multicenter randomized controlled trial, 162 patients were enrolled and stratified into one of four cohorts (52,53). There were two triple therapy groups: one consisted of either one-quarter fluence PDT (15 J/cm^2) plus 0.5 mg ranibizumab plus 0.5 mg intravitreal dexamethasone (IVDM) (n = 39) and the other with half fluence PDT (25 J/cm^2) plus 0.5 mg ranibizumab plus 0.5 mg IVDM (n = 39). The double therapy group consisted of half fluence PDT plus 0.5 mg ranibizumab (n = 43). The fourth cohort was ranibizumab monotherapy (n = 41). Patients qualified for this study if they had subfoveal CNV with visual acuity between 20/40 and 20/320, and lesion size ≤5400 μm. All patients in the combination groups received the double or triple therapy on day 0, then as needed every two months. The ranibizumab monotherapy group received three consecutive treatments, followed by monthly re-treatment as needed. Patients were studied for 24 months and the primary outcomes of interest were the mean number of re-treatments and mean change in visual acuity from baseline.

At 12 months, the triple therapy half fluence group had the fewest number of re-treatments (3) when compared with the triple therapy quarter fluence group (3.97), the double therapy half fluence group (4.05), and the ranibizumab monotherapy group (5.39). At month 24, this difference became more pronounced with the triple therapy half fluence group exhibiting a re-treatment average of 4.34 compared with 8.68 in the ranibizumab monotherapy group. All groups had a gain in visual acuity at 12 months, with the greatest gain seen in the triple therapy half fluence group (+6.8 letters) and the ranibizumab monotherapy group (+6.5 letters), though at 24 months, the group that showed the greatest gain in vision became the ranibizumab monotherapy group (+4.4 letters compared with +1.1 in the triple therapy half fluence group, and minimal change in the other two groups).

The proportion of patients who lost at least 15 letters was 7.7% and 15.4% in the triple therapy half fluence group, 7.3% and 14.6% in the monotherapy group, 12.8% and 20.5% in the triple therapy quarter fluence group, and 11.6% and 20.9% in the double therapy group at 12 months and 24 months, respectively. The proportion of patients who gained at least 15 letters was initially greatest in the triple therapy half fluence group (30.8%), followed by comparable gains in the triple therapy quarter fluence group and the double therapy half fluence groups (25.6%), followed by the monotherapy group (24.4%). However at 24 months, the proportion of patients who gained at least 15 letters was greatest in the monotherapy group (26.8%), compared with 20.5% in the triple therapy quarter fluence group, 16.3% in the double therapy group, and 15.4% in the triple therapy half fluence group. The mean change in central retinal thickness at 24 months was maximal in the triple therapy half fluence group (-123.9 µm) and double therapy half fluence group (-121 µm), followed by the triple therapy quarter fluence group (-110.3 µm) and the ranibizumab monotherapy group (-103.1 µm). There was a reduction in total CNV lesion size at 24 months in all groups (-103.3 µm in the triple therapy half fluence group, -205.3 µm in the monotherapy group, -112.5 µm in the double therapy group) with the exception of the triple therapy quarter fluence group (+94.8 µm). Adverse events were comparable to similar studies.

SUMMARY POINTS

Studies in Neovascular AMD

- Photodynamic therapy (PDT) with verteporfin is beneficial in predominantly classic or occult choroidal neovascularization (CNV) with evidence of disease progression when lesion size is ≤9 DA (TAP and VIP trials).
- PDT with verteporfin is beneficial in minimally classic CNV when lesion size is ≤6 DA (VIM trial).
- PDT with Verteporfin can retard the rate of visual loss, but does not confer gains in acuity, in contrast to anti-VEGF therapy (ANCHOR trial)
- To date, combination therapy with IVTA and PDT has not conferred gains in visual acuity; however, combination therapy may prolong the re-treatment interval.

- The value of combination therapy using ranibizumab with PDT remains unclear:
  - ○ DENALI Study: Combination therapy with ranibizumab and PDT (standard or reduced fluence) did not achieve noninferiority to ranibizumab monotherapy assessed by visual acuity. Combination therapy may lengthen the re-treatment interval.
  - ○ MONT BLANC Study: Combination therapy with ranibizumab and standard fluence PDT is noninferior to ranibizumab monotherapy. There was no difference between combination therapy and monotherapy in the proportion of patients with a treatment-free interval of at least 3 months.
- Combination therapy with PDT and ranibizumab is beneficial in polypoidal choroidal vasculopathy (EVEREST trial).
- Triple therapy with half fluence PDT, ranibizumab, and dexamethasone reduces the number of re-treatments over a 24-month period. However, monotherapy with ranibizumab confers the greatest visual benefit at 2 years (RADICAL trial).

REFERENCES

1. Henderson BW, Dougherty TJ. How does photodynamic therapy work? Photochem Photobiol 1992; 55: 145–57.
2. Dougherty TJ, Gomer CJ, Hender BW, et al. Photodynamic therapy. J Natl Cancer Inst 1998; 90: 889–905.
3. Hausmann W. Die sensibilisierende wirkung des hamatoporphyrins. Biochem Z 1911; 30: 276–316.
4. Castellani A, Page G, Concioli M. Photodynamic effect of haematoporphyrin on blood microcirculation. J Pathol Bacteriol 1963; 86: 99–102.
5. Fingar VH, Kik PK, Haydon PS, et al. Analysis of acute vascular damage after photodynamic therapy using benzoporphyrin derivative (BPD). Br J Cancer 1999; 79: 1702–8.
6. Husain D, Miller JW, Kenney AG, et al. Photodynamic therapy and digital angiography of experimental iris neovascularization using liposomal benzoporphyrin derivative. Ophthalmology 1997; 104: 1242–50.
7. Haimovici R, Kramer M, Miller JW, et al. Localization of lipoprotein-delivered benzoporphyrin derivative in the rabbit eye. Curr Eye Res 1997; 16: 83–90.
8. Husain D, Miller J. Photodynamic therapy of exudative age-related macular degeneration. Semin Ophthalmol 1997; 12: 14–25.
9. Husain D, Kramer M, Kenny AG, et al. Effects of photodynamic therapy using verteporfin on experimental choroidal neovascularization and normal retina and choroid up to 7 weeks after treatment. Invest Ophthalmol Vis Sci 1999; 40: 2322–31.
10. Mori K, Yoneya S, Ohta M, et al. Angiographic and histologic effects of fundus photodynamic therapy with a hydrophilic sensitizer (mono-L-aspartyl chlorin e6). Ophthalmology 1999; 106: 1384–91.
11. Kilman GH, Puliafito CA, Grossman GA, et al. Retinal and choroidal vessel closure using phthalocyanine photodynamic therapy. Lasers Surg Med 1994; 15: 11–18.

12. Kilman GH, Puliafito CA, Stern D, et al. Phthalocyanine photodynamic therapy: new strategy for closure of choroidal neovascularization. Lasers Surg Med 1994; 15: 2–10.

13. Asrani S, Zeimer R. Feasibility of laser targeted photo-occlusion of ocular vessels. Br J Ophthalmol 1995; 79: 766–70.

14. Obana A, Gohto Y, Kanai M, et al. Selective photodynamic effects of the new photosensitizer ATX-S10(Na) on choroidal neovascularization in monkeys. Arch Ophthalmol 2000; 118: 650–8.

15. Mang TS, Allison R, Hewson G, et al. A phase II/III clinical study of tin ethyl etiopurpurin (Purlytin)-induced photodynamic therapy for the treatment of recurrent cutaneous metastatic breast cancer. Cancer J Sci Am 1998; 4: 378–84.

16. Primbs GB, Casey R, Wamser K, et al. Photodynamic therapy for corneal neovascularization. Ophthalmic Surg Lasers 1998; 29: 832–8.

17. Blumenkranz MS, Woodburn KW, Quing F, et al. Lutetium texaphyrin (Lu-Tex): a potential new agent for ocular fundus angiography and photodynamic therapy. Am J Ophthalmol 2000; 129: 353–62.

18. Rockson SG, Lorenz DP, Cheong WF, et al. Photoangioplasty: an emerging clinical cardiovascular role for photodynamic therapy. Circulation 2000; 102: 591–6.

19. Kereiakes DJ, Szyniszewski AM, Whar D, et al. Phase I drug and light dose-escalation trial of motexafin lutetium and far red light activation (phototherapy) in subjects with coronary artery disease undergoing percutaneous coronary intervention and stent deployment: procedural and long-term results. Circulation 2003; 108: 1310–15.

20. Verigos K, Stripp H, Mick R, et al. Updated results of a phase I trial of motexafin lutetium-mediated interstitial photodynamic therapy in patients with locally recurrent prostate cancer. J Environ Pathol Toxicol Oncol 2006; 25: 373–87.

21. Graham KB, Arbor JD, Coonnolly EJ, et al. Digital angio¬graphy using lutetium texaphyrin in a monkey model of choroidal neovascularization. Invest Ophthalmol Vis Sci 1999; 40: 402.

22. Arbor JD, Connolly EJ, Graham K, et al. Photodynamic therapy of experimental choroidal neovascularization using intravenous infusion of lutetium texaphyrin. Invest Ophthalmol Vis Sci 1999; 40: 401.

23. Treatment of Age-Related Macular Degeneration with Photodynamic Therapy (TAP) Study Group. Photodynamic therapy of subfoveal choroidal neovascularization in age-related macular degeneration with verteporfin: one-year results of 2 randomized clinical trials-TAP Report. Arch Ophthalmol 1999; 117: 1329–45.

24. Miller JW, Schmidt-Erfurth U, Sickenberg M, et al. Photodynamic therapy with verteporfin for choroidal neovascularization caused by age-related macular degeneration: results of a single treatment in a phase 1 and 2 study. Arch Ophthalmol 1999; 117: 1161–73.

25. Schmidt-Erfurth U, Miller JW, Sickenberg M, et al. Photodynamic therapy with verteporfin for choroidal neovascularization caused by age-related macular degeneration: results of retreatments in a phase 1 and 2 study. Arch Ophthalmol 1999; 117: 1177–87.

26. Bressler NM. Photodynamic therapy of subfoveal choroidal neovascularization in age-related macular degeneration with verteporfin: two-year results of 2 randomized clinical trials-TAP report 2. Arch Ophthalmol 2001; 119: 198–207.

27. Bressler NM, Arnold J, Benchaboune M, et al. Verteporfin therapy of subfoveal choroidal neovascularization in patients with age-related macular degeneration: additional information regarding baseline lesion composition's impact on vision outcomes-TAP report no. 3. Arch Ophthalmol 2002; 120: 1443–54.

28. Kaiser P. Verteporfin therapy of subfoveal choroidal neovascularization in age-related macular degeneration: 5-year results of two randomized clinical trials with an open-label extension - TAP report no. 8. Graefe's Arch Clin Exp Ophthalmol 2006; 244: 1132–42.

29. Arnold J, Kilmartin D, Olson J, et al. Verteporfin therapy of subfoveal choroidal neovascularization in age-related macular degeneration: two-year results of a randomized clinical trial including lesions with occult with no classic choroidal neovascularization - verteporfin in photodynamic therapy report 2. Am J Ophthalmol 2001; 131: 541–60.

30. Azab M, Benchaboune M, Blinder KJ, et al. Verteporfin therapy of subfoveal choroidal neovascularization in age-related macular degeneration: meta-analysis of 2-year safety results in three randomized clinical trials: treatment of age-related macular degeneration with photodynamic therapy and verteporfin in photodynamic therapy study report no. 4. Retina 2004; 24: 1–12.

31. Kaiser PK, Visudyne In; Occult CNV (VIO) Study Group. Verteporfin PDT for subfoveal occult CNV in AMD: two-year results of a randomized trial. Curr Med Res Opin 2009; 25: 1853–60.

32. Azab M, Boyer DS, Bressler NM, et al. Verteporfin therapy of subfoveal minimally classic choroidal neovascularization in age-related macular degeneration: 2-year results of a randomized clinical trial. Arch Ophthalmol 2005; 123: 448–57.

33. Brown DM, Kaiser PK, Michels M, et al. Ranibizumab versus verteporfin for neovascular age-related macular degeneration. N Engl J Med 2006; 355: 1432–44.

34. Brown DM, Michels M, Kaiser PK, et al. Ranibizumab versus verteporfin photodynamic therapy for neovascular age-related macular degeneration: two-year results of the ANCHOR study. Ophthalmology 2009; 116: 57–65.e5.

35. Rosenfeld PJ, Boyer DS, Bressler NM, et al. Verteporfin therapy of subfoveal occult choroidal neovascularization in AMD using delayed light application: one-year results of the VALIO study. Am J Ophthalmol 2007; 144: 970–2.

36. Michels S, Wachtlin J, Gamulescu MA, et al. Comparison of early retreatment with the standard regimen in verteporfin therapy of neovascular age-related macular degeneration. Ophthalmology 2005; 112: 2070–5.

37. Schmidt-Erfurth U, Sacu S. Randomized multicenter trial of more intense and standard early verteporfin treatment of neovascular age-related macular degeneration. Ophthalmology 2008; 115: 134–40.

38. Arias L, Garcia-Arumi J, Ramon JM, et al. Photodynamic therapy with intravitreal triamcinolone in predominantly classic choroidal neovascularization: one-year results of a randomized study. Ophthalmology 2006; 113: 2243–50.

39. Maberley D. Photodynamic therapy and intravitreal triamcinolone for neovascular age-related macular degeneration: a randomized clinical trial. Ophthalmology 2009; 116: 2149–57.e1.

40. Heier JS, Boyer DS, Ciulla TA, et al. Ranibizumab combined with verteporfin photodynamic therapy in neovascular age-related macular degeneration: year 1 results of the FOCUS study. Arch Ophthalmol 2006; 124: 1532–42.

41. Antoszyk AN, Tuomi L, Chung CY, et al. Ranibizumab combined with verteporfin photodynamic therapy in neovascular age-related macular degeneration (FOCUS): year 2 results. Am J Ophthalmol 2008; 145: 862–74.

42. Potter MJ, Claudio CC, Szabo SM. A randomised trial of bevacizumab and reduced light dose photodynamic therapy in age-related macular degeneration: the VIA study. Br J Ophthalmol 2010; 94: 174–9.

43. Schmidt-Erfurth U, Wolf S. Same-day administration of verteporfin and ranibizumab 0.5 mg in patients with choroidal neovascularisation due to age-related macular degeneration. Br J Ophthalmol 2008; 92: 1628–35.

44. Larsen M, Schmidt-Erfurth U, Lanzetta P, et al. Verteporfin plus ranibizumab for choroidal neovascularization in age-related macular degeneration: twelve-month MONT BLANC study results. Ophthalmology 2012; 119: 992–1000.

45. QLT. QLT Announces 12-Month Results from Novartis Sponsored MONT BLANC Study. 2009. [Available from: http://www.qltinc.com/newsCenter/2009/090615.htm] (Cited 10 January 2012).

46. Novartis. Verteporfin Photodynamic Therapy Administered in Conjunction With Ranibizumab in Patients With Subfoveal Choroidal Neovascularization Secondary to Age-related Macular Degeneration (AMD). [database on the Internet]. 2011. [Available from: ClinicalTrials.gov, Web site http://clinicaltrials.gov/ct2/show/NCT00433017] (Cited 9 January 2012).

47. Kaiser PK, Boyer DS, Cruess AF, et al. Verteporfin plus ranibizumab for choroidal neovascularization in age-related macular degeneration: twelve-month results of the DENALI study. Ophthalmology 2012; 119: 1001–10.

48. Novartis. Efficacy/Safety of Verteporfin Photodynamic Therapy Administered and Ranibizumab compared with Ranibizumab in Patients With Subfoveal Choroidal Neo-vascularization. [database on the Internet]. 2011. [Available from: ClinicalTrials.gov, Web site http://clinicaltrials.gov/ct2/show/study/NCT00436553] (Cited 9 January 2012).

49. Koh A, Lee WK, Chen LJ, et al. EVEREST STUDY: Efficacy and safety of verteporfin photodynamic therapy in combination with ranibizumab or alone versus ranibizumab monotherapy in patients with symptomatic macular polypoidal choroidal vasculopathy. Retina 2012. [Epub ahead of print].

50. Drugs.com. 6-month results from EVEREST study evaluating Visudyne(R) therapy in patients with polypoidal choroidal vasculopathy [homepage on the Internet]. 2011. [Available from: http:/www.drugs.com/clinical_trials/6-month-results-everest-study-evaluating-visudyne-r-therapy-patients-polypoidal-choroidal-8636.html] (Cited 9 January 2012).

51. Novartis. Efficacy and safety of verteporfin added to ranibizumab in the treatment of symptomatic macular polypoidal choroidal vasculopathy (PCV). [database on the Internet]. 2011. [Available from: ClinicalTrials.gov, Web site http://clinicaltrials.gov/ct2/show/study/NCT00674323] (Cited 9 January 2012).

52. Drugs.com. QLT Announces Final Results from its RADI-CAL Study Evaluating Verteporfin PDT (Visudyne) Combination Therapy in Exudative AMD. [homepage on the Internet]. 2010. [Available from: http://www.drugs.com/clinical_trials/qlt-announces-final-results-radical-study-evaluating-verteporfin-pdt-visudyne-combination-therapy-9675.html] (Cited 9 January 2012).

53. QLT Inc. Reduced Fluence Visudyne-Anti-VEGF-Dexamethasone in Combination for AMD Lesions (RADI-CAL). [database on the Internet]. 2011. [Available from: ClinicalTrials.gov Web site http://clinicaltrials.gov/ct2/show/study/NCT00492284] (Cited 9 January 2012).

24

Photocoagulation of AMD-associated CNV feeder vessels: An optimized approach

Robert W. Flower, Rajiv Rathod, and Felix Y. Chau

INTRODUCTION

Within the last five years, the focus of treatment for age-related macular degeneration (AMD)-related choroidal neovascularization (CNV) has been dominated by drug-based approaches, and anti-VEGF therapy has prevailed as the most effective treatment thus far. However, pharmacologic therapies so far have had certain limitations and drawbacks, with the burden of repeat treatment at the top of the list, and there are patients who are refractory to anti-VEGF therapy. Consequently, alternative treatment modalities are still being explored and utilized, especially as part of a combination therapy approach. One such technique, called feeder vessel treatment (FVT), specifically targets the blood vessels supplying the CNV. FVT, which was introduced years ago and remains in limited use today, is an attractive approach because, unlike pharmacologic interventions, the treatment is directed and definitive. The effect of the treatment in theory should not diminish with time.

Although elegantly simple as a concept, successfully implementing a routine FVT method has been a protracted process. The history of its development spans a period of nearly 30 years, and the case can be made that its development has been coupled to the evolution of fundus angiography technology, especially choroidal angiography. Today FVT has been refined to take advantage of improvements not only in the devices used for angiogram acquisition and application of laser photocoagulation energy, but also in diagnostic angiogram analyses. In one method of FVT described here, even the method of applying laser energy to feeder vessels (FVs) has been optimized by the introduction of dye-enhanced photocoagulation (DEP), wherein indocyanine green (ICG) dye transiting targeted FVs at the instant of photocoagulation acts to selectively enhance absorption of the laser energy, thereby focusing the thermal tissue damage onto the targeted FV and sparing the surrounding tissues.

ORIGINS OF THE CONCEPT

Perhaps the earliest description of FVT in ophthalmology was in 1972 by Behrendt, who discussed argon laser photocoagulation of intraretinal and vitreous FVs of neovascular membranes associated with diabetic retinopathy (1). The recent availability of visible light wavelength lasers led to numerous such novel approaches aimed at controlling ocular neovascularization. Understandably, all of those were related to retinal and anterior segment neovascularization, since they could be directly visualized by means of readily available optical devices. The choroidal vasculature, on the other hand, was not a popular target of interest, since direct visualization of it was obscured by retinal and choroidal pigments, and in sodium fluorescein angiography images it appeared mostly only as a diffuse "choriocapillaris (CC) flush." The deeper-lying vascular layers remained obscured so far as routine clinical observations were concerned.

At about the same time, in the early 1970s, the concept of routine clinical angiography of the choroidal circulation using ICG dye was being developed. ICG fluorescence angiography initially had been explored as an investigative tool for studying choroidal blood flow in animal experiments. However, since ICG dye already had a long documented history of biocompatibility, exploring its use in human subjects as well was compelling. Since up to that time, relatively little attention had been paid to the choroidal circulation compared with the retina, there was no well-defined clinical goal at first in visualizing human choroidal blood flow beyond academic curiosity, so a rudimentary survey of both normal and diseased eyes was undertaken (2). One of the first groups of patients considered in the survey was those with macular degeneration.

Figure 24.1 shows the simultaneously acquired fluorescein and ICG angiogram images of the first patient successfully studied by that methodology. The greatly improved ability to visualize the angioarchitecture of AMD-associated CNV lesions afforded by ICG angiography, coupled with the concept of FV photocoagulation, led to the first attempts at ICG-guided photocoagulation of CNV-FVs. Unfortunately, the results of those first attempts were not encouraging: clear differentiation between CNV afferent and efferent vessels was not easy—or in most cases not possible—since both spatial and temporal resolution of the early ICG fluorescence angiogram images were limited, the spot size and aiming precision of the first visible light laser photocoagulation delivery systems also were limited, and perhaps most importantly, the laser light wavelengths available were not ideally suited to the task.

For some time thereafter, the concept of FV photocoagulation was not seriously pursued as a clinical tool. Instead, the dominant treatment approach for AMD-associated CNV came to be based on Macular

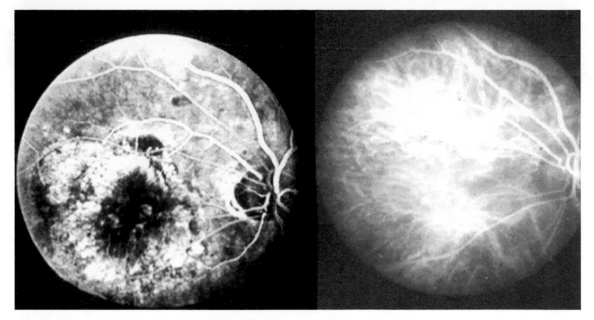

Figure 24.1 Simultaneously-acquired fluorescein (Left frame) and indocyanine green (1CG) (Right frame) angiogram images of the first patient with choroidal neovascularization studied using the ICG fluorescence angiography.

Photocoagulation Study (MPS) recommendations (3). These included destruction of the entire CNV membrane—as delineated by fluorescein angiography—along with an additional margin around the CNV, even when the procedure resulted in an immediate, non-recoverable additional loss of visual acuity (VA). The results of the MPS suggested that despite an immediate vision loss, three years later a patient so treated statistically would have better VA than if untreated. Those results notwithstanding, few ophthalmologists remained comfortable with the notion of having to destroy the retina in order to save it, preferring for the most part to avoid photocoagulation near the fovea.

REVISITING THE CONCEPT

The first notable clinical application of ICG fluorescence angiography was its use in guiding laser photocoagulation of CNV. This method was applied to patients whose clinical and fluorescein angiographic features did not meet the eligibility criteria for laser therapy defined by the MPS recommendations; generally it was applied to cases of poorly defined, or occult, CNV. In this application, use of ICG angiography resulted in improved localization of abnormal choroidal vessels, thereby making treatment by photocoagulation possible (4,5). While this clinical use of ICG undoubtedly contributed to sustaining interest in ICG angiography, arguably it was the commercial availability of the scanning laser ophthalmoscope (SLO) that contributed to the increasing interest in ICG angiography. Compared with the predominantly available commercial ICG angiography systems based on fundus camera optics capable of acquiring images at a rate of about one per second, the SLO afforded the ability to perform high-speed imaging. Ready access to high-speed ICG image acquisition systems was an important component of renewed interest in FV photocoagulation treatment.

The concept of FV photocoagulation was revisited as a treatment for AMD-associated CNV in February 1998 by Shiraga and coworkers; they reported the results of a pilot trial to assess the feasibility of extra-foveal photocoagulation of subfoveal CNV secondary to AMD (6). Their use of SLO ICG angiography resulted in the identification of FVs in 37 of 170 consecutive patients (22%). In 70% of those 37 cases (26 cases) extrafoveal photocoagulation of the FVs, using 575- to 630-nm wavelength light, resulted in the resolution of neovascular manifestations and improved or stabilized VA. The following December, Straurenghi and coworkers (7), also using SLO ICG angiography, reported finding treatable FVs in 15 of 22 patients having subfoveal CNV not amenable to the treatment suggested by the MPS (3). They successfully obliterated the FVs in 40% of the cases, resulting in improved or stabilized VA after more than two years. In a second group of 16 patients they reported a much higher success rate of 75%, attributed to the smaller FV diameters (less than 85 μm) found in this group. In December 1997, yet another series of FV treatments was begun using a high-speed, pulsed-laser (HSPL) fundus camera system for FV identification. (Flower RW, Glaser BM, Murphy RP, Macula Soc. Presentation, 1999.) The HSPL used in this study consisted of a Zeiss fundus camera modified to include a pulsed 805 nm-wavelength diode laser for excitation of ICG dye fluorescence in the choroidal circulation; images were acquired at a rate of 30 per second (8). In this latter study, a higher incidence (about 66%) of FV identification was achieved, apparently due to use of the HSPL system and different angiogram analysis techniques. Nevertheless, treatment success of the latter study appears to be equivalent to that of the other groups, even though the follow-up period was shorter and it focused on occult CNV, whereas the other studies appear to have focused on classic CNV.

The common experience of all these studies was that FV photocoagulation appeared to be a viable treatment approach and worthy of continued pursuit, even though the exact nature of the vessels being treated and the most efficacious application of laser energy remain to be determined. Clearly, there is a catch-22 associated with this methodology. There are no histological data on treated CNV-FVs, per se, and the only proof currently available of the accuracy of angiographic CNV-FV identification is improvement or stabilization of the patient's VA following treatment. But this standard of proof is biased toward failure, since conventional laser photocoagulation of CNV-FVs already has proven to be difficult or incomplete in some cases. Therefore, if the full potential of FV treatment is to be accurately assessed and eventually realized, a more consistently successful approach to laser photocoagulation must be devised. And at the same time, a much better understanding of the hemodynamic consequences of FV photocoagulation must be developed in order to facilitate a rational analysis of treatment successes and failures.

WHAT IS AN FV?

Properly characterizing CNV-FVs in terms of their locations within the choroid, their vessel wall structure, and the blood flow is a necessary step in developing the most efficacious photocoagulation method. In that regard, however, histological data about CNV angioarchitecture appear to be at odds with the angiographic appearance of the so-called FVs being treated.

Histological Appearance of CNV-FVs

The vessels passing through breaks in Bruch's membrane and connecting a CNV to the choroidal blood supply can be capillaries, arteries, or veins, as determined by the vessel wall structure. In general, CNV complexes up to 300 μm diameter have only one break containing a capillary-like vessel (9,10). Complexes on the order of 500 μm have two to four breaks, and at least one or two contain a capillary-like vessel; the others transmit only cells. CNV complexes of these dimensions consist of a single layer of capillary vessels on the inner surface of Bruch's membrane, and they arise from a layer of vessels which lies just beneath, instead of between, the intercapillary tissue pillars; so it is assumed these are new vessels replacing the choroidal capillaries. Because many tissue sections must be cut to find and track these vessels, there are only a few examples in which the vessels can actually be tracked in the choroid, and even then it is not always clear whether they lead to an artery or a vein. (Sarks JP and Sarks SH, written communication, March 14, 1999). Complexes on the order of 2000 μm have more than four breaks, and the vessels passing through are of medium size. These complexes usually are two layers thick, but still lie beneath the retinal pigment epithelium (RPE), and they can be served by well-formed arterial and venous vessels. Complexes from patients with disciform scars have breaks containing larger arteries and veins; these disrupt the RPE and invaded the retina. (Sarks SP and Sarks SH, written communication, March 14, 1999).

It has been suggested that on an average, there are 2.3 vessels passing through Bruch's membrane and connecting each CNV to the underlying choroidal vasculature (11). The frequency with which these vessels are capillaries, arteries, or veins has not yet been reported, but it is clear that the majority of penetrating vessels encountered are relatively short capillary-like vessels. It is clear also that such small vessels are not likely to be recognized in ICG angiogram images.

Angiographic Appearance of CNV-FVs

The most frequently identified and treated FVs reported in studies to date appear to be on the order of one to several millimeters long, a dimension quite large with respect to the penetrating vessels most frequently found in histological preparations. Figure 24.2 shows examples of FVs, identified using the HSPL fundus camera system, which have been successfully photocoagulated, resulting in improved or stabilized vision. In using that system, identification of FVs is made by first carefully examining the area surrounding the location of a known or suspected CNV complex in high-speed ICG angiogram images, since the most obvious characteristic of an FV is proximity to CNV. Some FVs are easily identified, as in Figure 24.2 (top left and right), when they are prominent and easily distinguishable from adjacent choroidal vessels. Often, however, FVs are less prominent, as in Figure 24.2 (bottom left and right), and identification requires use of an analytical technique such as phi-motion[a] angiography, which helps differentiate an FV from its surroundings by enhancing visualization of blood flow through it, toward the CNV. Determining direction of flow is essential to correctly identifying CNV-FVs—as opposed to their draining vessels—even when their angioarchitecture seems obvious.

Reconciling Histological and Angiographic Data

Clearly, the vessels identified in histological specimens as the conduits of blood from the CC to CNVs appear to be different from the so-called FVs identified in angiograms. Typically "FV" refers to an afferent vessel supplying blood to a particular vascular complex, one directly connected to the complex. To be precise, in the case of CNV that definition should apply to the short capillary-like vessels that penetrate Bruch's membrane and form a CNV/CC connection. The vessels in ICG angiograms dubbed FVs in the recently reported studies of CNV-FV photocoagulation, especially in the case of occult CNV; they meet the criterion of being afferent,

---

[a] Phi-motion is a phenomenon first identified by Wertheimer in 1912 (13); it refers to visual perception of motion where none exists. In a situation where there is a gap in visual information, the brain fills in what is missing. An example of the case in point is the appearance of two spatially separated points of light wherein first one is illuminated and, a finite time later, the second one is illuminated. The perception is that of a single point moving from the location of the first point to that of the second. By repeatedly viewing an appropriate segment of a high-speed angiogram image sequence in continuous loop fashion and at an appropriate speed, the phi-motion phenomenon accentuates perception of the movement of dye through vessels.

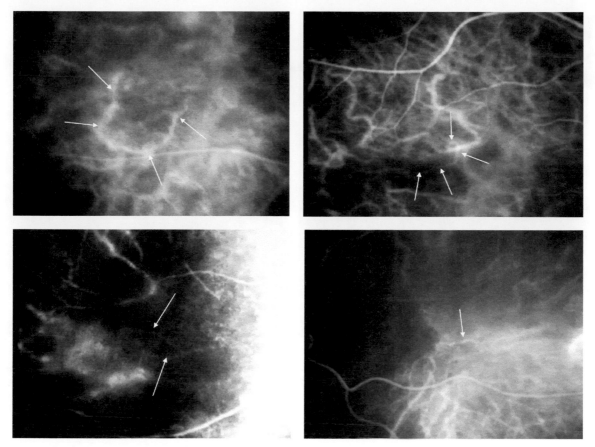

Figure 24.2 Examples of choroidal neovascularization feeder vessels, identified using the high-speed, pulsed-laser fundus camera system, that were successfully photocoagulated, resulting in improved or stabilized vision. In each case, arrows indicate the course of the feeder vessel. *Source*: From Ref. 12.

but they appear to be much larger than the capillary-like vessels seen in the histological specimens. Strictly speaking, therefore, the term "CNV-FV," as applied in angiographic descriptions, appears to be a misnomer for some other choroidal vessel; most likely Sattler's layer arterioles.

The so-called FVs seen in angiograms very much resemble vessels of the choroidal middle layer, or Sattler's layer, which lies just beneath the CC. A comparison of the ICG angiogram images of the FVs in Figure 24.2 with the scanning electron micrographs of corrosion casts of the anterior aspect of the CC in Figure 24.3 demonstrates this similarity. Therefore, it seems a reasonable assumption that the FVs identified in ICG angiograms and reported to have been successfully treated by photocoagulation are Sattler's layer arteriolar vessels. There is additional evidence to support the notion that the angiographically defined CNV-FVs are Sattler's layer vessels: a commonly observed characteristic of successfully treated FVs is their "beaded" appearance in ICG angiograms (RP Murphy, symposium presentation, Chicago, June 3, 2000); an example of that appearance is shown in Figure 24.4A. The most likely explanation for the beaded appearance is that the dye-filled FV is crossed throughout its length by smaller non-dye-filled choroidal vessels. This same phenomenon is more pronounced in high-speed ICG angiograms of rhesus monkey eyes following a carotid arterial dye injection, as

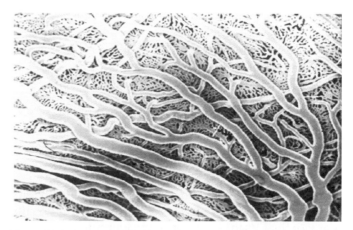

Figure 24.3 A scanning electron micrograph of a corrosion cast of the posterior (Sattler's) layer of small-diameter choroidal arteries and veins that feed and drain the choriocapillaris, which can be seen in the background. For the most part, the veins are oriented from the upper left-hand corner of the image toward the lower right-hand corner; they overlie the arteries. *Source*: From Ref. 12. Courtesy of Dr Andrzej W. Fryczkowski.

demonstrated in Figure 24.4B, wherein the carotid dye injection improves dye wave front definition, enhancing the observation of the temporal filling differences between various layers of choroidal vessels. When crossed by small non-dye-filled vessels, the crossings result in dark segments along the FV; when crossed by small dye-filled vessels, the crossings result in

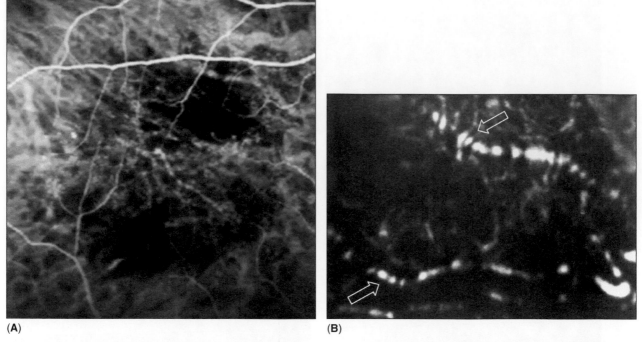

(A)   (B)

Figure 24.4 (**A**) Indocyanine green (ICG) angiogram demonstrating the commonly observed "beaded" appearance of choroidal neovascularization feeder vessels. (**B**) The same beaded appearance seen more prominently in the high-speed ICG angiograms of rhesus monkey eye following carotid arterial dye injection. When crossed by small non-dye-filled vessels, the intersections appear as dark segments along the feeder vessel (vessel indicated by the lower arrow); when crossed by small dye-filled vessels, the intersections appear hyperfluorescent due to additivity of fluorescence from the overlapping vessels (vessel indicated by the upper arrow). *Source*: From Ref. 14.

hyper-fluorescence, due to additivity of fluorescence from the overlapping vessels. The presence of small vessels between the FV and the CC fixes the FV location well below the CC, consistent with the notion that CNV-FVs are Sattler's layer vessels.

Additionally, Arnold and coworkers (15) have shown the choroids of AMD eyes to be as little as half the thickness of those in age-matched normal eyes (e.g., 90 µm compared with 180 g), primarily due to a significant decrease in the number of vessels that normally occupy the middle choroidal layers (Sattler's layer). So it is possible that the relatively high contrast of some FVs (Fig. 24.2) is a result of there being fewer than normal adjacent vessels in the same layer, and in the absence of the normal number of adjacent vessels, the FVs may have become preferential channels for blood flow through a diminished Sattler's layer. Therefore, the assumption that many of the FVs investigators have identified and photocoagulated are Sattler's layer arteriolar vessels is at least consistent with the evidence at hand.

THE RELATIONSHIP BETWEEN SATTLER'S LAYER VESSELS (FV$_s$) AND CNV

The explanation for an apparently successful photocoagulation treatment of so-called CNV-FVs (i.e., Sattler's layer vessels) lies in the hemodynamic relationship between the Sattler's layer vessels and the capillary-like vessels that form the CC/CNV communication.

An Anthropomorphic Model of the CC/CNV Connection

The relationship proposed to exist between these two types of vessels is modeled in Figure 24.5, wherein there

is no anatomical continuity between them, although functionally they behave as if there were. The figure also demonstrates how blood could move in a functionally contiguous manner from a Sattler's layer FV, into the CC, and then through a nearby capillary vessel leading to the CNV during the systolic phase of the intraocular pressure pulse.

By comparison to the sinusoid-like structure of the CC vascular plexus, it is likely that resistance to blood flow would be higher through a parallel CNV complex, connected to the CC by the capillary-like vessels that penetrate Bruch's membrane. In this model, blood flow through the CNV would occur, but it would not be as great as through the underlying CC. In keeping with the pulsatile nature of CC blood flow shown to exist as the result of the perpendicular interface of arterioles and the wide, flat choriocapillaries (8,16), a high hydrostatic pressure head must exist at the interface early during systole, relative to the surrounding CC (as indicated by the collapsed state of the choriocapillaries and the CNV vessels in Fig. 24.5A,B). In addition to pushing blood into the choriocapillaries, the pressure head would be partially dissipated in forcing some blood into the adjacent penetrating vessel. Thus, a small, pulsatile pressure gradient would be established through the CNV, even though the majority of flow would be through the CC. In this model, closure of the FV or even significant partial closure would have the effect of reducing the pressure head available at the penetrating vessel to a level so low that resistance to flow through the CNV could not be overcome, thereby effectively closing the CNV as well.

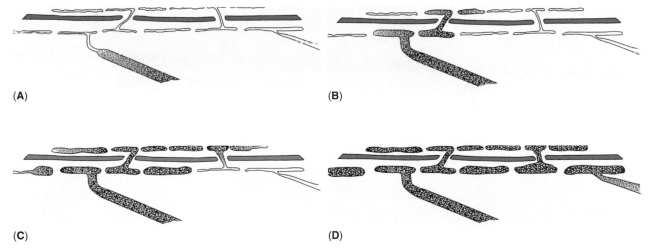

Figure 24.5 A schematic representation of the presumed relationship between a vessel penetrating Bruch's membrane (penetrating vessel) and connecting a choroidal neovascularization (CNV) membrane to the choriocapillaris (CC). The posterior margin of Bruch's membrane is represented by the dark horizontal line. A Sattler's layer choroidal arteriole (presumably a feeder vessel) is shown to be entering the CC from beneath. The four frames of the figure indicate how blood would move in a functionally contiguous manner from a Sattler's layer feeder vessel, into the CC, and then though a nearby penetrating vessel during the systolic phase of the intraocular pressure pulse even though the penetrating and feeder vessels are not anatomically contiguous: (**A**) At the onset of the blood pressure pulse, a high hydrostatic pressure head of blood (represented by the black dots) would develop at the perpendicular interface of arteriole and the wide, flat CC (as indicated by the collapsed state of the choriocapillaries and the CNV membrane). (**B**) Slightly later during the pulse, in addition to pushing blood into the choriocapillaries, part of the pressure head would be dissipated in forcing some blood into the adjacent penetrating vessel. Thus, a small pressure gradient would be established through the CNV. (**C**) Still later, blood flow through the CNV would occur, but it would not be as great as through the underlying CC, because by comparison to the sinusoid-like structure of the CC vascular plexus, it is likely that resistance to blood flow through a parallel CNV complex, connected to the CC by capillary-like penetrating vessels, would be higher. (**D**) Eventually, flow through the CNV would be complete. *Source*: From Ref. 12.

Thus, there is considerable evidence to support the hypothesis that ultimately the source of blood supplying a CNV is a Sattler's layer arteriole whose entry into the CC is situated near one of the capillary-like vessels that penetrate Bruch's membrane, forming a CC/CNV communication. That is, the FVs identified for focal photocoagulation treatment of CNV appear to be Sattler's layer arterioles that are functionally— but not directly physically—connected to the CNV. Throughout the rest of this discussion, the term CNV-FV is intended to imply a Sattler's layer vessel that is functionally contiguous with a CNV. This leads to the possibility that in some case a direct, anatomically contiguous connection between a Sattler's layer vessel and a CNV eventually could evolve, obviating any CC involvement at all; indeed, such an evolution might be the path leading from occult to classic CNV.

A Model of the FV/CC/CNV Hemodynamic Relationship

The simple anthropomorphic model of FV/CNV blood flow described above was conceived to account for the clinically observed resolution of retinal edema following FV photocoagulation, even when only partial FV vessel closure is achieved (12). However, since the submacular CC is a true vascular plexus—fed and drained by multiple interspersed arteries and veins— a much more sophisticated model is needed to describe the changes in CC blood flow beneath the CNV following FV photocoagulation. Therefore, a theoretical model for the human CC, based on available histologic and hemodynamic data, was developed to simulate the CC blood flow field before and after FV photocoagulation[b].

Known angioarchitectural and hemodynamic parameters for the CC and CNV from the literature were used to construct the theoretical model of a section of submacular CC and a small overlying CNV membrane shown in Figure 24.6. The CC plexus consists of two parallel sheets separated by 7.5 µm, between which 10 in. diameter columns are placed at regular intervals, leaving 15 µm wide channels in between to simulate the CC plexus. Isolated, but well-separated, precapillary arterioles and venules communicate with the CC plexus and perfuse it with blood. The cross-sectional dimensions of the arterioles and venules are of the same order as the CC thickness, h. The center-to-center spacing between adjacent arterioles and venules is much larger than h. Therefore, the CC was modeled as a planar porous medium containing a widely dispersed set of fluid inflows and outflows, simulating the feeding and draining vessels of Sattler's layer. Feeding arteriolar and draining venous vessels consist, respectively, of 7.5 and 15 µm diameter tubes entering the CC from beneath.

An overlying CNV membrane was modeled as a parallel miniature version of the CC, but with smaller dimensions that will result in a significantly higher resistance to fluid flow. The communication between the CNV and the CC is by way of two capillary-dimensioned

[b] This model was developed in collaboration with C. von Kerczek. L. Zhu, A. Ernest, C. Eggleton, and L.D.T. Topoleski from the Department of Mechanical Engineering University of Maryland, Baltimore, Maryland, USA.

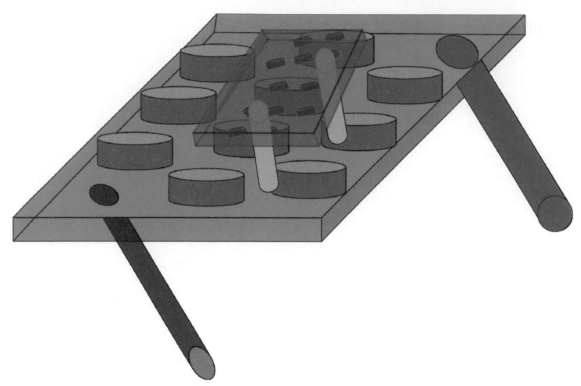

Figure 24.6 A Schematic representation of the computer simulated model of the choriocapillaris (CC) that would supply simulated overlying choroidal neovascularization (CNV). The CC segment is represented by the thin green rectangular box; the orange disks within the volume of the box represent the interstitial spaces surrounded by the network of choriocapillaries. One Sattler's layer arteriolar (*red cylinder*) vessel and one venous (*blue cylinder*) vessel are shown connected to the posterior CC. A CNV membrane is represented by the very thin purple rectangular box atop the orange discs. Two capillary-like vessels (green cylinders) that penetrate Bruch's membrane to form the CC/CNV connection (penetrating vessels) are shown. In the text, these are referred to as penetrating vessels. In the simulation, the positions of the penetrating vessels with respect to the Sattler's layer vessels were varied. *Source*: From Ref. 14.

vessels that penetrate Bruch's membrane. In the model, the position of the CNV could be changed in order to achieve various spatial relationships between the penetrating vessels and the Sattler's layer vessels that feed and drain the CC.

This theoretical model became the basis for computer simulation of blood flow distribution in a segment of human sub-foveal CC approximately 1300 × 1000 μm in area. The actual placement of the multiple Sattler's layer vessels to feed and drain blood from the simulated CC plexus segment was made according to the histologically determined locations of those vessels in one normal human eye (17). Figure 24.7 shows the anterior aspect of the computer simulated segment of that human submacular CC, marked with the actual locations of arteriolar and venous vessels, Sattler's layer vessels connected to its posterior aspect; the figure also shows the simulated CNV in two different locations. Blood flow rates in the feeding arterioles and venules were then estimated by matching the predicted precapillary arteriole and venule pressure difference to experimentally measured data; the experimentally measured maximum pressure difference between a feeding arteriole and venule was found to be 4.5 mmHg (18). Experimentally measured pressures and pressure differences were applied across the feeding and draining vessels in order to generate maps of blood flow through the computer-simulated model CC segment. Figure 24.8 shows the

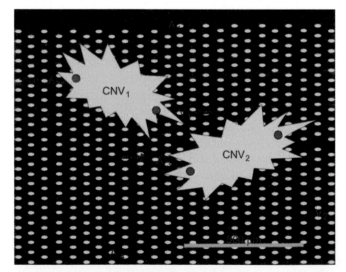

Figure 24.7 The anterior aspect of the computer simulated segment of a human submacular choriocapillaris, marked with the actual locations of arteriolar and venous vessels Sattler's layer vessels connected to its posterior aspect; the figure also shows the simulated choroidal neovascularization in two different locations. *Abbreviations*: CNV, choroidal neovascularization. *Source*: From Ref. 14.

normal isobar and iso-blood-speed distributions in the computer simulated segment of CC from Figure 24.7; it also shows how those distributions are altered when one of the Sattler's layer feeding arterioles is completely occluded.

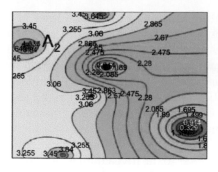
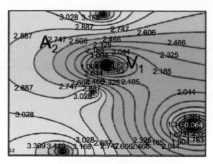
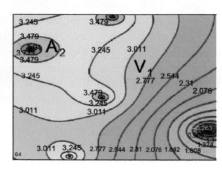
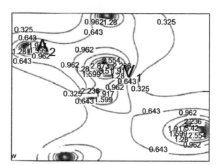
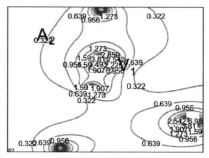
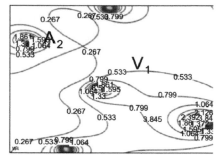

Figure 24.8 Isogramic maps of the blood pressure and blood speed fields of the choriocapillaris (CC) segment shown In Figure 24.7 under normal and simulated vascular photocoagulation conditions. The isogramic lines in the left-hand two frames identify the locations of constant pressure (upper frame) and flow (lower frame) throughout the CC segment under normal conditions. The pattern of these lines change, as shown in the other pairs of frames, when either the underlying Sattler's layer arteries (middle frames) or veins (right-hand frames) are occluded. The particular vessels occluded in these examples are arteriole A1, and venule V1, identified in Figure 24.7. *Source*: From Ref. 14.

A significant reduction in the local CC pressure probably results in significant changes in the blood flow through an overlying CNV network, since the driving force for CNV blood flow is the pressure difference between the capillary-like vessels that penetrate Bruch's membrane, forming the CC/CNV communication. Clinical observations indicate that partial—as well as complete—photocoagulation of the (presumed Sattler's layer) FV adjacent to a CNV's penetrating vessel(s) is an effective means of decreasing the blood flow in the CNV (BM Glaser, RP Murphy, G Staurenghi, personal communications, 1999). Therefore, the model also was used to simulate blood flow through a CNV before and after FV laser photocoagulation; the simulation was performed for the CNV membrane situated in two different locations, as indicated in Figure 24.7. The first location, CNV #1, was between arteriole #2 and venule #1, while the second, CNV #2, was between arteriole #3 and a point equidistant from venules #1 and #2. Photocoagulation of arteriole #2 and of venule #1 resulted in significant reduction of CNV #1 blood flow (71% and 79%, respectively), with similar results in CNV #2 when arteriole #3 was photocoagulated (84% reduction). On the other hand, even the complete closure of venules #1 or #2 produced less than 30% decrease in blood velocity through CNV #2.

Implications of the FV/CC/CNV Hemodynamic Relationship

This model predicts that even 50% closure of a blood vessel entering the posterior aspect of the CC in the vicinity of a capillary-like vessel leading to a CNV can be effective in reducing or possibly stopping CNV blood flow, regardless of whether that vessel is a feeding arteriole or a draining venule. In other words, the important hemodynamic event with respect to reducing or stopping CNV blood flow is a significant reduction of the blood pressure—hence, blood flow as well—in the local underlying CC. Thus, the predictions of the present computer-simulated model support the novel approach to CNV management made previously, namely that (i) rather than total obliteration of a CNV (which frequently results in recurrence), the end point of laser photocoagulation treatment can be reduction of CNV blood flow to the extent that undesirable manifestations of the CNV—most notably retinal edema—are halted or reversed and (ii) that CNV blood flow reduction can be mediated by reduction of blood flow through the underlying CC (12).

There are two important implications to that novel approach, one related to FV treatment and the other related to the mechanics of successful CNV treatments in general. Regarding FV photocoagulation treatment of CNV, the selection criterion for targeted FVs might be extended to include venous as well as arteriolar vessels entering the posterior CC in the vicinity of a CNV membrane. If, indeed, reduction of the underlying CC blood flow is the important treatment goal, then depending upon the orientation of the CNV's penetrating vessels with respect to the field of vessels feeding and draining the CC, targeting veins or veins in conjunction with arteries may yield the best results. After all, the ramifications of occluding a venous drainage channel to a true vascular plexus, like the posterior pole CC, is not the same as occlusion of the drainage vein of a true end-arteriolar vascular complex. In the former case, blood is diverted to adjacent venous channels, without excessive increase in capillary transmural pressure; whereas in the latter case, venous occlusion likely results in blood flow stasis and elevation of capillary transmural pressure to a level near that across the feeding arterial vessel wall.

Since the predicted relationship between CC and CNV blood flows actually is independent of the specific means by which CC blood flow is reduced, the second implication of the results is that reduction of CC blood flow underlying a CNV membrane may be a component mechanism common to successful CNV photocoagulation treatments, including photodynamic therapy (PDT), transpupillary thermal therapy (TTT), and drusen photocoagulation. It is well established that post-PDT angiograms routinely evidence reduced CC fluorescence (19), and that appears also to be the case following TTT (20). In the case of TTT, reduced CC blood flow may be due to increased resistance to plexus blood flow resulting from heat-induced interstitial tissue swelling and concomitant reduction of CC luninal space. Angiographic data specifically related to submacular blood flow following photocoagulation destruction of macular drusen have not been presented anywhere; however, it has been demonstrated that CC obliteration occurs with application of moderate to heavy laser burns and that loss of choriocapillaries can add significant resistance to blood flow through the CC plexus (8).

If reduced CC blood flow is a component mechanism of successful CNV treatment, regardless of the photocoagulation modality used, then FV photocoagulation arguably might be viewed as the most effective method. The difference between FV photocoagulation and the other methods is analogous to removing a weed from a lawn by pulling out its roots (FV) versus just cutting off the weed's leaves. It can be argued that FV photocoagulation is the most precise of the various methods in terms of manipulating CC blood flow, and it minimizes the area of tissue–laser interaction. Moreover, since blood flow through a particular CC area apparently can be manipulated by modulation of adjacent venous or as arteriolar vessels connected to the plexus' anterior side, it may be that the most precise manipulation of CC blood flow—and hence, treatment of CNV—will be by controlled, partial photocoagulation of carefully selected combinations of arterioles and venules in Sattler's layer vessels.

DEVELOPMENT OF A MORE EFFICACIOUS METHOD OF FV TREATMENT

The models of CNV-FVs are consistent with the clinical observation that often, even incomplete closure of an FV produces reduction of CNV dye filling, resolution of associated edema, and improved VA. Of course, partial closure of targeted FVs at present is an unintended endpoint of Argon and Krypton laser photocoagulation application. In such cases, failure to completely close the relatively deep-lying targeted vessels may be attributable to generation of an insufficiently high temperature

gradient, emanating from the RPE where laser light-to-heat transduction occurs. The temperature gradient that is produced does extend into the sensory retina and can produce significant damage there, so the location for FV photocoagulation must be chosen so as not to involve the fovea. It would be desirable, therefore, to avoid the concomitant retinal damage and to make FV photocoagulation more efficient and predictable. This would have the additional potential benefit of allowing such treatment to be applied much closer to the fovea than is presently possible, thereby increasing the number of patients who might benefit from CNV-FV treatment.

The Concept of ICG-DEP

An example of a successfully treated FV is shown in Figure 24.9, and it also shows an undesirable side effect as well: damage to the nerve fiber layer overlying the site of FV photocoagulation. Since CNV-FVs apparently lie below the plane of the CC, a method of photocoagulation that moves the epicenter of the laser-generated heat closer to those vessels and away from the sensory retina will be an improvement over the presently available method. The concept of ICG-DEP has that potential and, therefore, should be revisited for this application, bearing in mind that its use must be optimized to accommodate the characteristics of the targeted choroidal vasculature. The main premise of DEP is that application of laser light energy with a wavelength matched to the primary wavelength absorbed by a bolus of dye passing through the target blood vessel produces the most efficient photocoagulation burn in terms of vessel closure with minimum damage to surrounding tissue. Figure 24.10 demonstrates the main aspects of ICG-DEP and compares it with FV photocoagulation by conventional laser light photocoagulation. The concept of improving the efficiency of the photocoagulation process by ICG-dye enhancement is not new to the treatment of AMD-related CNV, as Reichel and coworkers utilized it for treating poorly defined subfoveal CNV. Eventually they reported their initial clinical investigation in 10 patients (21), but in terms of visual outcome, their results were equivocal, and the technique did not achieve widespread use. The particular dye-enhancement technique they used relied on the absorption of infrared laser light energy by dye-stained choroidal blood vessel walls minutes following dye injection. That apparently is a very inefficient process, compared with the one in which the same laser energy is absorbed by dye molecules within the target vessels during the transit of a high-concentration dye bolus (12).

A Combined ICG Angiography/DEP System

Performance of ICG-DEP requires the use of a laser delivery system that permits visualization of intravenously injected ICG dye as it traverses the vasculature. Such a system was constructed from a Zeiss fundus camera (Carl Zeiss, Oberkochen, Germany) modified to include a pulsed diode laser light source and a synchronized, gated CCD camera for performing high-speed ICG angiography, as previously described (8,22). The fundus camera was further modified so that the output

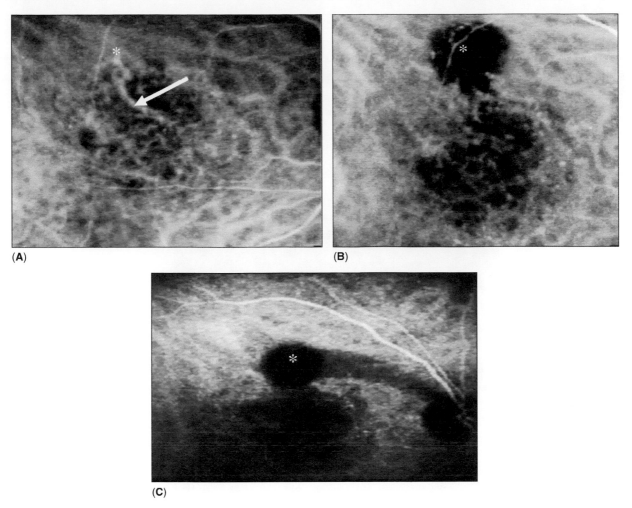

Figure 24.9 Post-treatment indocyanine green angiogram images of a successfully treated feeder vessel (FV). (**A**) Pretreatment: the FV is indicated by asterisk. (**B**) Post-treatment: note lack of CNV filling. (**C**) Image shows an undesirable side effect as well: damage to the nerve fiber layer overlying the site of FV photocoagulation. *Source*: From Ref. 12.

tip of the fiber optic of an 810 nm diode laser photocoagulator (Oculight SLx, Iris Medical Instruments, Mountain View, California, USA) can be positioned in the plane of the fundus illumination optics pathway normally occupied by the internal fixation pointer; that plane is conjugate to the fundus of the subject's eye. The He–Ne aiming beam emitted by the photocoagulator appears as a sharply focused spot when viewed through the fundus camera's video system, and the position of the fiber optic with respect to the subject's fundus can be controlled by the micromanipulator's X- and Y-adjustments. With this configuration, it is possible to deliver 810 nm photocoagulation light pulses to precisely located areas of the fundus while observing the fundus with visible light through the fundus camera eyepiece, making it possible to synchronize photocoagulation laser pulse delivery with arrival of a dye bolus at a targeted vessel site. The fundus camera/laser photocoagulation system is shown in Figure 24.11.

Clinical Application of ICG-DEP

Use of the ICG dye-enhanced camera system is demonstrated in the three frames of Figure 24.12, which show ICG angiogram images from a patient treated with ICG-DEP.

Incarceration of ICG dye immediately following laser photocoagulation (center frame) not only provides immediate feedback as to the success of the procedure, but constitutes as a strongly absorbing target for further laser application without the need to inject additional dye boluses. The reduction in retinal tissue damage concomitant to FV laser photocoagulation using ICG dye-enhancement is demonstrated in Figure 24.13, which compares the extent of RPE damage resulting from application of identical laser burns to identical choroidal arteries of a rabbit eye, one with and one without the presence of a transiting high-concentration dye bolus.

A single center, prospective, randomized study of FVT using ICG-DEP was conducted by Dr G. Staurenghi (University of Brescia, Italy) under the auspices of Novadaq Technologies, Inc. (Toronto, Canada). The objective of the study was to evaluate the safety and effectiveness of choroidal FV closure in the presence of ICG using the above described fundus camera/laser photocoagulation system. In the study, forty patients were evaluated for presence of visible FVs associated with CNV. Upon identification of the FVs, the patients were randomized into one of two treatment arms: one group of 20 patients was treated by choroidal FV photocoagulation during ICG dye

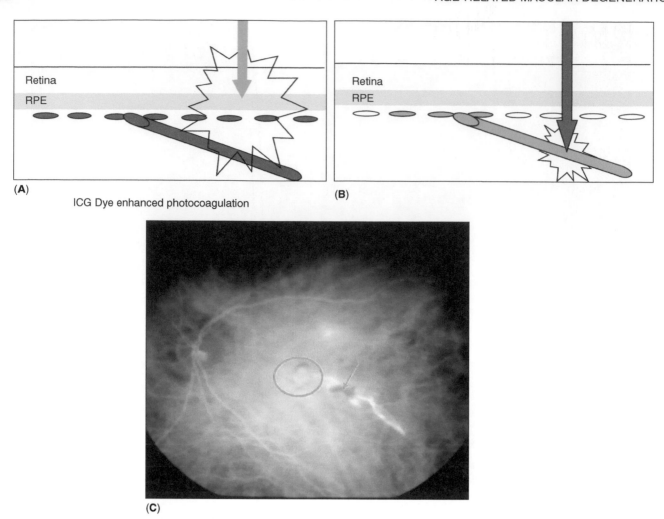

ICG Dye enhanced photocoagulation

Figure 24.10 Schematic comparison of choroidal vessel photocoagulation by (**A**) conventional laser, (**B**) ICG dye-enhanced laser, and (**C**) ICG angiogram image made immediately post-treatment with ICG-DEP demonstrating incarceration of ICG dye in the treated feeder vessel (arrow) and choroidal neovascularization membrane (circle). Abbreviations: ICG, indocyanine green; RPE, retinal pigment epithelium. *Source*: From Ref. 12. Courtesy of Dr B. Eric Jones, Baltimore, Maryland, USA.

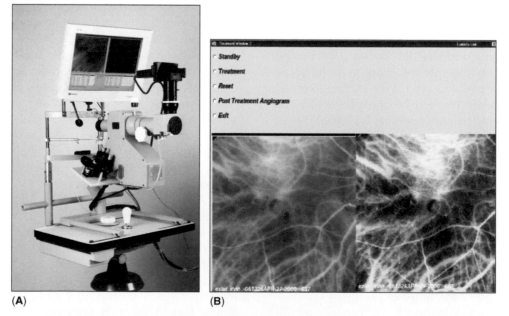

Figure 24.11 The fundus camera/photocoagulation system. (**A**) There is a joystick control on the left side of the fundus camera body for positioning the 810 nm wavelength photocoagulation laser beam on the patient's fundus. (**B**) The photocoagulation laser aiming beam (red spot) is visualized on the patient's live indocyanine green (ICG) angiogram, which is seen in the left pane of the monitor located above the patient's head. Reference ICG angiogram image from a previously made diagnostic study to determine the location of a treatable feeder vessel (FV); the targeted FV is indicated on the reference image by a white cross.

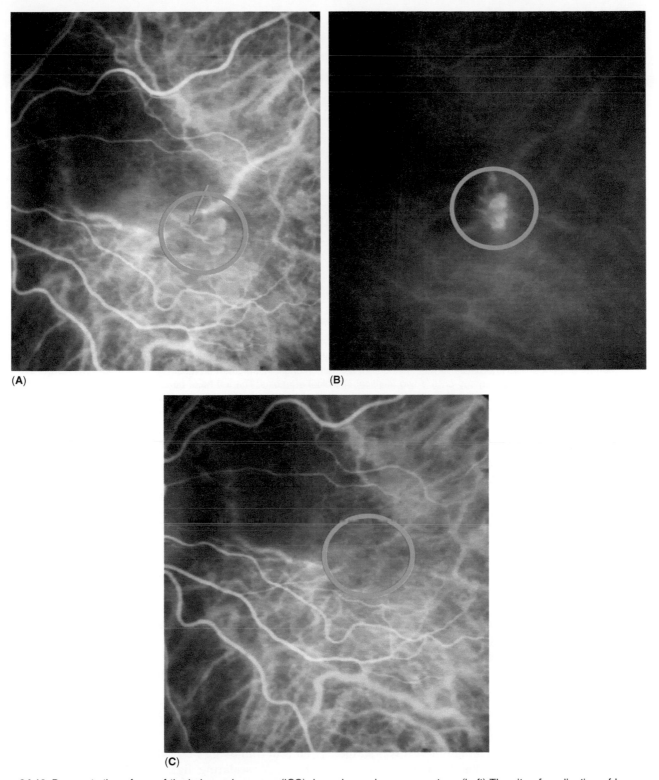

Figure 24.12 Demonstration of use of the indocyanine green (ICG) dye-enhanced camera system. (Left) The site of application of laser energy during subsequent transit of a high-concentration dye bolus (arrow). (Middle) Incarceration of ICG dye in the choroidal neovascularization (CNV) (circle) distal to the burn site. (Right) Validation of vessel closure by follow-up ICG angiography a week later (the circle indicates the location of the now non-perfused CNV).

transit (ICG-DEP arm); the other group of 20 patients (control arm) was identically using the same device system, but FV photocoagulation was done without ICG-DEP, using the laser energy alone. All patients were followed and/or treated at 2, 4, 8, 12 weeks, and 6 months; with one additional follow-up at 12 months post-first treatment.

The study demonstrated that the fundus camera/ laser photocoagulation system was easy to use, and that treatment session times decreased with experience with the system. The entire diagnostic, treatment, and post-treatment confirmation ICG angiography took 21–23 minutes; this was similar for both treatment

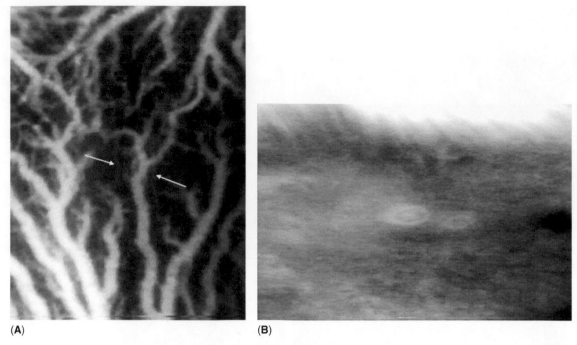

(A)   **(B)**

Figure 24.13 Showsthe reduction in retinal tissue damage concomitant to feeder vessel laser photocoagulation using indocyanine green (ICG) dye-enhancement, using identical choroidal arteries arising from a common origin in a pigmented rabbit eye as a model. (**A**) Arrows indicate the locations of laser burns of identical energy on the two identical choroidal arterioles. The left-hand burn was applied without use of ICG dye-enhancement, and the right-hand burn was placed during the transit of a high-concentration bolus of ICG dye. (**B**) Comparison of the extent of retinal pigment epithelium damage resulting from application of the identical laser burns inferior to the medullary rays.

arms. On average, four to five treatment sessions were required for complete treatment in both arms over the course of the study. And on average, the ICG-DEP arm used approximately seven times less energy/treatment session than the control arm (5.7 J per treatment session *vs.* 38.9 J per treatment session) to close targeted choroidal FVs.

Importantly, treatment was more effective and more durable in the ICG-DEP arm, as 90% of the patients were able to have their choroidal FVs closed or partially closed, with 70% of those vessels remaining closed at the last treatment assessment, compared with 77% and 44%, respectively, in the control arm. During the course of the study, 45% fewer patients in the ICG-DEP arm went on to require alternative treatments for their wet AMD than patients in the control arm. VA at the end of the treatment phase of this trial, as measured by the Early Treatment Diabetic Retinopathy Scale, showed that, for the whole treated population, on average the VA was stable, and 29% of all patients seen at this study milestone had an improvement in VA. Of those patients who completed the study as per the study-prescribed treatment regimen, at the last scheduled treatment visit, 67% had stable or improved VA, with 42% having 1–4 line improvement in VA, while 33% had a decrease of more than 3 lines of VA: none experienced severe vision loss (more than 6 lines of VA). Of the nine patients who followed the study-prescribed treatment regimen and had a VA equal or better than 20/100 at entry, seven (78%) had stable or improved VA at the last treatment visit, with four (44%) having a 1–4 line improvement in VA and two (22%) had more than 3 line decrease in VA.

Overall, the study added to the body of data demonstrating the efficacy of the concept of FVT of wet AMD. In addition, it demonstrated that the fundus camera/laser photocoagulation system simplifies FV treatment by allowing for real-time visualization of choroidal FVs during treatment. Moreover, FV photocoagulation with ICG-DEP produced a more effective and more durable treatment outcome than FV photocoagulation using laser only.

Photodynamic Therapy and CNV-FV Treatment

As an alternative to laser treatments of FVs using 630 nm red, 576 nm yellow, 514 nm argon green, and 810 nm diode laser, photodynamic therapy (PDT) has also been employed to occlude or reduce FV blood flow (23,24). The strategy behind this treatment is that verteporfin-mediated destruction of FVs may be accomplished with less collateral damage to the overlying retina. A phase 1 clinical trial using PDT with standard doses of verteporfin and escalating light doses of increasing duration ($50\ J/cm^2$, $100\ J/cm^2$, $125\ J/cm^2$, and $150\ J/cm^2$) directed at FVs was performed on nine patients with a single FV supplying a minimally classic CNV lesion on FA and high-speed ICG (23). The study found a mean increase on ETDRS visual acuity of 2.1 lines (p = 0.07) 3 months after treatment. Transient closure of the FV was achieved angiographically in 3 eyes at various light doses, hypoperfusion of the FV was achieved in 3 eyes, and neither closure nor hypoperfusion occurred in 3 eyes. At final follow-up, all FVs were reperfused. There was no evidence of retinal damage from the PDT. The authors concluded that verteporfin-enhanced FV therapy does not cause subfoveal retinal damage and may have the potential to improve central vision in subfoveal CNV in NVAMD, but this treatment was not recommended as monotherapy for CNV. This study was performed before anti-VEGF treatments were readily available.

THE FUTURE OF CNV-FV TREATMENT

The current anti-vascular endothelial growth factor (anti-VEGF) drugs, Avastin®, Lucentis®, or Eylea®, have experienced significant clinical success to date. It appears that these anti-VEGF drugs have such strong antipermeability effects on CNV membrane vessels that fluid outflow into surrounding tissues is reduced or stopped, resulting in stabilized or even improved VA. This can occur early, before the CNV angioarchitecture is substantially changed in the process, leaving some CNV blood flow intact; but repeated injections are needed. Interestingly, this is analogous to what happens in FVT, where only partial FV closure occurs or where reperfusion recurs following complete closure. Apparently, even partial FV closure results in reduced transmural pressure across CNV membrane vessels, which in turn reduces fluid outflow. In these cases, CNV angioarchitecture also appears substantially unchanged, and there is no concomitant recurrent edema, resulting in stabilized or improved VA. It has been postulated that during the period of reduced transmural pressure, neovascular membrane maturation progresses to a level of vessel structural integrity such that fluid outflow no longer occurs once the higher pre-FVT transmural pressures are reestablished.

If the foregoing understanding of the methods of action of the anti-VEGF and FVTs continues to hold true, then their use in combination might prove to be symbiotic in a way that leads to a very effective treatment approach, since both act to reduce edema resulting from CNV membrane fluid outflow, but by different pathways. However, as a stand-alone treatment, FVT ultimately still may prove to be the most desirable approach, because even when repeated treatments are applied, those treatments are totally noninvasive with respect to the peripheral retina and wall of the eye itself, and they are inexpensive. Moreover, consideration should be given to the long-term ramifications of successfully achieving the currently sought clinical treatment endpoint, namely CNV obliteration.

To the extent that CNV (especially "occult" CNV) serves to augment or replace functionally compromised choriocapillaries, successful destruction of the CNV ultimately will leave the adjacent sensory retina and RPE without adequate metabolic support from the choroidal circulation. In that situation, the RPE and retina likely will atrophy. It is for this reason that CNV blood flow obliteration as the treatment end point should be reconsidered in favor of modulating CNV blood flow just to the point that retinal edema is ameliorated, since that leaves a level of choroidal metabolic support for the RPE and retina in place. Owing to FVT's highly localized application and the ability it affords for immediate CNV blood flow assessment, DEP-FVT allows for a level of individual patient treatment titration that drug-based treatment cannot provide.

Aggressive CNV behavior, such as rapid membrane growth, edema formation, etc., has been viewed as a destructive event, and the conventional treatment aims to remedy such behavior by complete CNV obliteration. But the frequent recurrence of CNV following such treatment could be nature's continuing effort to compensate for the original—and perhaps now exacerbated—defect. Instead, such aggressive CNV behavior could be viewed as an overcompensation for some metabolic or other blood flow–related defect. And if laser treatment were to be applied in such a way as to just reduce the blood flow to aggressive CNV by an appropriate amount—perhaps until the CNV vasculature matures—then further aggressive behavior might be avoided; those cases of inadvertent incomplete FV closure resulting in improved vision are examples.

Photocoagulating the FVs supplying CNV associated with AMD can be not just a successful treatment method (6,7) especially for occult CNV. Indeed, there may be an important difference between the response of CNV evoked by direct application of laser energy, as in conventional treatment, and that evoked by reducing blood flow through the otherwise undisturbed membrane. If ultimately FV photocoagulation treatment were to be refined along these lines, the laser would become more a precision instrument to modulate blood flow than a weapon for destruction of the very retinal tissue whose function we are trying to conserve. Additionally, because of the pre- and post-treatment high-speed ICG angiograms the method requires, information about choroidal hemodynamics is being accrued that otherwise probably would never be available.

SUMMARY POINTS

- Identification of FVs is made by first carefully examining the area surrounding the location of a known or suspected CNV complex in high-speed ICG angiogram images.
- It is a reasonable assumption that the FVs identified in ICG angiograms and reported to have been successfully treated by photocoagulation are Sattler's layer arteriolar vessels.
- Clinical observations indicate that partial—as well as complete—photocoagulation of the (presumed Sattler's layer) FV adjacent to a CNV's penetrating vessel(s) is an effective means of decreasing the blood flow in the CNV.
- FV photocoagulation may be the most precise method of manipulating CC blood flow and minimizes the area of tissue/laser interaction.
- CNV blood flow eradication as the treatment endpoint should be reconsidered and replaced with modulation of the CNV blood flow just to the point that retinal edema is ameliorated, since that leaves a level of choroidal metabolic support for the RPE and retina in place.

REFERENCES

1. Behrendt T. Therapeutic vascular occlusions in diabetic retinopathy. Arch Ophthalmol 1972; 87: 629–33.
2. Patz A, Flower RW, Klein ML, et al. Clinical application of indocyanine green angiography. In: DeLaey JJ, ed. International Symposium on Fluorescein Angiography. Documenta Ophthalmologica Proceedings Series. Vol. 9. The Hague: Dr. W. Junk b.v, 1976: 245.
3. Macular Photocoagulation Study Group. Subfoveal neovascular lesions in age-related macular degeneration: guidelines for evaluation and treatment in the macular photocoagulation study. Arch Ophthalmol 1991; 109: 1242–57.
4. Slakter JS, Yannuzzi LA, Sorensen JS, et al. A pilot study of indocyanine green videoangiography-guided laser treatment of primary occult choroidal neovascularizaton. Arch Ophthalmol 1994; 112: 465–72.
5. Schwartz S, Guyer DR, Yannuzzi LA, et al. Indocyanine green videoangiography guided laser photocoagulation of primary occult choroidal neovascularizaton in age-related macular degeneration. Invest Ophthalmol Vis Sci 1995; 36: S244.
6. Shiraga F, Ojima Y, Matsuo T, et al. Feeder vessel photocoagulation of subfoveal choroidal neovascularization secondary to age-related macular degeneration. Ophthalmology 1998; 105: 662–9.
7. Staurenghi G, Orzalesi N, La Capria A, et al. Laser treatment of feeder vessels in subfoveal choroidal neovascular membranes: a revisitation using dynamic indocyanine green angiography. Ophthalmology 1998; 105: 2297–305.
8. Flower RW. Extraction of choriocapillaris hemodynamic data from ICG fluorescence angiograms. Invest Ophthalmol Vis Sci 1993; 34: 2720–9.
9. Sarks SH. Aging and degeneration in the macular region: a clinicopathological study. Br J Ophthalmol 1976; 60: 324–41.
10. Schneider S, Greven CM, Green WR. Photocoagulation of well-defined choroidal neovascularization in age-related macular degeneration. Retina 1998; 18: 242–50.
11. Green WR, Enger C. Age-related macular degeneration: histopathologic studies. the 1992 Lorenz E Zimmerman lecture. Ophthalmology 1993; 100: 1519–35.
12. Flower RW. Experimental studies of indocyanine green dye-enhanced photocoagulation of choroidal neovascularization feeder vessels. Am J Ophthalmol 2000; 129: 501–12.
13. Wertheimer M. Experimentelle Studien ueber das Sehen von Bewegung. Z Psychol 1912; 61: 161–265.
14. Flower RW, von Kerczek C, Zhu L, et al. A theoretical investigation of the role of choriocapillaris blood flow in treatment of sub-foveal choroidal neovascularization associated with age-related macular degeneration. Am J Ophthalmol 2001; 132: 85–93.
15. Arnold JJ, Sarks SH, Killingsworth MC, et al. Reticular pseudodrusen: a risk factor in age-related maculopathy. Retina 1995; 15: 183–91.
16. Flower RW. High-speed ICG angiography. In: Yannuzzi LA, Flower RW, Slakter JS, eds. Indocyanine Green Angiography. St. Louis: Mosby, 1997: 86–94.
17. Fryczkowski AW, Sherman MD. Scanning electron microscopy of human ocular vascular casts: the submacular choriocapillaris. Acta Anat (Basel) 1988; 132: 265–9.
18. Maepea O. Pressures in the anterior ciliary arteries, choroidal veins and choriocapillaris. Exp Eye Res 1992; 54: 731–6.
19. Flower RW, Snyder WA. Expanded hypothesis on the mechanism of photodynamic therapy action on choroidal neovascularization. Retina 1999; 19: 365–9.
20. Reichel E, Berrocal AM, Ip M, et al. Transpupillary thermotherapy (TTT) of occult subfoveal choroidal neovascularization in patients with age-related macular degeneration. Ophthalmology 1999; 106: 1908–14.
21. Reichel E, Puliafito CA, Duker JS, et al. Indocyanine green dye-enhanced diode laser photocoagulation of poorly defined subfoveal choroidal neovascularization. Ophthalmic Surg 1994; 25: 195–201.
22. Flower RW. Variability in choriocapillaris blood flow distribution. Invest Ophthalmol Vis Sci 1995; 36: 1247–58.
23. Kozak I, Cheng L, Cochran DE, Freeman WR. Phase I clinical trial results of verteporfin enhanced feeder vessel therapy in subfoveal choroidal neovascularisation in age related macular degeneration. Br J Ophthalmol 2006; 90: 1152–6.
24. Sickenberg M, Ballini JP, van den Bergh H. Photothera-pie dyamique a la Visudyne et occlusion du vasisseua afferent: rationnel d' une association synergique et options cliniques illustrees. J French Ophthalmol 2004; 27: 93–102.

25

Macular translocation and other surgical treatments

Francisco A. Folgar and Cynthia A. Toth

INTRODUCTION
Overview
With human lifespan rising in developed nations, age-related macular degeneration (AMD) continues to grow as the leading cause of central vision loss and legal blindness in elderly adults (1,2). Current medical treatment with vitamin and mineral supplementation lowers the risk of progression to neovascular advanced AMD, and it may potentially delay the onset of non-neovascular advanced AMD characterized by central geographic atrophy (GA) (3). Medical treatments for neovascular AMD include thermal laser photocoagulation, photodynamic therapy (PDT) with intravenous verteporfin, and intravitreal injection of antibodies targeting vascular endothelial growth factor (VEGF).

Prospective randomized clinical trials have shown that intravitreal delivery of anti-VEGF biologic agents achieve better clinical outcomes for patients with neovascular AMD than any previously available therapy (4–6). The Minimally classic/occult trial of anti-VEGF Antibody Ranibizumab in the treatment of neovascular AMD (MARINA) demonstrated that monthly injections of ranibizumab achieved a 95% rate of visual acuity maintenance and 34% rate of improvement of 3 lines or better for eyes with occult or type 1 choroidal neovascularization (CNV) after a two-year follow-up (4). The anti-VEGF ANtibody for the treatment of predominantly classic CNV in AMD (ANCHOR) trial demonstrated that ranibizumab achieved a 96% rate of visual acuity maintenance and 40% rate of improvement of 3 lines or better for eyes with predominantly classic or type 2 CNV after a one-year follow-up (5). The safety and efficacy reported in these trials established anti-VEGF intravitreal injections as the current standard for neovascular AMD treatment. Yet, other factors must also be weighed while treating patients with advanced AMD. The MARINA and ANCHOR trials excluded eyes with large submacular hemorrhages and large tears of the retinal pigment epithelium (RPE). A subset of patients who were enrolled in these trials did not respond to treatment, losing 3 or more lines of visual acuity after a two-year follow-up (7). Subretinal pathology such as fibrosis, atrophic scar, and central GA are unresponsive to VEGF signaling. Furthermore, medication tachyphylaxis and the burden of indefinite injection regimens also merit the consideration of alternatives to first-line medical therapy.

Surgical treatments for AMD were developed prior to the advent of anti-VEGF agents and they continue to play an important, albeit diminished, role in the treatment of advanced AMD. In this chapter, we will discuss the techniques, management, and outcomes of surgical treatment for AMD. We will primarily discuss the technique of macular translocation with 360-degree peripheral retinectomy (MT360), which achieves translocation of the macula by complete separation and rotation of the neurosensory retina from the original diseased RPE bed. Macular translocation surgery is indicated for the treatment of subfoveal CNV that is not amenable to laser photocoagulation and unresponsive to PDT or anti-VEGF agents. It may also treat vision loss in select cases of central GA. We will also discuss a variant of this technique known as limited macular translocation with scleral imbrication, submacular surgery for the removal of subfoveal CNV, the displacement of submacular hemorrhage secondary to AMD, and the transplantation of autologous RPE–choroid patch grafts. Although no multicenter prospective randomized clinical trials exist for macular translocation or RPE–choroid graft transplantation, the prospective Submacular Surgery Trials (SSTs) sponsored by the National Eye Institute failed to demonstrate favorable outcomes with early submacular surgery techniques (8,9). Thanks to significant advancements in vitreoretinal surgery and imaging, there has been renewed interest in adopting new techniques for the surgical treatment of AMD.

Clinical Rationale
Preservation or recovery of visual function can be achieved in eyes with subfoveal CNV by translocation of the neurosensory retina of the fovea over a healthier subretinal bed of RPE and choriocapillaris before permanent retinal damage occurs. The rationale for this outcome is that photoreceptors can be preserved if the fovea is placed above more normal subretinal tissues. The density of RPE cells and the pattern of circulation in the choriocapillaris are not uniform throughout the fundus. RPE cells are columnar and narrow (less than 14 μm in diameter and up to 30 μm in height) in the fovea and become flatter and wider (up to 60 μm in diameter) in the periphery (10). In the normal eye, the number of photoreceptors binding each RPE cell is roughly constant, regardless of the location in the fundus (10). Narrow, taller, and more tightly packed RPE cells accommodate a higher density of photoreceptors

and concentrate a greater amount of melanin pigmentation in the region of the fovea. The submacular choroid has a lobular architecture that allows for extremely fast circulation beneath the fovea, indeed the fastest circulation in the human body (11,12). The extramacular choroid of the equator and the periphery has parallel vasculature with capillaries in spindle and ladder-like configurations that circulate blood 5–10 times less rapidly than the submacular choroid (11). Despite these differences, successful outcomes after macular translocation surgery suggest that extrafoveal RPE and choriocapillaris can support translocated foveal photoreceptors. Transfer of the fovea onto a healthier bed of RPE and choriocapillaris, and beyond the borders of the CNV complex, allows for ablation or removal of CNV without damaging the fovea. Both preservation of visual function and permanent regression of CNV can be achieved.

Historical Background

The treatment of AMD with vitreoretinal surgery was first described in humans by Machemer and De Juan in 1988 (13). The first three human cases of macular translocation with 360-degree retinectomy were reported by Machemer and Steinhorst in 1993 (14). One patient had an uncomplicated translocation with significant improvement in vision, but the other two patients developed proliferative vitreoretinopathy (PVR) and postoperative retinal detachment (14). The original MT360 procedure has undergone numerous modifications that have reduced the duration of surgery, reduced postoperative complication rates, and improved clinical outcomes. Other modifications have been introduced and subsequently abandoned, due to worse patient outcomes. For example, 360-degree retinectomy was replaced with a 180-degree partial retinectomy in an attempt to decrease the risk of PVR and postoperative retinal detachment (15–17). Ninomiya et al., Akduman et al., and Ohji et al. separately reported increased rates of PVR and worse vision outcomes with partial retinectomy, leading to a return to full 360-degree retinectomy for macular translocation (15–17).

Surgical experience has led to the consensus that the macula should be rotated in the superior rather than inferior direction for various reasons. First, early cases of MT360 were complicated by PVR and retinal detachment, which was usually observed in the inferior retina (14). Although the overall rate of detachment has decreased, superior rotation of the fovea further reduces the chance of foveal detachment in the event of PVR formation. Second, gravity usually extends submacular hemorrhages inferiorly, thus damaging the inferior submacular RPE and making this site less fit to receive the displaced fovea (18,19). Likewise, the inferior macula is also predisposed to a greater risk from postoperative hemorrhage associated with recurrent CNV (20). Third, postoperative cyclotropia from superior translocation can be corrected by combined surgery which includes inferior oblique muscle advancement (21). This muscle surgery is far more effective and less challenging than the superior oblique tendon advancement that would be required after inferior macular translocation (21,22). Fourth, superior macular displacement places the scotoma from the inferiorly displaced CNV site into the superior visual field, where it is less likely to be a factor in ambulation and daily activities.

The original MT360 procedure did not involve extraocular muscle surgery, but this has become a cornerstone of the procedure. After MT360 without muscle correction, postoperative management was complicated by torsion of up to 55 degrees and binocular diplopia and cyclotropia (23,24). Current technique produces an upward rotation of 30 – 45 degrees, which exceeds the maximum adult amplitude of cyclofusion of 15 degrees (19). Eckardt introduced simultaneous extraocular muscle surgery with MT360 to counteract the induced excyclotropia, resulting in smaller degrees of residual cyclotorsion and less diplopia (24). While many continue to use this technique, it was modified by Freedman into a staged procedure with extraocular muscle surgery performed after MT360, which provides two advantages. First, it permits the clinician to measure the induced cyclotropia after MT360 to achieve more precise correction. Second, it allows for two separate and shorter translocation and extraocular muscle surgeries to be performed under local anesthesia (21).

PREOPERATIVE CONSIDERATIONS
Indications

The indications for MT360 in advanced AMD have changed in the era of anti-VEGF treatment, and the clinical and diagnostic criteria for performing MT360 may differ among experienced surgeons. Macular translocation is one of very few treatments shown to benefit patients with central GA in non-neovascular AMD; however, cases have been reported of rapid recurrence of GA at the displaced foveal site after translocation (25,26). Regardless of the characteristics of the AMD lesion and preoperative visual acuity, Uppal et al. have shown that the strongest indicators of foveal function after MT360 are the duration of vision loss and the degree of preoperative foveal fixation (27). The following general principles help to guide the evaluation of surgical candidates:

- Bilateral disease with significant vision loss in the fellow first eye at the time of evaluating the second affected eye. However, surgery should be contraindicated if either eye has no light perception (NLP) vision.
- Loss of central vision for less than three to six months in the second affected eye, moderate-to-good foveal fixation, and the potential for visual improvement based on diagnostic testing and clinical judgment.
- Pathology that is not responsive to anti-VEGF agents, including subretinal fibrosis, RPE tear, large submacular hemorrhage, and central GA without severe retinal thinning.
- Previous history of PDT, intravitreal anti-VEGF, and intravitreal corticosteroid are not contraindications.

- Previous extrafoveal or juxtafoveal laser photocoagulation for CNV is not a contraindication if there is no retinal thinning in the fovea on optical coherence tomography (OCT).
- Foveal laser photocoagulation and central neurosensory retinal atrophy on OCT are contraindications.
- In the presence of other diseases, such as diabetic retinopathy, optic neuropathy, glaucoma, and retinal vascular occlusions, surgery may be contraindicated.

Examination and Diagnostic Testing

A thorough examination and a diagnostic work-up are paramount to successful macular translocation for patients with advanced AMD. We recommend the following approach:

- Slit-lamp biomicroscopy to assess slit-beam foveal fixation, anterior segment anatomy, and lens status. Conjunctival scarring from previous surgery may influence the surgeon's approach to pars plana vitrectomy and subsequent extraocular muscle surgery. The cornea should be clear for proper wide field visualization during surgery, and phakic patients should undergo cataract surgery with phacoemulsification and posterior chamber intraocular lens placement either before or during MT360.
- Peripheral retinal examination with scleral depression to identify vitreoretinal tufts, retinal holes, and chorioretinal scars that may predispose to intraoperative retinal breaks and may impede formation of a total retinal detachment during MT360.
- Visual acuity, fixation, and microperimetry testing may provide information about foveal sensitivity and function before MT360; however, preoperative results have not been shown to correlate with foveal recovery and vision outcomes (28).
- Fundus photography including color, red-free, and infrared to assess pigmentary changes, subretinal hemorrhage, retinal vasculature, and preretinal membranes.
- Intravenous fluorescein angiography (with or without indocyanine green angiography) to determine leakage from submacular CNV, retinal angiomatous proliferation (RAP), transmission defects from RPE atrophy, and the degree of perfusion of the choroid and retinal capillaries.
- Fundus autofluorescence imaging captures the extent of inflammatory injury or atrophy of the RPE. It is useful to assess the metabolic health of the RPE at the new foveal site.
- Spectral domain OCT (SD-OCT) has dramatically improved our understanding of the ultrastructure of the retina and subretinal tissues in AMD. Examination with SD-OCT allows the clinician to evaluate the integrity of the outer nuclear layer, external limiting membrane (ELM), and photoreceptor outer segments of the fovea before and after MT360. It may reveal chorioretinal scarring and RPE atrophy otherwise masked by CNV, which may affect final vision outcomes.

SURGICAL TECHNIQUE AND MANAGEMENT
Macular Translocation with 360-Degree Peripheral Retinectomy

The original technique developed by Machemer started with a standard three-port pars plana vitrectomy under general anesthesia (14). A total retinal detachment was created by transscleral retinal hydrodissection with fluid infusion through multiple posterior sclerotomies. Returning into the vitreous cavity, a 360-degree peripheral retinectomy was performed and submacular CNV was removed. After a partial silicone oil fill, the entire retina was rotated in the superonasal direction around the attachment at the optic disc attachment. A complete silicone oil fill was performed, followed by 360-degree endolaser retinopexy to complete the procedure. Postoperative recurrence of CNV at the old foveal site was treated with laser photocoagulation. The first cases did not undergo extraocular muscle surgery, so patients with good visual recovery in the operated eye and some degree of functional vision in the contralateral eye often developed severe diplopia and cyclotropia (23). Proprioception did not adjust to the new perception of the environment, even when objects appeared straight from the newly translocated eye (with fellow eye patched), creating difficulty with daily activities (23). The current technique for MT360 is the result of major modifications to the Machemer technique that were developed soon after by Eckhardt (24), Tano (15,17), and Toth (19,21). Clinical outcomes have significantly improved with modern MT360, and the procedure will continue to evolve with advancements in pharmacology and vitreoretinal surgery.

The technique we describe here consists of three separate stages designed to allow each surgery to be performed without the need for general anesthesia: first, macular translocation with 360-degree retinectomy and silicone oil; second, extraocular muscle surgery to correct torsional diplopia; and third, removal of silicone oil. The first two stages may be combined into one procedure under general anesthesia, with muscle surgery performed first to correct the diplopia induced by translocation.

The high degree of postoperative cataract formation with pars plana vitrectomy in the elderly AMD population warrants cataract extraction before or during MT360. Under monitored anesthesia care with local retrobulbar block, all phakic eyes initially undergo cataract phacoemulsification and posterior chamber intraocular lens implantation. Then a standard pars plana vitrectomy is performed with complete separation of the posterior hyaloid and a thorough, meticulous shaving of the vitreous base. The procedure has been performed successfully with 20-gauge and small-gauge vitrectomy systems. Wide angle visualization is best achieved with a noncontact binocular indirect ophthalmic microscope (BIOM) system or a panoramic contact lens system.

After complete vitrectomy, an artificial retinal detachment is created by hydrodissection *ab interno*. In the method described by Toth, a single tiny round peripheral retinotomy is created at the level of the infero-nasal vitreous base with the vitrector. Enriched balanced salt solution (BSS Plus®, Alcon, Fort Worth, Texas, USA) vitrectomy infusion fluid is introduced into the subretinal space through a soft-tipped cannula over the peripheral retinotomy. Infusion continues until the neurosensory retina is detached from the RPE in all quadrants. Total retinal detachment is effectively created with a pressure gradient established by higher subretinal infusion pressure and lower vitreous cavity pressure. In order to achieve this gradient, the vitreous cavity infusion is lowered to just slightly above normal intraocular pressure while allowing outflow through an enlarged sclerotomy or cannula. For example, a 20-gauge outflow cannula will be used for a 23-gauge infusion cannula. If only a partial bullous retinal detachment forms, this may be caused by fluid outflow via a peripheral retinal break. A fluid air exchange will shift the subretinal fluid posteriorly and away from peripheral breaks, allowing for continued detachment. Alternately, multiple subretinal infusions via a 41-gauge flexible polyamide-tipped cannula will also produce the desired total retinal detachment. After complete detachment, partial fluid–air exchange again shifts subretinal fluid posteriorly to assure detachment of the macula and to avoid retinal breaks with the movement of instruments through the sclerotomies.

Placement of chandelier illumination is useful for the remainder of the surgery. Macular translocation proceeds with a retinectomy in the anterior vitreous base, nearly at the ora serrata, made with the vitrectomy cutter or scissors. If the vitrectomy cutter is used, perfluorooctane (PFO) heavy liquid is placed over the macula to displace subretinal fluid from the posterior pole, prevent blood from settling in the macula, and stabilize movement of the bullous detachment. The retinectomy is extended with either instrument around the ora serrata for 360 degrees until the peripheral retina is freed. Diathermy is seldom needed due to the anterior location of the incision. Perfluorooctane liquid is removed, and the temporal retina is reflected nasally in order to remove submacular hemorrhage, fibrosis, and CNV. If the decision is made to remove CNV, hemostasis is maintained by raising intraocular pressure, applying direct pressure, and diathermy to any sites of choroidal bleeding.

After placement of a small amount of preretinal PFO, Toth has shown that the retina can be rotated by catching the inner surface with a diamond-dusted soft silicone tip instrument and sliding the retina superiorly to displace the macula approximately 30–45 degrees. The old macular CNV bed is now centered under the inferotemporal arcade. With the macula in the desired position, more PFO is added to fill the vitreous cavity to the edges of the retinectomy. Several rows of continuous or tightly scattered endolaser photocoagulation are applied in a 360-degree circumference posterior to the retinectomy margins. A complete PFO–oil exchange is performed as would be typical for a giant retinal tear, to avoid retinal slippage. In the case of aphakia, the vitrectomy cutter may be used to create an inferior peripheral iridectomy prior to silicone oil (Fig. 25.1).

Extraocular Muscle Surgery

The aim of the second stage of surgery is to produce an excyclotorsion that will correct the intorsional diplopia induced by superior macular translocation. The technique described by Freedman involves the measurement of the cyclotropia by Maddox rod testing four to eight weeks after initial macular translocation (21). On average eight weeks after macular translocation, the operated eye undergoes extraocular muscle surgery. With the patient under monitored local anesthesia, the strabismus surgeon performs an inferior oblique resection with 5-mm myectomy (or alternatively, an inferior oblique advancement to the temporal edge of the superior rectus), followed by superior oblique tenotomy and recession. Larger angles of deviation greater than 35 degrees require, in addition, superior transposition of the lateral rectus muscle to the temporal border of the superior rectus and inferior transposition of the medial rectus muscle to the nasal border of the inferior rectus. Cases of refractory cyclotropia and diplopia after MT360 and extraocular muscle surgery are treated most often with muscle surgery of the contralateral eye (22).

The third and final stage involves removal of silicone oil. This procedure is performed on average three months after initial macular translocation. Silicone oil in the vitreous cavity is exchanged with BSS Plus fluid infusion though a standard pars plana approach. During this final operative stage, any eyes that remained aphakic should be treated with intraocular lens implantation. Eyes without lens capsule support may benefit from a number of techniques including anterior chamber placement, iris fixation, or external scleral fixation.

Postoperative Management and Complications

After completion of the first stage of MT360, patients alternate side-to-side positioning while lying down for one week, in order to tamponade the very peripheral retinectomy margin and diminish localized PVR formation. Patients should be examined for signs of PVR and retinal detachment, which may require repair with pars plana vitrectomy and replacement of silicone oil. Clinical studies for MT360 have reported retinal detachment with a prevalence of 8–43%, with earlier studies reporting higher detachment rates than later studies (17,19,24,29–35).

Fluorescein angiography and SD-OCT should be used to monitor for recurrent CNV at the old foveal site, and the appearance of CNV or GA threatening the relocated fovea and new RPE bed. As the prevalence of retinal detachment has decreased, recurrent CNV has become the most common complication after MT360 with a prevalence of 3–56% (17,19,24,29–35). This wide variability is likely in part due to the variety of approaches to treating CNV during MT360, including manual membrane removal, laser photocoagulation, anti-VEGF agents, and observation. Most reported cases of recurrent CNV originate from the old CNV

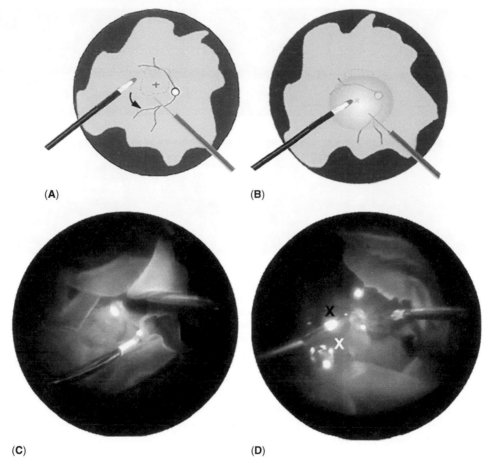

Figure 25.1 Macular translocation with 360-degree retinectomy with an inverted view of the left eye from the perspective of the vitreoretinal surgeon positioned at 12 o'clock, and instrument ports placed at 2 and 10 o'clock positions. Third and fourth ports for chandelier illumination and the fluid infusion line are not shown. **(A-B)** Diagrams show superior rotation of the detached retina and final positioning of the macula under perfluorooctane liquid. **(C-D)** Intraoperative video frames of the same steps, showing the new location of the fovea (*white X*) and the old site where the neovascular membrane was removed (*black X*), which now lies under the inferotemporal vascular arcade. *Source*: From Ref. 19.

bed and not *de novo* at the new foveal location (36). Recurrent CNV is managed with intravitreal anti-VEGF agents as first-line treatment and may be supplemented with laser photocoagulation, since these lesions have been shown to nearly always originate from the extrafoveal preoperative site of CNV (36). Residual CNV that has not been removed intraoperatively is accessible for treatment with laser photocoagulation or PDT as early as one week after macular translocation.

Cystoid macular edema (CME) is another frequently reported complication with a variable prevalence of 6–70%, but the use of SD-OCT has led to increased reporting of this complication and better understanding of why visual recovery may lag behind otherwise anatomically successful translocation (19,24,28,30,32–35). In a study of 84 eyes after MT360 for AMD, the effect of postoperative CME was evaluated in those eyes with successful preservation of the photoreceptor and RPE layers on SD-OCT. At one year after surgery, mean visual acuity improvement lagged by 1 line of vision in eyes with CME, compared with eyes without intraretinal fluid, but visual acuity improved over a longer follow-up when CME resolved (35). Cystoid macular edema is treated on an as-needed basis

with injections of periocular corticosteroids, intravitreal corticosteroids, or intravitreal anti-VEGF agents (32,33). Similarly, the 7–28% incidence of postoperative epiretinal membrane has been characterized by higher incidence reported in later studies due to SD-OCT (17,19,24,28,30–35).

Central RPE atrophy at the new foveal site after MT360 may be the result of the spread of an atrophic lesion created by juxtafoveal laser photocoagulation or RPE tear in neovascular AMD, as well as recurrence of central GA in non-neovascular AMD (25,26). There is currently no consensus on the management of recurrence of foveal GA after macular translocation (25). We emphasize the importance of preoperative diagnostic retinal imaging with SD-OCT to determine whether there is reasonable photoreceptor morphology in the fovea prior to translocation, and with fundus autofluorescence to evaluate the recipient RPE bed.

FUNCTIONAL OUTCOMES
Visual Function
Numerous clinical studies published over the last 10 years have demonstrated significant preservation or improvement of vision with MT360. Study results from the last 10 years are difficult to compare with one

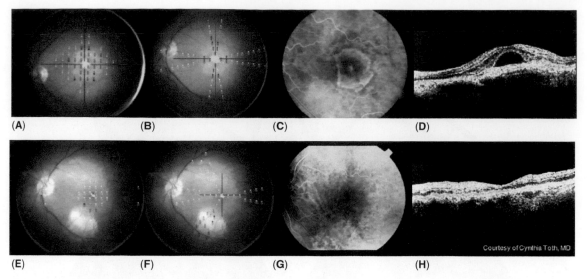

Courtesy of Cynthia Toth, MD

Figure 25.2 Color fundus photographs with superimposed microperimetry, fluorescein angiogram, and optical coherence tomography (from left to right) of a 76 year-old patient with 20/250 visual acuity in the left eye, decreased retinal sensitivity and loss of fixation on microperimetry (**A-B**), classic choroidal neovascularization (CNV) with distinct borders (**C**), subretinal fluid, and preserved outer retinal anatomy (**D**). Six months after MT360 with 20/64 visual acuity, improved macular sensitivity, recovery of central fixation and reading ability (**E-F**), staining at the inferior old CNV site without leakage (**G**), and improved foveal architecture with residual nasal folds (**H**).

another, as the introduction of anti-VEGF agents during this period has changed the disease profile of patients referred for surgical management. Across 10 published clinical studies enrolling at least 15 eyes with advanced AMD undergoing MT360, and at least 12 months of follow-up, the percentile of eyes with stable or better distance vision was 42–94% (17,19,24,29–34,37). The prevalence of eyes with final distance vision loss of 3 lines or worse was 7–35% (17,19,24,29–34,37). In the largest prospective studies of MT360, Aisenbrey et al. (n = 90 eyes) and Mruthyunjaya et al. (n = 64 eyes) have reported improvement of 3 lines or better in 27% and 30%, respectively, and vision loss of three lines or worse in 32% and 12%, respectively (30,32). In a prospective randomized interventional trial comparing MT360 with PDT, the MT360 group (n = 25 eyes) demonstrated stabilization of distance vision and improvement of near vision, whereas the PDT group had significant loss of both distance and near vision (34). Clinical studies testing near vision after MT360 have reported even greater improvement in near visual acuity and infrared-tracked reading function than distance visual function after translocation (24,28,32,34,37–40).

Visual Field and Electrophysiological Changes

Goldmann kinetic perimetry testing after MT360 shows good preservation of the visual field, but with 10–22% peripheral narrowing in all meridians due to 360-degree retinectomy and photocoagulation (41,42). The bed of CNV removed during surgery may manifest as a superotemporal extension of the blind spot on the Goldmann visual field (41). Microperimetry testing shows significant improvement in macular sensitivity after MT360, but still below the sensitivity of healthy controls, suggesting good recovery of retinal function despite structural damage from AMD (43). Microperimetry also

clearly reveals the superior scotoma corresponding to the inferior site of CNV removal (43). A pairwise analysis of microperimetry has failed to show a correlation between preoperative and postoperative macular sensitivity (28). Therefore, visual field testing and microperimetry are generally poor prognostic tests for MT360 (Fig. 25.2).

Electroretinography (ERG) studies after early cases of MT360 showed decreased scotopic and photopic full-field ERG amplitudes, which suggested retinal dysfunction secondary to artificial retinal detachment with 360-degree retinectomy (44,45). A subsequent multifocal ERG study showed increased macular ERG amplitudes and correlated vision improvement after MT360, arguing that foveal function does improve after surgery (46). A study of elecrooculography (EOG) recorded after MT360 showed a decrease of mean dark trough with normal Arden ratio after MT360, suggesting subnormal RPE function at the new foveal site (47). The postoperative mean dark trough on EOG appears to be correlated with vision outcomes (47).

Fundus Autofluorescence and Optical Coherence Tomography

Chen et al. first described fundus autofluorescence after MT360 in 33 eyes as a pattern of macular hyperautofluorescence that corresponded on SD-OCT to outer segment shortening and loss of the inner segment band (48). These eyes had central foveal variations: blocking hypoautofluorescence from CNV, hyperautofluorescence from CME, or a near-normal autofluorescent pattern (48). A larger series of 84 eyes showed that 23% had postoperative macular hypoautofluorescence and 8% had mixed or granular autofluorescence, both associated with nonsignificant vision improvement and SD-OCT features of photoreceptor layer thinning, loss of the ELM and outer segments, RPE atrophy, and

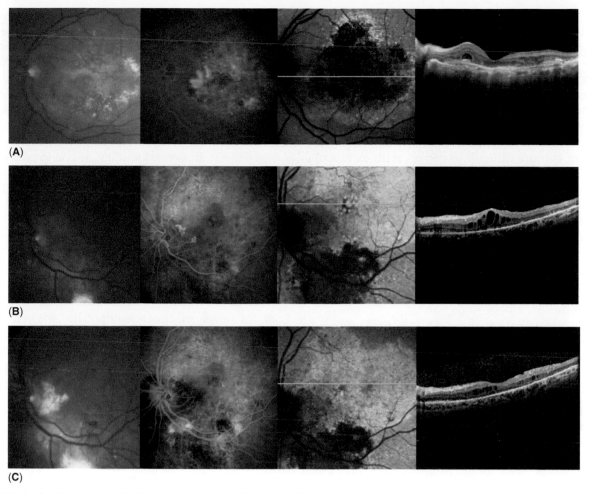

Figure 25.3 Color fundus photograph, fluorescein angiogram, fundus autofluorescence, and spectral domain optical coherence tomography (from left to right) of a 69-year-old patient at the following periods: **(A)** One month before MT360 with 20/200 visual acuity active choroidal neovascularization (CNV), diffuse macular edema, and atrophy of the retinal pigment epithelium in the left eye. **(B)** One year after MT360 with recurrent neovascularization at the superior edge of the old CNV site and cystoid macular edema (CME) in the translocated fovea. **(C)** Three years after MT360 with 20/80 visual acuity, quiescent CNV, and regressing CME after adjuvant laser and intravitreal anti-angiogenic treatments. *Source*: From Ref. 119.

increased choroidal reflectivity (35). Another 54% had uniform hyperautofluorescence and 16% had petaloid hyperautofluorescence patterns, similar to those described by Chen et al., and both correlated with significantly improved vision after surgery and SD-OCT features of outer segment shortening with loss of the inner segment band, but preserved ELM and RPE structures (35). These patterns were not correlated with preoperative vision or AMD phenotype. Autofluorescence imaging of this in-vivo model of photoreceptor transplantation suggests that retinal signaling factors induce the recipient RPE to proceed most often to a chronic hyperautofluorescent state associated with good functional outcomes, or occasionally to an atrophic hypoautofluorescent state with decreased vision (Fig. 25.3).

Sensorimotor Changes
The amount of torsion resulting from MT360 is usually greater than 30 degrees, which exceeds the maximum adult cyclofusion amplitude of 15 degrees (21). Improvements in extraocular muscle surgery techniques have greatly reduced symptomatic sensorimotor dysfunction

after MT360. The prevalence of residual diplopia was initially reported by 32% of patients after the combined procedure of compensatory muscle surgery at the same time as macular translocation described by Eckardt (24). The remainder of patients experienced the benefit of immediate cyclofusion after surgery. Modifications to the combined technique by Pertile and Claes resulted in residual diplopia after initial surgery being reported by only 6% of patients (29). Subjective patient reporting of diplopia, however, is not the only measure of successful muscle surgery. Other factors contribute to the long-term development of torsion and diplopia, including good vision in the contralateral eye with respect to the operated eye, suppression of one eye, and the natural cyclofusion amplitude of each person (49).

Quantitative measurement of strabismus and torsion is a more objective indicator of extraocular muscle surgery success. Freedman et al. published sensorimotor outcomes after MT360 and muscle surgery in patients with advanced AMD. In 53 patients, they measured residual hypertropia of 4 ± 10 prism diopters, exotropia of 13 ± 11 prism diopters, and intorsion of 4.5 ± 6.3 degrees postoperatively (21). In 63 patients, they reported that 41% were completely free of sensorimotor complaints, 32% experienced intermittent diplopia or cyclotropia, and 5% had constant postoperative diplopia and mild cyclotropia at 6 months which required correction with prism lenses or additional muscle surgery (21). In 32 patients without diplopia who underwent fusion testing, no patients demonstrated recovery of binocular fusion after MT360 (21).

Inferior macular translocation produces incyclotorsion that is more difficult to correct with extraocular muscle surgery than superior translocation. Freedman et al. have reported residual hypertropia of 11 ± 6 prism diopters, exotropia of 20 ± 24 prism diopters, and extorsion of 8.3 ± 4.8 degrees postoperatively in seven patients who required inferior rotation (22). These patients were more likely to have symptomatic diplopia and additional corrective muscle procedures (22).

Quality of Life
Patients with bilateral advanced AMD have significantly reduced quality of life (50). In two clinical studies, MT360 has been shown to dramatically improve quality of life as scored by the standardized National Eye Institute Vision Function Questionnaire (51,52). The quality-of-life score after MT360 is most strongly associated with improvement in reading ability, although it is also correlated with the magnitude of distance and near-vision improvement (51,52). Advanced AMD and MT360 have not been found to affect systemic health morbidity in standardized scoring studies (51).

LIMITED MACULAR TRANSLOCATION
Overview
Early studies of macular translocation surgery with 360-degree retinectomy reported complications of PVR and retinal detachment, which prompted investigators to develop macular translocation techniques that would not require the creation of a large retinectomy (14,53). In 1998, De Juan described the technique of limited macular translocation with scleral imbrication that subsequently has undergone several modifications (17,54–58). Regardless of which modified technique is used, the fundamental principles for achieving successful outcomes are careful patient selection and sufficient foveal displacement to reach healthier subretinal tissues and allow fovea-sparing ablation of CNV. The minimum required foveal displacement is the distance between the foveal center and a point on the border of the subfoveal lesion in the direction of the desired translocation (59). Consideration of the surgeon's median foveal displacement and a patient's minimum required displacement, allow the surgeon to have a good idea of the likelihood of achieving effective macular translocation in that patient.

Limited macular translocation for neovascular AMD was first reported by De Juan in a case series of three patients, in which all eyes gained three or more lines of vision (54). The study investigators reported a larger series of 102 eyes in which 48% had improvement

of two or more lines, 19% lost two or more lines of vision, and 62% achieved sufficient foveal displacement for complete postoperative laser photocoagulation of CNV (55). Median foveal displacement was 1200 μm at six months after inferior limited translocation (55). The distance of foveal displacement was one of the limitations in the use of this treatment for neovascular AMD. Subsequent studies, with infolding or outfolding of the sclera, produced an average foveal displacement of 1142–1576 μm (60–62). In several studies, at one to two years after surgery, 38–41% of eyes improved at least 2–3 lines, 24–40% of patients had lost approximately 3 or more lines, and 64–81% achieved effective foveal displacement (20,60–62).

Surgical Technique
Limited macular translocation begins with the exposure of bare sclera in the superotemporal quadrant and placement of imbrication mattress sutures through the sclera at the level of the equator. The original technique described by De Juan required a crescent-shaped scleral resection and apposition of the edges of the scleral defect, but this was discontinued as subsequent case series showed that the same effect can be achieved without tissue resection (20,54,55). Subtotal pars plana vitrectomy is performed with complete detachment of the posterior hyaloid. Steady subretinal infusion of BSS Plus with a very small gauge (39–41 gauge) flexible polyamide-tipped cannula produces a temporal retinal detachment. Although the macula often remains attached, partial fluid–air exchange is initiated once the retinal detachment has progressed anterior to the site of the imbrication sutures. During initial fluid–air exchange, subretinal fluid will shift to the posterior pole, separating the macula all the way to the temporal edge of the optic disc. Repeat fluid–air exchanges or addition of more subretinal fluid may be required to complete the macular and temporal retinal detachment.

Scleral imbrication under a partial retinal detachment achieves limited translocation of the fovea onto an adjacent bed of healthier RPE and choroid. The globe is softened by temporarily discontinuing fluid infusion or allowing outflow through a sclerotomy site. The preplaced scleral sutures are tightened to produce permanent infolding and anterior-posterior shortening of the scleral wall. Temporary scleral imbrication has also been described with the use of absorbable polyglactin sutures (63). Subtotal air fill is sufficient for tamponade, but retinal breaks may require laser retinopexy and isoexpansile gas tamponade. Evidence suggests that air/gas tamponades with upright positioning provide better displacement of subretinal fluid inferiorly by gravity, thus shifting the redundant retina downward (64). This explains why superior limited translocation is much more difficult to achieve (Fig. 25.4) (55).

Postoperative Management and Complications
After surgery, the patient is positioned sitting upright overnight. Upright positioning maximizes the amount of subretinal fluid that settles inferiorly with gravity,

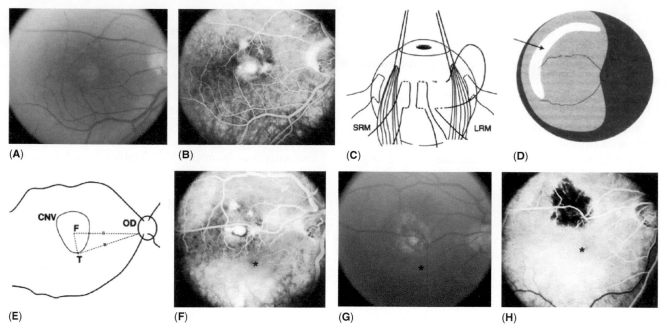

Figure 25.4 Limited macular translocation. **(A)** A color fundus photograph and **(B)** fluorescein angiogram of a 58-year-old patient with subfoveal choroidal neovascularization (CNV). **(C)** Scleral mattress sutures placed between superior rectus muscle (SRM) and lateral rectus muscle (LRM). **(D)** Choriosceral imbrication in the superotemporal quadrant (arrow) beneath a limited retinal detachment without peripheral retinectomy (light gray area). **(E)** Diagram showing the minimum required distance for inferior translocation from the foveal center ("F") to the edge of the CNV lesion ("T"). **(F)** Fluorescein angiogram taken 2 days postoperatively, showing 1800-μm inferior foveal displacement (*) and leakage from the old CNV site. **(G)** Color fundus photograph and **(H)** fluorescein angiogram taken 6 months after surgery, showing inferiorly translocated fovea (*) with 20/40 visual acuity, and ablated extrafoveal site of CNV. *Source*: From Ref. 120.

preventing macular folds (as long as the retinal detachment extends inferior to the macula) and increasing the distance of inferior foveal displacement. The removal of neovascular membranes at the time of limited macular translocation is generally avoided due to the unpredictable size of the RPE defect that may be created during excision (20,65). The CNV outside of the translocated fovea can be treated with further anti-VEGF agents at the time of surgery and with laser photocoagulation within one week after surgery. The most common complication is insufficient translocation with persistence of subfoveal CNV or early subfoveal recurrence, requiring additional treatment to prevent further vision loss (14,53,64).

Limited macular translocation carries similar intraoperative and postoperative risks inherent to other pars plana vitrectomy surgeries. Intraoperative retinal breaks may be caused by cutting with the vitrector, incarceration of vitreous or retina at the sclerotomies, or excessive manipulation of detached retina. During limited retinal detachment, complications such as macular hole, vitreous hemorrhage, and subretinal hemorrhage may occur. Scleral imbrication carries similar intraoperative risks to scleral buckling surgery. Full-thickness scleral perforation during the placement of imbrication sutures may lead to the formation of a retinal break or hemorrhage into the vitreous, subretinal, or suprachoroidal space. Increased pressure generated while tightening the imbrication sutures is a risk factor for retinal incarceration at the sclerotomies. The low-pressure state needed to permit choriosceral infolding is a risk factor for choroidal hemorrhage.

Another potential complication of translocation surgery is unintentional RPE or CNV transplantation. Diseased subfoveal RPE or CNV may adhere to and detach along with the neurosensory fovea and inhibit proper signaling between photoreceptors and the new RPE bed after translocation. Postmortem histological studies provide conflicting evidence on the incidence of unintentional RPE transplantation, and the effect of this phenomenon on functional outcomes remains controversial (66–69).

Retinal detachment after limited macular translocation is the most common postoperative complication (17,20,55,60,64). The risk and severity of PVR and subsequent tractional retinal detachment was significantly lower in early series of limited translocation compared with full translocation, but the risk increases with repeat surgical interventions (19,64). Cataract formation may require surgery if the media opacity prevents appropriate surveillance and treatment of recurrent CNV.

The degree of macular rotation after limited translocation is small, compared with MT360, therefore postoperative diplopia and cyclotropia are not as frequent. In all published series of patients undergoing limited macular translocation, the rates of diplopia and cyclotropia have been very low, and in almost all cases the symptoms resolve spontaneously within months after surgery (70). Correction with prism glasses has been found to treat symptoms satisfactorily until they resolve, and extraocular muscle surgery has only rarely been reported as necessary to correct persistent diplopia or to eliminate the permanent use of prisms (70). Other visual complications that are also rare but may be more difficult to manage are distortion due to macular fold and aniseikonia.

In summary, limited macular translocation surgery is an alternative surgical treatment for advanced AMD with unique benefits and shortcomings with respect to MT360. Limited translocation involves a small rotation angle of the macula that generally does not require a second stage of surgery for extraocular muscle adjustment. Formation of a smaller retinal detachment without retinectomy may reduce the incidence of postoperative PVR and may shorten recovery time. In addition, air tamponade is often sufficient for retinal attachment after limited translocation, avoiding the need for placement and removal of silicone oil. The limitations of this technique, however, have led to declined use among vitreoretinal surgeons. Limited macular translocation can only achieve small distances of foveal displacement, and single-surgeon outcomes are highly variable and unpredictable, with ranges of 200–2800 µm, 349 – 3391 µm, and 250 – 1900 µm in large published series (20,55,60). In cases of advanced AMD with large neovascular membranes or extensive foveal RPE damage, regardless of whether the lesions are within the scope of treatment with limited macular translocation, MT360 achieves better rates of effective foveal displacement and vision improvement with lower rates of fovea-threatening CNV (32,38).

SUBMACULAR SURGERY
Overview
Untreated subfoveal CNV and hemorrhage may lead to severe vision loss from non-resolving hemorrhage, fibrovascular proliferation, RPE tear, scarring, or chorioretinal atrophy (9,18,71). Hemorrhagic complications are also exacerbated by coagulopathies and anticoagulation therapy such as warfarin, clopidogrel, and aspirin (9). The aim of submacular surgery is primarily to remove the sequelae of neovascular AMD, and the procedure presents fewer technical challenges than macular translocation.

The SSTs were the largest multicenter prospective randomized clinical trials designed to find out whether submacular surgery could preserve or improve vision in patients with affected by CNV at a time when anti-VEGF intravitreal injections were not yet available (8,9,71). The SSTs were sponsored by the National Eye Institute, enrolled patients at 25 clinical sites from 1997 to 2003, and were divided into the following three trial arms: Group H for eyes with CNV secondary to presumed ocular histoplasmosis syndrome and idiopathic etiology, Group N for eyes with neovascular AMD and new-onset subfoveal CNV, and Group B for eyes with submacular blood due to primarily hemorrhagic CNV lesions in AMD (8,9). Group H did not enroll subjects with AMD and therefore will not be discussed in this chapter.

A fourth proposed trial was termed Group R for eyes with neovascular AMD and recurrent CNV after laser photocoagulation (72). Group R was discontinued after an initial pilot study showed that vision outcomes were superior with laser photocoagulation than with surgical removal of recurrent CNV (72). While Group R was designed to compare two different treatment regimens, Groups N and B were designed to compare submacular surgery against observation alone (8,9). In the following sections, various techniques of modern submacular surgery will be discussed, followed by the clinical outcomes from the SST Groups N and B, as well as other notable clinical trials.

Submacular Surgery for Removal of Choroidal Neovascularization
The goal of submacular surgery for CNV is to remove neovascular membranes and preserve the underlying RPE and choriocapillaris in order to reestablish foveal photoreceptor–RPE signaling. This surgery was thought to be most effective for type 2 CNV with classic lesions located between the RPE and neurosensory retina rather than for type 1 CNV lesions, between the RPE and choriocapillaris (8). However, SST Group N demonstrated a loss of RPE with submacular surgery for both types of lesions in AMD (8,73). Submacular surgery involves standard pars plana vitrectomy with complete detachment of the posterior hyaloid, an extrafoveal retinotomy created at the edge of the lesion, and localized retinal detachment created by fluid infusion into the subretinal space. Subretinal membranes are separated from surrounding tissues and then removed with caution to minimize further RPE detachment and prevent tearing of the retinotomy. During membrane removal, homeostasis is achieved by raising intraocular pressure and blood may be displaced using PFO liquid. Fluid–air exchange is generally a sufficient tamponade for the macular retinotomy.

Surgery for removal of subretinal CNV is associated with complications that may occur with any pars plana vitrectomy surgery and complications that are unique to this procedure. Since the area of retinal detachment is localized to the macula, postoperative PVR and retinal detachment occur more rarely than with macular translocation. Submacular surgery may be complicated specifically by vitreous or subretinal hemorrhage if intraoperative homeostasis is inadequate or if spontaneous bleeding arises from residual CNV. Most importantly, the RPE and Bruch's membrane are typically entangled within the CNV complex in neovascular AMD, not preserved as separate layers (73). Removal of RPE during CNV extraction very frequently produces permanent subfoveal RPE defects and poor vision outcomes. Delayed complications include cataract formation and recurrent CNV which require further treatment.

The SST Group N trial compared surgical removal versus observation for eyes with untreated subfoveal CNV and found no significant difference between surgery and observation after two-year follow-up (8). Among 226 eyes randomized to surgery, 12% had vision improvement of 2 lines or better, and 59% had vision loss of 2 lines or more from baseline. Among 228 eyes assigned to observation, 14% had vision improvement of 2 lines or better, and 56% had vision loss of 2 lines or worse (8). As expected, the surgery arm of the study reported more complications after two years: 52% had recurrent CNV, 80% of phakic eyes developed cataract, and there were 12 cases of retinal detachment. Among eyes with new subfoveal CNV assigned to observation, 66% had persistent CNV and 21% developed visually significant cataract after two years (8). In the current era of anti-VEGF agents, observation of new CNV falls below the standard of care for AMD, since these agents can recover vision. From this perspective, submacular surgery produced very poor outcomes in the Group N trial.

Submacular surgery has been explored for removal of RAP lesions associated with intraretinal neovascularization, chorioretinal anastomoses, and serous RPE detachment. Small studies suggest that excision of stage III membranes with chorioretinal anastomosis may stabilize vision, while subretinal lysis of feeder vessels in less advanced stage II lesions induces membrane regression and resolution of the RPE detachment (74–76). However, reperfusion of remnant lesions from new feeder vessels may lead to frequent recurrences (77).

Surgery for Displacement of Submacular Hemorrhage

Surgical evacuation of hemorrhage follows many of the same principles as surgery for subretinal CNV removal, with the addition of pharmacological adjuvants such as tissue plasminogen activator (tPA). Tissue plasminogen activator is a serine protease that cleaves plasminogen into plasmin. Early animal studies characterized dosage and technique of subretinal tPA injection for liquefaction of subretinal hemorrhage, lysis of fibrotic adhesions to RPE and neurosensory retina, and clearance of hemorrhage while minimizing damage to surrounding cellular layers (18,78–80). Initial case series by Lewis et al. and Lim et al. reported vision improvement in 83% and 68% of eyes, respectively, after subretinal tPA injection and evacuation of hemorrhage (81,82). Kamei et al. added PFO liquid after injection of subretinal tPA, in order to aid the evacuation of hemorrhage, resulting in short-term vision improvement in 82% of eyes (83).

The SST Group B trial compared surgical removal versus observation for eyes with predominantly hemorrhagic CNV due to AMD and found no improvement over observation after 2 years (9). In their technique, they begin with standard pars plana vitrectomy and then create a retinotomy adjacent to the hematoma. A localized retinal detachment is created by subretinal injection of fluid or a combination of fluid and tPA, followed by a pause to allow for thrombolysis. Blood is removed through the retinotomy with hemostasis by increased intraocular pressure and evacuation aided by PFO, followed by fluid–air exchange with air tamponade.

In both treatment arms, only 18% of eyes had vision improvement of 2 lines or better and 56–59% had vision loss of 2 lines or worse. There was a risk reduction of profound vision loss of more than 6 lines with

surgical intervention, but both treatment arms had equal number of eyes progress to NLP vision (9). As expected, complication rates were significantly higher in the surgery arm of the trial after two years: 55% had recurrent CNV, 44% of phakic eyes developed cataract, 8% developed PVR, and 16% had retinal detachment. In select cases of CNV removal in Group B, lesion size was reduced throughout follow-up, but lesion size had no effect on final visual acuity (9). As a result of these poor outcomes, removal of hemorrhage has largely been discontinued in clinical practice.

After the failures of CNV and hemorrhage removal, the next modifications were injection of tPA into the vitreous cavity in the outpatient setting (84) or at the time of pars plana vitrectomy (85–88), with or without a gas bubble, or even displacement of clot with a gas bubble and no tPA (89). Haupert et al. reported a pilot study of vitrectomy surgery with subretinal tPA injection and intravitreal gas with complete inferior displacement of hemorrhage in all 11 eyes and vision improvement in 73% (86). Olivier et al. reported a series of 29 eyes with complete displacement in 86% and vision improvement of two lines or better in 62% (87). All of these displacement procedures included prone positioning. Rather than evacuating blood through a retinotomy, both techniques described by Haupert et al. and Olivier et al. inject submacular tPA until the hemorrhagic lesion is completely bathed in low-dose tPA of 12.5–50 micrograms per 0.1 mL solution (86,87). High-dose tPA between 50–100 micrograms per 0.1 mL has been implicated with toxic retinal effects, including hyperpigmentary RPE changes, reduced photopic and scotopic ERG amplitudes, and neovascular retinal detachment (78,84,90–92).

Displacement surgery is completed with a 75–100% fluid–gas exchange and then prone positioning. The gas bubble subsequently displaces the hemorrhage from the foveal center, usually achieving total displacement into the subretinal space of the inferior quadrant. We recommend maintaining supine positioning for the first hour after surgery to allow tPA clot lysis to progress, followed by upright positioning until the gas bubble dissolves. Stopa and Linkoff demonstrated that an upright head position is more appropriate for blood displacement than prone positioning, since it recruits the force of gravity to produce a downward subretinal fluid shift similar to limited translocation (Fig. 25.5) (93).

When we compare the results of tPA intravitreal injection to submacular tPA, there are higher rates of vitreous hemorrhage and slightly worse functional outcomes, with the former, and higher rates of recurrent submacular hemorrhage with the latter (84–88). In addition, the incorporation of anti-VEGF agents into treatment of subretinal hemorrhage is gaining widespread adoption. Anti-VEGF adjuvants may reduce vitreous hemorrhage complications and treat hemorrhagic CNV located in the sub-RPE space. Comparison studies of submacular hemorrhage displacement with vitrectomy and co-application of intravitreal anti-VEGF and tPA

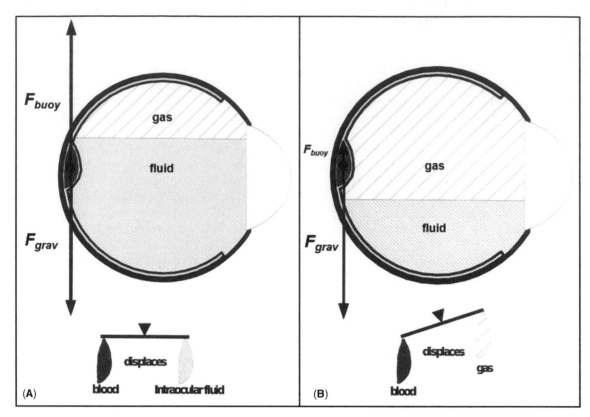

Figure 25.5 A diagram representing the pneumatic displacement for submacular hemorrhage (SMH). **(A)** Below the fluid level, SMH displaces fluid of equal density and generates a force of buoyancy (buoy) equal to its force of gravity. Blood cannot be displaced from the submacular space. **(B)** Above the fluid level, SMH displaces isoexpansile gas that is 830 times less dense than fluid, generating a force of buoyancy that is 830 times smaller. In the upright position, blood is displaced downward by the force of gravity (grav), which remains unchanged. *Source*: From Ref. 93.

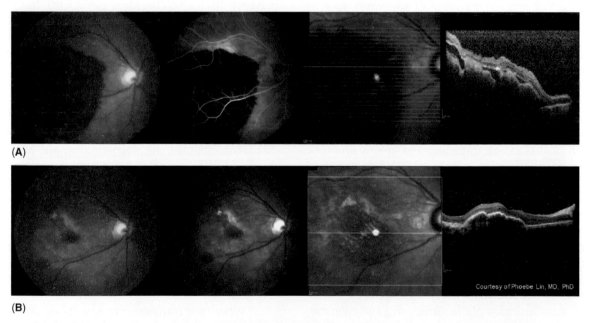

Figure 25.6 Displacement of submacular hemorrhage. **(A)** From left to right: Color fundus photography, fluorescein angiography, and near-infrared photography, followed by spectral domain optical optical coherence tomography (SD-OCT), of a patient with counting-fingers visual acuity in the right eye and large submacular hemorrhage with preserved macular perfusion and outer retinal anatomy. **(B)** From left to right: Color, red-free, and near-infrared photography, followed by SD-OCT, of the right eye 5 months after vitrectomy, subretinal injection of tissue plasminogen activator combined with bevacizumab, and fluid–gas exchange. Despite residual subfoveal material, most of the hemorrhage was displaced inferiorly, the foveal architecture was restored, and visual acuity improved to 20/25.

(94,95), and co-applicaton of subretinal anti-VEGF and tPA (96,97), have found that combined administration of tPA and anti-VEGF agents lead to significantly better vision outcomes than tPA alone (Fig. 25.6).

RPE–CHOROID GRAFT TRANSPLANTATION
Overview
Transplantation of autologous RPE and choroid follows the same principle as macular translocation surgery:

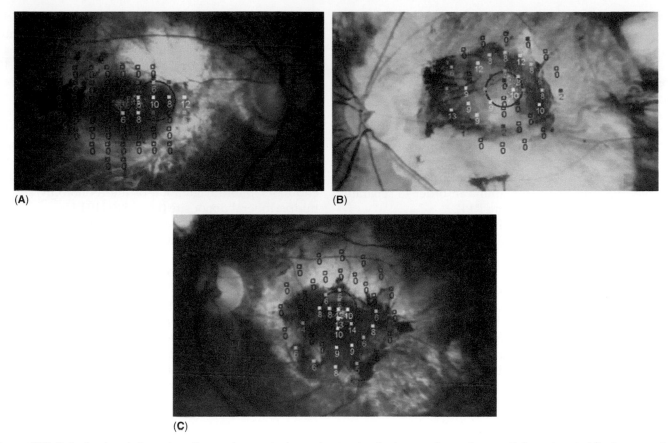

Figure. 25.7 Color fundus photographs with superimposed microperimetry showing improved macular sensitivity and central fixation on autologous retinal pigment epithelium—choroid grafts over long-term follow-up after transplantation: **(A)** Seven years after surgery with visual acuity 20/32; **(B)** four years after surgery with visual acuity 20/80; **(C)** six years after surgery with visual acuity 20/50. *Source*: From Ref. 114.

preservation of viable macular photoreceptors by providing healthier subretinal tissues. This objective is achieved in reverse, however, by transplanting a full-thickness patch of RPE, Bruch's membrane, choriocapillaris, and choroid from the periphery to the subfoveal area without rotation of the neurosensory retina. In 1991, Peyman reported the first autologous and homologous pedicles of RPE and Bruch's membrane transplanted in patients with advanced AMD (98). This report was followed by studies transplanting fetal RPE cells in culture or autologous RPE cell monolayers into the subretinal space for neovascular AMD. These procedures were complicated by graft atrophy, fibrotic encapsulation, cystoid macular edema, and failure of the RPE to form a functional monolayer (99–101).

Aylward developed a full-thickness RPE–choroid patch graft that was harvested from the macular area at the edge of the RPE defect after submacular CNV extraction (102). These grafts were small and difficult to position, and they failed to demonstrate sustained visual function (103). This technique was modified by Van Meurs, who showed that larger RPE–choroid grafts harvested from the midperiphery were able to remain viable and preserve visual function over long-term follow-up (104,105). Variations of this procedure with successful visual outcomes and graft survival have been described by Van Meurs, Wong, Pertile, and other groups (106–111). In an early series of 45 eyes

with advanced AMD, 47% had severe visual loss of more than two lines and 53% were hindered by severe graft fibrosis (112). A smaller series of 12 eyes reported 58% with visual loss of more than two lines and 17% with improvement of more than two lines after six 6 months (110). In another series of 12 eyes with geographic atrophy, 33% had loss of more than 2 lines and 58% had stable vision at one year (113). Maaijwee et al. reported a study of 84 eyes in which 24% had visual loss of more than 2 lines after one year, and mean visual acuity of the entire cohort over four years of follow-up was not statistically different than baseline (105).

More recent studies by Ma et al. and Cereda et al. have shown better clinical outcomes: only 8–12% developed visual loss of more than 2 lines, while 62–76% demonstrated visual acuity improvement of one or more lines (108,111). In the largest prospective study published to date, Van Zeeburg et al. followed 133 eyes after RPE–choroid graft transplantation and reported the frequency of achieving their visual acuity end point of 20/200 (1.0 logMAR) or better (114). At one year after surgery, 35% of eyes achieved or surpassed 20/200 visual acuity. At four years, 43% of eyes with available follow-up (n = 46) had visual acuity of 20/200 or better. In their subgroup analysis, eyes with classic or occult subfoveal CNV had slightly better functional outcomes than eyes with predominantly hemorrhagic lesions (Fig. 25.7) (114).

Surgical Technique

At the time of RPE–choroid transplantation, phakic eyes should undergo cataract phacoemulsification and posterior chamber intraocular lens implantation. Transplantation proceeds with a complete pars plana vitrectomy, including elevation of the posterior hyaloid, complete posterior vitreous detachment, and thorough shaving of the vitreous base. The retina is detached as described with macular translocation: a small peripheral retinotomy is created with the vitrectomy cutter, followed by subretinal infusion of BSS Plus vitrectomy fluid with a flexible polyamide-tipped cannula in order to separate the macula from the underlying RPE.

After detachment of the macula, two separate methods have been shown to successfully harvest and transplant the RPE–choroid graft. Van Meurs has described a technique in which a paramacular temporal retinotomy is made in the horizontal raphe (104). Hemorrhage and CNV membranes are removed with subretinal forceps through the retinotomy. In the midperiphery, diathermy is applied around the area of the graft donor site. A full-thickness circular graft of retina, RPE, and choroid is cut with vitreous scissors within the diathermy margins and then mobilized with forceps

grasping the choroid side. The retina is gently peeled from the graft, and then the RPE–choroid graft is introduced through the paramacular retinotomy into the subretinal space with a customized spatula (104,110). Heavy PFO liquid is injected over the macula to assist with centering and releasing the free graft under the fovea. The most frequently reported intraoperative complications are difficulty with release of the graft after subfoveal placement and inadequate positioning or flattening of the graft, which may result in subfoveal folds or wrinkles. Successful transplantation is followed by endolaser photocoagulation of the retinotomy and the midperipheral donor site (Fig. 25.8) (104,110).

Wong and Pertile have described a modified technique with a 180-degree temporal retinectomy (107,108). After separation of the macula and temporal retina, fluid–air exchanges are performed to achieve a bullous peripheral retinal detachment to the ora serrata. The temporal retinectomy is extended around the ora serrata with the vitrectomy cutter or curved scissors. The neurosensory retinal flap is reflected over the nasal retina, and the exposed CNV membrane is slowly removed with forceps while carefully maintaining hemostasis. In the temporal midperiphery, diathermy is applied directly to

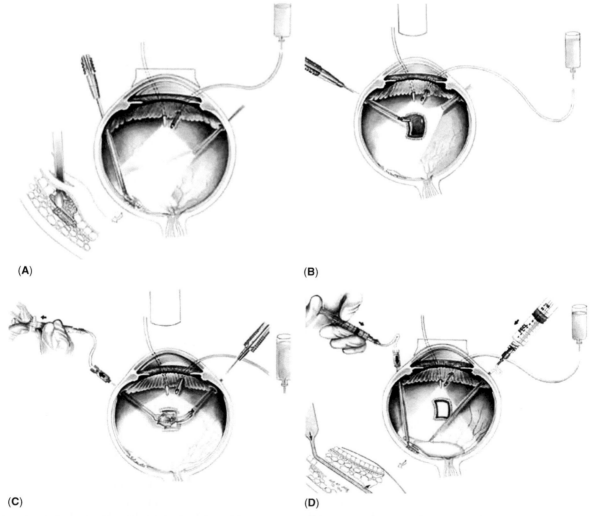

(A)   **(B)**

(C)   **(D)**

Figure 25.8 A diagram showing autologous patch graft transplantation: **(A)** Removal of subfoveal neovascular membrane. **(B)** Excision of full-thickness patch graft from the midperiphery. **(C)** Extraction from the scleral bed and removal of overlying neurosensory retina. **(D)** Subfoveal placement of patch graft under perfluorooctane liquid. *Source*: From Ref. 105.

the uveal bed around the donor site. The RPE–choroid patch is cut within the diathermy margins and harvested under high intraocular pressure. While stabilized under PFO liquid, the free graft is slid from the donor site to the subfoveal space with customized forceps. After PFO–fluid exchange, the temporal retina is folded back into place, followed by preretinal PFO injection and endolaser photocoagulation to the retinectomy margin (107–109,111). With both RPE–choroid transplantation techniques, PFO is exchanged with silicone oil for intraocular tamponade, and then oil is removed three months later in a second procedure.

Postoperative Management and Complications

Postoperative management of autologous RPE–choroid grafts requires multimodal imaging to monitor graft revascularization. Clinicians may also find benefit in microperimetry for monitoring macular sensitivity and central fixation. In the early arterial filling phase of fluorescein angiography, diffuse filling of the graft choriocapillaris produces a characteristic capillary flush that can be compared with the surrounding area to assess graft revascularization (106,108). Indocyanine green (ICG) angiography is a superior method for evaluating choroidal circulation. Differences in the choroidal vascular patterns between macular choroid and the midperipheral choroid of the patch graft allow more accurate evaluation of graft revascularization with ICG angiography. Graft perfusion is identified first by large feeder vessels entering vertically from the underlying uveal bed, and then by parallel ladder-like choroidal vessels within the graft (106,108). In addition, SD-OCT is a less-invasive imaging technology that can be used to monitor revascularization with cross-sectional measurements of graft thickness, vessel quantity, and vascular lumen size (109). Grafts usually manifest increased fundus autofluorescence after surgery, which does not appear to correlate with graft perfusion status. Absence of autofluorescence may point to areas on the graft where RPE was damaged during surgical manipulation (102,104,108,112,115).

Failure of revascularization is the primary complication associated with autologous RPE–choroid graft transplantation. Graft failure has been reported with a prevalence of 5 – 25% based on small angiographic case series of 4–30 eyes (102,104–111,113–116). Successful graft vascularization has been shown to follow stages equivalent to wound healing in free skin grafts (109). The first stage occurs within the first week after surgery and consists of a thin patch without any perfusion of choroidal graft vessels on fluorescein or ICG angiography. The patch is supported instead by plasma exudation from the vasculature of the recipient uveal bed (serum imbibition). The second stage, between the first and second weeks after surgery, is characterized by increased graft thickness and increased caliber of graft vessels on SD-OCT, and by the appearance of peripheral afferent vessels connecting to the graft on ICG angiography. After three weeks, the third stage leads to the establishment of efferent choroidal circulation, complete graft perfusion with on fluorescein and ICG angiography, decreased

graft edema, and filling of the lumen of all graft vessels on SD-OCT. Normal RPE–choroid graft revascularization is complete within two months after surgery (109).

Secondary complications include PVR, retinal detachment, and subretinal hemorrhage affecting the fovea. Retinal detachment secondary to PVR formation has been reported in 8–42% of cases (101,102,105,106,108,110,111,113–115). Van Zeeburg and Van Meurs have published the largest series to date, reporting retinal detachment in 13 of 133 eyes after transplantation (114). The incidence of postoperative submacular hemorrhage ranged from 8 to 33% in early studies (105,108,110,113); however, subsequent reports have reported no cases with this complication (111,115). Improvements in intraoperative techniques for hemostasis and graft positioning have decreased hemorrhagic events. Other less common complications of this surgical treatment include epiretinal membrane, macular hole, and recurrence of subfoveal CNV. In some rare cases, graft failure or atrophy had led to an angiogenic stimulus that may form an anastomosis with the retinal vasculature. These RAP-like neovascular lesions appear simultaneously as focal intraretinal staining on fluorescein and focal hyperfluorescence on ICG angiography (108).

In 2009, Chen et al. published a comparative review of outcomes for MT360 versus RPE–choroid patch graft without 180-degree retinectomy (117). Postoperative outcomes favored MT360: retinal detachment in 25% and 33%, recurrent extrafoveal CNV in 25% and 33%, cystoid macular edema in 67% and 100%, and severe vision loss of more than 2 lines in 25% and 50% of eyes in the MT360 and patch graft groups, respectively (117). Based on clinical evidence, we recommend MT360 over RPE–choroid transplantation for the second eye affected by advanced AMD unresponsive to other treatment. Patch graft transplantation, however, does not require macular rotation, and therefore poses little risk of diplopia after surgery. This distinct advantage could make this procedure suitable for the first non–responder eye with advanced AMD and functional vision in the contralateral eye.

CONCLUSION

In the current era of anti-VEGF treatment, the indications for surgical treatments have changed dramatically. Nevertheless, modern surgical techniques for MT360 and submacular hemorrhage displacement have been demonstrated to preserve or improve vision with very low rates of severe complications. The Submacular Surgery Trials yielded dismal results, with outcomes for CNV removal and submacular hemorrhage removal that were no better than observation alone. From these trials we learned that surgical removal of neovascular lesions alone produces excessive damage to the fovea and RPE. In summary, modern surgical techniques have evolved to avoid this pitfall and achieve meaningful functional outcomes in eyes with advanced AMD. First, the macular recovery surgeries, including macular translocation and RPE–choroid graft transplantation, restore the photoreceptor–RPE–choriocapillaris complex by transferring the macula to a healthier bed of RPE or by transplanting a patch of RPE and choroid beneath the fovea. Second, the displacement of submacular hemorrhage with tPA and isoexpansile gas, with or without anti-VEGF adjuvants, can restore vision without hazardous removal of blood and CNV.

In 2005, Falker et al. conducted a comprehensive meta-analysis summarizing the results of surgical treatment studies for advanced AMD reported through 2004, and they compared these results with the SST reports (118). A multivariate logistic regression model found that vision improvement of two lines or better occurred in 31% of all reported macular translocation surgeries, 28% of submacular surgeries for CNV removal, 62% of surgeries for submacular hemorrhage, and 22% of patch graft transplantations (118). Vision deterioration of two lines or worse occurred in 27% of macular translocations, 25% of surgeries for CNV removal, 13% of surgeries for submacular hemorrhage, and 21% of patch graft transplantations (118). Although MT360 and limited macular translocation were analyzed together in one category by Falkner et al., the combined results were better than the dismal outcomes for both treatment arms in the SST Group N trial (8,9,118). The outcomes of surgery for submacular hemorrhage displacement were also far better than the outcomes in both treatment arms of the SST Group B trial (9,118).

There are many potential venues for the evolution of surgical treatments for AMD. Patients may benefit from a combination of MT360 and cellular replacement strategies such as RPE transplantation, photoreceptor transplantation, and pluripotent stem cell delivery. Improvements in surgical instrumentation will continue to facilitate the manipulation of the neurosensory retina, reduce the risk of iatrogenic retinal breaks, and reduce cellular trauma to photoreceptors and RPE.

In order to improve functional outcomes, it is important to identify those patients that will benefit the most from surgical treatment. Poor vision outcomes often may be associated with the treatment of eyes that simply do not have the potential to recover vision after translocation of the fovea. Therefore, there is a need to better define and standardize the indications for the macular recovery surgeries of MT360 and RPE–choroid transplantation. Analysis of retinal architecture with SD-OCT, imaging of the choroid with enhanced depth SD-OCT, classification of the state of RPE viability with fundus autofluorescence, and quantification of photoreceptor and RPE cell populations with adaptive optics are all arenas of ongoing investigation that may improve our risk stratification of candidates for MT360.

From a basic science perspective, MT360 serves as an in-vivo human model of autologous transplantation of the neurosensory retina. This provides the opportunity to study the photoreceptor–RPE signaling interactions in a host of different maculopathies.

Unique observations seen after MT360, such as new-onset subfoveal RPE atrophy after translocation for GA, vision recovery despite photoreceptor outer segment degeneration, and CNV migration toward the relocated fovea, provide the opportunity to unravel the mechanisms involved in intercellular signaling and AMD progression.

SUMMARY POINTS

- Anti-VEGF intravitreal agents are the current first-line treatment for neovascular age-related macular degeneration (AMD); however, the surgical treatment of AMD continues to play an important role in selected cases of neovascular AMD and non-neovascular AMD with central geographic atrophy.
- The multicenter randomized prospective Submacular Surgery Trials did not demonstrate any clinical benefit to submacular surgery for new subfoveal CNV, submacular hemorrhage, or recurrent CNV in AMD.
- Since neovascular AMD was first treated by Machemer with macular translocation surgery with 360-degree retinectomy (MT360), clinical outcomes have significantly improved with numerous surgical advancements over the last 20 years.
- Limited macular translocation with scleral imbrication is a less invasive procedure that creates less torsional diplopia, but the reduced foveal displacement significantly limits its applications.
- Autologous RPE–choroid patch graft transplantation provides vital RPE and uveal support to foveal photoreceptors without macular rotation and induced diplopia. Although functional and anatomic outcomes currently lag behind MT360, patch grafts may be the preferred surgical approach for the first eye with advanced AMD.
- Macular recovery surgeries such as MT360 and RPE–choroid transplantation continue to demonstrate significant preservation or improvement of vision in patients with advanced AMD in numerous prospective clinical studies.
- Retinal imaging with fluorescein angiography, spectral domain optical coherence tomography, and fundus autofluorescence are important for proper diagnostic evaluation and postoperative management in the macular recovery surgeries.
- Surgical treatment with subretinal tissue plasminogen activator injection and pneumatic displacement has led to a significant improvement in visual outcomes for large submacular hemorrhages.

REFERENCES

1. Klein R, Klein BE, Linton KL, THE Beaver Dam Eye Study. Prevalence of age-related maculopathy. Ophthalmology 1992; 99: 933–43.
2. Klaver CC, Wolfs RC, Vingerling JR, Hofman A, de Jong PT. Age-specific prevalence and causes of blindness and

visual impairment in an older population: the Rotterdam Study. Arch Ophthalmol 1998; 116: 653–8.

3. Bressler NM, Bressler SB, Congdon NG, et al. Potential public health impact of age-related eye disease study results: AREDS report no. 11. Arch Ophthalmol 2003; 121: 1621–4.

4. Rosenfeld PJ, Brown DM, Heier JS, et al. Ranibizumab for neovascular age-related macular degeneration. N Engl J Med 2006; 355: 1419–31.

5. Brown DM, Kaiser PK, Michels M, et al. Ranibizumab versus verteporfin for neovascular age-related macular degeneration. N Engl J Med 2006; 355: 1432–44.

6. Martin DF, Maguire MG, Ying GS, et al. Ranibizumab and bevacizumab for neovascular age-related macular degeneration. N Engl J Med 2011; 364: 1897–908.

7. Rosenfeld PJ, Shapiro H, Tuomi L, et al. Characteristics of patients losing vision after 2 years of monthly dosing in the phase III ranibizumab clinical trials. Ophthalmology 2011; 118: 523–30.

8. Hawkins BS, Bressler NM, Miskala PH, et al. Surgery for subfoveal choroidal neovascularization in age-related macular degeneration: ophthalmic findings: SST report no. 11. Ophthalmology 2004; 111: 1967–80.

9. Bressler NM, Bressler SB, Childs AL, et al. Surgery for hemorrhagic choroidal neovascular lesions of age-related macular degeneration: ophthalmic findings: SST report no. 13. Ophthalmology 2004; 111: 1993–2006.

10. Ts'o MO, Friedman E. The retinal pigment epithelium. I. comparative histology. Arch Ophthalmol 1967; 78: 641–9.

11. Yoneya S, Tso MO. Angioarchitecture of the human choroid. Arch Ophthalmol 1987; 105: 681–7.

12. Bill A, Sperber G, Ujiie K. Physiology of the choroidal vascular bed. Int Ophthalmol 1983; 6: 101–7.

13. de Juan E Jr, Machemer R. Vitreous surgery for hemorrhagic and fibrous complications of age-related macular degeneration. Am J Ophthalmol 1988; 105: 25–9.

14. Machemer R, Steinhorst UH. Retinal separation, retinotomy, and macular relocation: I. Experimental studies in the rabbit eye. Graefes Arch Clin Exp Ophthalmol 1993; 231: 629–34.

15. Ninomiya Y, Lewis JM, Hasegawa T, Tano Y. Retinotomy and foveal translocation for surgical management of subfoveal choroidal neovascular membranes. Am J Ophthalmol 1996; 122: 613–21.

16. Akduman L, Karavellas MP, MacDonald JC, Olk RJ, Freeman WR. Macular translocation with retinotomy and retinal rotation for neovascular age-related macular degeneration. Retina 1999; 19: 418–23.

17. Ohji M, Fujikado T, Kusaka S, et al. Comparison of three techniques of foveal translocation in patients with subfoveal choroidal neovascularization resulting from age-related macular degeneration. Am J Ophthalmol 2001; 132: 888–96.

18. Toth CA, Morse LS, Hjelmeland LM, Landers MB 3rd. Fibrin directs early retinal damage after experimental subretinal hemorrhage. Arch Ophthalmol 1991; 109: 723–9.

19. Toth CA, Freedman SF. Macular translocation with 360-degree peripheral retinectomy impact of technique and surgical experience on visual outcomes. Retina 2001; 21: 293–303.

20. Fujii GY, de Juan E Jr, Pieramici DJ, et al. Inferior limited macular translocation for subfoveal choroidal neovascularization secondary to age-related macular degeneration: 1-year visual outcome and recurrence report. Am J Ophthalmol 2002; 134: 69–74.

21. Freedman SF, Holgado S, Enyedi LB, Toth CA. Management of ocular torsion and diplopia after macular translocation for age-related macular degeneration: prospective clinical study. Am J Ophthalmol 2003; 136: 640–8.

22. Holgado S, Enyedi LB, Toth CA, Freedman SF. Extraocular muscle surgery for extorsion after macular translocation surgery new surgical technique and clinical management. Ophthalmology 2006; 113: 63–9.

23. Seaber JH, Machemer R. Adaptation to monocular torsion after macular translocation. Graefes Arch Clin Exp Ophthalmol 1997; 235: 76–81.

24. Eckardt C, Eckardt U, Conrad HG. Macular rotation with and without counter-rotation of the globe in patients with age-related macular degeneration. Graefes Arch Clin Exp Ophthalmol 1999; 237: 313–25.

25. Cahill MT, Mruthyunjaya P, Bowes Rickman C, Toth CA. Recurrence of retinal pigment epithelial changes after macular translocation with 360 degrees peripheral retinectomy for geographic atrophy. Arch Ophthalmol 2005; 123: 935–8.

26. Khurana RN, Fujii GY, Walsh AC, et al. Rapid recurrence of geographic atrophy after full macular translocation for non-neovascular age-related macular degeneration. Ophthalmology 2005; 112: 1586–91.

27. Uppal G, Milliken A, Lee J, et al. New algorithm for assessing patient suitability for macular translocation surgery. Clin Exp Ophthalmol 2007; 35: 448–57.

28. Mettu PS, Sarin N, Stinnett SS, Toth CA. Recovery of the neurosensory retina after macular translocation surgery is independent of preoperative macular sensitivity in neovascular age-related macular degeneration. Retina 2011; 31: 1637–49.

29. Pertile G, Claes C. Macular translocation with 360 degree retinotomy for management of age-related macular degeneration with subfoveal choroidal neovascularization. Am J Ophthalmol 2002; 134: 560–5.

30. Aisenbrey S, Bartz-Schmidt KU, Walter P, et al. Long-term follow-up of macular translocation with 360 degrees retinotomy for neovascular age-related macular degeneration. Arch Ophthalmol 2007; 125: 1367–72.

31. Abdel-Meguid A, Lappas A, Hartmann K, et al. One year follow up of macular translocation with 360 degree retinotomy in patients with age related macular degeneration. Br J Ophthalmol 2003; 87: 615–21.

32. Mruthyunjaya P, Stinnett SS, Toth CA. Change in visual function after macular translocation with 360 degrees retinectomy for neovascular age-related macular degeneration. Ophthalmology 2004; 111: 1715–24.

33. Chen FK, Patel PJ, Uppal GS, et al. Long-term outcomes following full macular translocation surgery in neovascular age-related macular degeneration. Br J Ophthalmol 2010; 94: 1337–43.

34. Luke M, Ziemssen F, Volker M, et al. Full macular translocation (FMT) versus photodynamic therapy (PDT) with verteporfin in the treatment of neovascular age-related macular degeneration: 2-year results of a prospective, controlled, randomised pilot trial (FMT-PDT). Graefes Arch Clin Exp Ophthalmol 2009; 247: 745–54.

35. Folgar FA, Maldonado RS, Sarin N, Toth CA. Variations in photoreceptor-RPE morphology and function are manifest in distinct fundus autofluorescence patterns after macular translocation surgery for advanced AMD. Invest Ophthalmol Vis Sci 2012; 53: ARVO E-Abstract 2687.

36. Baer CA, Rickman CB, Srivastava S, et al. Recurrent choroidal neovascularization after macular translocation

surgery with 360-degree peripheral retinectomy. Retina 2008; 28: 1221–7.

37. Fujikado T, Asonuma S, Ohji M, et al. Reading ability after macular translocation surgery with 360-degree retinotomy. Am J Ophthalmol 2002; 134: 849–56.

38. Lai JC, Lapolice DJ, Stinnett SS, et al. Visual outcomes following macular translocation with 360-degree peripheral retinectomy. Arch Ophthalmol 2002; 120: 1317–24.

39. Toth CA, Lapolice DJ, Banks AD, Stinnett SS. Improvement in near visual function after macular translocation surgery with 360-degree peripheral retinectomy. Graefes Arch Clin Exp Ophthalmol 2004; 242: 541–8.

40. Uppal G, Feely MP, Crossland MD, et al. Assessment of reading behavior with an infrared eye tracker after 360 degrees macular translocation for age-related macular degeneration. Invest Ophthalmol Vis Sci 2011; 52: 6486–96.

41. Kubota A, Ohji M, Kusaka S, et al. Evaluation of the peripheral visual field after foveal translocation. Am J Ophthalmol 2001; 132: 581–4.

42. Takeuchi K, Kachi S, Iwata E, Ishikawa K, Terasaki H. Visual function 5 years or more after macular translocation surgery for myopic choroidal neovascularisation and age-related macular degeneration. Eye (Lond) 2012; 26: 51–60.

43. Chieh JJ, Stinnett SS, Toth CA. Central and pericentral retinal sensitivity after macular translocation surgery. Retina 2008; 28: 1522–9.

44. Luke C, Aisenbrey S, Luke M, et al. Electrophysiological changes after 360 degrees retinotomy and macular translocation for subfoveal choroidal neovascularisation in age related macular degeneration. Br J Ophthalmol 2001; 85: 928–32.

45. Terasaki H, Miyake Y, Suzuki T, et al. Change in full-field ERGs after macular translocation surgery with 360 degrees retinotomy. Invest Ophthalmol Vis Sci 2002; 43: 452–7.

46. Terasaki H, Ishikawa K, Niwa Y, et al. Changes in focal macular ERGs after macular translocation surgery with 360 degrees retinotomy. Invest Ophthalmol Vis Sci 2004; 45: 567–73.

47. Luke C, Alteheld N, Aisenbrey S, et al. Electro-oculographic findings after 360 degrees retinotomy and macular translocation for subfoveal choroidal neovascularisation in age-related macular degeneration. Graefes Arch Clin Exp Ophthalmol 2003; 241: 710–15.

48. Chen FK, Patel PJ, Coffey PJ, Tufail A, Da Cruz L. Increased fundus autofluorescence associated with outer segment shortening in macular translocation model of neovascular age-related macular degeneration. Invest Ophthalmol Vis Sci 2010; 51: 4207–12.

49. Freedman SF, Gearinger MD, Enyedi LB, Holgado S, Toth CA. Measurement of ocular torsion after macular translocation: disc fovea angle and maddox rod. J AAPOS 2003; 7: 103–7.

50. Cahill MT, Banks AD, Stinnett SS, Toth CA. Vision-related quality of life in patients with bilateral severe age-related macular degeneration. Ophthalmology 2005; 112: 152–8.

51. Cahill MT, Stinnett SS, Banks AD, Freedman SF, Toth CA. Quality of life after macular translocation with 360 degrees peripheral retinectomy for age-related macular degeneration. Ophthalmology 2005; 112: 144–51.

52. Luke M, Ziemssen F, Bartz-Schmidt KU, Gelisken F. Quality of life in a prospective, randomised pilot-trial of photodynamic therapy versus full macular translocation in treatment of neovascular age-related macular degeneration–a report of 1 year results. Graefes Arch Clin Exp Ophthalmol 2007; 245: 1831–6.

53. Wolf S, Lappas A, Weinberger AW, Kirchhof B. Macular translocation for surgical management of subfoveal choroidal neovascularizations in patients with AMD: first results. Graefes Arch Clin Exp Ophthalmol 1999; 237: 51–7.

54. de Juan E Jr, Loewenstein A, Bressler NM, Alexander J. Translocation of the retina for management of subfoveal choroidal neovascularization II: a preliminary report in humans. Am J Ophthalmol 1998; 125: 635–46.

55. Pieramici DJ, De Juan E Jr, Fujii GY, et al. Limited inferior macular translocation for the treatment of subfoveal choroidal neovascularization secondary to age-related macular degeneration. Am J Ophthalmol 2000; 130: 419–28.

56. Benner JD, Meyer CH, Shirkey BL, Toth CA. Macular translocation with radial scleral outfolding: experimental studies and initial human results. Graefes Arch Clin Exp Ophthalmol 2001; 239: 815–23.

57. Fujii GY, de Juan E Jr, Au Eong KG, Harlan JB Jr. Effective nasal limited macular translocation. Am J Ophthalmol 2001; 132: 124–6.

58. Sullivan P, Filsecker L, Sears J. Limited macular translocation with scleral retraction suture. Br J Ophthalmol 2002; 86: 434–9.

59. Au Eong KG, Pieramici DJ, Fujii GY, et al. Macular translocation: unifying concepts, terminology, and classification. Am J Ophthalmol 2001; 131: 244–53.

60. Pawlak D, Glacet-Bernard A, Papp M, et al. Limited macular translocation compared with photodynamic therapy in the management of subfoveal choroidal neovascularization in age-related macular degeneration. Am J Ophthalmol 2004; 137: 880–7.

61. Kamei M, Tano Y, Yasuhara T, Ohji M, Lewis H. Macular translocation with chorioscleral outfolding: 2-year results. Am J Ophthalmol 2004; 138: 574–81.

62. Lewis H. Macular translocation with chorioscleral outfolding: a pilot clinical study. Am J Ophthalmol 2001; 132: 156–63.

63. Deramo VA, Meyer CH, Toth CA. Successful macular translocation with temporary scleral infolding using absorbable suture. Retina 2001; 21: 304–11.

64. Fujii GY, Pieramici DJ, Humayun MS, et al. Complications associated with limited macular translocation. Am J Ophthalmol 2000; 130: 751–62.

65. Fujii GY, de Juan E, Thomas MA, et al. Limited macular translocation for the management of subfoveal retinal pigment epithelial loss after submacular surgery. Am J Ophthalmol 2001; 131: 272–5.

66. Albini TA, Rao NA, Li A, et al. Limited macular translocation: a clinicopathologic case report. Ophthalmology 2004; 111: 1209–14.

67. Bereczki A, Toth J, Suveges I. Histological examination of the pigment epithelium-bruch membrane-choriocapillaris complex after macular translocation. Br J Ophthalmol 2000; 84: 550–1.

68. Roig-Melo EA, Afaro DV 3rd, Heredia-Elizondo ML, et al. Macular translocation: histopathologic findings in swine eyes. Eur J Ophthalmol 2000; 10: 297–303.

69. Wickham L, Lewis GP, Charteris DG, Fisher SK, Da Cruz L. Histological analysis of retinas sampled during translocation surgery: a comparison with normal and transplantation retinas. Br J Ophthalmol 2009; 93: 969–73.

70. Buffenn AN, de Juan E, Fujii G, Hunter DG. Diplopia after limited macular translocation surgery. J AAPOS 2001; 5: 388–94.

71. Skaf AR, Mahmoud T. Surgical treatment of age-related macular degeneration. Semin Ophthalmol 2011; 26: 181–91.

72. Bressler NM, Bressler SB, Hawkins BS, Marsh MJ, Sternberg P Jr, Thomas MA. Submacular surgery trials randomized pilot trial of laser photocoagulation versus surgery for recurrent choroidal neovascularization secondary to age-related macular degeneration: I. ophthalmic outcomes submacular surgery trials pilot study report number 1. Am J Ophthalmol 2000; 130: 387.407.

73. Grossniklaus HE, Green WR, Trials Research Group. Histopathologic and ultrastructural findings of surgically excised choroidal neovascularization. submacular surgery. Arch Ophthalmol 1998; 116: 745–9.

74. Borrillo JL, Sivalingam A, Martidis A, Federman JL. Surgical ablation of retinal angiomatous proliferation. Arch Ophthalmol 2003; 121: 558–61.

75. Shimada H, Mori R, Arai K, Kawamura A, Yuzawa M. Surgical excision of neovascularization in retinal angiomatous proliferation. Graefes Arch Clin Exp Ophthalmol 2005; 243: 519–24.

76. Nakata M, Yuzawa M, Kawamura A, Shimada H. Combining surgical ablation of retinal inflow and outflow vessels with photodynamic therapy for retinal angiomatous proliferation. Am J Ophthalmol 2006; 141: 968–70.

77. Shiragami C, Iida T, Nagayama D, Baba T, Shiraga F. Recurrence after surgical ablation for retinal angiomatous proliferation. Retina 2007; 27: 198–203.

78. Benner JD, Morse LS, Toth CA, Landers MB 3rd, Hjelmeland LM. Evaluation of a commercial recombinant tissue-type plasminogen activator preparation in the subretinal space of the cat. Arch Ophthalmol 1991; 109: 1731–6.

79. Toth CA, Benner JD, Hjelmeland LM, Landers MB 3rd, Morse LS. Ultramicrosurgical removal of subretinal hemorrhage in cats. Am J Ophthalmol 1992; 113: 175–82.

80. Lewis H, Resnick SC, Flannery JG, Straatsma BR. Tissue plasminogen activator treatment of experimental subretinal hemorrhage. Am J Ophthalmol 1991; 111: 197–204.

81. Lewis H. Intraoperative fibrinolysis of submacular hemorrhage with tissue plasminogen activator and surgical drainage. Am J Ophthalmol 1994; 118: 559–68.

82. Lim JI, Drews-Botsch C, Sternberg P Jr, Capone A Jr, Aaberg TM Sr. Submacular hemorrhage removal. Ophthalmology 1995; 102: 1393–9.

83. Kamei M, Tano Y, Maeno T, et al. Surgical removal of submacular hemorrhage using tissue plasminogen activator and perfluorocarbon liquid. Am J Ophthalmol 1996; 121: 267–75.

84. Hesse L, Schmidt J, Kroll P. Management of acute submacular hemorrhage using recombinant tissue plasminogen activator and gas. Graefes Arch Clin Exp Ophthalmol 1999; 237: 273–7.

85. Hassan AS, Johnson MW, Schneiderman TE, et al. Management of submacular hemorrhage with intravitreous tissue plasminogen activator injection and pneumatic displacement. Ophthalmology 1999; 106: 1900–6; discussion 6-7.

86. Haupert CL, McCuen BW 2nd, Jaffe GJ, et al. Pars plana vitrectomy, subretinal injection of tissue plasminogen activator, and fluid-gas exchange for displacement of thick submacular hemorrhage in age-related macular degeneration. Am J Ophthalmol 2001; 131: 208–15.

87. Olivier S, Chow DR, Packo KH, MacCumber MW, Awh CC. Subretinal recombinant tissue plasminogen activator injection and pneumatic displacement of thick submacular hemorrhage in age-related macular degeneration. Ophthalmology 2004; 111: 1201–8.

88. Hillenkamp J, Surguch V, Framme C, Gabel VP, Sachs HG. Management of submacular hemorrhage with intravitreal versus subretinal injection of recombinant tissue plasminogen activator. Graefes Arch Clin Exp Ophthalmol 2010; 248: 5–11.

89. Ohji M, Saito Y, Hayashi A, Lewis JM, Tano Y. Pneumatic displacement of subretinal hemorrhage without tissue plasminogen activator. Arch Ophthalmol 1998; 116: 1326–32.

90. Hrach CJ, Johnson MW, Hassan AS, et al. Retinal toxicity of commercial intravitreal tissue plasminogen activator solution in cat eyes. Arch Ophthalmol 2000; 118: 659–63.

91. Irvine WD, Johnson MW, Hernandez E, Olsen KR. Retinal toxicity of human tissue plasminogen activator in vitrectomized rabbit eyes. Arch Ophthalmol 1991; 109: 718–22.

92. Johnson MW, Olsen KR, Hernandez E, Irvine WD, Johnson RN. Retinal toxicity of recombinant tissue plasminogen activator in the rabbit. Arch Ophthalmol 1990; 108: 259–63.

93. Stopa M, Lincoff A, Lincoff H. Analysis of forces acting upon submacular hemorrhage in pneumatic displacement. Retina 2007; 27: 370–4.

94. Arias L, Mones J. Transconjunctival sutureless vitrectomy with tissue plasminogen activator, gas and intravitreal bevacizumab in the management of predominantly hemorrhagic age-related macular degeneration. Clin Ophthalmol 2010; 4: 67–72.

95. Guthoff R, Guthoff T, Meigen T, Goebel W. Intravitreous injection of bevacizumab, tissue plasminogen activator, and gas in the treatment of submacular hemorrhage in age-related macular degeneration. Retina 2011; 31: 36–40.

96. Klettner A, Puls S, Treumer F, Roider J, Hillenkamp J. Compatibility of recombinant tissue plasminogen activator and bevacizumab co-applied for neovascular age-related macular degeneration with submacular hemorrhage. Arch Ophthalmol 2012. [Epub ahead of print].

97. Treumer F, Roider J, Hillenkamp J. Long-term outcome of subretinal coapplication of rtPA and bevacizumab followed by repeated intravitreal anti-VEGF injections for neovascular AMD with submacular haemorrhage. Br J Ophthalmol 2012; 96: 708–13.

98. Peyman GA, Blinder KJ, Paris CL, et al. A technique for retinal pigment epithelium transplantation for age-related macular degeneration secondary to extensive subfoveal scarring. Ophthalmic Surg 1991; 22: 102–8.

99. Algvere PV, Berglin L, Gouras P, Sheng Y. Transplantation of fetal retinal pigment epithelium in age-related macular degeneration with subfoveal neovascularization. Graefes Arch Clin Exp Ophthalmol 1994; 232: 707–16.

100. Algvere PV, Gouras P, Dafgard Kopp E. Long-term outcome of RPE allografts in non-immunosuppressed patients with AMD. Eur J Ophthalmol 1999; 9: 217–30.

101. Binder S, Krebs I, Hilgers RD, et al. Outcome of trans-
      plantation of autologous retinal pigment epithelium in
      age-related macular degeneration: a prospective trial.
      Invest Ophthalmol Vis Sci 2004; 45: 4151–60.
102. Stanga PE, Kychenthal A, Fitzke FW, et al. Retinal pig-
      ment epithelium translocation after choroidal neovas-
      cular membrane removal in age-related macular
      degeneration. Ophthalmology 2002; 109: 1492–8.
103. MacLaren RE, Bird AC, Sathia PJ, Aylward GW. Long-
      term results of submacular surgery combined with
      macular translocation of the retinal pigment epithelium
      in neovascular age-related macular degeneration. Oph-
      thalmology 2005; 112: 2081–7.
104. van Meurs JC, Van Den Biesen PR. Autologous retinal
      pigment epithelium and choroid translocation in
      patients with neovascular age-related macular degen-
      eration: short-term follow-up. Am J Ophthalmol 2003;
      136: 688–95.
105. Maaijwee K, Heimann H, Missotten T, et al. Retinal pig-
      ment epithelium and choroid translocation in patients
      with neovascular age-related macular degeneration:
      long-term results. Graefes Arch Clin Exp Ophthalmol
      2007; 245: 1681–9.
106. Maaijwee K, Van Den Biesen PR, Missotten T, Van
      Meurs JC. Angiographic evidence for revascularization
      of an rpe-choroid graft in patients with age-related mac-
      ular degeneration. Retina 2008; 28: 498–503.
107. Gibran SK, Romano MR, Wong D. Perfluorocarbon liq-
      uid assisted large retinal epithelium patching in sub-
      macular hemorrhage secondary to age related macular
      degeneration. Graefes Arch Clin Exp Ophthalmol 2009;
      247: 187–91.
108. Cereda MG, Parolini B, Bellesini E, Pertile G. Surgery for
      CNV and autologous choroidal RPE patch transplanta-
      tion: exposing the submacular space. Graefes Arch Clin
      Exp Ophthalmol 2010; 248: 37–47.
109. van Zeeburg EJ, Cereda MG, van der Schoot J, Pertile G,
      van Meurs JC. Early perfusion of a free RPE-choroid
      graft in patients with neovascular macular degenera-
      tion can be imaged with spectral domain-OCT. Invest
      Ophthalmol Vis Sci 2011; 52: 5881–6.
110. MacLaren RE, Uppal GS, Balaggan KS, et al. Autolo-
      gous transplantation of the retinal pigment epithelium
      and choroid in the treatment of neovascular age-
      related macular degeneration. Ophthalmology 2007;
      114: 561–70.
111. Ma Z, Han L, Wang C, et al. Autologous transplantation
      of retinal pigment epithelium-Bruch's membrane com-
      plex for hemorrhagic age-related macular degeneration.
      Invest Ophthalmol Vis Sci 2009; 50: 2975–81.
112. Joussen AM, Heussen FM, Joeres S, et al. Autologous
      translocation of the choroid and retinal pigment epithe-
      lium in age-related macular degeneration. Am J Oph-
      thalmol 2006; 142: 17–30.
113. Joussen AM, Joeres S, Fawzy N, et al. Autologous trans-
      location of the choroid and retinal pigment epithelium
      in patients with geographic atrophy. Ophthalmology
      2007; 114: 551–60.
114. van Zeeburg EJ, Maaijwee KJ, Missotten TO, Heimann
      H, van Meurs JC. A free retinal pigment epithelium-cho-
      roid graft in patients with neovascular age-related mac-
      ular degeneration: results up to 7 years. Am J
      Ophthalmol 2012; 153: 120–7; e2.
115. Caramoy A, Liakopoulos S, Menrath E, Kirchhof B.
      Autologous translocation of choroid and retinal pig-
      ment epithelium in geographic atrophy: long-term
      functional and anatomical outcome. Br J Ophthalmol
      2010; 94: 1040–4.
116. Treumer F, Bunse A, Klatt C, Roider J. Autologous reti-
      nal pigment epithelium-choroid sheet transplantation
      in age related macular degeneration: morphological
      and functional results. Br J Ophthalmol 2007; 91:
      349–53.
117. Chen FK, Patel PJ, Uppal GS, et al. A comparison of
      macular translocation with patch graft in neovascular
      age-related macular degeneration. Invest Ophthalmol
      Vis Sci 2009; 50: 1848–55.
118. Falkner CI, Leitich H, Frommlet F, Bauer P, Binder S.
      The end of submacular surgery for age-related macular
      degeneration? A meta-analysis. Graefe's Arch Clin Exp
      Ophthalmol 2007; 245: 490–501.
119. Ehlers PA, Toth CA. Macular translocation. In: Stephen
      J, Ryan VA. editors. Retina, 5th edn. Philadelphia, PA:
      Elsevier, 2012.
120. De Juan E Jr, Fujii GY. Limited macular translocation.
      Eye 2001; 15: 413–23.

26

Prophylactic treatment: The AREDS study results

Benjamin P. Nicholson, Catherine A. Cukras, and Emily Y. Chew

INTRODUCTION

Age-related macular degeneration (AMD) is the leading cause of blindness in the developed world (1,2). There are two forms of advanced AMD: central geographic atrophy and neovascular AMD. While new treatments have shown improved outcomes for patients with neovascular AMD over the last decade, there remains no proven treatment for central geographic atrophy. Therapies that focus on prevention by addressing modifiable risk factors such as diet and nutritional status are key approaches to reducing the burden of disease. Such preventive strategies are especially important as life expectancy in the United States and Europe continues to increase.

The exact pathogenesis of macular degeneration remains unknown but aging, genetic factors, and environmental factors play important roles. Oxidative damage is implicated as an end effector in the pathogenesis of AMD. The retina is uniquely susceptible to oxidative damage given its high metabolic activity and daily exposure to light (3,4). Pathologic examination and proteome analysis of retinas of eyes with AMD reveal more protein adducts resulting from oxidative modification of carbohydrate and lipid than control eyes (5). The consistent association of smoking with AMD across many different epidemiologic studies and clinical trials provides further evidence that oxidative stress contributes to the disease process. The increasing incidence of macular degeneration with advancing age may be related to gradual dysfunction and degeneration of retinal tissues as oxidative damage accumulates. A growing body of evidence also implicates inflammatory processes in the pathogenesis and progression of macular degeneration (4). Together, these findings provide the biologic plausibility for a role for supplements such as antioxidants and omega-3 fatty acids for prevention and treatment of AMD.

The Age-Related Eye Disease Study (AREDS), a large, randomized, controlled trial of nutritional supplements for AMD, has demonstrated the role of supplements in patients at risk for advanced AMD. This trial and other studies that have investigated the relationship between nutrition and AMD are discussed herein.

THE AGE-RELATED EYE DISEASE STUDY

The Age Related Eye Disease Study (AREDS) is a multicenter, randomized, placebo-controlled trial that was designed to study the natural history of AMD and age-related cataract and to assess the impact of antioxidant vitamins and zinc supplementation on these conditions (6). The intervention incorporated both antioxidants and zinc for two main reasons (6). First, several epidemiologic studies and clinical trials at that time had suggested that antioxidants had a role in reducing the risk of cancer, cardiovascular disease, and eye disease. A small trial also suggested that pharmacologic doses of zinc reduced the risk of vision loss in AMD (7). The second reason was the growing use of commercially available antioxidants and zinc supplements among AMD patients, despite a paucity of clinical evidence. A large, randomized trial was needed to evaluate whether these supplements help in reducing the risks involved in AMD.

The AREDS trial randomized 3640 participants with AMD to antioxidant supplements, zinc, combined antioxidants and zinc, or placebo (Table 26.1). The combined AREDS supplement contained 15 mg beta-carotene, 500 mg vitamin C, 400 international units vitamin E, 80 mg zinc oxide, and 2 mg of copper as cupric oxide. The individual components are discussed separately later in this chapter. Participants were stratified into four categories of AMD based on clinical appearance:

Category 1: No drusen to few drusen; 0.44% developed advanced AMD by year 5.

Category 2: Extensive small drusen, pigment abnormalities, or at least one intermediate druse in at least one eye; 1.3% probability of progression to advanced AMD by year 5.

Category 3: Extensive intermediate drusen, large drusen, or noncentral GA in at least one eye; 18% probability of progression to advanced AMD by year 5. Patients within category 3 who had bilateral large drusen or noncentral GA in at least one eye at enrollment were four times more likely to progress to advanced AMD than the remaining participants in category 3 (27% *vs.* 6% at five years).

Category 4: Advanced AMD or vision loss due to non advanced AMD in one eye; 43% probability of progression to advanced AMD in five years.

The interventional AMD study results were published in 2001 (8). The combination of antioxidant vitamins with zinc was protective against the development of advanced AMD for category 3 and 4 participants (OR 0.66, 95% CI 0.47–0.91, P = 0.001). Those with category 1 or 2 AMD had a very low risk of progression to advanced AMD, and a much larger sample size and longer follow-up would be required to evaluate for a treatment effect for the AREDS formulation for these patients.

Table 26.1 AREDS Treatment Groups

Formulations	Beta-Carotene	Vitamin C	Vitamin E	Zinc Oxide	Cupric Oxide
Placebo	–	–	–	–	–
Antioxidants	15 mg	500 mg	400 IU	–	–
Zinc	–	–	–	80 mg	2 mg
Antioxidants + Zinc	15 mg	500 mg	400 IU	80 mg	2 mg

Abbreviations: AREDS, Age-Related Eye Disease Study; IU international units.

CAROTENOIDS

Carotenoids are organic pigments synthesized by plants and bacteria but not by animals. Carotenoids can be further classified into carotenes (e.g. beta-carotene) and xanthophylls (e.g. lutein, zeaxanthin), which are oxidized derivatives of carotenes. Lutein and zeaxanthin are the only two carotenoids that are naturally found in macular pigment, while beta-carotene is a provitamin A carotenoid studied in AREDS (9). Carotenoids are efficient free-radical scavengers and function as antioxidants in biologically relevant systems. Furthermore, macular pigment absorbs short wavelength light and is thought to protect the outer retina and RPE from light-induced damage.

Beta-Carotene

Beta-carotene is not found in high concentrations in the macula. Major sources of beta-carotene in the diet include cantaloupe, citrus fruits, carrots, and broccoli (10). Beta-carotene was the major carotenoid used in AREDS because other trials were underway at the time investigating the impact of beta-carotene supplementation on cancer and cardiovascular disease (8). Moreover, beta-carotene, unlike lutein and zeaxanthin, was commercially available. AREDS, as reviewed above, showed that supplementation with a combination of high dose zinc, 15 mg beta-carotene, vitamins C and E, and copper was associated with a significant reduction in the risk of progression to advanced AMD in category 3 and 4 participants (OR, 0.72; 99% CI, 0.52–0.98) (8). The antioxidants-only group had a nonsignificant reduction in risk (OR 0.80; 99% CI, 0.59–1.09).

Since beta-carotene was studied in AREDS in combination with other nutrients, it is informative to review other studies of beta-carotene to assess its individual effect. Other available data on the therapeutic role of beta-carotene in AMD have been mixed. A nested case–control study within the Rotterdam Study examining dietary intake of beta-carotene showed a significant reduction in risk of incident early AMD for patients homozygous for *CFH* Y402H in the upper tertile of dietary beta-carotene intake (11). A significant effect was not detected in carriers of the *LOC387715* genotype. In an analysis of the entire Rotterdam cohort, an above-average intake of beta-carotene, vitamin C, vitamin E, and zinc showed a protective effect on incident AMD (35% risk reduction). In univariate analysis, beta-carotene alone was not shown to have a significant effect (12).

Several studies have not shown a benefit for beta-carotene supplementation in AMD. A cross-sectional study of the Alpha-Tocopherol, Beta-Carotene Cancer prevention study (ATBC) cohort in which male smokers were randomized to either 20 mg of beta-carotene, 50 mg of alpha-tocopherol, or a combination for six years failed to demonstrate a significant effect on the final prevalence of AMD (13). Similarly, a complex analysis of the baseline dietary data from the AREDS cohort found no relationship between beta-carotene intake and early or late prevalent AMD. The Blue Mountains Eye Study was an observational, population-based study of common eye diseases in Australia (14). In this study, beta-carotene consumption was a risk factor for the development of incident neovascular AMD (RR 2.40, 95% CI 0.98–5.91, when comparing top tertile of intake with bottom tertile) (15).

Two large, randomized, controlled clinical trials have reported an increased lung cancer risk with beta-carotene supplementation (16,17). Both trials studied primarily smokers and former smokers or asbestos workers. They used higher doses (20–30 mg) of beta-carotene than the AREDS formulation (15 mg), and participants in the Beta-Carotene and Retinol Efficacy Trial also took retinol supplements. The Physicians Health Study, a randomized controlled trial of beta-carotene, did not show a significant difference in mortality or incidence of lung cancer between the treated and untreated groups (18).

The ideal role for beta-carotene in the treatment of AMD remains to be determined. The Age Related Eye Disease Study 2 (AREDS2) will further assess the role of beta-carotene in the AREDS formula by including two formulations without beta-carotene in the secondary randomization of the study (Tables 26.2 and 26.3).

Xanthophylls

Lutein and zeaxanthin are macular pigments that absorb short wavelength light and are thought to thereby protect the outer retina and retinal pigment epithelium (RPE) from damage. They are the primary xanthophylls of interest for preventive treatment of AMD, and AREDS2 has been designed to study the clinical relevance of lutein and zeaxanthin supplements for AMD. Macular pigment levels are decreased in AMD donor eyes when compared with control eyes (19), so lutein and zeaxanthin supplements may help to correct a deficiency in AMD patients. Participants in AREDS2 were randomized to four groups in the primary randomization: placebo, lutein (10 mg)

Table 26.2 Treatment Groups in the Primary Randomization in AREDS2 (3)

Supplement	Daily dose
Placebo	–
Lutein/zeaxanthin	10 mg/2 mg
DHA/EPA	350 mg/650 mg
Lutein/zeaxanthin + DHA/EPA	10 mg/2 mg + 350 mg/650 mg

Abbreviations: AREDS, Age-Related Eye Disease Study; DHA, docosahexaenoic acid; EPA, eicosapentaenoic acid.

Table 26.3 Treatment Groups in the Secondary Randomization in AREDS2 (3)

Formulations	Vitamin C	Vitamin E	Beta-Carotene	Zinc Oxide	Cupric Oxide
1	500 mg	400 IU	15 mg	80 mg	2 mg
2	500 mg	400 IU	**0 mg**	80 mg	2 mg
3	500 mg	400 IU	15 mg	**25 mg**	2 mg
4	500 mg	400 IU	**0 mg**	**25 mg**	2 mg

Abbreviations: AREDS, Age-Related Eye Disease Study; IU, international units.

and zeaxanthin (2 mg), omega-3 long-chain polyunsaturated fatty acids (LC PUFA, 1 g), or a combination treatment (Table 26.2) (3).

Lutein and zeaxanthin are attractive targets for study because of the results of several observational studies. In the AREDS cohort, dietary lutein and zeaxanthin were the only dietary nutrients that were inversely associated with early AMD, geographic atrophy, or neovascular AMD (20). Several other studies have found similar observational results for dietary xanthophylls. In the Eye Disease Case Control Study, greater intake was associated with a reduced risk for AMD (14). The Blue Mountains Eye Study found that those in the upper tertile for dietary lutein and zeaxanthin had a reduced 10-year risk of incident neovascular AMD (RR 0.35, 95% CI 0.13–0.92), but there was no effect on incident early AMD (15). Similarly, data from the Nurses' Health Study and Health Professionals Follow-Up Study suggest that lutein and zeaxanthin are protective for neovascular AMD but not for early AMD (21).

Studies of serum lutein and zeaxanthin levels have suggested that higher levels may be protective against AMD. Baseline data from the Pathologies Oculaires Liées à l'Age (POLA) Study showed that patients with AMD had significantly lower plasma lutein and zeaxanthin levels (22), while a similar study of Chinese participants showed lower plasma lutein and zeaxanthin levels in neovascular AMD patients than in controls (23).

Other studies have not found an association between AMD and the macular xanthophylls. The Rotterdam Study found no correlation between baseline intake data and incident AMD (12), although subgroup analyses of *CFH* Y402H homozygotes and *LOC387715* carriers found that lutein and zeaxanthin intake was protective (11). A nested case–control study within the Beaver Dam Eye Study also found no difference in serum levels between cases and controls (24).

The Food and Drug Administration (FDA) in 2006 reviewed the literature on lutein and zeaxanthin supplementation and concluded that the available data at the time was not strong enough to support their use for treatment of AMD (25). The results of AREDS2 should help clarify their role in treatment.

VITAMIN C

Vitamin C is a water soluble, glucose-derived molecule which plays an important role in collagen, catecholamine, and neurohormone synthesis. It also functions as an antioxidant by scavenging free radicals and detoxifying them in the retina and other neural tissue (26). Vitamin C plays an important role in immune function, iron absorption, and vitamin E regeneration. It is entirely derived from the diet and is abundant in citrus fruits, tomatoes, potatoes, red and green peppers, broccoli, kiwi, and strawberries (12).

Vitamin C, found in rod outer segments and Muller cells, protects vitamin E, an important retinal cell membrane component, from ultraviolet irradiation-induced oxidation (26). Vitamin C also allows vitamin E regeneration, thus improving antioxidant activity in the retina. Vitamin C supplementation has been shown to protect rat eyes from light toxicity (27), and animals exposed to more light have higher concentrations of vitamin C in the retina (28). For these reasons, vitamin C and other antioxidants are thought to protect the retina from oxidative damage.

As discussed above, vitamin C is one of the components of the protective AREDS formulation. In the Rotterdam Study, an above median intake of vitamin C, vitamin E, beta-carotene, and zinc was associated with a 35% reduced risk of incident AMD (12). No prospective trials of vitamin C alone for AMD have been conducted. Most observational studies of vitamin C and AMD have not detected a benefit. The majority of these studies rely upon patient surveys of dietary vitamin C intake. This includes the AREDS Case Control Study (20), the Blue Mountains Eye Study (15), the Eye Disease Case Control Study (14), the Beaver Dam Eye Study (29), the Nurses' Health Study, and Health Professionals Follow-up Study (21). Studies of serum levels of vitamin C have not revealed a relationship with AMD status (30).

VITAMIN E

"Vitamin E" refers to a group of both tocopherols and tocotrienols, and the most abundant form in the retina is alpha-tocopherol (31). Vitamin E is a potent antioxidant and free-radical scavenger. Dietary sources include whole grains, fortified cereals, and nuts (32). Oxidative damage to the retina and RPE is thought to contribute to the pathogenesis of AMD, leading to the investigation of vitamin E and other antioxidant supplements to be used for treatment and prevention of AMD.

The AREDS formulation, as discussed above, contained 400 international units of vitamin E and was protective for patients at the highest risk for the development of advanced AMD (8). However, three randomized, controlled trials of vitamin E have not shown a significant effect for vitamin E alone. The Women's Health Study, which studied 600 international units of vitamin E on alternate days in 39,876 healthy female health professionals, showed no effect on incident, visually significant AMD over 10 years (33). Similarly, the ATBC study found no protective effect in 29,000 male smokers over six years of follow-up (13). The Vitamin E, Cataract, and Age-Related Maculopathy (VECAT) study examined the effect of 500 IU vitamin E on the incidence of AMD in 1193 Australians. It showed no effect of vitamin E supplementation on the incidence of early or late AMD (34).

On the other hand, data from the Rotterdam Study support the findings from AREDS. Analysis of dietary surveys found that an above median intake of vitamin E, vitamin C, beta-carotene, and zinc was associated with a 35% reduced risk of incident AMD (12). Furthermore, an analysis of vitamin E intake alone in this study found a protective effect for incident AMD. Data from other observational studies including POLA (30) and the Beaver Dam Eye Study (24) have suggested a beneficial effect on AMD.

Some studies have called into question the safety of vitamin E supplementation. The Selenium and Vitamin E Cancer Prevention Trial (SELECT) found an increased risk of prostate cancer in the treatment group taking 400 IU of vitamin E daily compared with placebo (35). There were one to two more cases of prostate cancer per 1000 taking daily vitamin E, but this effect was not found in the group that took both vitamin E and selenium. Furthermore, other randomized trials of vitamin E supplementation including the ATBC trial (36), the Physicians Health Study II (37), and AREDS have not found an increased risk of prostate cancer. A large meta-analysis examining the impact of vitamin E on mortality showed a minimally increased risk of mortality with vitamin E supplementation both when used alone or in combination with beta-carotene and vitamin A (RR 1.04, 95% CI 1.01–1.07) (38). This meta-analysis also found a small increased mortality risk for beta-carotene (RR 1.07, 95%

CI 1.02–1.11). AREDS mortality analyses did not show any effect of AREDS supplements on mortality (39).

ZINC

Zinc is an essential micronutrient. Important dietary sources include shellfish, beef, fortified cereals, pork, beans, and chicken (40). Deficiency is rare in North America, and it tends to occur in populations that consume large quantities of unleavened grain products that contain phytates, which are proteins that chelate zinc.

Numerous proteins found in the retina require zinc as a co-factor (41). For example, zinc is a co-factor for Cu/Zn superoxide dismutase, which converts superoxide to oxygen and hydrogen peroxide. Human RPE cells are more susceptible to hydrogen peroxide-induced oxidative damage in zinc-deficient culture media, and this may be due to a zinc-related reduction in catalase activity (42). Zinc levels are relatively high in human retina, and deficiency has been linked to night blindness and impaired dark adaptation (43). Furthermore, zinc levels in the neural retina and choroid have been shown to vary with age (41). Zinc levels decline with age in the neural retina and increase with age in the choroid. No age-related change has been demonstrated in the RPE.

Zinc (80 mg) is a component of the protective AREDS supplement for AMD. The zinc without antioxidants treatment group in AREDS had a suggestive, but not statistically significant, reduction in risk of progression to advanced disease (OR 0.75; 99% CI, 0.55–1.03). A small, randomized, controlled trial of 100 mg of oral zinc sulfate for a wide range of AMD patients was concluded in 1988. This trial provided the first clinical evidence of a beneficial effect of zinc supplementation in AMD (7). Since 1988, AREDS and several other studies have provided further evidence of a relationship between zinc status and AMD. In the Rotterdam Study, an above-median intake of vitamin E, vitamin C, beta-carotene, and zinc was associated with a 35% reduced risk of incident AMD (12). Furthermore, analysis of dietary zinc intake in the Rotterdam cohort showed a protective effect for zinc on incident AMD. Analyses from the Blue Mountains Eye Study also found a higher dietary zinc intake to have a favorable effect on incident AMD (15). In the Beaver Dam Eye Study, dietary zinc had a moderate favorable effect on incident pigmentary changes but not on overall incident AMD (44).

There are also several studies that have not detected a relationship between zinc status and AMD. Stur and colleagues performed a randomized, controlled trial of 200 mg of oral zinc sulfate over two years in patients with unilateral neovascular AMD (n = 112) (45). Only 14 patients developed new neovascularization during the two-year study, and there was no apparent treatment benefit. The Nurses' Health Study and Health Professionals Follow-up Study found no relationship between dietary zinc and incident AMD (21), and the Eye Disease Case Control Study showed no relationship between serum zinc levels and prevalent neovascular AMD (14).

Oral zinc supplements are generally well tolerated, but toxicities can occur. Zinc can interfere with the absorption of dietary copper and iron (6). Zinc chloride is a gastrointestinal irritant (8). In AREDS, patients taking zinc were hospitalized more often for genitourinary complaints than controls (7.5% *vs.* 4.9%; P = 0 001) (8). In AREDS2, a lower zinc dose (25 mg) will be tested because 80 mg doses are now thought to overload the gastrointestinal tract's capacity for zinc absorption.

FATTY ACIDS

As discussed previously, LC PUFAs, docosahexaenoic acid (DHA), and eicosapentaenoic acid (EPA) are being investigated for AMD in AREDS2. DHA is present in high concentrations in the outer segments of photoreceptors (46). It is an important structural component of retinal membranes, and tissue DHA status affects retinal cell signaling and photo transduction. Humans synthesize DHA from the essential fatty acids alpha-linoleic acid (ALA) and EPA (46). Dietary sources of ALA include flaxseed oil, soybeans, and canola oil. Oily fish such as tuna, halibut, and salmon are excellent sources of EPA and DHA (46).

DHA and EPA are hypothesized to be protective agents in AMD, and protective effects could be mediated via effects on gene expression, retinal cell differentiation, and cell survival (47). DHA activates a number of nuclear hormone receptors that operate as transcription factors for molecules that modulate redox-sensitive and proinflammatory genes. Omega-3 LC PUFAs also affect the production and activation of angiogenic growth factors, arachidonic acid-based proangiogenic eicosanoids, and matrix metalloproteinases involved in vascular remodeling (46).

While not all studies have detected a salutary effect of omega-3 LC PUFAs for AMD, a great majority of evidence suggests a benefit for those with higher omega-3 intake. Evidence to date comes from numerous observational studies, and no randomized trials of omega-3 supplementation for AMD have yet been completed. The Women's Health Study followed over 38,000 female health professionals for an average of 10 years, finding that the risk of incident AMD was significantly lower in the highest tertile of DHA intake (RR 0.62, 95% CI 0.44–0.87 when compared with lowest tertile) (48). In AREDS, at-risk participants in the highest quintile of EPA plus DHA intake were less likely to progress to central geographic atrophy or neovascular AMD than those in the lowest quintile (RR 0.65 for central geographic atrophy, 95% CI 0.45–0.92; RR 0.68 for neovascular AMD, 95% CI 0.49–0.94) (49). In the Blue Mountains Eye Study, those who consumed at least one serving of fish weekly were less likely to develop early AMD over 10 years (RR 0.69, 95% CI 0.49–0.98) (50). AREDS2 is currently evaluating 1 g of omega-3 LC PUFAs in the treatment of AMD.

SUMMARY POINTS

- Although data in the literature are mixed with regards to each of the Age-Related Eye Disease Study (AREDS) and AREDS2 micronutrients, the AREDS results demonstrate the role of the specific AREDS antioxidant with zinc formulation in the prevention of advanced AMD.

- The AREDS formulation is recommended as a treatment for nonsmokers with extensive intermediate drusen, large drusen, noncentral geographic atrophy, or unilateral advanced AMD. Observational data for the macular xanthophylls and for omega-3 fatty acids are promising, but in the absence of data from a large, randomized clinical trial these supplements cannot yet be recommended for AMD.
- AREDS2 has been designed to resolve these questions, and AREDS2 study results are eagerly anticipated.

REFERENCES

1. Congdon N, O'Colmain B, Klaver CC, et al. Causes and prevalence of visual impairment among adults in the united states. Arch Ophthalmol 2004; 122: 477–85.
2. Kocur I, Resnikoff S. Visual impairment and blindness in Europe and their prevention. Br J Ophthalmol 2002; 86: 716–22.
3. Krishnadev N, Meleth AD, Chew EY. Nutritional supplements for age-related macular degeneration. Curr Opin Ophthalmol 2010; 21: 184–9.
4. Ding X, Patel M, Chan CC. Molecular pathology of age-related macular degeneration. Prog Retin Eye Res 2009; 28: 1–18.
5. Crabb JW, Miyagi M, Gu X, et al. Drusen proteome analysis: an approach to the etiology of age-related macular degeneration. Proc Natl Acad Sci U S A 2002; 99: 14682–7.
6. The Age-Related Eye Disease Study (AREDS): design implications. AREDS report no. 1. Control Clin Trials 1999; 20: 573–600.
7. Newsome DA, Swartz M, Leone NC, Elston RC, Miller E. Oral zinc in macular degeneration. Arch Ophthalmol 1988; 106: 192–8.
8. A randomized. placebo-controlled, clinical trial of high-dose supplementation with vitamins C and E, beta carotene, and zinc for age-related macular degeneration and vision loss: AREDS report no. 8. Arch Ophthalmol 2001; 119: 1417–36.
9. Khoo HE, Prasad KN, Kong KW, Jiang Y, Ismail A. Carotenoids and their isomers: color pigments in fruits and vegetables. Molecules 2011; 16: 1710–38.
10. Nebeling LC, Forman MR, Graubard BI, Snyder RA. Changes in carotenoid intake in the United States: the 1987 and 1992 national health interview surveys. J Am Diet Assoc 1997; 97: 991–6.
11. Ho L, van Leeuwen R, Witteman JC, et al. Reducing the genetic risk of age-related macular degeneration with dietary antioxidants, zinc, and omega-3 fatty acids: the Rotterdam study. Arch Ophthalmol 2011; 129: 758–66.
12. van Leeuwen R, Boekhoorn S, Vingerling JR, et al. Dietary intake of antioxidants and risk of age-related macular degeneration. JAMA 2005; 294: 3101–7.
13. Teikari JM, Laatikainen L, Virtamo J, et al. Six-year supplementation with alpha-tocopherol and beta-carotene and age-related maculopathy. Acta Ophthalmol Scand 1998; 76: 224–9.
14. Seddon JM, Ajani UA, Sperduto RD, et al. Eye Disease Case-Control Study Group. Dietary carotenoids, vitamins A, C, and E, and advanced age-related macular degeneration. JAMA 1994; 272: 1413–20.

15. Tan JS, Wang JJ, Flood V, et al. Dietary antioxidants and the long-term incidence of age-related macular degeneration: the Blue Mountains Eye Study. Ophthalmology 2008; 115: 334–41.

16. The Alpha-Tocopherol, Beta Carotene Cancer Prevention Study Group. The effect of vitamin E and beta carotene on the incidence of lung cancer and other cancers in male smokers. N Engl J Med 1994;330:1029–35.

17. Omenn GS, Goodman GE, Thornquist MD, et al. Effects of a combination of beta carotene and vitamin A on lung cancer and cardiovascular disease. N Engl J Med 1996; 334: 1150–5.

18. Hennekens CH, Buring JE, Manson JE, et al. Lack of effect of long-term supplementation with beta carotene on the incidence of malignant neoplasms and cardiovascular disease. N Engl J Med 1996; 334: 1145–9.

19. Bone RA, Landrum JT, Mayne ST, et al. Macular pigment in donor eyes with and without AMD: a case-control study. Invest Ophthalmol Vis Sci 2001; 42: 235–40.

20. SanGiovanni JP, Chew EY, Clemons TE, et al. The relationship of dietary carotenoid and vitamin A, E, and C intake with age-related macular degeneration in a case-control study: AREDS report no. 22. Arch Ophthalmol 2007; 125: 1225–32.

21. Cho E, Seddon JM, Rosner B, Willett WC, Hankinson SE. Prospective study of intake of fruits, vegetables, vitamins, and carotenoids and risk of age-related maculopathy. Arch Ophthalmol 2004; 122: 883–92.

22. Delcourt C, Carriere I, Delage M, Barberger-Gateau P, Schalch W. Plasma lutein and zeaxanthin and other carotenoids as modifiable risk factors for age-related maculopathy and cataract: the POLA study. Invest Ophthalmol Vis Sci 2006; 47: 2329–35.

23. Zhou H, Zhao X, Johnson EJ, et al. Serum carotenoids and risk of age-related macular degeneration in a Chinese population sample. Invest Ophthalmol Vis Sci 2011; 52: 4338–44.

24. Mares-Perlman JA, Brady WE, Klein R, et al. Serum antioxidants and age-related macular degeneration in a population-based case-control study. Arch Ophthalmol 1995; 113: 1518–23.

25. Trumbo PR, Ellwood KC. Lutein and zeaxanthin intakes and risk of age-related macular degeneration and cataracts: an evaluation using the food and drug administration's evidence-based review system for health claims. Am J Clin Nutr 2006; 84: 971–4.

26. Friedman PA, Zeidel ML. Victory at C. Nat Med 1999; 5: 620–1.

27. Organisciak DT, Wang HM, Li ZY, Tso MO. The protective effect of ascorbate in retinal light damage of rats. Invest Ophthalmol Vis Sci 1985; 26: 1580–8.

28. Penn JS, Naash MI, Anderson RE. Effect of light history on retinal antioxidants and light damage susceptibility in the rat. Exp Eye Res 1987; 44: 779–88.

29. Mares-Perlman JA, Klein R, Klein BE, et al. Association of zinc and antioxidant nutrients with age-related maculopathy. Arch Ophthalmol 1996; 114: 991–7.

30. Delcourt C, Cristol JP, Tessier F, et al. POLA Study Group. Age-related macular degeneration and antioxidant status in the POLA study. Pathologies Oculaires Liees a l'Age. Arch Ophthalmol 1999; 117: 1384–90.

31. Katz ML, Robison WG Jr. Light and aging effects on vitamin E in the retina and retinal pigment epithelium. Vision Res 1987; 27: 1875–9.

32. Dietary Supplement Fact Sheet: Vitamin E. Office of Dietary Supplements, National Institutes of Health. (Accessed

August 2, 2012, at http://ods.od.nih.gov/factsheets/VitaminE-HealthProfessional/.)

33. Christen WG, Glynn RJ, Chew EY, Buring JE. Vitamin E and age-related macular degeneration in a randomized trial of women. Ophthalmology 2010; 117: 1163–8.

34. Taylor HR, Tikellis G, Robman LD, McCarty CA, McNeil JJ. Vitamin E supplementation and macular degeneration: randomised controlled trial. BMJ 2002; 325: 11.

35. Klein EA, Thompson IM Jr, Tangen CM, et al. Vitamin E and the risk of prostate cancer: the selenium and vitamin E cancer prevention trial (SELECT). JAMA 2011; 306: 1549–56.

36. Albanes D, Heinonen OP, Huttunen JK, et al. Effects of alpha-tocopherol and beta-carotene supplements on cancer incidence in the alpha-tocopherol beta-carotene cancer prevention study. Am J Clin Nutr 1995; 62: 1427S–30S.

37. Gaziano JM, Glynn RJ, Christen WG, et al. Vitamins E and C in the prevention of prostate and total cancer in men: the physicians' health study II randomized controlled trial. JAMA 2009; 301: 52–62.

38. Bjelakovic G, Nikolova D, Gluud LL, Simonetti RG, Gluud C. Mortality in randomized trials of antioxidant supplements for primary and secondary prevention: systematic review and meta-analysis. JAMA 2007; 297: 842–57.

39. Clemons TE, Kurinij N, Sperduto RD. Associations of mortality with ocular disorders and an intervention of high-dose antioxidants and zinc in the age-related eye disease study: AREDS report no. 13. Arch Ophthalmol 2004; 122: 716–26.

40. Dietary Supplement Fact Sheet: Zinc. Office of Dietary Supplements, National Institutes of Health. (Accessed March 5, 2012, at http://ods.od.nih.gov/FactSheets/Zinc/.)

41. Wills NK, Ramanujam VM, Kalariya N, Lewis JR, van Kuijk FJ. Copper and zinc distribution in the human retina: relationship to cadmium accumulation, age, and gender. Exp Eye Res 2008; 87: 80–8.

42. Tate DJ Jr, Miceli MV, Newsome DA. Zinc protects against oxidative damage in cultured human retinal pigment epithelial cells. Free Radic Biol Med 1999; 26: 704–13.

43. Grahn BH, Paterson PG, Gottschall-Pass KT, Zhang Z. Zinc and the eye. J Am Coll Nutr 2001; 20: 106–18.

44. VandenLangenberg GM, Mares-Perlman JA, Klein R, et al. Associations between antioxidant and zinc intake and the 5-year incidence of early age-related maculopathy in the beaver dam eye study. Am J Epidemiol 1998; 148: 204–14.

45. Stur M, Tittl M, Reitner A, Meisinger V. Oral zinc and the second eye in age-related macular degeneration. Invest Ophthalmol Vis Sci 1996; 37: 1225–35.

46. SanGiovanni JP, Chew EY. The role of omega-3 long-chain polyunsaturated fatty acids in health and disease of the retina. Prog Retin Eye Res 2005; 24: 87–138.

47. Gordon WC, Bazan NG. Retina. In: Harding JJ, ed. Biochemisttry of the Eye, 1st edn. London: Chapman & Hall, 1997.

48. Christen WG, Schaumberg DA, Glynn RJ, Buring JE. Dietary omega-3 fatty acid and fish intake and incident age-related macular degeneration in women. Arch Ophthalmol 2011; 129: 921–9.

49. Sangiovanni JP, Agron E, Meleth AD, et al. {omega}-3 Long-chain polyunsaturated fatty acid intake and 12-y incidence of neovascular age-related macular degeneration and central geographic atrophy: AREDS report 30, a prospective cohort study from the age-related eye disease study. Am J Clin Nutr 2009; 90: 1601–7.

50. Tan JS, Wang JJ, Flood V, Mitchell P. Dietary fatty acids and the 10-year incidence of age-related macular degeneration: the blue mountains eye study. Arch Ophthalmol 2009; 127: 656–65.

27

Visual cycle modulation

Ravi S. J. Singh and Judy E. Kim

Age-related macular degeneration (AMD) is the most common cause of irreversible vision loss in patients over the age of 60 in developed countries (1). With the expected increase in the aged population and age-related eye diseases due to increased life expectancies, significant efforts are being made to better understand and treat AMD. While anti-vascular endothelial growth factor agents have been successfully utilized to combat neovascular AMD, there is still much need for improved management of non-neovascular AMD.

Under physiological conditions, the retinal pigment epithelium (RPE) maintains photoreceptor homeostasis by providing nutrients and disposal of shed outer segments. While the exact pathogenesis of AMD is not fully understood, genetic, immunological, and environmental factors play a role to disrupt this homeostasis. A prominent early feature of AMD is accumulation of toxic by-products of photoreceptor outer-segment metabolism, such as lipofuscin and A2E in the Bruch's membrane and RPE (2–4). The disease is clinically characterized by the deposition of drusen along the Bruch's membrane with dysfunction and degeneration of RPE, photoreceptors and, in some cases, development of choroidal neovascularization (CNV). Fundus autofluorescence imaging of non-neovascular AMD may demonstrate increased autofluorescence, especially along the edge of geographic atrophy (GA), consistent with excess lipofuscin accumulation and over time, enlargement of GA occurs into these areas of excess lipofuscin accumulation (5). Therefore, it is reasonable to assume that if the accumulation of the lipofuscin and other toxic by-products can be reduced, it should be possible to reduce RPE and photoreceptor degeneration and potentially slow down the progression of non-neovascular AMD (6,7).

The retina converts light stimuli into neuronal impulse by a process called visual transduction. Rods and cones contain light-receptive proteins called opsins that are members of the G-protein linked receptor family linked to a chromophore which is 11-*cis*-retinaldehyde for most opsins (8). Visual transduction begins with light absorption by opsin pigment that causes isomerization of the associated chromophore (8). This initiates a complex cascade of events leading to hyperpolarization of the photoreceptor membrane and generation of a synaptic impulse. Following a light impulse, 11-*cis*-retinaldehyde is photoisomerized to all-*trans*-retinaldehyde to initiate phototransduction; it is regenerated by a sequence of reactions referred to as the visual cycle.

Besides regenerating 11-*cis*-retinaldehyde, the visual cycle also generates toxic by-products of chromophores such as lipofuscin and A2E, which accumulate in minimal amounts in the RPE with normal aging, but in patients with AMD these accumulate and reach retinotoxic levels (9).

VISUAL CYCLE

In order to understand the therapeutic approaches with visual cycle modulators, it is prudent to understand various steps of the visual cycle and how defects in some of these steps manifest clinically. The main steps of the visual cycle are highlighted in Figure 27.1. Light-induced isomerization of 11-*cis*-retinaldehyde to all-*trans*-retinaldehyde induces a short-lived change in rhodopsin conformation to an activated state called metarhodopsin II (10). Metarhodopsin II stimulates the visual transduction cascade with closure of cGMP-gated cation channels and hyperpolarization of the photoreceptor cell. Then, metarhodopsin is inactivated to apo-opsin and releases all-*trans*-retinaldehyde. Free all-*trans*-retinaldehyde then undergoes a series of enzymatic reactions to regenerate 11-*cis*-retinaldehyde. This pathway, called the visual cycle or retinoid cycle, ensures an optimal supply of chromophore to the photoreceptors for maintaining vision and requires close interaction between the RPE and photoreceptor outer segments. Free all-*trans*-retinaldehyde is cleared from the interior of photoreceptor discs by an ATP-binding cassette transporter (ABCA4) (11). Under physiological conditions, some of the retinaldehyde combines with phosphatidylethanolamine (PE), in the disc lipid bilayer, to form *N-retinylidene-PE* (N-ret-PE) that is not readily cleared by ABCA4. Mice with a knockout mutation in the *abcr* gene show delayed clearance of all-*trans*-retinaldehyde and elevated *N-ret-PE* in the retina. Patients with Stargardt's disease have a mutation in the ABCA4 gene and have increased levels of N-ret-PE and all-*trans*-retinaldehyde in the retina (11,12). Elevated levels of N-ret-PE and all-*trans*-retinaldehyde undergo a secondary non-enzymatic condensation to yield toxic A2PE-H2. The distal outer photoreceptor segments containing A2PE-H2 and elevated levels of all-*trans*-retinaldehyde and *N-ret-PE* are phagocytosed by the RPE as part of the normal disc-renewal process (13,14). However, in this pathologic state, the RPE is unable to fully degrade the non-physiologic load and thus toxic retinal fluorophores A2E and lipofuscin accumulate. This produces the characteristic clinical phenotype of Stargardt's disease (11,12).

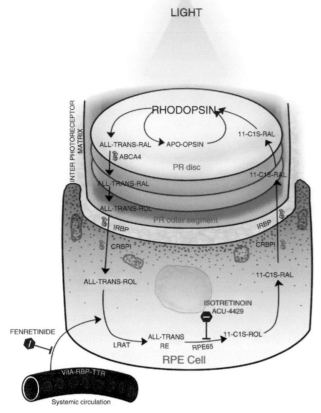

Figure 27.1 Light-induced photoisomerization of 11-cis-retinaldehyde to all-trans-retinaldehyde leads to visual transduction. Visual cycle involves a series of reactions to replenish the spent chromophore and regenerate 11-cis-retinaldehyde. Therapeutic strategies to modulate the visual cycle propose to reduce the flux through the visual cycle by blocking specific steps as illustrated above. *Abbreviations*: CRBP1, cellular retinol-binding protein 1; IRBP, interphotoreceptor-binding protein; PR, Photoreceptor; RAL, retinaldehyde; RE, retinyl ester; ROL, retinol; RBP, retinol binding protein; TTR, transthyretin; VitA, vitamin A.

Accumulation of A2E and lipofuscin in the RPE also occurs with age but the amount is low and does not cause significant toxicity (14).

After transport from the photoreceptor discs to the outer segments, all-*trans*-retinaldehyde is enzymatically reduced to all-*trans*-retinol (vitamin A) by retinol dehydrogenases (14,15). All-*trans*-retinol is rapidly released by photoreceptor cells to the interphotoreceptor matrix, where it binds to interphotoreceptor-binding protein (IRBP) which promotes further release of all-*trans*-retinol from bleached photoreceptors (16). RPE cells contain cellular retinol-binding protein-1 (CRBP1) that has a 100-fold higher affinity for all-*trans*-retinol than IRBP (17) and CRBP1 promotes the uptake of all-*trans*-retinol into the RPE. The RPE also receives all-*trans*-retinol from the blood where it is complexed with the retinol-binding protein (RBP) and transthyretin.

Within the RPE cells, CRBP1-bound all-*trans*-retinol is enzymatically esterified to all-*trans*-retinyl ester by the enzyme, lecithin:retinol acyl transferase (LRAT) (18). The all-*trans*-retinyl ester is then isomerized to 11-*cis*-configuration by RPE65 isomerase (18–20). Mice with a knockout mutation in the *rpe65* gene contain no detectable 11-*cis*-retinoids (19) and children with RPE65 mutation develop Leber's congenital amaurosis (21).

The final step of the visual cycle involves oxidation of the 11-*cis*-retinol to 11-*cis*-retinaldehyde. The newly formed 11-*cis*-retinaldehyde has a much higher affinity for IRBP than CRBP1 (17,22) that promotes its release from RPE cells to the interphotoreceptor matrix. The photoreceptor opsins then take up the 11-*cis*-retinaldehyde from the interphotoreceptor matrix to generate another visual transduction cycle.

Photoreceptor outer segments are continually formed and the distal ends are shed intermittently that are phagocytosed by the RPE (13). The RPE lysosomal system efficiently degrades the phagocytosed retinoids including chromophores, *N-ret-PE*, A2PE-H2, and other by-products. While only minimal amounts of A2E and lipofuscin accumulate in the RPE in normal aging process, in pathologic states such as AMD, the RPE phagolysosomal system becomes less efficient and this inefficient clearing leads to accumulation of lipofuscin, A2E and other toxic by-products (9,14). This sets up a vicious cycle as lipofuscin and A2E-mediated cytotoxicity further compromises RPE function; A2E impairs the degradative capacity of RPE (23), initiates blue-light-induced phototoxicity in RPE cells (24), causes loss of membrane integrity, and induces apoptosis in RPE cells (25–27) with a secondary photoreceptor loss (23,28).

The pathogenesis of AMD is most likely multifactorial. It includes underlying mutations in the complement pathways, increased susceptibility to oxidative damage and inflammation, accumulation of cytotoxic undegradable waste products in RPE such as A2E and lipofuscin, and environmental factors such as cigarette smoking, light exposure, and lack of antioxidants in diet (7,29,30). One strategy to treat AMD would be to reduce or prevent the formation of toxic lipofuscin and A2E (7) which could slow down the progression of photoreceptor degeneration and vision loss. Proposed approaches to modulate the visual cycle aim to limit flux through the visual cycle and delay the accumulation of lipofuscin and A2E. Some of the current efforts and approaches to visual cycle modulation are discussed in the following section.

ISOTRETINOIN

Isotretinoin (Accutane®, Hoffmann-La Roche, Inc., Nutley, New Jersey, USA) is an oral retinoid drug used for treating severe acne vulgaris. It was noted that some of the patients on this medication experienced reduced night vision and had depression of scotopic ERG (31). Isotretinoin decreases the formation of 11-*cis*-retinaldehyde by inhibiting retinol dehydrogenases and RPE65 isomerase (31,32) and in animal studies, it blocked the age-dependent accumulation of lipofuscin and A2E in wild-type mice and the synthesis of toxic fluorophores in abcr/knockout mice (33–35). This spurred interest in using isotretinoin as a potential treatment for AMD. It was evaluated in human patients with neovascular AMD, but failed to show any notable visual benefits and patients had frequent adverse reactions including muscle aches, labile mood, and mucus membrane dryness (36).

N-(4-HYDROXYPHENYL) RETINAMIDE

N-(4-hydroxyphenyl) retinamide (Fenretinide®, ReVision Therapeutics, San Diego, California, USA) is an oral synthetic retinoid analog that is used as a chemotherapeutic agent to treat cancer. It is effective against a variety of cancer cells because it is antiangiogenic, induces apoptosis, and enhances production of reactive oxygen (37). It also lowers serum RBP (38) and thereby reduces transport of vitamin A to RPE. By limiting the supply of vitamin A to retina, it is expected to downregulate the visual cycle and thus reduce the accumulation of toxic fluorophores. Normally, all-trans-retinol is transported to the RPE as a complex with RBP and transthyretin. The large size of the retinol–RBP–transthyretin complex resists glomerular filtration in the kidney and provides a steady state concentration of retinol for uptake by the RPE. Fenretinide binds to RBP and prevents its interaction with transthyretin; kidneys readily excrete RBP that is not complexed with transthyretin. Fenretinide treatment causes a dose-dependent reduction in circulating RBP and thus decreases the level of RBP-bound retinol that is available for uptake by the RPE (39). When administered to abcr/knockout mice, fenretinide caused dose-dependent reductions in serum retinol and RBP, and arrested accumulation of A2E and lipofuscin in the RPE with modest delays in dark adaptation (39). Results from a two-year, randomized, multicenter phase 2 study suggest that fenretinide may reduce the progression of GA. In this study, the effect of 100 mg or 300 mg per day of fenretinide was evaluated in 246 patients with GA. Results not only suggest a beneficial effect of delaying the progression of GA as measured by lesion growth, but also the possible use of RBP levels as a surrogate marker for efficacy since sustained reduction in RBP seemed to be predictive of a positive treatment response to fenretinide (40,41). Results also show a possible decrease in the incidence of CNV with treatment (42). This may not be entirely surprising given the antiangiogenic properties of fenretinide (37).

Fenretinide has been extensively used for cancer therapy and prevention of malignant neoplasms across a wide range of patient population and appears to be well tolerated (43–45). Acquired night blindness and dry eye symptoms were rarely symptomatic and reversible changes in dark adaptation and ERG were noted with use of high doses in some studies (45,46). However, these studies were performed on subjects having no ocular pathology and the effect of long-term use of fenretinide in patients with AMD, where the RPE is already diseased, is not yet known.

ACU-4429

ACU-4429 (Acucela Inc., Bothell, Washington, USA) is another visual cycle modulator being evaluated for use in AMD. It is an orally administered small non-retinoid molecule that inhibits RPE65 isomerase and prevents the conversion of all-trans-retinyl ester to 11-cis-retinol (47). By slowing down the regeneration of visual chromophore, the drug is expected to decrease the rate of accumulation of A2E. It was shown to be safe and well tolerated as a single dose of up to 75 mg in healthy volunteers. Side effects include reversible dyschromatopsia and delayed dark adaptation (47). Since the drug was expected to affect rod function only and the cone ERG was unaltered in the study, dyschromatopsia noted in subjects on a higher dose was attributed to a possible secondary effect of rod inhibition on cone function. Further trials of this medication are underway.

Therapeutic modulation of the visual cycle holds promise as a possible future AMD treatment. By reducing the flux through the visual cycle, this approach arrests the accumulation of lipofuscin and A2E in mice (35,39) and appears to be well tolerated in healthy human volunteers (47). However, the obvious downside of downregulating the visual cycle is delayed dark adaptation (45–47), which may have minimal bearing on present day predominantly photopic lifestyles. Moreover, modest reductions in scotopic vision may be a tolerable trade off, if these medications do indeed prove beneficial in preserving central visual acuity in patients with AMD by decelerating the progression of dry AMD. However, numerous questions remain unanswered. While visual cycle modulation is well tolerated in healthy volunteers, patients with already diseased RPE and retina could have clinically relevant adverse manifestations. Many patients with AMD already have reduced dark adaptation at baseline (48–50) and it is possible that visual cycle modulators may further worsen it to a significant degree. Additionally, the present recommendation of dietary supplementation for patients with category 3 and 4 AMD with Age-Related Eye Disease Study (AREDS) formulation that includes beta-carotene (51,52), seems contradictory to reducing the flux through the visual cycle, as beta-carotene gets metabolized to all-trans-retinol in the RPE (53). However, the beneficial role of high doses of beta-carotene may be an antioxidant effect (7,54) and not antagonistic to visual cycle modulators. Future studies will elucidate this relationship further.

The goal of treating dry AMD is to prevent vision loss by anatomic and physiological preservation of photoreceptors and the RPE–choriocapillaris complex. Since vision loss in AMD is multifactorial, it is likely that a multimodal therapeutic approach would have a better chance of succeeding and preserving vision in this condition. Visual cycle modulation holds promise as a therapeutic approach for patients with dry AMD and possibly retinal dystrophies such as Stargardt disease for which no treatment is currently available. The ongoing research and clinical trials will provide valuable new insights and hope for our patients over the years to come.

SUMMARY POINTS

- Light-induced photoisomerization of 11-cis-retinaldehyde initiates phototransduction in the retina and the spent 11-cis-retinaldehyde is regenerated by a sequence of reactions called visual cycle.

- A prominent early feature of AMD is the accumulation of toxic by-products of the visual cycle, such as lipofuscin and A2E, in the Bruch's membrane and RPE.
- Therapeutic strategies to modulate the visual cycle aim to limit flux through the visual cycle and slow down the accumulation of toxic lipofuscin and A2E.
- Drugs that modulate visual cycle such as ACU-4429 and fenretinide are being evaluated in clinical trials for treating non-neovascular AMD.
- Visual cycle modulation may reduce scotopic vision as an adverse effect.
- Future studies will help elucidate the role of visual cycle modulation in the treatment of non-neovascular AMD.

REFERENCES

1. Klein R, Klein BE, Linton KL. Prevalence of age-related maculopathy. The Beaver Dam Eye Study. Ophthalmology 1992; 99: 933–43.
2. Leveziel N, Tilleul J, Puche N, et al. Genetic factors associated with age-related macular degeneration. Ophthalmologica 2011; 226: 87–102.
3. Fazelat A, Bahrani H, Buzney S, et al. Autoimmunity and age-related macular degeneration: a review of the literature. Semin Ophthalmol 2011; 26: 304–11.
4. Galor A, Lee DJ. Effects of smoking on ocular health. Curr Opin Ophthalmol 2011; 22: 477–82.
5. Schmitz-Valckenberg S, Fleckenstein M, Scholl HP, et al. Fundus autofluorescence and progression of age-related macular degeneration. Surv Ophthalmol 2009; 54: 96–117.
6. Yehoshua Z, Rosenfeld PJ, Albini TA. Current clinical trials in dry amd and the definition of appropriate clinical outcome measures. Semin Ophthalmol 2011; 26: 167–80.
7. Zarbin MA, Rosenfeld PJ. Pathway-based therapies for age-related macular degeneration: an integrated survey of emerging treatment alternatives. Retina 2010; 30: 1350–67.
8. Filipek S, Stenkamp RE, Teller DC, et al. G protein-coupled receptor rhodopsin: a prospectus. Annu Rev Physiol 2003; 65: 851–79.
9. Kinnunen K, Petrovski G, Moe MC, et al. Molecular mechanisms of retinal pigment epithelium damage and development of age-related macular degeneration. Acta Ophthalmol 2012; 90: 299–309.
10. Okada T, Ernst OP, Palczewski K, et al. Activation of rhodopsin: new insights from structural and biochemical studies. Trends Biochem Sci 2001; 26: 318–24.
11. Tsybovsky Y, Molday RS, Palczewski K. The ATP-binding cassette transporter ABCA4: structural and functional properties and role in retinal disease. Adv Exp Med Biol 2010; 703: 105–25.
12. Allikmets R. A photoreceptor cell-specific ATP-binding transporter gene (ABCR) is mutated in recessive Stargardt macular dystrophy. Nat Genet 1997; 17: 122.
13. Young RW, Bok D. Participation of the retinal pigment epithelium in the rod outer segment renewal process. J Cell Biol 1969; 42: 392–403.
14. Travis GH, Golczak M, Moise AR, et al. Diseases caused by defects in the visual cycle: retinoids as potential therapeutic agents. Annu Rev Pharmacol Toxicol 2007; 47: 469–512.
15. Rattner A, Smallwood PM, Nathans J. Identification and characterization of all-trans-retinol dehydrogenase from photoreceptor outer segments, the visual cycle enzyme that reduces all-trans-retinal to all-trans-retinol. J Biol Chem 2000; 275: 11034–43.
16. Gonzalez-Fernandez F, Ghosh D. Focus on Molecules: interphotoreceptor retinoid-binding protein (IRBP). Exp Eye Res 2008; 86: 169–70.
17. Edwards RB, Adler AJ. Exchange of retinol between IRBP and CRBP. Exp Eye Res. 1994; 59: 161–70.
18. Gollapalli DR, Rando RR. All-trans-retinyl esters are the substrates for isomerization in the vertebrate visual cycle. Biochemistry 2003; 42: 5809–18.
19. Redmond TM, Yu S, Lee E, et al. Rpe65 is necessary for production of 11-cis-vitamin A in the retinal visual cycle. Nat Genet 1998; 20: 344–51.
20. Moiseyev G, Chen Y, Takahashi Y, et al. RPE65 is the isomerohydrolase in the retinoid visual cycle. Proc Natl Acad Sci USA 2005; 102: 12413–18.
21. Gu SM, Thompson DA, Srikumari CR, et al. Mutations in RPE65 cause autosomal recessive childhood-onset severe retinal dystrophy. Nat Genet 1997; 17: 194–7.
22. Chen Y, Noy N. Retinoid specificity of interphotoreceptor retinoid-binding protein. Biochemistry 1994; 33: 10658–65.
23. Finnemann SC, Leung LW, Rodriguez-Boulan E. The lipofuscin component A2E selectively inhibits phagolysosomal degradation of photoreceptor phospholipid by the retinal pigment epithelium. Proc Natl Acad Sci USA 2002; 99: 3842–7.
24. Sparrow JR, Nakanishi K, Parish CA. The lipofuscin fluorophore A2E mediates blue light-induced damage to retinal pigmented epithelial cells. Invest Ophthalmol Vis Sci 2000; 41: 1981–9.
25. Schutt F, Davies S, Kopitz J, et al. Photodamage to human RPE cells by A2-E, a retinoid component of lipofuscin. Invest Ophthalmol Vis Sci 2000; 41: 2303–8.
26. Suter M, Reme C, Grimm C, et al. Age-related macular degeneration. The lipofusion component N-retinyl-N-retinylidene ethanolamine detaches proapoptotic proteins from mitochondria and induces apoptosis in mammalian retinal pigment epithelial cells. J Biol Chem 2000; 275: 39625–30.
27. De S, Sakmar TP. Interaction of A2E with model membranes. Implications to the pathogenesis of age-related macular degeneration. J Gen Physiol 2002; 120: 147–57.
28. Steinberg RH. Interactions between the retinal pigment epithelium and the neural retina. Doc Ophthalmol 1985; 60: 327–46.
29. Kennedy CJ, Rakoczy PE, Constable IJ. Lipofuscin of the retinal pigment epithelium: a review. Eye (Lond) 1995; 9: 763–71.
30. Kopitz J, Holz FG, Kaemmerer E, et al. Lipids and lipid peroxidation products in the pathogenesis of age-related macular degeneration. Biochimie 2004; 86: 825–31.
31. Law WC, Rando RR. The molecular basis of retinoic acid induced night blindness. Biochem Biophys Res Commun 1989; 161: 825–9.
32. Gollapalli DR, Rando RR. The specific binding of retinoic acid to RPE65 and approaches to the treatment of macular degeneration. Proc Natl Acad Sci USA 2004; 101: 10030–5.

33. Nencini C, Barberi L, Runci FM, et al. Retinopathy induced by drugs and herbal medicines. Eur Rev Med Pharmacol Sci 2008; 12: 293–8.

34. Weleber RG, Denman ST, Hanifin JM, et a-l. Abnormal retinal function associated with isotretinoin therapy for acne. Arch Ophthalmol 1986; 104: 831–7.

35. Radu RA, Mata NL, Nusinowitz S, et al. Isotretinoin treatment inhibits lipofuscin accumulation in a mouse model of recessive Stargardt's macular degeneration. Novartis Found Symp 2004; 255: 51–63; discussion 63–7, 177–8.

36. Lim JI, Walonker AF, Levin L, et al. One-year results of a pilot study using oral 13-cis retinoic acid as a treatment for subfoveal predominantly occult choroidal neovascularization in patients with age-related macular degeneration. Retina 2006; 26: 314–21.

37. Sogno I, Vene R, Ferrari N, et al. Angioprevention with fenretinide: targeting angiogenesis in prevention and therapeutic strategies. Crit Rev Oncol Hematol 2010; 75: 2–14.

38. Berni R and Formelli F. In vitro interaction of fenretinide with plasma retinol-binding protein and its functional consequences. FEBS Lett 1992; 308: 43–5.

39. Radu RA, Han Y, Bui TV, et al. Reductions in serum vitamin A arrest accumulation of toxic retinal fluorophores: a potential therapy for treatment of lipofuscin-based retinal diseases. Invest Ophthalmol Vis Sci 2005; 46: 4393–401.

40. Regeneron Therapeutics. Fenritinide. 2010. [Available from: http://www.revisiontherapeutics.com/research/fenretinide.htm]

41. Slakter J. Two-year analysis of the efficacy and safety of fenretinide vs. placebo in the treatment of geographic atrophy. Presented at AAO Annual Meeting. Chicago, 2010.

42. Mata NL, Tsivkovskaia N, Bui TV. Fenretinide reduces the incidence of choroidal neovascularization in patients with geographic atrophy. Presented at ARVO Annual Meeting. Ft. Lauderdale, 2011.

43. Decensi A, Fontana V, Fioretto M, et al. Long-term effects of fenretinide on retinal function. Eur J Cancer 1997; 33: 80–4.

44. Camerini T, Mariani L, De Palo G, et al. Safety of the synthetic retinoid fenretinide: long-term results from a controlled clinical trial for the prevention of contralateral breast cancer. J Clin Oncol 2001; 19: 1664–70.

45. Kaiser-Kupfer MI, Peck GL, Caruso RC, et al. Abnormal retinal function associated with fenretinide, a synthetic retinoid. Arch Ophthalmol 1986; 104: 69–70.

46. Decensi A, Torrisi R, Polizzi A, et al. Effect of the synthetic retinoid fenretinide on dark adaptation and the ocular surface. J Natl Cancer Inst 1994; 86: 105–10.

47. Kubota R, Boman NL, David R, et al. Safety and effect on rod function of acu-4429, a novel small-molecule visual cycle modulator. Retina 2012; 32: 183–8.

48. Haimovici R, Owens SL, Fitzke FW, et al. Dark adaptation in age-related macular degeneration: relationship to the fellow eye. Graefes Arch Clin Exp Ophthalmol 2002; 240: 90–5.

49. Owsley C, Jackson GR, White M, et al. Delays in rod-mediated dark adaptation in early age-related maculopathy. Ophthalmology 2001; 108: 1196–202.

50. Brown B, Adams AJ, Coletta NJ, et al. Dark adaptation in age-related maculopathy. Ophthalmic Physiol Opt 1986; 6: 81–4.

51. Snodderly DM. Evidence for protection against age-related macular degeneration by carotenoids and antioxidant vitamins. Am J Clin Nutr 1995; 62: 1448S–61S.

52. Age-Related Eye Disease Study Research Group. A randomized, placebo-controlled, clinical trial of high-dose supplementation with vitamins C and E, beta carotene, and zinc for age-related macular degeneration and vision loss. Arch Ophthalmol 2001; 119: 1417–36.

53. Chichili GR, Nohr D, Schaffer M, et al. beta-Carotene conversion into vitamin A in human retinal pigment epithelial cells. Invest Ophthalmol Vis Sci 2005; 46: 3562–9.

54. Burton GW, Ingold KU. Beta-Carotene: an unusual type of lipid antioxidant. Science 1984; 224: 569–73.

28

Cellular transplantation for advanced age-related macular degeneration

Lucian V. Del Priore, Henry J. Kaplan, George N. Magrath, and Tongalp H. Tezel

INTRODUCTION

Age-related macular degeneration (AMD) is the leading cause of blindness in the elderly population in the Western world (1), and severe vision loss occurs due to the development of choroidal neovascularization or geographic atrophy. Ninety percent of AMD patients who experience severe vision loss do so as a result of choroidal neovascularization (2), which represents the growth of neovascular tissue from the choriocapillaris, within Bruch's membrane, and eventually into the subretinal pigment epithelial and/or subretinal space. Developing new treatments that prevent or reverse vision loss in AMD is of paramount importance due to the severe visual loss that occurs with this condition and the knowledge that disease prevalence will increase with a shift in the demographics of western populations to older ages. Geographic atrophy accounts for the remainder of the vision loss due to AMD. The Beaver Dam studies have placed the incidence of pure geographic atrophy at 1.3% (2). Geographic atrophy refers to loss of the retinal pigment epithelium, choriocapillaris, and the overlying outer retina (3). While the risk factors of geographic atrophy have been identified (4), there is currently a lack of approved therapies for geographic atrophy.

The last decade has witnessed significant advances in the management of neovascular AMD. Several drugs have become available for treatment of this condition, including photosensitizers and compounds targeting vascular endothelial growth factor, or VEGF. The first approved therapy in the United States was photodynamic therapy with verteporfin (5). This was followed very rapidly by the approval of the first compound that targeted VEGF, namely, the anti-VEGF aptamer pegaptanib (Macugen®, Pfizer, New York, USA) (6–17). Although photodynamic therapy and intravitreal administration of pegaptanib dramatically altered the landscape in the treatment of neovascular AMD, the most important advances in disease management over the last decade have been the introduction of anti-VEGF drugs, including the anti-VEGF antibody fragment ranibizumab (18–23) (Lucentis®, Genentech/Roche, South San Francisco, California, USA), the widespread off-label use of intravitreal bevacizumab (24–31), and the recent approval of aflibercept (Eylea®, Regeneron) which acts as a trap for VEGF (32,33).

While the last decade has brought about a revolution in the treatment of neovascular AMD, there are currently no therapies to reverse vision loss in patients with geographic atrophy that have received Food and Drug Administration approval in the United States, or a CE mark in Europe. Numerous investigational therapies are in various stages of clinical trials. These include ciliary neurotrophic factor, complement inhibitors, glatiramer acetate, and OT-551 (34–37). These therapies are promising, but none have progressed past clinical trials, leaving a large void in the current therapy of geographic atrophy. There is some evidence suggesting that nutritional supplementation may delay the progression of geographic atrophy (38), and many physicians recommend supplements to non-neovascular AMD patients with and without geographic atrophy.

Despite these significant advances in the management of neovascular AMD, there is a large unmet need for many patients with loss of vision from either the neovascular or the non- neovascular form of this disease. More than 50% of patients do not respond to therapy with anti-VEGF drugs, and many patients with advanced disease have loss of vision due to scar formation and altered subretinal architecture. No treatments exist to reverse vision for patients in geographic atrophy. These limitations have led to the investigation of alternative treatment modalities for advanced AMD, including subfoveal membranectomy with and without RPE transplantation or translocation, macular translocation, and subretinal injection of human embryonic stem cells (39–44). Initial efforts to improve vision with adult or fetal cell transplantation alone have not met with success; reconstitution of the normal subretinal architecture is necessary for visual improvement in these individuals. Ultimately this may require maculoplasty, which is defined as reconstruction of macular anatomy in patients with advanced vision loss in neovascular AMD (45). In our view, successful maculoplasty will require replacing or repairing damaged cells (using transplantation, translocation or stimulation of autologous cell proliferation); immune suppression (if allografts are used to replace damaged cells); and reconstruction or replacement of Bruch's membrane (to restore the integrity of the substrate for proper cell attachment). Successful maculoplasty will build upon prior development of surgical techniques for managing severe vision loss in AMD patients with advanced subfoveal exudation. These techniques include surgical excision of choroidal neovascularization (39–43,46–48); surgical excision combined with allograft transplantation of adult or fetal RPE (49–60) or iris pigment epithelium (61–72) or macular translocation with or without choroidal membrane excision (73–91).

In advanced geographic atrophy, the host Bruch's membrane is devoid of native RPE and there is atrophy of the outer retina and choriocapillaris. In advanced wet AMD, excision of the subfoveal neovascular membrane in AMD leaves a large RPE defect under the fovea due to the removal of native RPE along with the surgically removed neovascular complex (92).Resulting persistent RPE defects lead to the development of progressive choriocapillaris and photoreceptor atrophy (93). Histopathology after subfoveal membranectomy alone shows absence of large swatches of native RPE, combined with damage to the outer retina, choriocapillaris atrophy, and absence or damage to the inner aspects of native Bruch's membrane (94,95). In both circumstances, repopulation of host Bruch's membrane with replacement cells will require attachment and proliferation of donor RPE on areas on Bruch's membrane that are damaged by disease and/or surgical manipulation (96). We have previously shown that the status of host Bruch's membrane has a profound effect on the behavior of RPE transplanted after subfoveal membranectomy (45,97–104). Thus, reconstruction of Bruch's membrane is a necessary component for successful maculoplasty (105). Herein we review the current status of efforts directed at macular reconstruction in neovascular AMD.

RATIONALE FOR RPE TRANSPLANTATION IN AMD

In 1991, Thomas and Kaplan reported two patients who experienced significant visual improvement after surgical excision of subfoveal choroidal neovascularization from presumed ocular histoplasmosis syndrome (POHS, although now known simply as ocular histoplasmosis syndrome, OHS) (40). One patient improved from 20/200 preoperatively to 20/40, whereas the other patient improved from 20/200 to 20/25. De Juan and Machemer (46) had previously performed disciform scar excision in four patients with end-stage AMD, but the manuscript by Thomas and Kaplan was the first to demonstrate that excellent visual acuity was possible after submacular surgery. After these initial publications, several authors reported small, uncontrolled series of patients undergoing submacular surgery for AMD (40–42,106,107). The Subfoveal Surgery Trial demonstrated that subfoveal membranectomy alone was better than observation for patients with OHS and an initial visual acuity better than 20/100, but was not better than observation for AMD patients with subfoveal neovascularization (47). Examination of the results of prior nonrandomized studies of submacular surgery suggests that significant visual improvement is limited after submacular surgery for AMD, and that RPE removal may be an important factor limiting postoperative visual recovery. There appear to be significant differences in the postoperative visual recovery after submacular surgery for patients with AMD versus OHS. There could be many factors responsible for this observed difference, including advanced patient age in AMD, disease within

Bruch's membrane in AMD, the size of the choroidal neovascular complex (larger in AMD eyes compared with OHS), the location of the ingrowth site, and the relationship of the choroidal neovascular membrane to the native RPE (108). Patients with OHS and other disorders may have a better prognosis because the choroidal neovascular membrane lies anterior to the RPE and can thus be removed while leaving the native RPE intact (108). However in AMD eyes, the choroidal neovascular complex is frequently deep to the native RPE, so that surgical membrane excision denudes Bruch's membrane of native RPE.

The consequences of RPE removal during submacular surgery are significant because removal of the native RPE leads to progressive choriocapillaris atrophy and limits visual recovery after submacular surgery (109–112). The subfoveal choriocapillaris can be perfused one to two weeks after submacular surgery in AMD eyes but become nonperfused without further surgery or laser photocoagulation (109). Thach et al. examined the choroidal perfusion after surgical removal of subfoveal membranes in 12 eyes of 11 AMD patients (113). Stereoscopic fluorescein and indocyanine green angiograms of the excision bed revealed hypofluorescence with visible perfusion in the underlying median and large choroidal vessels in all eyes. On the basis of these observations the authors concluded that the choriocapillaris and small choroidal vessels were frequently abnormal or absent in the bed of the removed neovascular membrane. We cannot exclude the possibility of some nonperfusion of the subfoveal choriocapillaris being present in patients before submacular surgery. However, patients who develop subfoveal choroidal neovascularization experience sudden and severe visual loss, demonstrating that the perfusion of the choriocapillaris is sufficient to support good visual function even if it is not normal.

Experimental evidence suggests that the native RPE is removed with the choroidal neovascularization in AMD. Grossniklaus et al. (114) examined specimens removed from the subretinal space as part of the Submacular Surgery Trial. Most of these patients (61 out of 78) had AMD and the balance had OHS or idiopathic neovascularization. The specimens contained fibrovascular tissue, fibrocellular tissue, and hemorrhage. Vascular endothelium and RPE were the most common cellular constituents. As expected, the membranes from AMD patients were more likely to be beneath the RPE and the size of the RPE defect was larger in AMD eyes. Histopathologic examination of an eye from a patient who had undergone surgical excision of a choroidal neovascular membrane in AMD revealed an RPE defect in the center of the dissection bed with incomplete resurfacing of the RPE defect after surgery (95). Thus, AMD patients are more likely to have a bare area of Bruch's membrane after surgery and the RPE defect is more likely to persist after surgery in these eyes.

RPE removal at the time of submacular surgery would lead to progressive atrophy of the subfoveal choriocapillaris. Destruction of the RPE with sodium iodate leads to changes in the RPE and choriocapillaris within one week and marked choriocapillaris atrophy within one month (115). In contrast, the choriocapillaris has a normal appearance in areas where the RPE still appeared healthy. Similar changes are seen after intravitreal ornithine injection and in an experimental model of thioridazine retinopathy (116–119). Repopulation of Bruch's membrane occurs after RPE removal in the cat with choriocapillaris preservation under the areas of healed RPE and choriocapillaris atrophy in unhealed areas (120). RPE removal in the non-tapetal porcine eye yields similar results (93,121,122). Bruch's membrane becomes repopulated with a monolayer or multilayer of variably pigmented cells one month after surgical debridement of the RPE. In these regions, the outer nuclear layer and outer limiting membrane remained intact and the choriocapillaris appeared patent. In regions of poor RPE healing the lumen of the choriocapillaris was collapsed and the choriocapillaris endothelium was separated from its basement membrane (93,121,122).

Thus, a combination of experimental and clinical studies suggests that the following sequence of events occurs after choroidal neovascular membrane excision (Fig. 28.1). Subfoveal surgery can be performed without disturbing the native RPE in some eyes, but choroidal neovascular membrane excision results in a focal RPE defect in AMD eyes and in some younger eyes with other

diseases. If the native RPE is not disturbed, the underlying choriocapillaris will not undergo secondary atrophy. If the native RPE is removed, the defect will heal by migration and proliferation of new RPE from the edge of the epithelial defect if the native basal lamina is intact. The proliferating RPE are hypopigmented, making it difficult to visualize these cells in vivo. There are no changes in the choriocapillaris if the area of the RPE defect is completely and rapidly repopulated by hypopigmented RPE. Incomplete or delayed healing of the RPE defect will lead to atrophy of the choriocapillaris although the medium and large vessels of the choroid can remain patent.

In geographic atrophy eyes there is already atrophy of the RPE, as well as atrophy of the outer retina and superficial choriocapillaris in regions devoid of native RPE. The inner aspects of human Bruch's membrane are maintained by the RPE, and normal RPE is required for healthy basement membrane turnover and maintenance. Prior authors have shown that the basement membrane from elderly individuals with geographic atrophy do not support transplanted RPE. Thus, the disease present within the host bed of patients with advanced geographic atrophy is similar to the situation present after removal of the native RPE during submacular surgery (123). In both circumstances it will be necessary to repopulate bare, diseased Bruch's membrane with donor RPE.

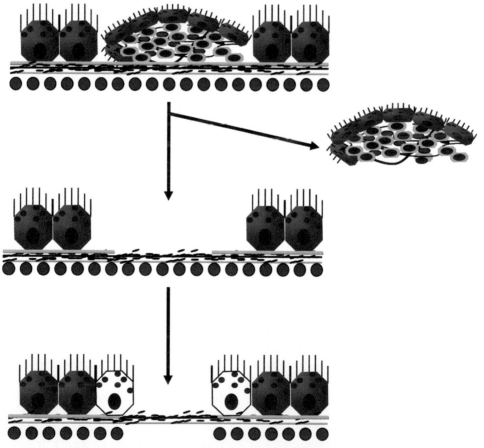

Figure 28.1 (*Top*) A schematic representation of sub-retinal pigment epithelium (RPE) choroidal neovascular membrane typical in age-related macular degeneration. (*Middle*) Membrane removal denudes the native RPE from Bruch's membrane and excises fragment of the inner aspects of Bruch's membrane. Native RPE cannot heal the epithelial defect completely in the absence of native basal lamina. (*Bottom*) Non-pigmented RPE may heal the defect partially in the presence of residual basal lamina, but will not heal the epithelial defect completely in the absence of basal lamina. An RPE defect leads to an atrophy of the subfoveal choriocapillaris.

RPE HARVESTING TECHNIQUE

We have used the following method for harvesting and storage of intact adult human RPE sheets prior to transplantation (104). Briefly, human cadaver eyes are cleaned of extraocular tissue and the suprachoroidal space is sealed with cyanoacrylate glue (124). A small scleral incision is made 3 mm posterior to the limbus until the choroidal vessels are exposed. Tenotomy scissors are introduced through this incision into the suprachoroidal space and the incision is extended circumferentially. Four radial relaxing incisions are made in the sclera and the sclera is peeled away from the periphery to the optic nerve with care not to tear the choroid. The eye cup is then incubated with 25 U/mL of Dispase® (Gibco, Grand Island, New York, USA) for 30 minutes, rinsed with a carbon dioxide free medium, and a circumferential incision is made into the subretinal space along the ora serrata. The loosened RPE sheets are separated from the rest of the ocular tissue and placed on a slice of 50% gelatin on a 25 mm x 75 mm x 1 mm glass slide (Fisher Scientific, Pittsburgh, Pennsylvania, USA) with the apical RPE surface facing upward. Contamination with choroidal cells is avoided by directly visualizing the RPE sheets under a dissecting microscope while they are being harvested. The glass slide containing the gelatin film with the RPE sheet is then placed in a 100 mm x 15 mm polystyrene dish and incubated in a humidified atmosphere of 5% CO2 and 95% air at 37°C for five minutes to allow the gelatin to melt and encase the RPE sheet. The specimen is kept at 4°C for five minutes to solidify the liquid gelatin and then stored in a carbon dioxide-free medium (pH = 7.4) at 4°C. Harvested sheets are stained with cytokeratin to ensure purity of the cell population.

Transmission electron microscopy shows intact RPE cells with well-developed microvilli, basal infoldings, and intercellular connections. The initial viability of intact RPE sheets is 86% with a progressive decline in viability with increased storage time. Cells harvested within 24 hours after death maintain greater viability than those harvested after 24 hours (p < 0.05) and maintain 82% viability for as long as 48 hours if stored at 4°C.

Advance Cell Technology: Phase 1 Clinical Trial

Human embryonic stem cells (hESC) have been differentiated into RPE cells. Prior to tissue transplantation, single blastomere hESC lines, MA01 and MA09, were dissociated from the primary mouse embryonic fibroblast layer by treating with 0.05% trypsin. They were then seeded in low attachment plates to allow embryoid body formation in minimal essential medium with B-27 supplementation. After 7 days' incubation they were plated on gelatin-coated dishes until RPE colonies were visible. RPE was purified by exposure to Type IV collagenase and isolated using glass pipette. Purified RPE was seeded onto gelatin-coated tissue culture plates in EGM02 medium until the desired density of RPE cells was obtained. The cells were then transferred back to minimal essential medium and cultured to the desired phenotype. RPE was dissociated from culture using trypsin and Hanks-based cell dissociation buffer and cryopreserved in fetal bovine serum (125).

BRUCH'S MEMBRANE CHANGES IN AMD

At the light microscope level Bruch's membrane appears to be a continuous structure that extends from the peripapillary area to the peripheral ora serrata. This anatomic structure was recognized by light microscopists in the nineteenth century on the basis of the staining pattern on light microscopy. The development of transmission and scanning electron microscopy revealed that human Bruch's membrane is a pentalaminar structure composed of a central elastin membrane, surrounded by collagen layers bordered externally by the basement membrane of the RPE and choriocapillaris (Fig. 28.2). From internal to external, Bruch's membrane has five anatomic layers with known structure and function. The innermost (i.e., closest to the RPE and furthest from the external sclera) layer of Bruch's membrane is the RPE basal lamina, which serves as the anchoring surface for the RPE. Throughout the human body, basal laminae are thin acellular membranes, approximately 50 nm in thickness, that line one side of epithelia (126). The inner aspect of the RPE basal lamina is bordered by the RPE plasma membrane; the outer surface borders the inner collagen layer and fibers from the inner collagen layer extend into the basal laminar layer of Bruch's membrane. Next comes the inner collagen layer, which is a dense collagen matrix that interconnects the basal lamina and elastin layers of Bruch's membrane. Most of the dysfunction within AMD starts in the inner collagen layer. For example, drusen-like material can accumulate either on the inner or outer aspect of the basal lamina layer; soft drusen, which represent accumulation of abnormal material within the inner collagen layer, will split the inner collagen layer from the basal lamina layer. Choroidal neovascularization often invades this tissue plane, essentially splitting the inner collagen layer from the basal lamina as it grows and progresses (127). Proceeding externally, the elastin layer is not continuous in humans from the optic nerve to the ora. In advanced AMD, the elastin layer becomes fragmented (92). The outer collagen layer is similar to the inner collagen layer at the ultrastructural level. Structural changes occur within the outer collagen layer as a function of advancing patient age, including collagen cross-linking. However extracellular deposits, including drusen and lipid deposits, appear to spare this layer and accumulate mainly within the inner collagen layer as described above. Lastly, the basal lamina of the choriocapillaris separates the choriocapillaris from the outer collagen layer. Unlike the basal lamina of the RPE, there is no evidence of deposit formation on either side of the choriocapillaris basal lamina as a function of advancing patient age (128–130).

Basal laminae are typically thin acellular membranes, approximately 50 nm in thickness, composed of collagen IV and XVIII, laminin, nidogen, agrin, and perlecan (126). Collagen I, collagen III, and fibronectin are

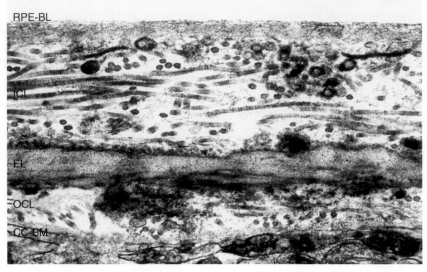

Figure 28.2 Anatomic layers of human Bruch's membrane. *Abbreviations*: CC-BL, basal lamina of the choriocapillaris; EL, elastin layer; ICL, inner collagen layer; OCL, outer collagen layer; RPE–BL, basal lamina of the retinal pigment epithelium .

present within the inner and outer collagen layer; the RPE and choriocapillaris basal lamina are composed largely of laminin and collagen IV (131), but also contain collagen V and heparan sulfate proteoglycan (132). The elastin layer contains elastin and collagen VI (132). Fibronectin is associated with basement membranes, collagen fibers, and elastic fibers throughout Bruch's membrane, although precise immunolocalization of fibronectin is hampered by the fact that this is a soluble serum protein. There is differential distribution of different collagen IV alfa chain isoforms within human Bruch's membrane; alfa1 (IV) and alfa2 (IV) chains were identified in 55% of RPE basement membranes and 100% of choriocapillaris basement membranes, respectively (133). RPE basement membranes also contained alfa3 (IV), alfa4 (IV), and alfa5 (IV) chains, but these chains were not present within choriocapillaris basal lamina. The alfa6 (IV) chain was not identified in any sections (133). Collagen XVIII is also present within the inner aspects of human Bruch's membrane; interestingly, endostatin, which is the C-terminal fragment of collagen XVIII, is typically released from collagen XVIII via proteolysis (134). Administration of intravitreal endostatin can inhibit experimental choroidal neovascularization (135) and gene therapy to increase levels of endostatin can prevent the development of choroidal neovascularization in AMD (136). Mice lacking basement membrane collagen XVIII/endostatin have massive accumulation of sub-RPE deposits with striking similarities to basal laminar deposits, abnormal RPE, and age-dependent loss of vision (137).

CLINICAL RESULTS OF RPE TRANSPLANTATION, RPE AND MACULAR TRANSLOCATION

The goal of RPE transplantation is to repopulate Bruch's membrane with donor RPE prior to the development of widespread atrophy of the choriocapillaris. There is some preliminary experimental evidence suggesting that

RPE transplanted into a debrided bed will support the native choriocapillaris and healthy RPE may reverse choriocapillaris atrophy after it develops (138). To date all human studies of RPE transplantation for neovascular AMD have been performed at the same time as submacular surgery, rather than after subfoveal choriocapillaris atrophy has progressed. Much can be learned from clinical trials of macular translocation as well, since this surgery tests the hypothesis that rotation of the fovea over areas of healthy RPE *and* choriocapillaris can lead to significant visual recovery. The following studies have been reported to date:

- Van Zeeburg et al. reported the results of 133 eyes with AMD which underwent RPE–choroid graft translocation between 2001 and 2006. All the patients had a subfoveal choroidal neovascular membrane. The mean preoperative best corrected visual acuity (BCVA) was 20/250. Four years after surgery 15% of the patients had a BCVA greater than 20/200 and 5% had a BCVA greater than 20/40. They reported complications which included 13 patients with proliferative vitreoretinopathy,13 with recurrent neovascularization, and 2 with hypotony (139).

- Falkner-Radler et al. performed RPE–choroid sheet transplantation and RPE cell-suspension transplantation on 14 consecutive patients with advanced neovascular AMD. They reported a gain of 3 or more lines of visual acuity in two patients in the sheet transplantation group and one patient in the suspension group. One patient in each group had a loss of vision of 3 or more lines (140).

- Radtke et al. performed transplantation of neural retinal progenitor cell layers with RPE in patients with geographic atrophy or retinitis pigmentosa. Four of the ten patients enrolled in the trial were treated due to geographic atrophy. All four of these patients had improvement in visual acuity; however, two of these patients had improvement in the vision of both eyes. They noted that the survival of the transplant at one year was not correlated with the visual outcome (141).

- Heussen et al. performed autologous translocation of the choroid and RPE in 30 patients with neovascular AMD. The full-thickness graft donor site was chosen outside the arcades. The visual outcomes included stabilization of vision in six eyes, increase in vision in five eyes, and a decrease in vision in 19 eyes. They had no evidence of the patch graft failure at one year, but there was significant risk of late CNV formation (142).

- MacLaren et al. performed a full-thickness patch graft of RPE and choroid harvested from the superior equatorial retina into the subfoveal space in 12 patients with neovascular AMD. A viable graft was seen in 11 of the 12 patients and three patients had a good visual outcome. The mean logMAR visual acuity improved from 0.88 to 0.79 in these patients. Operative complications occurred in eight patients, including five retinal detachments and hemorrhage in four patients. The mean logMAR visual acuity for the cohort fell from 0.86 to 1.16 (143).

- Peyman et al. performed a submacular scar excision with translocation of an autologous RPE pedicle flap or transplantation of an allogeneic RPE–Bruch's membrane explant in two patients (59). The final visual acuity was 20/400 in the first patient and count fingers at 2 feet in the second patient. Neither of these patients was immune suppressed.

- Algvere et al. initially reported subretinal membrane removal with transplantation of fetal human RPE patches in five AMD patients and subsequently reported on a larger series of 17 eyes (49,144,145). Cystoid macular edema developed and the grafts became encapsulated by white fibrous tissue within several months after surgery but none of these patients received systemic immune suppression. Scanning laser ophthalmoscopic microperimetry demonstrated that patients were able to fixate over the area of the RPE graft immediately after surgery, but an absolute scotoma developed in this region several months after surgery. These results are not surprising because the patients were not immune suppressed, and RPE transplanted into the subretinal space will be rejected (54,146–148). The authors observed better integrity of the graft margins in geographic atrophy patients, suggesting that rejection may be more common in neovascular AMD. In the long term, there is continued deterioration of function and graft integrity in all cases of neovascular AMD and 5/9 eyes with non-neovascular AMD (49,144,145).

- Subfoveal membranectomy with transplantation of adult human RPE sheets has been performed in 11 AMD patients who were immune suppressed postoperatively with prednisone, cyclosporine, and immuran. Eligibility criteria included the presence of drusen, patient age more than 60 years, a BCVA of <20/63 (Bailey–Lovie chart), and subfoveal neovascularization

<9 disc area on preoperative fluorescein angiography. The mean visual acuity, contrast sensitivity, and reading speed did not change significantly for six months postoperatively. Transplants showed no signs of rejection in patients who were able to continue immune suppression for the first six months after surgery, but patients who discontinued immune suppression developed signs of graft rejection two weeks later. Histopathology is available of an 85-year-old woman who died four months after RPE sheet transplantation (53). A complete autopsy showed the cause of death to be congestive heart failure. A patch of hyperpigmentation was visible at the transplant site under the foveola after surgery. Mound-like clusters of individual round, large densely pigmented cells were present in the subretinal space and outer retina in this area, and the transplant site did not contain a uniform monolayer in most areas. There was loss of the photoreceptor outer segments and native RPE in the center of the transplant bed, with disruption of the outer nuclear layer predominantly over regions of multilayered pigmented cells. Cystic spaces were present in the inner and outer retina. A residual intra-Bruch's membrane component of the original choroidal neovascular complex was present under the transplant site. The poor morphology at the transplant site was consistent with the lack of visual improvement seen after surgery in this patient.

- Weisz et al. delivered a patch of fetal RPE under the retina in one patient with geographic atrophy (149). Visual acuity remained stable at 20/80 one month after surgery but deteriorated to 20/500 by five months postoperatively. Mild subretinal fibrosis developed after surgery. The patient demonstrated a systemic immune response to phosducin and rhodopsin postoperatively in the absence of systemic immune suppression.

- Binder and coworkers have reported on 53 eyes undergoing subfoveal surgery for choroidal neovascularization in AMD (14 undergoing subfoveal membranectomy alone and 39 undergoing membranectomy with transplantation of autologous RPE suspensions) (51,150). There was no difference in visual acuity postoperatively between the groups, but postoperative reading vision was better in the transplant eyes and the recurrence rate of choroidal neovascularization was low (51,150).

- Van Meurs reported short-term results with patch transplantation techniques in which a free pedicle graft was harvested from the midperiphery and placed under the fovea immediately after subfoveal membranectomy. Their initial report concluded that surgery was technically feasible but was associated with a high surgical complication rate, with retinal detachment due to proliferative vitreoretinopathy in three of eight eyes (151,152). Wolf et al. reported temporary improvement in vision in only one of seven patients (153). In a larger series, Joussen et al. reported on autologous translocation of RPE and choroid in 45 eyes of 43 patients with subfoveal AMD. Surgical complications were significant, with half the eyes requiring additional procedures due to retinal detachment, proliferative vitreoretinopathy, macular pucker, or vitreous hemorrhage. Only four eyes achieved a 15-letter increase in BCVA. The authors claimed that the graft was revascularized on indocyanine green angiography in most eyes (154).

- Stanga et al. reported on nine eyes with neovascular AMD undergoing subfoveal surgery combined with patch RPE transplantation (91,155). Their initial paper reported transient fixation over the graft by scanning laser ophthalmoscopy. However, a long-term follow-up of four of these patients demonstrated that recovery of fixation is temporary, with a decline in fixation ability long-term, despite the fact that areas of hyperpigmentation, interpreted by the authors as representing a healthy graft, could still be seen ophthalmoscopically.

- Schwartz et al. reported a safety and tolerability study of subretinal transplantation of human embryonic stem cell–derived retinal pigment epithelium in patients with either Stargardt's macular dystrophy or dry AMD. The authors were able to show 99% embryonic stem cell differentiation to RPE prior to transplantation; there was structural evidence that the RPE had attached and continued to persist up to four months. Their study showed no signs of hyperproliferation, tumorigenicity, ectopic tissue formation, or host rejection at the four-month time point (96).

- Prior workers have emphasized the fact that much can be learned about the potential of RPE transplantation from studying macular translocation results. For neovascular AMD, the macular translocation series suggests that approximately 20% of patients can achieve a final vision of 20/50 or better (73–76,86,153,156–173). However, several facts should be considered before inferring the results of RPE transplantation on the basis of macular translocation studies alone. First, the surgical complication rate of macular translocation surgery is initially quite high, with a steep learning curve that appears to be surgeon-dependent. Second, in macular translocation surgery the fovea is shifted to a new location over healthy RPE *and* choriocapillaris; the native RPE is already attached to host Bruch's membrane, thus avoiding issues that arise when RPE is translocated or transplanted to a new location. Third, macular translocation surgery causes a significant decline in the global ERG that may reflect the significant effects of this surgery on overall retinal function (89,174,175). The situation is further complicated by the observation that subfoveal atrophy recurred in three of four patients with geographic atrophy in AMD, thus implying that changes in the outer retina may be responsible for the development of geographic atrophy (158,176). This finding has significant implications for RPE transplantation in geographic atrophy, since one will expect a similar rapid loss of RPE in AMD with geographic atrophy after

transplantation. Rapid recurrence of geographic atrophy was also observed by Khurana et al. after macular translocation (177).

MECHANISM OF RPE ATTACHMENT TO HUMAN BRUCH'S MEMBRANE

RPE Attachment in Tissue Culture

Several investigators have characterized the ligands available for surface attachment of human RPE. The basal surface of RPE cells contain a β_1-subunit of integrin (178,179) and the inner aspect of Bruch's membrane contains laminin, fibronectin, heparan sulfate, and collagen (132). Attachment of RPE to coated artificial surfaces can be mediated by an interaction between the β_1-subunit of integrin and known extracellular matrix molecules. For example, RPE cells bind to Petri dishes coated with laminin or fibronectin but do not attach to untreated, uncoated Petri dishes (179). The synthetic tetrapeptide RGDS (arginine-glycine-aspartate serine), which is derived from the cell-binding domain of fibronectin, decreases RPE binding to laminin-coated or fibronectin-coated dishes (180). Thus, *in-vitro* binding studies suggest that RPE can attach to laminin or fibronectin coating a plastic surface via an interaction between the β_1-integrin subunit and laminin and fibronectin.

Molecular binding studies demonstrate a role for integrins and extracellular matrix ligands in mediating RPE attachment to RPE–derived extracellular matrix and human Bruch's membrane in a more direct fashion (Fig. 28.3) (181). The attachment rate of human RPE cells to RPE–derived extracellular matrix was $66.0 \pm 6.0\%$. Coating the surface with albumin or an irrelevant anti-IgG antibody did not change the attachment rates significantly ($64.5 \pm 3.0\%$ and $63.5 \pm 3.4\%$, respectively; $p > 0.05$ for each compared with extracellular matrix alone). The addition of fibronectin, laminin, type IV collagen, or vitronectin increased the attachment rates to $79.0 \pm 7.0\%$, $76.0 \pm 6.0\%$, $80.3 \pm 9.0\%$, or $81.3 \pm 6.3\%$, respectively ($p < 0.05$ for each compared with extracellular matrix alone). The addition of anti-fibronectin, anti-laminin, anti-collagen IV, or anti-vitronectin (1:100 dilution) decreased the attachment rates to $56.2 \pm 3.0\%$, $49.4 \pm 5.0\%$, $55.2 \pm 4.1\%$, or $51.0 \pm 7.3\%$, respectively ($p < 0.05$ for each compared with extracellular matrix alone). Increasing the concentration of antibodies to a 1:10 dilution did not inhibit RPE reattachment further (data not shown). Simultaneous addition of anti-fibronectin, anti-laminin, anti-collagen IV, and anti-vitronectin antibodies (1:100 dilution) markedly decreased the attachment rates further to $25.3 \pm 9.0\%$ ($p < 0.05$). Treatment with RGDS, a tetrapeptide known to block the interaction between the β_1-subunit of integrin and extracellular matrix proteins, markedly decreased the RPE reattachment rate to $21.0 + 6.3\%$ ($p < 0.05$). Treatment of RPE cells with anti-β_1 integrin antibodies before plating the cells decreased the attachment rate to $15.0 \pm 7.0\%$ ($p < 0.05$). The reattachment rate of RPE to uncoated tissue culture plastic was $24.6 \pm 3.2\%$. The mechanism of attachment of RPE to human Bruch's membrane explants is similar (181).

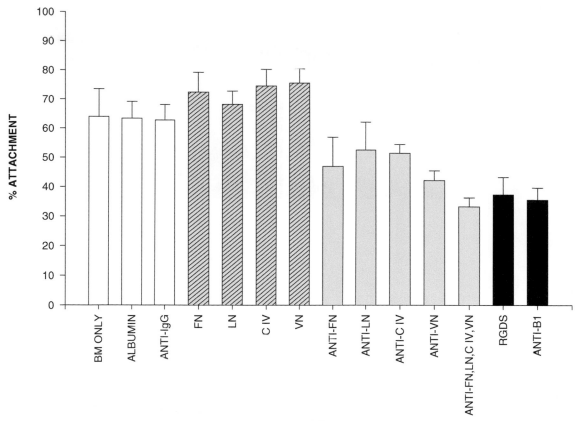

Figure 28.3 Human RPE cell attachment rate to Bruch's membrane in tissue culture. Data were divided into four groups: (1) Group 1, open bars: The attachment rate on extracellular matrix alone (64.0 ± 9.5%) was not altered by the addition of albumin (63.4 ± 5.7%) or an irrelevant anti-IgG antibody (62.8 ± 5.3%). (2) Group 2, shaded diagonal stripes: The addition of extracellular matrix components increased the attachment rate over baseline. The attachment rate after the addition of fibronectin (72.4 ± 6.8%), laminin (68.2 ± 4.6%), collagen type IV (74.6 ± 5.7%), or vitronectin (75.6 + 4.9%) was always higher than the attachment rate to Bruch's membrane alone (64.0 ± 9.5%; p < 0.05 for all comparisons). (3) Group 3, solid gray: The addition of antibodies against Bruch's membrane components decreased the attachment rate over baseline. The attachment rate after the addition of anti-fibronectin (47.0 ± 10.0%), anti-laminin (52.6 ± 9.6%), anti-collagen type IV (51.5 ± 3.0%), or anti-vitronectin (42.2 ± 3.3%) was always lower than the attachment rate to Bruch's membrane alone. Simultaneous addition of anti-fibronectin, anti-laminin, anti-collagen IV, and anti-vitronectin markedly decreased RPE reattachment to extracellular matrix (35.6 ± 4.1%; p, 0.05). (4) Group 4, black: Striking inhibition of cell reattachment was produced by addition of the synthetic peptide RGDS or by preincubating the cells with anti-β_1-integrin (33.3 ± 3.0% and 37.4 ± 5.9%, respectively). Cell attachment to uncoated tissue culture plastic was 25.8 ± 4.5%. Data presented as mean ± standard deviation, n, 9. *Abbreviations*: anti-β_1, antibody to β_1-subunit of integrin; anti-IgG, an irrelevant IgG antibody; C IV, type IV collagen; FN, fibronectin; LM, laminin; RGDS, (arginine-glycine-aspartate-serine); VN, vitronectin; . *Source*: From Ref. 181.

Importance of RPE Attachment for Cell Survival

We have previously demonstrated that RPE that are harvested for transplantation must be allowed to reattach to a substrate to prevent RPE apoptosis (102). Second passage human RPE cells were plated onto tissue culture plastic precoated with extracellular matrix, fibronectin, laminin, uncoated tissue culture plastic, untreated plastic, and untreated plastic coated with 4% agarose. Reattachment rates were determined for each substrate 24 hours after plating. The TUNEL (terminal deoxynucleotidyl transferase-mediated dUTP nick end labeling) technique was used to determine apoptosis rates in attached cells, unattached cells, and the entire cell population. Attachment rates were as follows: extracellular matrix-coated tissue culture plastic > fibronectin-coated tissue culture plastic > laminin-coated tissue culture plastic > uncoated tissue culture plastic > untreated plastic > agarose-coated untreated plastic. Apoptosis rates for the entire cell population were increased as the RPE cell attachment rate decreased, and the proportion of apoptotic cells in the entire population was inversely

related to the percent attached cells (r = –0.95). These results imply that RPE cells that are removed from their substrate prior to transplantation must reattach rapidly to a substrate to prevent apoptosis.

EFFECTS OF AGE-RELATED CHANGES WITHIN BRUCH'S MEMBRANE ON RPE ATTACHMENT AND BEHAVIOR

Importance of Bruch's Membrane Layer and Age in RPE Attachment

The anatomic layers of Bruch's membrane are not intact after submacular membranectomy in AMD eyes (182,183). Histopathologic evidence suggests that the RPE basal lamina is excised with the choroidal neovascular membrane greater than 90% of the time, thus exposing the inner collagen layer of Bruch's membrane, and the dissection plane is not uniform throughout the excision bed (92,114). In addition, aging of human Bruch's membrane causes numerous changes within this structure such as collagen cross-linking, elastin fragmentation, and deposition of abnormal material with in

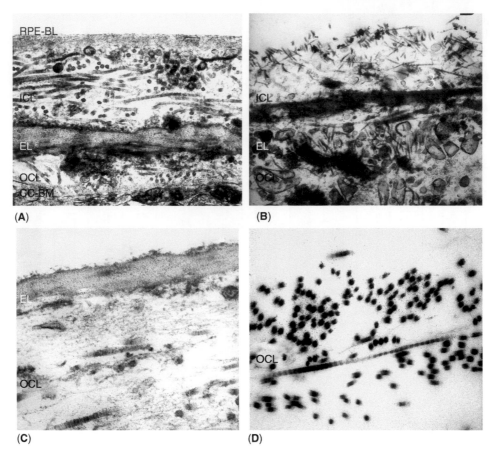

Figure 28.4 Preparation of Bruch's membrane explants. Native RPE cells are removed by treatment with ammonium hydroxide (**A**), yielding a preparation with the RPE basal lamina (RPE–BL) on the uppermost surface (**B**). RPE–BL is removed mechanically, exposing the inner collagen layer (ICL) (**C**). Addition of collagenase exposes the elastin layer (EL) (4); treatment with elastase exposes the outer collagen layer (OCL) (**D**). *Abbreviations*: CC-BM, choriocapillaris basement membrane.

Bruch's membrane as outlined above (184); survival of transplanted cells is substrate dependent, and thus the age/presence of disease within Bruch's membrane plus surgical removal of the inner aspects of human Bruch's membrane will have a profound and detrimental impact on transplant survival. In view of these considerations, we have examined the effects of Bruch's membrane age and the layer available for cell attachment on RPE behavior (55,100,103).

We have determined the effects of Bruch's membrane layer on RPE attachment by isolating individual layers of human Bruch's membrane in the laboratory as described previously (Fig. 28.4) (100). Human Bruch's membrane explants were prepared from 10 human cadaver eyes by removing native RPE with 0.02 N ammonium hydroxide. Six mm punches of peripheral Bruch's membrane were stabilized on 4% agarose and placed in a 96-well plate with the Bruch's membrane facing upward. The RPE basal lamina, inner collagen layer, elastin layer, and outer collagen layer were exposed by removing each apical layer sequentially by mechanical or enzymatic means. First passage human RPE cells harvested from a single donor were plated onto the surface (15,000 viable cells/explant) and the RPE reattachment rate to each layer of Bruch's membrane was determined. The RPE reattachment rate was highest to the inner aspects of Bruch's membrane and decreased as deeper layers of Bruch's membrane were exposed (i.e., basal

lamina > inner collagen layer > elastin layer > outer collagen layer). The reattachment rate to the inner collagen layer, elastin layer and outer collagen layer harvested from elderly donors (age > 60 years) was less than that of the corresponding layers harvested from younger (age < 50 years) donors (Fig. 28.5). These results demonstrate that the ability of harvested RPE to reattach to human Bruch's membrane depends on the anatomic layer of Bruch's membrane present in the host tissue. The layer of Bruch's membrane available also affects the morphology of the grafted RPE (Fig. 28.6) and their subsequent behavior. The apoptosis rate of attached cells increased as deeper layers of Bruch's membrane were exposed (103). Both the proliferation rate and mitotic index (103) of the grafted cells were higher on basal lamina than on deeper layers. RPE cells plated onto basal lamina repopulated the explant surface within 14 ± 3 days, whereas cells plated onto inner collagen layer and elastin layer eventually died and never reached confluence. These findings suggest that the ability of transplanted RPE cells to repopulate bare Bruch's membrane will depend on the layer of Bruch's membrane available for RPE cell reattachment (185).

Aged Bruch's membrane does not support transplanted RPE cells readily. Fetal RPE cells were transplanted onto aged Bruch's membrane and bovine corneal endothelial cell extracellular matrix. The fetal RPE cells were also transplanted onto the superficial

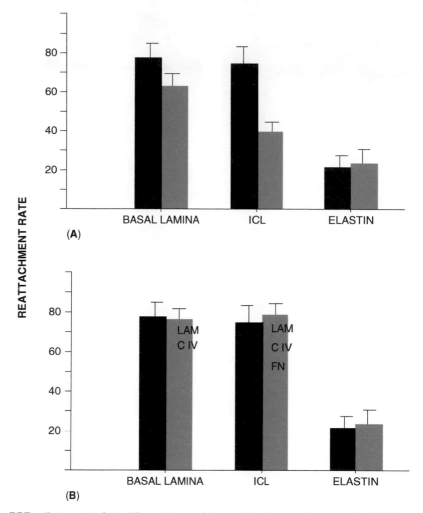

Figure 28.5 Ability of human RPE cells to reattach to different layers of human Bruch's membrane explants (4 donors' age >50 yrs, 3 donors' age <50 yrs) 24 hours after plating. (**A**) RPE reattachment rates on younger and older basal lamina were comparable (p = 0.13). However the reattachment to older inner collagen layer (ICL) was significantly lower than to younger inner collagen layer (p = 0.02). The RPE reattachment rate to inner collagen layer was lower than to basal lamina in older donors (p < 0.01) but was similar in younger donors (p > 0.05). The reattachment to elastin was significantly lower than to basal lamina and inner collagen layer in both younger and older donors (p < 0.05). (**B**) Addition of laminin (LAM) and collagen IV (C IV) to young basal lamina has no effect, but addition to older basal lamina increases the attachment rate on older Bruch's membrane to same level seen on younger Bruch's membrane. Similarly, addition of laminin, collagen IV, and fibronectin (FN) has no effect on young inner collagen layer, but increases attachment onto older inner collagen layer to same level as young inner collagen layer. Addition of ligands to young or older elastin layer has no effect. *Source*: From Ref. 55. Black bars = Bruch's donor age <50; Grey bars = Bruch's donor age >50.

inner collagenous layer and deep inner collagenous layer of aged Bruch's membrane. Nuclear density counts were decreased on all surfaces of Bruch's membrane and decreased with time over 14 days. This indicates a need to reconstruct Bruch's membrane to enhance RPE survival (186).

ANATOMIC RECONSTRUCTION OF HUMAN BRUCH'S MEMBRANE

As mentioned earlier there are two major factors related to Bruch's membrane status that influence the ability of grafted RPE to survive after subretinal transplantation, namely, the layer of Bruch's membrane available after subretinal membranectomy and the presence of age-related changes within Bruch's membrane. Several authors have suggested replacing Bruch's membrane with a basement membrane substrate, such as thin silicone rubber, lens capsule, amniotic membrane, or a more complex bioengineered artificial structure

(187,188). Although there is some appeal to this notion, it should be remembered that cells are exquisitely sensitive to all aspects of their substrate including chemical composition as well as mechanical substrate properties. Finding a substrate that mimics Bruch's membrane chemically and mechanically presents a significant challenge; in addition, it will be difficult to secure the artificial substrate to Bruch's membrane itself and to establish a stable, long-term interface between biologic and synthetic tissues.

We have taken a different approach to this problem by reconstructing Bruch's membrane to make it a more hospitable substrate for RPE attachment (45). These efforts have involved deposition of exogenous attachment ligands on the inner aspects of Bruch's membrane; cleaning deposits from an aged Bruch's membrane by treating it with sodium citrate and detergents; and a combined approach in which debris is removed from the Bruch's membrane, followed by

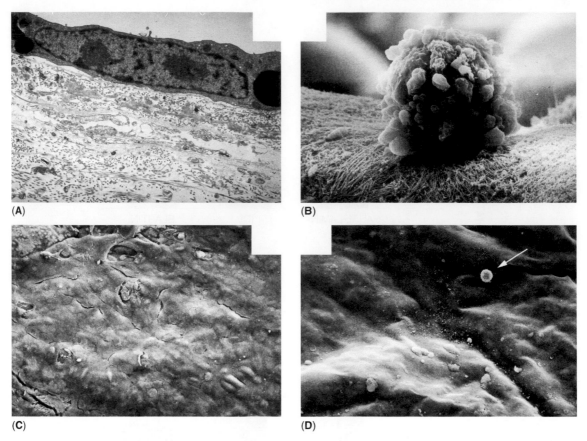

Figure 28.6 Morphology of human RPE cells (donor age = 80) after seeding onto different layers of human Bruch's membrane explants (6 donors). **(A, B)** RPE plated onto basal lamina reached confluence within 14 ± 3 days in over 90% of the wells. **(C, D)** Cells plated onto inner collagen layer detached from the surface, and only a few rare cells (arrow) could be seen on the surface 21 days after plating. Cells plated onto elastin exhibited a similar behavior (not shown). *Source*: From Ref. 103.

resurfacing with extracellular matrix ligands (45). Specifically, we determined the effects of cleaning and/or extracellular matrix protein coating on the reattachment, apoptosis, proliferation, and final surface coverage of the transplanted RPE. Explants of aged Bruch's membrane with inner collagen layer exposed were prepared from five human cadaver eyes (donor age = 69–84 years) and treated with Triton-X and/or coated with a mixture of laminin (330 µg/mL), fibronectin (250 µg/mL), and vitronectin (33 µg/mL); 15,000 viable human fetal and ARPE-19 cells were plated onto the surface and the RPE reattachment, apoptosis, and proliferation ratios were determined on the modified surfaces. Cells were cultured up to 17 days to determine the surface coverage. Ultrastructure of the modified Bruch's membrane and RPE morphology were studied with transmission and scanning electron microscopy. The reattachment ratios of fetal human RPE and ARPE-19 cells were similar on aged inner collagen layer (41.5 ± 1.7% and 42.9 ± 2.7%, p > 0.05). The reattachment ratio increased with extracellular matrix-protein coating and decreased with detergent treatment. Combined cleaning and coating restored the reattachment ratio of fetal RPE cells, but failed to increase the reattachment ratio of ARPE-19 cells. The highest apoptosis was observed on untreated inner collagen layer. Cleaning and the combined procedure of cleaning and extracellular matrix-protein coating decreased the fetal RPE apoptosis. Only

RPE cells plated on a cleaned or a cleaned and extracellular matrix-protein coated inner collagen layer demonstrated proliferation that led to substantial surface coverage at day 17. Thus, these results demonstrate that age-related changes that impair RPE repopulation of Bruch's membrane can be significantly reversed by combined cleaning and extracellular matrix-protein coating of the inner collagen layer. Development of biologically tolerant techniques for modifying the inner collagen layer *in vivo* may be able to enhance the ability of the RPE to reattach and repopulate aged inner collagen layer. Figure 28.7 shows the effect of different treatments on the ultrastructural features of the inner collagen layer (45).

Zarbin et al. have proposed using conditioned media to achieve better RPE survival. Bovine corneal endothelial cells were seeded into the inner collagenous layer (ICL) of Bruch's membrane in explants of human donor eyes to resurface the ICL with extracellular matrix. Fetal RPE cells were then transplanted onto the new extracellular matrix. The donor eyes with the BCL extracellular matrix showed higher nuclear densities than control eyes after transplantation (189).

IRIS PIGMENT EPITHELIAL TRANSPLANTATION FOR AMD

Within the last decade several investigators have pioneered the use of iris pigment epithelium as a replacement for RPE in retinal degenerations, including

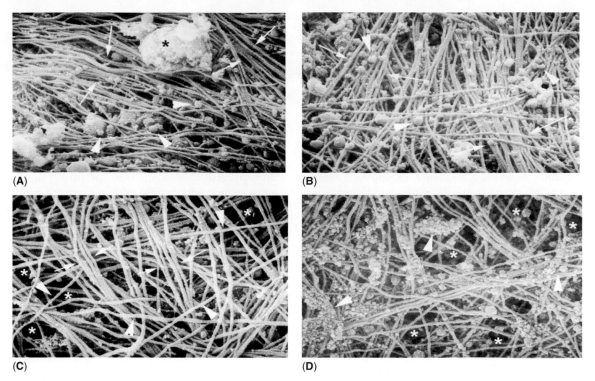

Figure 28.7 Scanning electron microscopy of inner collagen layer modification with cleaning and resurfacing in an 84-year-old donor. (**A**) Untreated inner collagen layer revealed replacement of fine interdigitating structure of the collagen framework by unidirectionally running cross-linked bundles of collagen (white arrows). Small globular structures on the collagen fibers probably represent aggregates of extracellular matrix-proteins (white arrowheads). Macro deposits of lipoprotein debris filled interfibrillar spaces (asterisk). (**B**) Extracellular matrix-protein coating without cleaning yielded an increased amount of extracellular matrix-protein aggregates on the collagen matrix. Cross-linking of collagen fibers was not affected by the coating (white arrows). (**C**) Cleaning with Triton-X and sodium citrate removed the debris and resulted in gaps between collagen fibers (white asterisk). Along with debris most of the globular extracellular matrix-proteins disappeared. Note that cross-links between collagen fibers were broken yielding individual fibers (white arrowheads) and rare incompletely separated macrofibers (white arrows). (**D**) Cleaning and subsequent extracellular matrix-protein coating not only broke the cross-links between collagen fibers but also allowed extracellular matrix-proteins to diffusely attach on the regenerated collagen framework. Note that extracellular matrix proteins were smaller in size and did not form multimeric aggregates as on the native matrix. Removal of macroaggregates also created spaces between collagen fibers that may help to restore the hydraulic conductivity across Bruch's membrane. (Bars = 0.5 μm). *Source*: From Ref. 45.

age-related macular degeneration (AMD) (190). This use of iris pigment epithelium is based upon the common embryological origin of these two cell lines, the ready availability of autologous iris pigment epithelium via iris biopsy, and the need to replace RPE in various disease states. Application of iris pigment epithelium transplantation for treatment of tapetoretinal degenerations due to a known gene defect, such as Leber's congenital amaurosis and RPE–dependent forms of retinitis pigmentosa, are not likely to be fruitful since autologous iris pigment epithelium and RPE would have the same genetic defect. The largest clinical application for autologous iris pigment epithelium transplantation may be in repair of age-related cell and tissue loss in AMD; here transplanted iris pigment epithelium could replace native RPE removed during submacular surgery for neovascular AMD or lost during the development of geographic atrophy in non-neovascular AMD.

To date a handful of laboratory and clinical studies have been performed to determine the ability of iris pigment epithelium to survive after subretinal transplantation and perform RPE functions, including outer segment phagocytosis, recycling of visual pigment, and release of cytokines and other growth factors (67). Prior authors have concluded that iris pigment epithelium

can survive at least six months after subretinal transplantation but proper interpretation of these results is confounded by the difficulty in identifying transplanted cells unequivocally (61,64,65,71,191). Initial studies suggested that subretinal or choroidal iris pigment epithelium transplants may slow down the rate of photoreceptor degeneration in the Royal College of Surgeons (RCS) rat for several months compared with untreated controls (67,68). However iris pigment epithelium is inferior at rescue compared to RPE, and iris pigment epithelium is no better than sham surgery (192).

Iris pigment epithelium function in vitro and after subretinal transplantation in vivo has also been investigated by previous workers. Iris pigment epithelium is capable of retinol metabolism (193) and the transplanted iris pigment epithelium can ingest outer segments (192). The ability of cultured iris pigment epithelium to phagocytose latex beads is 76% of the activity of RPE (67). Cultured iris pigment epithelium maintains melanogenesis for up to 5 passages in tissue culture (62). Iris pigment epithelium and RPE form monolayers on Descemet's membrane (194,195) and exhibit similar growth on native and micro patterned human lens capsule (196). Iris pigment epithelium can form tight junctions thus raising the possibility that the transplanted iris pigment epithelium could reestablish the blood-retinal barrier normally formed by RPE (67).

To date a handful of clinical studies have been performed on subretinal transplantation of iris pigment epithelium to replace surgically excised RPE in patients with neovascular AMD. Autologous iris pigment epithelium transplantation has been performed in 35 patients after removal of subfoveal choroidal neovascular membranes with no significant difference in vision between transplanted patients versus those who underwent choroidal neovascularization removal alone. Autologous iris pigment epithelium translocation after submacular membranectomy can preserve foveal function at a low level but does not improve visual acuity (197). These poor functional results are consistent with the poor attachment and survival of iris pigment epithelium and RPE on aged Bruch's membrane (198). Despite the lack of visual improvement, subretinal iris pigment epithelium transplants in AMD patients may prevent recurrence of subretinal neovascularization (68,190).

We have demonstrated that there are major differences in the gene expression profile of primary RPE versus iris pigment epithelium harvested from the same donor eye, including the lack of expression in iris pigment epithelium of genes known to be critical for RPE function. For example, iris pigment epithelium do not express the gene for retinol dehydrogenase, whose gene product is necessary for recycling visual pigments. Recoverin is a visual cycle protein expressed in abundance in the RPE but not iris pigment epithelium although its role in the RPE function is not known. Iris pigment epithelium does not express other major functional RPE genes, including angiopoietin 1, S-antigen, and a transcriptional regulator of the c-fos promoter. Numerous cell adhesion genes and additional genes related to RPE phagocytosis, tight junction formation, and vitamin A metabolism are missing in iris pigment epithelium cells, including thrombospondin 1 and ras-related C3 botulinum toxin substrate (Cai et al., personal communication).

In order for iris pigment epithelium to replace surgically excised or dysfunctional RPE, the transplanted iris pigment epithelium should probably develop an expression profile that closely resembles native RPE. Our results suggest that the native iris pigment epithelium expression profile may be a potential obstacle to successful subretinal transplantation. Since the microenvironment of cells influences their behavior and gene expression, we cannot exclude the possibility that the expression profile of iris pigment epithelium may change after subretinal transplantation to more closely resemble native RPE. However, our data suggest that the expression level of many genes must change for iris pigment epithelium to resemble RPE. Some authors have suggested that transplanted iris pigment epithelium can serve as a potential reservoir for a single growth factor or cytokine and thereby rescue adjacent cells from the effects of progressive tapetoretinal degeneration (199). For example, iris pigment epithelium induced to transcribe the BNDF gene could protect against retinal damage due to N-methyl-D-aspartate-induced neuronal death and light toxicity (66,200). Iris pigment epithelium genetically modified to express pigment epithelial derived factor inhibits choroidal neovascularization in a rat model of laser-induced choroidal neovascularization, and increase the survival and preserve rhodopsin expression in photoreceptor cells in the RCS rat (201). For such applications the striking difference in the gene expression profile between RPE and iris pigment epithelium may be less of an obstacle to successful cell-based therapy. Additional studies, including determining the gene expression profile of iris pigment epithelium and RPE *after* subretinal transplantation, are needed to determine whether the microenvironment of the subretinal space will have a marked effect on the iris pigment epithelium gene profile.

FUTURE DIRECTIONS

At the current time there are many unresolved issues that may influence the ability of transplanted cells to repopulate Bruch's membrane and numerous questions need to be addressed before successful cell transplantation can occur. In the absence of an animal model for AMD the approach to this problem must rely on a mixture of in vivo studies of cell transplantation in healthy animals, *in vitro* studies of cell reattachment to human Bruch's membrane diseased with AMD, and a small number of clinical trials on AMD patients. There are several important variables that need to be investigated.

Source of Cells

The ideal cell source for human transplantation studies is not known. Adult human RPE cells are readily available from donor Eye Bank eyes but it is not known if these cells are the best source or whether the age of the donor RPE makes any difference. Fetal human RPE may be able to repopulate Bruch's membrane better than adult RPE but there are ethical and legal issues involved with the use of human fetal cells, and fetal cells cannot be autologous. Use of immortalized human RPE cells lines has been proposed, but the effects of immortalization or passaging in tissue culture on the distribution of cell surface receptors necessary for cell attachment to Bruch's membrane may be an issue. We have shown that there are significant differences in the gene expression profile of native and immortalized human RPE, thus raising the important question of whether the immortalized cells can replace all aspects of cell function (in press). There is some concern about tumorigenic potential if immortalized cells are used. Several authors have already used iris pigment epithelial cells because these cells are related embryologically to the RPE, are readily available, and will not be rejected immunologically (71,202). However, iris pigment epithelial transplantation combined with subfoveal surgery has not led to a dramatic improvement in vision to better than 20/200 (70,71,203), and there are significant differences in the gene expression profile of these cells compared with RPE cells.

Several other cell sources that may be useful for RPE transplantation have not been investigated fully. First, the isolation of retinal progenitor cells (stem cells) raises the interesting possibility of using these cells to repopulate denuded areas of Bruch's membrane (202). This is an attractive possibility because a small population of such retinal progenitor cells could yield a large population of cells for transplantation, and isolation of progenitors from adults could avoid problems of immune rejection. Second, xenotransplantation of porcine cells has already been performed in the management of central nervous system disease including stroke, Parkinson's disease, and Alzheimer's disease. These cells have been well tolerated after transplantation into the central nervous system in patients and the possibility of using fetal xenografts could provide an attractive alternative to the use of human tissue (204).

Immune Suppression

A second issue that needs to resolved is related to the immune suppression necessary to ensure graft survival. In the original paper by Algvere et al., (49), sequential fundus photograph strongly suggested that immune rejection developed in these non-suppressed individuals since the grafts became encapsulated and cystoid macular edema developed within three months. Systemic immune suppression appeared to be sufficient to prevent ophthalmic signs of graft rejection but local suppression with slow release devices (intravitreal cyclosporine implants, for example) would be preferable (49).

Status of Bruch's Membrane After Submacular Surgery

As mentioned above, the status of Bruch's membrane after submacular surgery is important for the ultimate success of cell transplantation. Disease within Bruch's membrane and iatrogenic removal of the inner layers of Bruch's membrane during submacular surgery affect the ability of transplanted RPE to repopulate this structure. There are several approaches that could be used to rectify this problem including cleaning of Bruch's membrane surface deposits, deposition of soluble extracellular matrix ligands, addition of conditioned media to the cells suspension, or placement of an artificial substrate such as lens capsule, extracellular matrix or healthy Bruch's membrane, into the subretinal space (123). Successful application of these techniques in vivo has yet to be demonstrated.

Timing of Surgery/Identification of Surgical Candidates

The issue regarding the timing of surgery is still to be resolved. Patients with disciform scars have evidence of significant atrophy of the outer retina over the neovascular tissue. Thus, prompt intervention may be necessary to improve the visual prognosis. Also choriocapillaris atrophy may develop under the fovea in patients with chronic subfoveal neovascularization, so that prompt surgery may improve preservation of this vascular supply as well.

SUMMARY POINTS

- The development of techniques to surgically excise choroidal neovascular membranes has introduced the possibility of surgically reconstructing the subretinal space in patients who have subfoveal choroidal neovascularization in AMD, OHS, and other disorders.
- Early attempts at reconstructing the anatomy of the subretinal space were focused on simple surgical excision of choroidal neovascularization.
- Subfoveal membrane excision can lead to good visual results if the subfoveal RPE is not removed at the time of surgery, or if the RPE is removed and adjacent RPE then repopulates the subfoveal area of Bruch's membrane within one week after surgery.
- The presence of native or regenerated RPE is required to prevent postoperative atrophy of the subfoveal choriocapillaris, because the subfoveal choriocapillaris will undergo atrophy if Bruch's membrane remains devoid of RPE for more than 1 week after subfoveal surgery.
- Persistent bare areas of Bruch's membrane will be present in patients who have large defects in the RPE monolayer, or in whom advanced patient age or disease to the inner aspects of Bruch's membrane prevents complete RPE resurfacing by migration and proliferation of adjacent RPE.
- Initial studies on RPE cell transplantation have not led to dramatic visual improvements, but the presence of disease within Bruch's membrane, iatrogenic removal of the inner layers of Bruch's membrane, and immune rejection of the transplant have limited visual recovery after surgery.
- The next challenges in submacular surgery is to deliver RPE or stem cells differentiated into the subretinal space as an organized monolayer, ensure the rapid attachment of these cells to Bruch's membrane, and prevent immunologic rejection of these cells.
- Cell survival immediately after transplantation is important to prevent atrophy of the subfoveal choriocapillaris.
- Development of an elusive animal model would facilitate progress in this field, because in the absence of an animal model, conclusions must be drawn from a combination of in vitro studies studying cell attachment to normal and diseased Bruch's membrane, in vivo studies of cell transplantation in normal animals, and a limited number of in vivo studies of RPE transplantation in individuals with age-related macular degeneration.

REFERENCES

1. Defoe DM, Ahmad A, Chen W, et al. Membrane polarity of the Na(+)-K+ pump in primary cultures of Xenopus retinal pigment epithelium. Exp Eye Res 1994; 59: 587–96.
2. Smith W, Assink J, Klein R, et al. Risk factors for age-related macular degeneration: Pooled findings from three continents. Ophthalmology 2001; 108: 697–704.

3. Klein R, Peto T, Bird A, et al. The epidemiology of age-related macular degeneration. Am J Ophthalmol 2004; 137: 486–95.

4. Age-Related Eye Disease Study Research Group. Risk factors associated with age-related macular degeneration: a case-control study in the age-related eye disease study: age-related eye disease study report number 3. Ophthalmology 2000; 107: 2224–32.

5. Treatment of Age-related Macular Degeneration With Photodynamic Therapy Study Group. Photodynamic therapy of subfoveal choroidal neovascularization in age-related macular degeneration with verteporfin: one-year results of 2 randomized clinical trials–TAP report 1. Arch Ophthalmol 1999; 117: 1329–45.

6. Pegaptanib sodium (Macugen) for macular degeneration. Med Lett Drugs Ther 2005; 47: 55–6.

7. Adamis AP, Altaweel M, Bressler NM, et al. Changes in retinal neovascularization after pegaptanib (Macugen) therapy in diabetic individuals. Ophthalmology 2006; 113: 23–8.

8. Cunningham ET Jr, Adamis AP, Altaweel M, et al. A phase II randomized double-masked trial of pegaptanib, an anti-vascular endothelial growth factor aptamer, for. diabetic macular edema. Ophthalmology 2005; 112: 1747–57.

9. D'Amico DJ, Masonson HN, Patel M, et al. Pegaptanib sodium for neovascular age-related macular degeneration: two-year safety results of the two prospective, multicenter, controlled clinical trials. Ophthalmology 2006; 113: 1001 e1–6.

10. Fraunfelder FW. Pegaptanib for wet macular degeneration. Drugs Today (Barc) 2005; 41: 703–9.

11. Gonzales CR. Enhanced efficacy associated with early treatment of neovascular age-related macular degeneration with pegaptanib sodium: an exploratory analysis. Retina 2005; 25: 815–27.

12. Gragoudas ES, Adamis AP, Cunningham ET, et al. Pegaptanib for neovascular age-related macular degeneration. N Engl J Med 2004; 351: 2805–16.

13. Moshfeghi AA, Puliafito CA. Pegaptanib sodium for the treatment of neovascular age-related macular degeneration. Expert Opin Investig Drugs 2005; 14: 671–82.

14. Ng EW, Shima DT, Calias P, et al. Pegaptanib, a targeted anti-VEGF aptamer for ocular vascular disease. Nat Rev Drug Discov 2006; 5: 123–32.

15. Rakic JM, Blaise P, Foidart JM. Pegaptanib and age-related macular degeneration. N Engl J Med 2005; 352: 1720–1; author reply 1720–1.

16. Sullivan F. Pegaptanib was effective and safe without a dose-response relation in neovascular, age-related, macular degeneration. ACP J Club 2005; 143: 18.

17. Tobin KA. Macugen treatment for wet age-related macular degeneration. Insight 2006; 31: 11–14.

18. Gaudreault J, Fei D, Rusit J, et al. Preclinical pharmacokinetics of Ranibizumab (rhuFabV2) after a single intravitreal administration. Invest Ophthalmol Vis Sci 2005; 46: 726–33.

19. Husain D, Kim I, Gauthier D, et al. Safety and efficacy of intravitreal injection of ranibizumab in combination with verteporfin PDT on experimental choroidal neovascularization in the monkey. Arch Ophthalmol 2005; 123: 509–16.

20. K, Kim IK, Husain D, Michaud N, et al. Effect of intravitreal injection of ranibizumab in combination with verteporfin PDT on normal primate retina and choroid. Invest Ophthalmol Vis Sci 2006; 47: 357–63.

21. Michels S, Rosenfeld PJ. Treatment of neovascular age-related macular degeneration with Ranibizumab/Lucentis. Klin Monatsbl Augenheilkd 2005; 222: 480–4.

22. Rosenfeld PJ. Intravitreal avastin: the low cost alternative to lucentis? Am J Ophthalmol 2006; 142: 141–3.

23. Rosenfeld PJ, Heier JS, Hantsbarger G, et al. Tolerability and efficacy of multiple escalating doses of ranibizumab (Lucentis) for neovascular age-related macular degeneration. Ophthalmology 2006; 113: 632 e1.

24. Avery RL, Pieramici DJ, Rabena MD, et al. Intravitreal bevacizumab (Avastin) for neovascular age-related macular degeneration. Ophthalmology 2006; 113: 363–372 e5.

25. Bakri SJ, Cameron JD, McCannel CA, et al. Absence of histologic retinal toxicity of intravitreal bevacizumab in a rabbit model. Am J Ophthalmol 2006; 142: 162–4.

26. Luke M, Warga M, Ziemssen F, et al. Effects. of bevacizumab ((R)) on retinal function in isolated vertebrate retina. Br J Ophthalmol 2006; 90: 1178–82.

27. Manzano RP, Peyman GA, Khan P, et al. Testing intravitreal toxicity of bevacizumab (Avastin). Retina 2006; 26: 257–61.

28. Maturi RK, Bleau LA, Wilson DL. Electrophysiologic findings after intravitreal bevacizumab (Avastin) treatment. Retina 2006; 26: 270–4.

29. Michels S, Rosenfeld PJ, Puliafito CA, et al. Systemic bevacizumab (Avastin) therapy for neovascular age-related macular degeneration twelve-week results of an uncontrolled open-label clinical study. Ophthalmology 2005; 112: 1035–47.

30. Rosenfeld PJ, Fung AE, Puliafito CA. Optical coherence tomography findings after an intravitreal injection of bevacizumab (avastin) for macular edema from central retinal vein occlusion. Ophthalmic Surg Lasers Imaging 2005; 36: 336–9.

31. Shahar J, Avery RL, Heilweil G, et al. Electrophysiologic and retinal penetration studies following intravitreal injection of bevacizumab (Avastin). Retina 2006; 26: 262–9.

32. Stewart MW, Rosenfeld PJ, Penha FM, et al. Pharmacokinetic rationale for dosing every 2 weeks versus 4 weeks with intravitreal ranibizumab, bevacizumab, and aflibercept (Vascular Endothelial Growth Factor Trap-Eye). Retina 2012; 32: 434–57.

33. Stewart MW, Rosenfeld PJ. Predicted biological activity of intravitreal. VEGF TraBr J Ophthalmol 2008; 92: 667–8.

34. Zhang K, Hopkins JJ, Heier JS, et al. Ciliary neurotrophic factor delivered by encapsulated cell intraocular implants for treatment of geographic atrophy in age-related macular degeneration. Proc Natl Acad Sci USA 2011; 108: 6241–5.

35. Rohrer B, Long Q, Coughlin B, et al. A targeted inhibitor of the complement alternative pathway reduces RPE injury and angiogenesis. In: Lambris JD, Adamis A, eds. Models of Age-Related Macular Degeneration Inflammation and Retinal Disease: Complement Biology and Pathology. New York: Springer, 2010: 137–49.

36. Landa G, et al. Weekly Vaccination with Copaxone (Glatiramer Acetate) as a potential therapy for dry age-related macular degeneration. Curr Eye Res 2008; 33: 1011–13.

37. Wong WT, Kam W, Cunningham D, et al. Treatment of geographic atrophy by the topical administration of OT-551: results of a phase II clinical trial. Invest Ophthalmol Vis Sci 2010; 51: 6131–9.

38. Age-Related Eye Disease Study Research Group. A randomized, placebo-controlled, clinical trial of high-dose supplementation with vitamins C and E, beta carotene, and zinc for age-related macular degeneration and vision loss: AREDS report no. 8. Arch Ophthalmol 2001; 119: 1417–36.

39. Berger AS, Kaplan HJ. Clinical experience with the surgical removal of subfoveal neovascular membranes. Short-term postoperative results. Ophthalmology 1992; 99: 969–75; discussion 975–6.

40. Thomas MA, Kaplan HJ. Surgical removal of subfoveal neovascularization in the presumed ocular histoplasmosis syndrome. Am J Ophthalmol 1991; 111: 1–7.

41. Thomas MA, Grand MG, Williams DF, et al. Surgical management of subfoveal choroidal neovascularization. Ophthalmology 1992; 99: 952–68; discussion 975–6.

42. Lambert HM, Capone A, Aaberg TM, et al. Surgical excision of subfoveal neovascular membranes in age-related macular degeneration. Am J Ophthalmol 1992; 113:257–62.

43. Coscas G, Meunier I. Surgery of macular neovascular subretinal membranes. J Fr Ophthalmol 1993; 16: 633–41.

44. Hsiue GH, Lai JY, Lin PK. Absorbable sandwich-like membrane for retinal-sheet transplantation. J Biomed Mater Res 2002; 61: 19–25.

45. Tezel TH, Del Priore LV, Kaplan HJ. Reengineering of aged Bruch's membrane to enhance retinal pigment epithelium repopulation. Invest Ophthalmol Vis Sci 2004; 45: 3337–48.

46. de Juan E Jr, Machemer R. Vitreous surgery for hemorrhagic and fibrous complications of age-related macular degeneration. Am J Ophthalmol 1988; 105: 25–9.

47. Submacular surgery trials randomized pilot trial of laser photocoagulation versus surgery for recurrent choroidal neovascularization secondary to age-related macular degeneration: II. Quality of life outcomes submacular surgery trials pilot study report number 2. Am J Ophthalmol 2000; 130: 408–18.

48. Bressler NM, Bressler SB, Hawkins BS, et al. Submacular surgery trials randomized pilot trial of laser photocoagulation versus surgery for recurrent choroidal neovascularization secondary to age-related macular degeneration: I. Ophthalmic outcomes submacular surgery trials pilot study report number 1. Am J Ophthalmol 2000; 130: 387–407.

49. Algvere PV, Berglin L, Gouras P, et al. Transplantation of fetal retinal pigment epithelium in age-related macular degeneration with subfoveal neovascularization. Graefes Arch Clin Exp Ophthalmol 1994; 232: 707–16.

50. Berger AS, Tezel TH, Del Priore LV, et al. Photoreceptor transplantation in retinitis pigmentosa: short-term follow-u. Ophthalmology 2003; 110: 383–91.

51. Binder S, Stolba U, Krebs I, et al. Transplantation of autologous retinal pigment epithelium in eyes with foveal neovascularization resulting from age-related macular degeneration: a pilot study. Am J Ophthalmol 2002; 133: 215–25.

52. Del Priore LV. Effect of sham surgery on retinal function after subretinal transplantation of the artificial silicone retina. Arch Ophthalmol 2005; 123: 1156; author reply 1156–7.

53. Del Priore LV, Kaplan HJ, Tezel TH, et al. Retinal pigment epithelial cell transplantation after subfoveal membranectomy in age-related macular degeneration: clinicopathologic correlation. Am J Ophthalmol 2001; 131: 472–80.

54. Del Priore LV, Tezel TH, Kaplan HJ. Survival of allogeneic porcine retinal pigment epithelial sheets after subretinal transplantation. Invest Ophthalmol Vis Sci 2004; 45: 985–92.

55. Kaplan HJ, Tezel TH, Berger AS, et al. Retinal transplantation. Chem Immunol 1999; 73: 207–19.

56. Kaplan HJ, Tezel TH, Berger AS, et al. Human photoreceptor transplantation in retinitis pigmentosa. A safety study. Arch Ophthalmol 1997; 115: 1168–72.

57. Kaplan HJ, et al. RPE Transplantation in Age-Related Macular Degeneration. In First International Conference on New Developments in the Treatment of Age-related Macular Degeneration, 1998.

58. Lois N. Transplantation of autologous retinal pigment epithelium in eyes with foveal neovascularization. Am J Ophthalmol 2002; 134: 468; author reply 468–9.

59. Peyman GA, Blinder KJ, Paris CL, et al. A technique for retinal pigment epithelium transplantation for age-related macular degeneration secondary to extensive subfoveal scarring. Ophthalmic Surg 1991; 22: 102–8.

60. Stur M. Transplantation of autologous retinal pigment epithelium in eyes with foveal neovascularization. Am J Ophthalmol 2002; 134: 469–70; author reply 470–2.

61. Abe T, Tomita H, Kano T, et al. Autologous iris pigment epithelial cell transplantation in monkey subretinal region. Curr Eye Res 2000; 20: 268–75.

62. Abe T, Takeda Y, Yamada K, et al. Cytokine gene expression after subretinal transplantation. Tohoku J Exp Med 1999; 189: 179–89.

63. Abe T, Yoshida M, Tomita H, et al. Functional analysis after auto iris pigment epithelial cell transplantation in patients with age-related macular degeneration. Tohoku J Exp Med 1999; 189: 295–305.

64. Crafoord S, Geng L, Seregard S, et al. Experimental transplantation of autologous iris pigment epithelial cells to the subretinal space. Acta Ophthalmol Scand 2001; 79: 509–14.

65. Crafoord S, Geng L, Seregard S, et al. Photoreceptor survival in transplantation of autologous iris pigment epithelial cells to the subretinal space. Acta Ophthalmol Scand 2002; 80: 387–94.

66. Hojo M, Abe T, Sugano E, et al. Photoreceptor protection by iris pigment epithelial transplantation transduced with AAV-mediated brain-derived neurotrophic factor gene. Invest Ophthalmol Vis Sci 2004; 45: 3721–6.

67. Rezai KA, Kohen L, Wiedemann P, et al. Iris pigment epithelium transplantation. Graefes Arch Clin Exp Ophthalmol 1997; 235: 558–62.

68. Schraermeyer U, Kayatz P, Thumann G, et al. Transplantation of iris pigment epithelium into the choroid slows down the degeneration of photoreceptors in the RCS rat. Graefes Arch Clin Exp Ophthalmol 2000; 238: 979–84.

69. Jordan JF, Semkova I, Kociok N, et al. Iris pigment epithelial cells transplanted into the vitreous accumulate at the optic nerve head. Graefes Arch Clin Exp Ophthalmol 2002; 240: 403–7.

70. Thumann G, Aisenbrey S, Schraermeyer U, et al. Transplantation of autologous iris pigment epithelium after removal of choroidal neovascular membranes. Arch Ophthalmol 2000; 118: 1350–5.

71. Thumann G, Bartz-Schmidt KU, El Bakri H, et al. Transplantation of autologous iris pigment epithelium to the subretinal space in rabbits. Transplantation 1999; 68: 195–201.

72. Williams KA. Transplantation of autologous iris pigment epithelial cells as a treatment for age-related macular degeneration? Transplantation 1999; 68: 171–2.

73. Aisenbrey S, Bartz-Schmidt U. Macular translocation with 360-degree retinotomy for management of age-related macular degeneration with subfoveal choroidal neovascularization. Am J Ophthalmol 2003; 135: 748–9; author reply 749.

74. Chang AA, Tan W, Beaumont PE, et al. Limited macular translocation for subfoveal choroidal neovascularization in age-related macular degeneration. Clin Exp Ophthalmol 2003; 31: 103–9.

75. D'Amico DJ, Friberg TR. Limited inferior macular translocation for the treatment of subfoveal choroidal neovascularization secondary to age-related macular degeneration. Am J Ophthalmol 2001; 132: 289–90.

76. Fujii GY, de Juan E, Humayun MS, et al. Limited macular translocation for the management of subfoveal choroidal neovascularization after photodynamic therapy. Am J Ophthalmol 2003; 135: 109–12.

77. Fujii GY, Au Eong KG, Humayun MS, et al. Limited macular translocation: current concepts. Ophthalmol Clin North Am 2002; 15: 425–36.

78. Fujii GY, Humayun MS, Pieramici DJ, et al. Initial experience of inferior limited macular translocation for subfoveal choroidal neovascularization resulting from causes other than age-related macular degeneration. Am J Ophthalmol 2001; 131: 90–100.

79. Glacet-Bernard A, Simon P, Hamelin N, et al. Translocation of the macula for management of subfoveal choroidal neovascularization: comparison of results in age-related macular degeneration and degenerative myopia. Am J Ophthalmol 2001; 131: 78–89.

80. Hamelin N, Glacet-Bernard A, Brindeau C, et al. Surgical treatment of subfoveal neovascularization in myopia: macular translocation vs surgical removal. Am J Ophthalmol 2002; 133: 530–6.

81. Lewis H, Kaiser PK, Lewis S, et al. Macular translocation for subfoveal choroidal neovascularization in age-related macular degeneration: a prospective study. Am J Ophthalmol 1999; 128: 135–46.

82. Ng EW, Fujii GY, Au Eong KG, et al. Macular translocation in patients with recurrent subfoveal choroidal neovascularization after laser photocoagulation for nonsubfoveal choroidal neovascularization. Ophthalmology 2004; 111: 1889–93.

83. Ohji M, Fujikado T, Kusaka S, et al. Comparison of three techniques of foveal translocation in patients with subfoveal choroidal neovascularization resulting from age-related macular degeneration. Am J Ophthalmol 2001; 132: 888–96.

84. Park CH, Toth CA. Macular translocation surgery with 360-degree peripheral retinectomy following ocular photodynamic therapy of choroidal neovascularization. Am J Ophthalmol 2003; 136: 830–5.

85. Pawlak D, Glacet-Bernard A, Papp M, et al. Limited macular translocation compared with photodynamic therapy in the management of subfoveal choroidal neovascularization in age-related macular degeneration. Am J Ophthalmol 2004; 137: 880–7.

86. Pertile G, Claes C. Macular translocation with 360 degree retinotomy for management of age-related macular degeneration with subfoveal choroidal neovascularization. Am J Ophthalmol 2002; 134: 560–5.

87. Pieramici DJ, De Juan E, Fujii GY, et al. Limited inferior macular translocation for the treatment of subfoveal choroidal neovascularization secondary to age-related macular degeneration. Am J Ophthalmol 2000; 130: 419–28.

88. Roth DB, Estafanous M, Lewis H. Macular translocation for subfoveal choroidal neovascularization in angioid streaks. Am J Ophthalmol 2001; 131: 390–2.

89. Terasaki H. Rescue of retinal function by macular translocation surgery in age-related macular degeneration and other diseases with subfoveal choroidal neovascularization. Nagoya J Med Sci 2001; 64: 1–9.

90. Stanga PE, Kychenthal A, Fitzke FW, et al. Retinal pigment epithelium translocation and central visual function in age related macular degeneration: preliminary results. Int Ophthalmol 2001; 23: 297–307.

91. Stanga PE, Kychenthal A, Fitzke FW, et al. Retinal pigment epithelium translocation after choroidal neovascular membrane removal in age-related macular degeneration. Ophthalmology 2002; 109: 1492–8.

92. Grossniklaus HE, Hutchinson AK, Capone A, et al. Clinicopathologic features of surgically excised choroidal neovascular membranes. Ophthalmology 1994; 101: 1099–111.

93. Del Priore LV, Kaplan HJ, Silverman MS, et al. Experimental and surgical aspects of retinal pigment epithelial cell transplantation. Eur J Implant Ref Surg 1993; 5: 128–32.

94. Rosa RH, Thomas MA, Green WR. Clinicopathologic correlation of submacular membranectomy with retention of good vision in a patient with age-related macular degeneration. Arch Ophthalmol 1996; 114: 480–7.

95. Hsu JK, Thomas MA, Ibanez H, et al. Clinicopathologic studies of an eye after submacular membranectomy for choroidal neovascularization. Retina 1995; 15: 43–52.

96. Schwartz SD, Hubschman JP, Heilwell G, et al. Embryonic stem cell trials for macular degeneration: a preliminary report. Lancet 2012; 379: 713–20.

97. Del Priore LV, et al. Extracellular matrix ligands promote RPE attachment to inner Bruch's membrane. Curr Eye Res 2002; 25: 79–89.

98. Del Priore LV, Kaplan HJ, Berger A. Retinal pigment epithelial trnasplantation inthe magagement of subfoveal choroidal neovascularization. Semin Ophthalmol 1997; 12: 45–55.

99. Akduman L, Del Priore LV, Kaplan HJ. Spontaneous resolution of retinal detachment occurring after macular hole surgery. Arch Ophthalmol 1998; 116: 465–7.

100. Del Priore LV, Tezel TH. Reattachment rate of human retinal pigment epithelium to layers of human Bruch's membrane. Arch Ophthalmol 1998; 116: 335–41.

101. Del Priore LV, Tezel TH, Ho TC, Kaplan HJ. Retinal Pigment epithelial transplantation in exudative age-related macular degeneration: what do in vivo and in vitro studies teach us?, In: Coscas G, Piccolino CF, eds. Retinal Pigment Epithelium and. Macular Diseases, Documenta Ophthalmologica Proceeedings Series 62. Boston: Kluwere Academic Publishers, 1999: 125–34.

102. Tezel TH, Del Priore LV. Reattachment to a substrate prevents apoptosis of human retinal pigment epithelium. Graefes Arch Clin Expe Ophthalmol 1997; 235: 41–7.

103. Tezel TH, Del Priore LV. Repopulation of different layers of host human Bruch's membrane by retinal pigment epithelial cell grafts. Invest Ophthalmol Vis Sci 1999; 40: 767–74.

104. Tezel TH, Del Priore LV, Kaplan HJ. Harvest and storage of adult human retinal pigment epithelial sheets. Curr Eye Res 1997; 16: 802–9.

105. Tezel TH, Bora NS, Kaplan HJ. Pathogenesis of age-related macular degeneration. Trends Mol Med 2004; 10: 417–20.

106. Berger A, Del Priore LV, Kaplan HJ. Surgery for subfoveal choroidal neovascularization vitreo-retinal and uveitis update. In the 47th Annual Symposium of the New Orleans Academy of Ophthalmology. Kugler Publications, the Hague, the Netherlands, 1998.

107. Berger AS, Conway M, Del Priore LV, et al. Submacular surgery for subfoveal choroidal neovascular membranes in patients with presumed ocular histoplasmosis. Arch Ophthalmol 1997; 115: 991–6.

108. Gass JD. Biomicroscopic and histopathologic considerations regarding the feasibility of surgical excision of subfoveal neovascular membranes. Am J Ophthalmol 1994; 118: 285–98.

109. Akduman L, Del Priore LV, Desai VN, et al. Perfusion of the subfoveal choriocapillaris affects visual recovery after submacular surgery in presumed ocular histoplasmosis syndrome. Am J Ophthalmol 1997; 123: 90–6.

110. Desai VN, Del Priore LV, Kaplan HJ. Choriocapillaris atrophy after submacular surgery in presumed ocular histoplasmosis syndrome. Arch Ophthalmol 1995; 113: 408–9.

111. Nasir MA, Sugino I, Zarbin MA. Decreased choriocapillaris perfusion following surgical excision of choroidal neovascular membranes in age-related macular degeneration. Br J Ophthalmol 1997; 81: 481–9.

112. Pollack JS, Del Priore LV, Smith ME, et al. Postoperative abnormalities of the choriocapillaris in exudative age-related macular degeneration. Br J Ophthalmol 1996; 80: 314–18.

113. Thach AB, Marx JL, Frambach DA, et al. Choroidal hypoperfusion after surgical excision of subfoveal neovascular membranes in age-related macular degeneration. Int Ophthalmol 1996; 20: 205–13.

114. Grossniklaus HE, Green WR. Histopathologic and ultrastructural findings of surgically excised choroidal neovascularization. Submacular Surg Trials Res Group. Arch Ophthalmol 1998; 116: 745–9.

115. Korte GE, Reppucci V, Henkind P. RPE destruction causes choriocapillary atrophy. Invest Ophthalmol Vis Sci 1984; 25: 1135–45.

116. Henkind P, Gartner S. The relationship between retinal pigment epithelium and the choriocapillaris. Trans Ophthalmol Soc UK 1983; 103: 444–7.

117. Kuwabara T, Ishikawa Y, Kaiser-Kupfer MI. Experimental model of gyrate atrophy in animals. Ophthalmology 1981; 88: 331–5.

118. Miller FS 3rd, Bunt-Milam AH, Kalina RE. Clinical-ultrastructural study of thioridazine retinopathy. Ophthalmology 1982; 89: 1478–88.

119. Takeuchi M, Itagaki T, Takahashi K, Ohkuma H, Uyama M. Changes in the intermediate stage of retinal degeneration after intravitreal injection of ornithine. Nippon Ganka Gakkai Zasshi 1993; 97: 17–28.

120. Leonard DS, Zhang XG, Panozzo G, et al. Clinicopathologic correlation of localized retinal pigment epithelium debridement. Invest Ophthalmol Vis Sci 1997; 38: 1094–109.

121. Del Priore LV, Kaplan HJ, Hornbeck R, Jones Z, Swinn M. Retinal pigment epithelial debridement as a model for the pathogenesis and treatment of macular degeneration. Am J Ophthalmol 1996; 122: 629–43.

122. Valentino TL, Kaplan HJ, Del Priore LV, et al. Retinal pigment epithelial repopulation in monkeys after submacular surgery. Arch Ophthalmol 1995; 113: 932–8.

123. Sugino IK, Rapista A, Sun Q, et al. A method to enhance cell survival on Bruch's membrane in eyes affected by age and age-related macular degeneration. Invest Ophthalmol Vis Sci 2011; 52: 9598–609.

124. Pfeffer B. Improved methodology for cell culture of human and monkey retinal pigment epoithelium. Prog Retina Res 1991; 10: 251–91.

125. Lu B, Malcuit C, Wang S, et al. Long-term safety and function of RPE from human embryonic stem cells in preclinical models of macular degeneration. Stem Cells 2009; 27: 2126–35.

126. Halfter W, Dong S, Schurer B, et al. Composition, synthesis, and assembly of the embryonic chick retinal basal lamina. Dev Biol 2000; 220: 111–28.

127. Green WR, McDonnell PJ, Yeo JH. Pathologic features of senile macular degeneration. Ophthalmology 1985; 92: 615–27.

128. Green WR, Enger C. Age-related macular degeneration histopathologic studies. The 1992 Lorenz E. Zimmerman Lecture. Ophthalmology 1993; 100: 1519–35.

129. Green WR, Key SN 3rd. Senile macular degeneration: a histopathologic study. Trans Am Ophthalmol Soc 1977; 75: 180–254.

130. Green WR, McDonnell PJ, Yeo JH. Pathologic features of senile macular degeneration. Ophthalmology 1985; 92: 615–27.

131. Lin WL. Immunogold localization of extracellular matrix molecules in Bruch's membrane of the rat. Curr Eye Res 1989; 8: 1171–8.

132. Das A, Frank RN, Zhang NL, et al. Ultrastructural localization of extracellular matrix components in human retinal vessels and Bruch's membrane. Arch Ophthalmol 1990; 108: 421–9.

133. Chen L, Miyamura N, Ninomiya Y, et al. Distribution of the collagen IV isoforms in human Bruch's membrane. Br J Ophthalmol 2003; 87: 212–15.

134. Bhutto IA, Kim SY, McLeod DS, et al. Localization of collagen XVIII and the endostatin portion of collagen XVIII in aged human control eyes and eyes with age-related macular degeneration. Invest Ophthalmol Vis Sci 2004; 45: 1544–52.

135. Shang QL, Ma JX, Wei JS, et al. Experimental choroidal neovascularization is inhibited by subretinal administration of Endostatin. Zhonghua Yan Ke Za Zhi 2004; 40: 266–71.

136. Mori K, Ando A, Gehlbach P, et al. Inhibition of choroidal neovascularization by intravenous injection of adenoviral vectors expressing secretable endostatin. Am J Pathol 2001; 159: 313–20.

137. Marneros AG, Keene DR, Hansen U, et al. Collagen XVIII/endostatin is essential for vision and retinal pigment epithelial function. EMBO J 2004; 23: 89–99.

138. Korte GE, Bellhorn RW, Burns MS. Remodelling of the retinal pigment epithelium in response to intraepithelial capillaries: evidence that capillaries influence the polarity of epithelium. Cell Tissue Res 1986; 245: 135–42.

139. van Zeeburg EJT, Maaijwee KJ, Missotten TO, Heimann H, van Meurs JC. A free retinal pigment epithelium–choroid graft in patients with exudative age-related macular degeneration: results up to 7 years. Am J Ophthalmol 2012; 153: 120–127, e2.

140. Falkner-Radler CI, Krebs I, Glittenberg C, et al. Human retinal pigment epithelium (RPE) transplantation: outcome after autologous RPE-choroid sheet and RPE cell-suspension in a randomised clinical study. Br J Ophthalmol 2011; 95: 370–5.

141. Radtke ND, Aramant RB, Petry HM, et al. Vision improvement in retinal degeneration patients by implantation of retina together with retinal pigment epithelium. Am J Ophthalmol 2008; 146: 172–82.

142. Heussen FM, Fawzy NF, Joeres S, et al. Autologous translocation of the choroid and RPE in age-related macular degeneration: 1-year follow-up in 30 patients and recommendations for patient selection. Eye (Lond) 2008; 22: 799–807.

143. MacLaren RE, Uppal GS, Balaggan KS, et al. Autologous transplantation of the retinal pigment epithelium and choroid in the treatment of neovascular age-related macular degeneration. Ophthalmology 2007; 114: 561–70.

144. Algvere PV, Berglin L, Gouras P, et al. Transplantation of RPE in age-related macular degeneration: observations in disciform lesions and dry RPE atrophy. Graefes Arch Clin Exp Ophthalmol 1997; 235: 149–58.

145. Algvere PV, Gouras P, Dafgard Kopp E. Long-term outcome of RPE allografts in non-immunosuppressed patients with AMD. Eur J Ophthalmol 1999; 9: 217–30.

146. Jiang LQ, Jorquera M, Streilein JW. Immunologic consequences of intraocular implantation of retinal pigment epithelial allografts. Exp Eye Res 1994; 58: 719–28.

147. Ye J, Li W, Ryan SJ. Long-term studies on allotransplantation of rabbit retinal pigment epithelial cells double-labelled with 5-bromodeoxyuridine and natural pigment. Chin Med J (Engl) 1998; 111: 736–40.

148. Ye J, Wang HM, Ogden TE, et al. Allotransplantation of rabbit retinal pigment epithelial cells double-labelled with 5-bromodeoxyuridine (BrdU) and natural pigment. Curr Eye Res 1993; 12: 629–39.

149. Weisz JM, Humayun MS, De Juan E, et al. Allogenic fetal retinal pigment epithelial cell transplant in a patient with geographic atrophy. Retina 1999; 19: 540–5.

150. Binder S, Krebs I, Hilgers RD, et al. Outcome of transplantation of autologous retinal pigment epithelium in age-related macular degeneration: a prospective trial. Invest Ophthalmol Vis Sci 2004; 45: 4151–60.

151. van Meurs JC, ter Averst E, Hofland LJ, et al. Autologous peripheral retinal pigment epithelium translocation in patients with subfoveal neovascular membranes. Br J Ophthalmol 2004; 88: 110–13.

152. van Meurs JC, Van Den Biesen PR. Autologous retinal pigment epithelium and choroid translocation in patients with exudative age-related macular degeneration: short-term follow-u. Am J Ophthalmol 2003; 136: 688–95.

153. Wolf S, Lappas A, Weinberger AW, et al. Macular translocation for surgical management of subfoveal choroidal neovascularizations in patients with AMD: first results. Graefes Arch Clin Exp Ophthalmol 1999; 237: 51–7.

154. Joussen AM, Heussen FM, Joeres S, et al. Autologous translocation of the choroid and retinal pigment epithelium in age-related macular degeneration. Am J Ophthalmol 2006; 142: 17–30.

155. Stanga PE, Kychenthal A, Fitzke FW, et al. Retinal pigment epithelium translocation and central visual function in age related macular degeneration: preliminary results. Int Ophthalmol 2001; 23: 297–307.

156. Abdel-Meguid A, Lappas A, Hartmann K, et al. One year follow up of macular translocation with 360 degree retinotomy in patients with age related macular degeneration. Br J Ophthalmol 2003; 87: 615–21.

157. Benner JD, Meyer CH, Shirkey BL, et al. Macular translocation with radial scleral ouffolding: experimental studies and initial human results. Graefes Arch Clin Exp Ophthalmol 2001; 239: 815–23.

158. Cahill MT, Mruthyunjaya P, Bowes Rickman C, et al. Recurrence of retinal pigment epithelial changes after macular translocation with 360 degrees peripheral retinectomy for geographic atrophy. Arch Ophthalmol 2005; 123: 935–8.

159. de Juan E Jr, Fujii GY. Limited macular translocation. Eye 2001; 15: 413–23.

160. Eckardt C, Eckardt U. Macular translocation in non exudative age-related macular degeneration. Retina 2002; 22: 786–94.

161. Haller JA, Hartranft CD, Fujii GY, et al. Limited macular translocation for neovascular maculopathy. Semin Ophthalmol 2000; 15: 81–7.

162. Koh SS, Arroyo J. Macular translocation with 360-degree retinotomy for treatment of exudative age-related macular degeneration. Int Ophthalmol Clin 2004; 44: 73–81.

163. Lai JC, Lapolice DJ, Stinnett SS, et al. Visual outcomes following macular translocation with 360-degree peripheral retinectomy. Arch Ophthalmol 2002; 120: 1317–24.

164. Lewis H. Macular translocation with choriosceral outfolding: a pilot clinical study. Am J Ophthalmol 2001; 132: 156–63.

165. Luke C, Alteheld N, Aisenbrey S, et al. Electro-oculographic findings after 360 degrees retinotomy and macular translocation for subfoveal choroidal neovascularisation in age-related macular degeneration. Graefes Arch Clin Exp Ophthalmol 2003; 241: 710–15.

166. Machemer R. Macular translocation. Am J Ophthalmol 1998; 125: 698–700.

167. McLeod D. Foveal translocation for exudative age related macular degeneration. Br J Ophthalmol 2000; 84: 344–5.

168. Mruthyunjaya P, Stinnett SS, Toth CA. Change in visual function after macular translocation with 360 degrees retinectomy for neovascular age-related macular degeneration. Ophthalmology 2004; 111: 1715–24.

169. Ninomiya Y, Lewis JM, Hasegawa T, et al. Retinotomy and foveal translocation for surgical management of subfoveal choroidal neovascular membranes. Am J Ophthalmol 1996; 122: 613–21.

170. Oyagi T, Fujikado T, Hosohata J, et al. Foveal sensitivity and fixation stability before and after macular translocation with 360-degree retinotomy. Retina 2004; 24: 548–55.

171. Pieramici DJ, de Juna E Jr. Limited inferior macular translocation for the treatment of subfoveal choroidal neovascularization secondary to age-related macular degeneration. Am J Ophthalmol 2001; 132: 139–40.

172. Toth CA, Freedman SF. Macular translocation with 360-degree peripheral retinectomy impact of technique and surgical experience on visual outcomes. Retina 2001; 21: 293–303.

173. Toth CA, Lapolice DJ, Banks AD, et al. Improvement in near visual function after macular translocation surgery with 360-degree peripheral retinectomy. Graefes Arch Clin Exp Ophthalmol 2004; 242: 541–8.

174. Terasaki H, Ishikawa K, Niwa Y, et al. Changes in focal macular ERGs after macular translocation surgery with

360 degrees retinotomy. Invest Ophthalmol Vis Sci 2004; 45: 567–73.

175. Terasaki H, Miyake Y, Suzuki T, et al. Change in full-field ERGs after macular translocation surgery with 360 degrees retinotomy. Invest Ophthalmol Vis Sci 2002; 43: 452–7.

176. Cahill MT, Freedman SF, Toth CA. Macular transloca-tion with 360 degrees peripheral retinectomy for geo-graphic atrophy. Arch Ophthalmol 2003; 121: 132–3.

177. Khurana RN, Fujii GY, Walsh AC, et al. Rapid recur-rence of geographic atrophy after full macular translo-cation for non exudative age-related macular degeneration. Ophthalmology 2005; 112: 1586–91.

178. Chu P, Grunwald GB. Identification of the 2A10 antigen of retinal pigment epithelium as a beta 1 subunit of inte-grin. Invest Ophthalmol Vis Sci 1991; 32: 1757–62.

179. Chu PG, Grunwald GB. Functional inhibition of retinal pigment epithelial cell-substrate adhesion with a mono-clonal antibody against the beta 1 subunit of integrin. Invest Ophthalmol Vis Sci 1991; 32: 1763–9.

180. Avery RL, Glaser BM. Inhibition of retinal pigment epi-thelial cell attachment by a synthetic peptide derived from the cell-binding domain of fibronectin. Arch Oph-thalmol 1986; 104: 1220–2.

181. Ho TC, Del Priore LV. Reattachment of cultured human retinal pigment epithelium to extracellular matrix and human Bruch's membrane. Invest ophthalmol Vis Sci 1997; 38: 1110–18.

182. Deberg M, Labasse A, Christgau S, et al. New serum biochemical markers (Coll 2-1 and Coll 2-1 NO2) for studying oxidative-related type II collagen network degradation in patients with osteoarthritis and rheuma-toid arthritis. Osteoarthritis Cartilage 2005; 13: 258–65.

183. Paik DC, Dillon J, Galicia E, et al. The nitrite/collagen reaction: non-enzymatic nitration as a model system for age-related damage. Connect Tissue Res 2001; 42: 111–22.

184. Spraul CW, Roth HJ, Moller P, et al. Histologic and mor-phometric analysis of the choroid, Bruch's membrane, and retinal pigment epithelium in postmortem eyes with age-related macular degeneration and histologic examination of surgically excised choroidal neovascular membranes. Surv Ophthalmol 1999; 44: S10–32.

185. Tezel TH, Kaplan HJ, Del Priore LV. Fate of human reti-nal pigment epithelial cells seeded onto layers of human Bruch's membrane. Invest Ophthalmol Vis Sci 1999; 40: 467–76.

186. Gullapalli VK, Sugino IK, Van Patten Y, et al. Impaired RPE survival on aged submacular human Bruch's mem-brane. Exp Eye Res 2005; 80: 235–48.

187. Lee CJ, Vroom JA, Fishman HA, et al. Determination of human lens capsule permeability and its feasibility as a replacement for Bruch's membrane. Biomaterials 2006; 27: 1670–8.

188. Sheridan C, Williams R, Grierson I. Basement mem-branes and artificial substrates in cell transplantation. Graefes Arch Clin Exp Ophthalmol 2004; 242: 68–75.

189. Sugino IK, Gullapalli VK, Sun Q, et al. Cell-Deposited Matrix Improves Retinal Pigment Epithelium Survival on Aged Submacular Human Bruch's Membrane. Invest Ophthalmol Vis Sci 2011; 52: 1345–58.

190. Thumann G, Kirchhof B. Transplantation of iris pigment epithelium. Ophthalmologe 2004; 101: 882–5.

191. Steinhorst UH, et al. Autologous subretinal transplanta-tion of cultivated porcine iris pigment epithelial cells (IPE)]. Klin Monatsbl Augenheilkd 2001; 218: 192–6.

192. Schraermeyer U, Kociok N, Heimann K. Rescue effects of IPE transplants in RCS rats: short-term results. Invest Ophthalmol Vis Sci 1999; 40: 1545–56.

193. Schraermeyer U, Thumann G, Luther T, et al. Subreti-nally transplanted embryonic stem cells rescue photore-ceptor cells from degeneration in the RCS rats. Cell Transplant 2001; 10: 673–80.

194. Hartmann U, Sistani F, Steinhorst UH. Human and por-cine anterior lens capsule as support for growing and grafting retinal pigment epithelium and iris pigment epithelium. Graefes Arch Clin Exp Ophthalmol 1999; 237: 940–5.

195. Thumann G, Schraermeyer U, Bartz-Schmidt KU, et al. Descemet's membrane as membranous support in RPE/IPE transplantation. Curr Eye Res 1997; 16: 1236–8.

196. Lee CJ, Huie P, Leng T, et al. Microcontact printing on human tissue for retinal cell transplantation. Arch Oph-thalmol 2002; 120: 1714–18.

197. Lappas A, Foerster AM, Weinberger AW, et al. Translo-cation of iris pigment epithelium in patients with exu-dative age-related macular degeneration: long-term results. Graefes Arch Clin Exp Ophthalmol 2004; 242: 638–47.

198. Itaya H, Gullapalli V, Sugino IK, et al. Iris pigment epi-thelium attachment to aged submacular human Bruch's membrane. Invest Ophthalmol Vis Sci 2004; 45: 4520–8.

199. Zhang C, Tang S, Luo Y, et al. Adeno-associated virus mediated LacZ gene transfect to cultured human iris pigment epithelium cells. Yan Ke Xue Bao 2003; 19. 49–53.

200. Kano T, Abe T, Tomita H, et al. Protective effect against ischemia and light damage of iris pigment epithelial cells transfected with the BDNF gene. Invest Ophthal-mol Vis Sci 2002; 43: 3744–53.

201. Semkova I, Kreppel F, Welsandt G, et al. Autologous transplantation of genetically modified iris pigment epi-thelial cells: a promising concept for the treatment of age-related macular degeneration and other disorders of the eye. Proc Natl Acad Sci USA 2002; 99: 13090–5.

202. Tropepe V, Coles BL, Chiasson BJ, et al. Retinal stem cells in the adult mammalian eye. Science 2000; 287: 2032–6.

203. Thumann G. Potential of pigment epithelium transplan-tation in the treatment of AMD. Graefes Arch Clin Exp Ophthalmol 2002; 240: 695–7.

204. Deacon T, Schumacher J, Dinsmore J, et al. Histological evidence of fetal pig neural cell survival after transplan-tation into a patient with Parkinson's disease. Nat Med 1997; 3: 350–3.

29

Novel therapeutic interventions: Stem cells

Pearse A. Keane and Srinivas R. Sadda

INTRODUCTION

In recent years, the introduction of ranibizumab (Lucentis®, Genentech, South San Francisco, California, USA), bevacizumab (Avastin®, Genentech), and aflibercept (Eylea®, Regeneron, Tarrytown, New York, USA) has revolutionized the treatment of patients with neovascular age-related macular degeneration (AMD) (1). In contrast, no pharmacotherapy has yet proven successful for the treatment of patients with the advanced atrophic form of AMD—geographic atrophy (GA) (2). A large number of therapeutic approaches are under development with a view to rectifying this situation; of these, stem cell–based therapies are among the most promising (3). In fact, the human eye has a number of desirable features for the application of stem cells and the first human trials of embryonic stem cells have recently been performed in patients with retinal degenerative disease (4). In this chapter, we provide an overview of work performed to date in the development of stem cell therapies for AMD; perhaps more importantly however, we provide a framework for clinicians by which the rapid advances that are likely to occur in the coming years can be easily understood.

STEM CELLS: AN OVERVIEW

Stem cells are biological cells, found in all multicellular organisms, which demonstrate two important properties (5,6). First, they are capable of self-renewal (i.e., they can divide indefinitely while still maintaining their undifferentiated state). Second, they have the capacity to differentiate into specialized cell types. The "potency" of a stem cell refers to its differentiation capability. Pluripotent stem cells can differentiate into nearly all cell types (i.e., cells derived from all three embryonic germ layers), whereas multipotent stem cells can differentiate into a number of different cell types, but only those from a closely related family of cells.

In mammals, there are two principal categories of stem cells: (i) embryonic stem cells, which are isolated from the inner cell mass of blastocysts (i.e., early-stage embryos), and (ii) adult stem cells, which are found in various tissues around the body (5,6). Embryonic stem cells are pluripotent, and are thus responsible for the generation of all cell types in the adult, that is, more than 220 types are derived from all three germ layers (ectoderm, endoderm, and mesoderm). Adult stem cells (also known as "somatic stem cells") are multipotent, and act as a repair system for the organs in which they originate. Adult stem cells that undergo a further stage of differentiation are commonly referred to as progenitor cells; these cells are oligopotent (i.e., they can differentiate into only a few cell types) and can divide only a limited number of times (in the literature, these terms are sometimes equated).

Numerous types of adult stem cells have been described (5,6). Hematopoietic stem cells are found in the bone marrow (and in umbilical cord blood) and give rise to all blood cell types. Endothelial stem cells are a rare form of adult stem cell, found in the bone marrow, which give rise to endothelial cells lining blood vessels (endothelial progenitor cells have also been found circulating in the blood). Mesenchymal stem cells (also referred to as multipotent stromal cells) are found in adipose tissue, placenta, umbilical cord tissue, deciduous ("baby") teeth, adult muscle, and bone marrow. These stem cells are capable of differentiating into mesoderm-like cells (e.g., osteoblast, adipocytes, and chondrocytes). The presence of neural stem cells has also been described in recent decades [prior to this, the human central nervous system (CNS) was considered fixed and incapable of regeneration]. Neural stem cells are of particular interest in the context of retinal degenerative diseases as the retina is a constituent of the CNS, and retinal progenitor/stem cells have recently been described (6).

Finally, an entirely new form of stem cell has recently been generated: induced pluripotent stem cells (5,6). These cells are pluripotent cells artificially derived from adult tissues (prior to their discovery, pluripotent stem cells could only be derived from embryos). In this process, terminally differentiated adult (somatic) cells are "reprogrammed" by retroviral transduction of transcription factors (i.e., viruses are used to genetically alter the cells and force expression of certain genes) or through the use of small molecules. Induced pluripotent stem cells are of considerable interest, as they do not involve the use of human embryos.

STEM CELL–BASED THERAPEUTIC STRATEGIES FOR AGE-RELATED MACULAR DEGENERATION

As highlighted earlier, the human eye has a number of advantages for the application of stem cell therapies (7). First, the human retina is readily accessible using well-established, and routinely performed, surgical techniques. In addition, transplantation of non-neuronal tissues is performed in most large ophthalmic centers (e.g., human corneas from deceased donors). Second, the retina is relatively small in size, reducing the number of cells required for any transplantation strategy, and relatively isolated from the rest of the body, reducing the risk of systemic adverse effects. Third, the human eye has a degree of immune privilege that may reduce the risk of rejection for many transplanted stem cell types. Finally, sophisticated tools exist for evaluation of ocular structure (e.g., with adaptive optics it is possible to visualize individual photoreceptors within the eye) and ocular function (e.g., multiple forms of psychophysical testing that are likely to permit detection of even subtle improvements in vision) (8,9).

AMD, as a disease, may also be well suited to the application of stem cell–based therapies. The clinical hallmark of early AMD is the deposition of acellular, polymorphous material, termed drusen, between the retinal pigment epithelium (RPE) and Bruch's membrane (10,11). Drusen formation is commonly accompanied by abnormalities of the overlying RPE, including focal loss, focal proliferation, and intraretinal migration. Patients with early AMD are frequently asymptomatic; however, the development of late AMD is typically associated with severe visual loss. In one form of late AMD, that is geographic atrophy, alterations in the RPE accumulate and lead ultimately to confluent areas of RPE atrophy. Loss of the RPE in this manner is then accompanied by loss of the overlying photoreceptors, as well as varying degrees of loss of the underlying choroidal blood supply (choriocapillaris) (12). Thus, the advanced atrophic form of AMD may be thought of as a retinal neurodegenerative disease that broadly affects the outer retina (i.e., the inner retina is largely intact, with a functioning connection to visual centers in the brain). As such, strategies aimed at replacing the damaged tissue with physiologically intact retinal cells seem particularly attractive. This concept is not new; however, it has received a new impetus with the recognition of the idea that stem cells may serve as a potentially limitless source of such physiologically intact cells.

Broadly speaking, stem cell–based therapies involve two main approaches: (i) generation of RPE cells for replacement of degenerate RPE and rescue of overlying photoreceptors and (ii) generation of photoreceptor precursors for integration into, and repair of, degenerating outer retina. Even before the introduction of stem cell–based technologies, both approaches have been explored, albeit in a somewhat primitive manner, and with limited efficacy. In human clinical studies, these attempts have typically been via autologous transplantation of human tissue (e.g., grafting a full-thickness patch of RPE and choroid from the retinal periphery to the macula in a single patient) (13–15), or allogeneic transplantation of fetal tissue (16,17). In the future, such transplantation approaches are likely to be stem cell based.

Retinal Progenitor Cells

In the developing embryo, the retina first becomes recognizable with the evagination of the neural tube to form paired optic vesicles (18). Each vesicle then undergoes a series of morphological changes resulting in the formation of a two-layered optic cup, the inner layer of which develops into the neurosensory retina, and the outer layer of which develops into the RPE. Once the optic cup has formed, the cells within this structure become known as retinal progenitor cells, generating all forms of retinal neurons and supporting cells in a sequence highly conserved across vertebrates. As a result, retinal progenitor cells, obtained from fetal or neonatal retinas, have been employed in a number of retinal transplantation studies (6,7).

In both fetal and neonatal rodents, the retina has been shown to consist of a mix of retinal progenitor cells, differentiating neurons, and photoreceptors. These cell types have been transplanted into the subretinal space of both rodents and humans in the form of intact retinal sheets or microaggregates (i.e., small pieces containing tens to hundreds of retinal cells) (19–21). In these studies, the transplanted material has been shown to both survive and differentiate. However, only very limited integration of transplanted material has been shown. Furthermore, restoration of visual function has not been well established—in those studies with functional improvement, but lack of demonstrable integration, any improvement is likely attributable to neuroprotective effects of trophic factors released from the grafted tissue (21,22). Therefore, alternative strategies, utilizing suspensions of retinal cells enzymatically dissociated from fetal or neonatal eyes, have been developed (23).

In 2006, MacLaren et al. reported the successful integration of neonatal dissociated retinal cells following transplantation into the subretinal space of mice (24). In this report, successful integration was critically dependent on the age of the donor cells—those donor cells most effective at integration were derived from retinas of animals in their first postnatal week. This corresponds to a stage of retinal development when the majority of rod photoreceptors are generated, and thus the authors suggest that newly formed postmitotic rod photoreceptors, rather than progenitor cells have the greatest potential for successful integration. In this seminal work, transplanted cells were found to migrate into the outer nuclear layer, develop the morphology of differentiated photoreceptors, and make synaptic connections in the outer plexiform layer with host bipolar cells. Using pupillometry and extracellular field potential recording from the ganglion cell layer, they also provided evidence for functional integration. Despite this, the total number of integrated cells remained small (300–1000 cells per eye). A later work from the same team has shown that pharmacological reduction of Muller cell reactivity—and thus disruption of the external limiting membrane (ELM)—can enhance outer retinal integration (25). While this and other work have demonstrated the feasibility of, and defined a strategy for, photoreceptor replacement therapies, the requirement for fetal donor tissue raises serious ethical concerns and places practical limitations on the quantity of cells available. Therefore, an alternate approach would involve the generation of immortal stem cell lines with the resulting prospect of unlimited quantities of retinal precursors for transplantation—such immortal stem cell lines could conceivably be generated from (i) adult stem cells, (ii) embryonic stem cells, (iii) or from a new cell type namely, induced pluripotent stem cells.

Adult Stem Cells

In the developing eye, the two layers of the optic cup give rise to the neurosensory retina and the RPE respectively (18). At a slightly later stage in development, the iris and ciliary epithelium become distinct, with a region of undifferentiated, mitotically active progenitor cells located between the ciliary epithelium and the developing neural retina. In amphibians, this region is maintained in mature animals and is commonly referred to as the ciliary marginal zone. The ocular regenerative powers displayed by amphibians arise from the persistence of this zone (as far back as the 1700s, the Swiss naturalist, Charles Bonnet, was able to demonstrate ocular regeneration in newts). In mammals, by contrast, this zone is inactive, with only a limited capacity for ocular regeneration. In 2000, Tropepe et al. reported that single pigmented ciliary margin cells, obtained from mice, can proliferate and differentiate in vitro to form retinal specific cell types, including rod photoreceptors, bipolar neurons, and Muller glia (26). In 2004, Coles et al. reported identification of a small population (approx. 10,000) of similar cells in human eyes ranging from early postnatal to seventh decade (27). These so-called "retinal stem cells" can be expanded in vitro to increase cell number, but evidence suggests their ability to generate new differentiated retinal neurons is limited, both in vitro and in vivo (28,29).

In addition to ciliary epithelium cells, a number of other putative adult stem cell sources have been studied as potential sources of cells for retinal transplantation (30). For example, neural stem cells capable of differentiating into oligodendrocytic, astrocytic, and neuronal phenotypes have been identified in adult mouse and human brains (31). These neural stem cells have also been differentiated into retinal type cells, such as opsin positive cells and RPE, both in vitro and in vivo (32,33). It has also been suggested that mesenchymal stem cells are capable of differentiation into other tissue types, including retinal type cells (6). While generation of photoreceptors from adult stem cells—be they retinal, neural, or mesenchymal—is of considerable interest, it has become increasingly clear that use of pluripotent stem cells is likely to be more effective (34). As a consequence, most early-stage clinical studies for diseases like AMD are now focused on the use of embryonic stem cells and/or induced pluripotent stem cells.

Embryonic Stem Cells

Embryonic stem cells are pluripotent stem cells isolated from early-stage embryos (blastocysts) (6). Initial work in this area began in the 1960s with the study of teratocarcinomas in mice (35). Growth of these tumors was induced by surgical transplantation of normal, early-stage mouse embryos to extrauterine sites in histocompatible hosts. Cells isolated from teratocarcinomas could be grown in culture and were found to demonstrate the properties required of stem cells (i.e., self-renewal and potency). This early version of embryonic stem cell thus came to be known as an embryonic carcinoma cell.

Direct isolation of embryonic stem cells was first performed in mice, and reported in 1981, by two independent groups. First, Evans and Kaufman, working in the University of Cambridge, developed a technique to delay uterine implantation of early-stage mouse embryos; this delay allowed an increase in blastocyst cell number and greatly facilitated subsequent culture of these cells in vitro (36). Later that year, Gail Martin, working in the University of California, San Francisco, described a different technique where embryonic stem cells were derived from mouse blastocysts specifically cultured in media conditioned by an established teratocarcinoma stem cell line (37). At this point, the term "embryonic stem cell" was first coined.

In 1998, James Thompson and coworkers, working in the University of Wisconsin-Madison, developed a technique to isolate and grow embryonic stem cells in humans (38). In this work, fresh (or frozen) cleavage-stage human embryos, produced by in-vitro fertilization (IVF) for fertility purposes, were utilized (in IVF, multiple embryos are generated, not all of which can be implanted; the surplus embryos, which will otherwise be discarded, may be donated with consent). These embryos were cultured to the blastocyst stage and their inner cell masses isolated. As a result, five embryonic stem cell lines, originating from five embryos, were derived. After undifferentiated proliferation in vitro for four to five months, these cells were found to maintain the potential to form derivatives of all three embryonic germ layers, including gut epithelium (endoderm), cartilage, bone, smooth muscle, and striated muscle (mesoderm), and neural epithelium, embryonic ganglia, and stratified squamous epithelium (ectoderm). In the decade following publication of this seminal work, stem cell research has increased exponentially.

For a number of reasons, embryonic stem cells are attractive for the treatment of retinal neurodegenerative and other disorders. In particular, embryonic stem cells offer the potential for generation of unlimited number of healthy young cells—for example, retinal photoreceptors—for transplantation into diseased eyes (34). By comparison, many forms of adult stem cells are rare, difficult to isolate, and difficult to grow in culture. Differentiation of embryonic stem cells in vitro can also be tightly controlled to ensure optimum safety, purity, potency, and a myriad of other parameters (39). Conversely, use of embryonic stem cells has significant barriers to clinical translation. First, transplantation of embryonic stem cells may result in teratoma formation (as described above, transplantation of early-stage mice embryos onto a histocompatible host has been shown to result in teratocarcinoma formation) (40). Second, immunological rejection of embryonic stem cells may be a significant barrier, although a work suggests that it may be possible to reduce immunogenicity in the differentiation process [e.g., through reducing the complexity of the human leucocyte antigen (HLA) complex] or by somatic cell nuclear transfer techniques (41). Finally, as embryonic stem cells are derived from discarded human embryos—with destruction of the embryo—their use has formidable ethical and regulatory barriers (42,43).

As described above, the first step in the development of embryonic stem cell–based therapies is isolation and culture of an embryonic stem cell line. The next step is successful differentiation of such cells into functional adult cell types. To date, adult cell types generated include neurons, cardiomyocytes, hepatocytes, lung epithelium, and pancreatic β-cells (6). Embryonic stem cells have also been successfully differentiated into photoreceptors, photoreceptor progenitors, and RPE cells, both in mice and in humans (44–49). Furthermore, in 2011, Eiraku and coworkers were able to demonstrate that a population of homogenous mouse embryonic stem cells could be used to generate synthetic retinas in vitro, with the complex process of optic vesicle formation appearing to occur spontaneously when cultured in the presence of extracellular matrix components (50). Until recently, the efficiency of retinal cell differentiation in vitro has been low, so this technique represents an exciting opportunity to increase the efficiency of production of photoreceptor precursors.

Transplantation of naïve embryonic stem cells into the subretinal space of rats has been shown to result in tumor formation (40); however, predifferentiation of cells before transplantation may reduce this risk. In 2004, Haruta et al. reported survival—and absence of tumor formation—when pigment epithelium cells derived from non–human primate embryonic stem cells were transplanted into the subretinal space of Royal College of Surgeons (RCS) rats (51). In 2006, Lund et al. were also able to demonstrate improvements in visual function following transplantation of human embryonic stem cell–derived RPE lines into the subretinal space of RCS rats (a rodent model of retinal degeneration) (52). In 2009, Lamba et al. were able to demonstrate improved visual function following transplantation of human embryonic stem cell–derived retinal cells into the subretinal space of Crx(-/-) mice (a model of Leber's Congenital Amaurosis) (53).

In 2012, the preliminary results of the first human embryonic stem cell trial, carried out by Advanced Cell Technology (Marlborough, MA) at the Jules Stein Eye Institute in Los Angeles, were reported (4). In this work, human embryonic stem cells (cell line MA09) were used to generate RPE cells with greater than 99% purity. A single patient with advanced atrophic AMD, and a single patient with Stargardt's disease, were initially enrolled. Pars plana vitrectomy was performed and then, 5×10^4 (50,000) cells, suspended in 150 μL of balanced salt solution (BSS) were injected into the subretinal space (the location of macular injection was chosen to avoid completely atrophic areas). Following surgery, patients were immunosuppressed using low-dose tacrolimus for six weeks and mycophenolate mofetil for 12 weeks. After surgery, the transplanted RPE cells could be clearly seen on color fundus photography and optical coherence tomographyimaging, with no evidence of hyperproliferation, tumorigenicity, ectopic tissue formation, or immune mediated transplant rejection. Four

months after surgery, modest gains in visual acuity were also reported: from 0 to 5 ETDRS letters for the patient with Stargardt's disease, and from 21 to 28 letters for the patient with AMD. While these results are promising, these are very preliminary, involving only two patients and a short-term follow-up. Furthermore, assessment of visual endpoints in patients with low vision remains a controversial area. As a result, Advanced Cell Technology is currently performing larger clinical trials in the United States (NCT01344993—12 patients with AMD, receiving between 50,000 and 200,000 cells, at the Jules Stein Eye Institute and Wills Eye Hospital) and United Kingdom (NCT01469832—12 patients with Stargardt's disease, receiving between 50,000 and 200,000 cells, at Moorfields Eye Hospital and the Aberdeen Royal Infirmary Eye Unit). Imminent clinical trials are also being planned by a number of other groups, including the London Project to Cure Blindness at University College, London, in conjunction with Pfizer Regenerative Medicine, and by Cell Cure Neurosciences Ltd. in Israel (7).

Induced Pluripotent Stem Cells

As described above, considerable barriers exist to the clinical application of embryonic stem cells, in particular ethical concerns regarding use of human embryos, and issues related to immune rejection of unmatched tissue. Therefore, an ideal solution will involve the generation of stem cells with pluripotent potential from fully differentiated adult somatic cells (i.e., "reprogramming" of adult cells). Major steps toward such a solution have been made in recent years (34).

The first major breakthrough in the reprogramming of somatic cells occurred in 1996, with the production of "Dolly, the sheep" by transfer of the nuclear content of an adult sheep somatic cell into an enucleated, unfertilized sheep egg ("somatic cell nuclear transfer") (54). Following stimulation with an electric shock, this hybrid cell was then shown to develop into an embryo (and, ultimately, the first cloned animal). This seminal work demonstrated that terminally differentiated adult cells are capable of being reverted back to an embryonic totipotent state (i.e., a single cell which can divide and produce all the differentiated cells in an organism). In 2004, researchers in Korea claimed to have replicated this work in humans, that is, transferred nuclear content from an adult cell into an enucleated, unfertilized egg; stimulated the resulting hybrid to develop into a human embryo; and then cultured the resulting human embryonic stem cells (55). Unfortunately however, much of this work is now known to be a fabrication and the associated papers have been retracted.

An alternative approach, where somatic cells are reprogrammed by fusion with embryonic stem cells, has subsequently been described (56). Collectively, these works demonstrated that both unfertilized eggs and embryonic stem cells contain factors that can confer totipotency or pluripotency on somatic cells. As a consequence, Takahashi and Yamanaka examined 24 different factors for their ability to induce pluripotency in somatic cells. In this work, reported in 2006, they demonstrated that only four transcription factors (Oct4, Sox2, Klf4, and c-Myc), introduced via retroviral expression, were required to reprogram adult mouse skin fibroblasts into pluripotent stem cells—the so-called "induced pluripotent stem cells" (57,58). These cells were found to possess a similar developmental potential as embryonic stem cells, with similar morphology, proliferation, and teratoma formation. The first generation of induced pluripotent stem cells differed from embryonic stem cells in gene expression and epigenetic patterns. This issue has been largely rectified in newer generations, and mouse-induced pluripotent cells have been shown to sustain the development of an entire mouse (59). Subcutaneous grafting of human-induced pluripotent stem cells in rodents has also been shown to give rise to teratomas giving rise to all three embryonic germ layers (34,60).

Induced pluripotent stem cells have been demonstrated to differentiate into a broad range of adult cell types, such as different neural cells, cardiomyocytes, neural crest cells, and muscle cells. Following differentiation, the therapeutic benefit of induced pluripotent stem cells has also been demonstrated in mouse models of sickle cell anemia (61), amyotrophic lateral sclerosis (62), and Parkinson disease (63). Thus, it is now widely accepted that human-induced pluripotent stem cells are genuinely pluripotent. Despite this, due to epigenetic memory, subtle differences may remain between induced pluripotent and embryonic stem cells (64)—in particular, as suggested in literature that differentiation of induced pluripotent stem cells may be biased towards their tissue of origin (65). An additional consideration is that the transcription factors used to generate induced pluripotent stem cells include well-known oncogenes (e.g., c-Myc) that could be reactivated during transcription and, thus, increase the potential for tumor formation (66). In 2008, it was demonstrated that oncogenes could be removed after the induction of pluripotency; in 2009, generation of induced pluripotent cells was demonstrated without genetic alterations of these cells, via channeling of certain proteins into the cells, the so-called protein-induced pluripotent stem cells (67).

To date, a number of groups have shown differentiation of induced pluripotent stem cells into retinal cell types. In 2009, Carr et al. reported the differentiation of induced pluripotent stem cells into cells morphologically similar to RPE cells, and expressing numerous markers of developing and mature RPE cells (68). These differentiated cells were then found to be capable of phagocytosing photoreceptor outer segments in vitro, and in vivo following transplantation into RCS rats. Long-term visual function was also maintained in animals receiving transplantation of these cells. In 2009, Hirami et al. also reported generation of retinal progenitor cells (69), while Meyer et al. demonstrated that human-induced pluripotent stem cells were able to acquire features of advanced retinal differentiation in a sequence and time course that mimics normal retinal development (69). In 2010, Lamba et al. reported differentiation of induced pluripotent stem cells into

photoreceptors, and the integration of these cells into the outer nuclear layer after transplantation into the subretinal space of adult mice (70). In 2010, Parameswaran et al. further reported generation of retinal ganglion cells, cone photoreceptors, and rod photoreceptors, from mouse-induced pluripotent stem cells (71). Much of the current work on induced pluripotent stem cells is focused on establishing whether these cells are truly indistinguishable from embryonic stem cells and free from detrimental epigenetic or genetic modifications. When these issues can be clarified, it seems likely that human clinical trials will follow shortly thereafter.

CONCLUSION

AMD, the commonest cause of irreversible visual loss in the developed world (72), is characterized by loss of the RPE and degeneration of the overlying photoreceptors (12). Therefore, transplantation of healthy photoreceptors and/or RPE cells is an exciting option for future treatment of this disease. In the past, clinical studies employing this approach have involved autologous or allogeneic transplantation of retinal tissue. However, the former involves technical challenging surgery, while the latter involves use of fetal tissue, and thus both practical and ethical concerns. Moreover, both strategies have demonstrated only limited functional integration of transplanted tissue. In recent years, it has become clear that functional integration of transplanted retinal photoreceptors is possible, but is highly dependent on the differentiation stage of the cells in question (24). Since 1998, the advent of human embryonic stem cells offers the prospect of unlimited supplies of cells for transplantation, with tight control of their differentiation state (38). Since 2007, the development of human-induced pluripotent stem cells raises the prospect of retinal transplantation with all the advantages of embryonic cell technologies, but without fears regarding immunological rejection, or ethical concerns (58). In 2012, preliminary results from the first human clinical trial of embryonic stem cells were reported in a single patient with AMD, with larger trials under way. Therefore, it is clear that stem cell–based therapies are at the cutting edge of new therapeutic interventions for AMD, with many exciting breakthroughs likely in the coming years.

SUMMARY POINTS

- Age-related macular degeneration (AMD) is characterized by loss of the retinal pigment epithelium (RPE) and overlying photoreceptors and, therefore, transplantation of healthy photoreceptors and/or RPE is an attractive treatment option.
- Retinal transplantation has previously been explored, in humans, using both autologous and allogeneic tissue (i.e., tissue transplanted from a different location within the same individual, or from an individual of the same species). However, as a result of technical and ethical challenges, each of these approaches has demonstrated only limited success.

- An alternate approach to retinal transplantation would involve the use of stem cells to generate unlimited quantities of healthy photoreceptors and/or RPE.
- Human embryonic stem cell-derived RPE cells have recently entered clinical trials for the treatment of AMD and Stargardt's disease, with promising initial results. However, generation of embryonic stem cell lines faces considerable barriers due to its requirement for human embryos at outset, and the possibility of immune rejection of non-matched tissue.
- The recent development of induced pluripotent stem cells raises the prospect of retinal transplantation with all the advantages of embryonic cell technologies, but without fears regarding immunological rejection, or ethical concerns.

REFERENCES

1. Martin DF, Maguire MG, Ying GS, et al. Ranibizumab and bevacizumab for neovascular age-related macular degeneration. N Engl J Med 2011; 364: 1897–908.

2. Zarbin MA, Rosenfeld PJ. Pathway-based therapies for age-related macular degeneration: an integrated survey of emerging treatment alternatives. Retina 2010; 30: 1350–67.

3. Chiang A, Haller JA. Vitreoretinal disease in the coming decade. Curr Opin Ophthalmol 2010; 21: 197–202.

4. Schwartz SD, Hubschman JP, Heilwell G, et al. Embryonic stem cell trials for macular degeneration: a preliminary report. Lancet 2012; 379: 713–20.

5. Slack J. Stem Cells: A Very Short Introduction. New York, NY: Oxford University Press, 2012.

6. Huang Y, Enzmann V, Ildstad ST. Stem cell-based therapeutic applications in retinal degenerative diseases. Stem Cell Rev 2011; 7: 434–45.

7. Bull ND, Martin KR. Concise review: toward stem cell-based therapies for retinal neurodegenerative diseases. Stem Cells 2011; 29: 1170–5.

8. Keane PA, Sadda SR. Imaging chorioretinal vascular disease. Eye 2010; 24: 422–7.

9. Neelam K, Nolan J, Chakravarthy U, Beatty S. Psychophysical function in age-related maculopathy. Surv Ophthalmol 2009; 54: 167–210.

10. de Jong PT. Age-related macular degeneration. N Engl J Med 2006; 355: 1474–85.

11. Jager RD, Mieler WF, Miller JW. Age-related macular degeneration. N Engl J Med 2008; 358: 2606–17.

12. Green WR, Enger C. Age-related macular degeneration histopathologic studies. the 1992 Lorenz E. Zimmerman Lecture. Ophthalmology 1993; 100: 1519–35.

13. MacLaren RE, Uppal GS, Balaggan KS, et al. Autologous transplantation of the retinal pigment epithelium and choroid in the treatment of neovascular age-related macular degeneration. Ophthalmology 2007; 114: 561–70.

14. Joussen AM, Joeres S, Fawzy N, et al. Autologous translocation of the choroid and retinal pigment epithelium in patients with geographic atrophy. Ophthalmology 2007; 114: 551–60.

15. Binder S, Krebs I, Hilgers RD, et al. Outcome of transplantation of autologous retinal pigment epithelium in age-related macular degeneration: a prospective trial. Invest Ophthalmol Vis Sci 2004; 45: 4151–60.

16. Weisz JM, Humayun MS, De Juan E Jr, et al. Allogenic fetal retinal pigment epithelial cell transplant in a patient with geographic atrophy. Retina 1999; 19: 540–5.

17. Humayun MS, de Juan E Jr, del Cerro M, et al. Human neural retinal transplantation. Invest Ophthalmol Vis Sci 2000; 41: 3100–6.

18. Lamba D, Karl M, Reh T. Neural regeneration and cell replacement: a view from the eye. Cell Stem Cell 2008; 2: 538–49.

19. Seiler M, Aramant RB, Ehinger B, Adolph AR. Transplantation of embryonic retina to adult retina in rabbits. Exp Eye Res 1990; 51: 225–8.

20. Ghosh F, Ehinger B. Full-thickness retinal transplants: a review. Ophthalmologica 2000; 214: 54–69.

21. Gouras P, Du J, Kjeldbye H, et al. Long-term photoreceptor transplants in dystrophic and normal mouse retina. Invest Ophthalmol Vis Sci 1994; 35: 3145–53.

22. Klassen HJ, Ng TF, Kurimoto Y, et al. Multipotent retinal progenitors express developmental markers, differentiate into retinal neurons, and preserve light-mediated behavior. Invest Ophthalmol Vis Sci 2004; 45: 4167–73.

23. Qiu G, Seiler MJ, Mui C, et al. Photoreceptor differentiation and integration of retinal progenitor cells transplanted into transgenic rats. Exp Eye Res 2005; 80: 515–25.

24. MacLaren RE, Pearson RA, MacNeil A, et al. Retinal repair by transplantation of photoreceptor precursors. Nature 2006; 444: 203–7.

25. West EL, Pearson RA, Tschernutter M, et al. Pharmacological disruption of the outer limiting membrane leads to increased retinal integration of transplanted photoreceptor precursors. Exp Eye Res 2008; 86: 601–11.

26. Tropepe V, Coles BL, Chiasson BJ, et al. Retinal stem cells in the adult mammalian eye. Science 2000; 287: 2032–6.

27. Coles BL, Angenieux B, Inoue T, et al. Facile isolation and the characterization of human retinal stem cells. Proc Natl Acad Sci USA 2004; 101: 15772–7.

28. Cicero SA, Johnson D, Reyntjens S, et al. Cells previously identified as retinal stem cells are pigmented ciliary epithelial cells. Proc Natl Acad Sci USA 2009; 106: 6685–90.

29. Gualdoni S, Baron M, Lakowski J, et al. Adult ciliary epithelial cells, previously identified as retinal stem cells with potential for retinal repair, fail to differentiate into new rod photoreceptors. Stem Cells 2010; 28: 1048–59.

30. West EL, Pearson RA, MacLaren RE, et al. Cell transplantation strategies for retinal repair. Prog Brain Res 2009; 175: 3–21.

31. Clarke DL, Johansson CB, Wilbertz J, et al. Generalized potential of adult neural stem cells. Science 2000; 288: 1660–3.

32. Dong X, Pulido JS, Qu T, Sugaya K. Differentiation of human neural stem cells into retinal cells. Neuroreport 2003; 14: 143–6.

33. Enzmann V, Howard RM, Yamauchi Y, et al. Enhanced induction of RPE lineage markers in pluripotent neural stem cells engrafted into the adult rat subretinal space. Invest Ophthalmol Vis Sci 2003; 44: 5417–22.

34. Boucherie C, Sowden JC, Ali RR. Induced pluripotent stem cell technology for generating photoreceptors. Regen Med 2011; 6: 469–79.

35. Andrews PW, Matin MM, Bahrami AR, et al. Embryonic stem (ES) cells and embryonal carcinoma (EC) cells: opposite sides of the same coin. Biochem Soc Trans 2005; 33(Pt 6): 1526–30.

36. Evans MJ, Kaufman MH. Establishment in culture of pluripotential cells from mouse embryos. Nature 1981; 292: 154–6.

37. Martin GR. Isolation of a pluripotent cell line from early mouse embryos cultured in medium conditioned by teratocarcinoma stem cells. Proc Natl Acad Sci USA 1981; 78: 7634–8.

38. Thomson JA, Itskovitz-Eldor J, Shapiro SS, et al. Embryonic stem cell lines derived from human blastocysts. Science 1998; 282: 1145–7.

39. Cowan CA, Klimanskaya I, McMahon J, et al. Derivation of embryonic stem-cell lines from human blastocysts. N Engl J Med 2004; 350: 1353–6.

40. Arnhold S, Klein H, Semkova I, et al. Neurally selected embryonic stem cells induce tumor formation after long-term survival following engraftment into the subretinal space. Invest Ophthalmol Vis Sci 2004; 45: 4251–5.

41. Lanza RP, Chung HY, Yoo JJ, et al. Generation of histocompatible tissues using nuclear transplantation. Nat Biotechnol 2002; 20: 689–96.

42. Bahadur G, Morrison M, Machin L. Beyond the 'embryo question': human embryonic stem cell ethics in the context of biomaterial donation in the UK. Reprod Biomed Online 2010; 21: 868–74.

43. Murdoch A, Braude P, Courtney A, et al. The procurement of cells for the derivation of human embryonic stem cell lines for therapeutic use: recommendations for good practice. Stem Cell Rev 2012; 8: 91–9.

44. Lamba DA, Karl MO, Ware CB, Reh TA. Efficient generation of retinal progenitor cells from human embryonic stem cells. Proc Natl Acad Sci USA 2006; 103: 12769–74.

45. Zhao X, Liu J, Ahmad I. Differentiation of embryonic stem cells into retinal neurons. Biochem Biophys Res Comms 2002; 297: 177–84.

46. Vugler A, Carr AJ, Lawrence J, et al. Elucidating the phenomenon of HESC-derived RPE: anatomy of cell genesis, expansion and retinal transplantation. Exp Neurol 2008; 214: 347–61.

47. Ikeda H, Osakada F, Watanabe K, et al. Generation of Rx+/Pax6+ neural retinal precursors from embryonic stem cells. Proc Natl Acad Sci USA 2005; 102: 11331–6.

48. Osakada F, Ikeda H, Mandai M, et al. Toward the generation of rod and cone photoreceptors from mouse, monkey and human embryonic stem cells. Nat Biotechnol 2008; 26: 215–24.

49. Klimanskaya I, Hipp J, Rezai KA, et al. Derivation and comparative assessment of retinal pigment epithelium from human embryonic stem cells using transcriptomics. Cloning Stem Cells 2004; 6: 217–45.

50. Eiraku M, Takata N, Ishibashi H, et al. Self-organizing optic-cup morphogenesis in three-dimensional culture. Nature 2011; 472: 51–6.

51. Haruta M, Sasai Y, Kawasaki H, et al. In vitro and in vivo characterization of pigment epithelial cells differentiated from primate embryonic stem cells. Invest Ophthalmol Vis Sci 2004; 45: 1020–5.

52. Lund RD, Wang S, Klimanskaya I, et al. Human embryonic stem cell-derived cells rescue visual function in dystrophic RCS rats. Cloning Stem Cells 2006; 8: 189–99.

53. Lamba DA, Gust J, Reh TA. Transplantation of human embryonic stem cell-derived photoreceptors restores some visual function in Crx-deficient mice. Cell Stem Cell 2009; 4: 73–9.

54. Wilmut I, Schnieke AE, McWhir J, et al. Viable offspring derived from fetal and adult mammalian cells. Nature 1997; 385: 810–13.

55. Hwang WS, Ryu YJ, Park JH, et al. Evidence of a pluripotent human embryonic stem cell line derived from a cloned blastocyst. Science 2004; 303: 1669–74.

56. Cowan CA, Atienza J, Melton DA, Eggan K. Nuclear reprogramming of somatic cells after fusion with human embryonic stem cells. Science 2005; 309: 1369–73.

57. Takahashi K, Yamanaka S. Induction of pluripotent stem cells from mouse embryonic and adult fibroblast cultures by defined factors. Cell 2006; 126: 663–76.

58. Takahashi K, Tanabe K, Ohnuki M, et al. Induction of pluripotent stem cells from adult human fibroblasts by defined factors. Cell 2007; 131: 861–72.

59. Boland MJ, Hazen JL, Nazor KL, et al. Adult mice generated from induced pluripotent stem cells. Nature 2009; 461: 91–4.

60. Gutierrez-Aranda I, Ramos-Mejia V, Bueno C, et al. Human induced pluripotent stem cells develop teratoma more efficiently and faster than human embryonic stem cells regardless the site of injection. Stem Cells 2010; 28: 1568–70.

61. Hanna J, Wernig M, Markoulaki S, et al. Treatment of sickle cell anemia mouse model with iPS cells generated from autologous skin. Science 2007; 318: 1920–3.

62. Dimos JT, Rodolfa KT, Niakan KK, et al. Induced pluripotent stem cells generated from patients with ALS can be differentiated into motor neurons. Science 2008; 321: 1218–21.

63. Wernig M, Zhao JP, Pruszak J, et al. Neurons derived from reprogrammed fibroblasts functionally integrate into the fetal brain and improve symptoms of rats with parkinson's disease. Proc Natl Acad Sci USA 2008; 105: 5856–61.

64. Stadtfeld M, Apostolou E, Akutsu H, et al. Aberrant silencing of imprinted genes on chromosome 12qF1 in mouse induced pluripotent stem cells. Nature 2010; 465: 175–81.

65. Polo JM, Liu S, Figueroa ME, et al. Cell type of origin influences the molecular and functional properties of mouse induced pluripotent stem cells. Nat Biotechnol 2010; 28: 848–55.

66. Nakagawa M, Koyanagi M, Tanabe K, et al. Generation of induced pluripotent stem cells without Myc from mouse and human fibroblasts. Nat Biotechnol 2008; 26: 101–6.

67. Zhou H, Wu S, Joo JY, et al. Generation of induced pluripotent stem cells using recombinant proteins. Cell Stem Cell 2009; 4: 381–4.

68. Carr AJ, Vugler AA, Hikita ST, et al. Protective effects of human iPS-derived retinal pigment epithelium cell transplantation in the retinal dystrophic rat. PLoS One 2009; 4: e8152.

69. Hirami Y, Osakada F, Takahashi K, et al. Generation of retinal cells from mouse and human induced pluripotent stem cells. Neurosci Lett 2009; 458: 126–31.

70. Lamba DA, McUsic A, Hirata RK, et al. Generation, purification and transplantation of photoreceptors derived from human induced pluripotent stem cells. PLoS One 2010; 5: e8763.

71. Parameswaran S, Balasubramanian S, Babai N, et al. Induced pluripotent stem cells generate both retinal ganglion cells and photoreceptors: therapeutic implications in degenerative changes in glaucoma and age-related macular degeneration. Stem Cells 2010; 28: 695–703.

72. Bressler NM. Age-related macular degeneration is the leading cause of blindness. JAMA 2004; 291: 1900–1.

30

Clinical considerations for visual rehabilitation

Susan A. Primo and Cheryl Frueh

INTRODUCTION

While the trauma of macular degeneration is difficult enough for some patients to cope with, the visual impairment left afterwards is even tougher. Patients must not only learn to accept the fate of retinal disease, but must also summon the strength to accept the fact that they will have to surrender a certain degree of independence as visual acuity declines. The visual rehabilitative process helps the visually impaired patient to regain a satisfactory level of independence and can be achieved by assisting the patient in learning to cope with the psychological, emotional, and economic aspects of vision loss through the use of optical, non-optical, and electronic devices and where there are some exciting new technologies available. Typically, this type of integrated, multidisciplinary rehabilitative process is necessary for patients with severe and profound visual impairment, that is, legal blindness.

The term legal blindness is defined as a visual acuity of 20/200 or worse in the best-corrected better eye or a visual field of 20° or less in the widest diameter of vision. A patient cannot have poor vision in one eye only and be considered legally blind. This classification becomes a part of the patient's permanent record and has implications for eligibility for state financial assistance, tax benefits, reduced public transportation fares, and other circumstances. In addition, in many states that have "commissions" for the blind, reporting of legal blindness may cause a driver's license to be revoked. For many people, having a driver's license, whether actually driving or not, has significant meaning and serves as a form of identification. The practitioner should be aware of these issues when designating this classification.

THE LOW VISION EVALUATION
Clinical Considerations

The examiner should notice head and body movements as the patient initially walks into the examination room as these seemingly minor observations provide information not only about visual status, but also about a patient's level of adaptation to the vision loss. In addition, before visual acuity testing begins, any auxiliary testing is performed, which may include contrast sensitivity, microperimetry visual fields, Amsler grid, or standard visual fields. These tests can shed light on the size and extent of the central scotoma as well as on other subjective aspects of the acuity loss.

The evaluation then begins with a complete and thorough understanding of the patient's ocular history.

Detailed documentation of surgical history and stage of pathology are important components. Typically, a low vision evaluation should commence bearing in mind whether or not a patient has undergone all surgical and nonsurgical attempts at restoring visual function. First, the low vision examiner is concerned with performing an extensive evaluation often using the state-of-the-art devices, which can be quite expensive. If the patient's final visual acuity is in question, these devices may not be suitable once the visual acuity has reached its final level and has stabilized. Secondly, the "mourning process" of losing sight must be kept in mind with the patient understanding (or beginning to understand) that the next step must be taken to begin the visual rehabilitative process. This is not to say that if miracle breakthroughs become available, then a patient should not have access to any possibility of restoring sight. However, success with low vision devices is completely dependent upon (i) patients' full acceptance of their visual impairment and (ii) the ability and desire to move on. In some cases, the evaluation will be the first step in this process.

During the history, the patient is asked about aspects of vision loss. These aspects include duration, symmetry, fluctuations, stability, loss of ability to discriminate color, effects of various illuminations or lighting conditions, loss of independence with activities of daily living, and mobility concerns. These questions assist patients in learning to talk about the effects of the visual impairment on their lifestyle, an important step in beginning the rehabilitative process. While ascertaining this information, the low vision examiner also documents any current devices including glasses, which may already be in the patient's possession. Frequently, a well-meaning spouse or relative has already offered the patient a magnifier of some sort. It is important to categorize all such devices for type, style, and power. It is also important to determine the usefulness of these devices. For example, can the patient read large print or headlines of a newspaper with glasses and/or a magnifier? Oftentimes, patients will say that all devices are useless, but in reality, they may be able to see large print and not regular print. While this may be considered useless to them, it is important to the examiner.

Perhaps, the last and most important part of the history is an expression by patients of their goals and expectations. During this portion, the examiner determines whether the patient has realistic goals and expectations or whether the desire is to "just see again."

A detailed list of desired activities is recorded in order of importance to the patient. Sometimes it takes a little prodding, but virtually all patients' primary desire is to be able to read again. It is important to determine whether patients simply want to read mail or bills in order to handle their own finances and/or want to continue leisurely reading printed materials such as newspaper, novels, etc. The advent of e-readers has been a plus to many visually impaired patients. Second to a desire to read, is usually improvement of distance vision. Again, specific distant activities (watching television, bird-watching, or driving) need to be discussed. The driving issue is an extremely sensitive area and the examiner should exercise compassion and sensitivity in discussing this topic. A more detailed discussion of driving will follow later in this chapter. Using a checklist approach is a quick and easy method for determining the patient's current level of vision and, subsequently, any special material the patient wishes to read or certain activities the patient wishes to engage in, like sewing, drawing, or painting; or cardgames, golf, etc. (Fig. 30.1). Finally, maximizing an education environment is critical for young children or adults, as is attention to patients' workplace if they are employed or seeking gainful employment.

Checklist for current level of vision/goals

	YES	NO	DESIRES
Headlines	____	____	____
Magazines	____	____	____
Regular Newsprint	____	____	____
Labels, price tags	____	____	____
Money	____	____	____
Recognize faces	____	____	____
Watch TV	____	____	____
Cooking	____	____	____
Sew, knit, etc.	____	____	____
Housekeeping	____	____	____
Hygiene	____	____	____
Handiwork	____	____	____
Garden/yard work	____	____	____
Sports (golf, etc.)	____	____	____
Play cards	____	____	____
Driving	____	____	____
Other	____	____	____
Glare	____	____	

Figure 30.1 Checklist for current level of vision/goals.

Although there is a standard format to the low vision evaluation, the examiner always bears in mind a goal-orientated approach. For example, if a patient expresses the desire to read only, the focus will be on achieving this goal. The examiner might explain possibilities for improvement in distance vision, but if a patient is still uninterested, the telescopic evaluation is probably unnecessary. Likewise, if a patient's only desire is to drive, a short near evaluation may be performed to demonstrate possibilities, but clearly the emphasis in this case would be on the telescopic evaluation.

As clear-cut as it may seem, visual acuity testing is an extremely important (and often long) part of the rehabilitative examination. Evaluating a patient with reduced visual acuity requires that basic examination techniques be modified. It is generally recommended that vision testing be done at 2 m (10 ft equivalent) with a self-illuminated, portable eye chart. The Early Treatment Diabetic Retinopathy Study (ETDRS) chart is the most widely used. A projector chart is the least favorable means of measuring acuity in a patient with reduced vision. Not only is contrast not constant with a projector chart depending on the level of room illumination, but a patient would also have to be moved closer to the chart if vision was worse than 20/400. Moving a visually impaired patient only reinforces awareness of the vision loss and causes stress and negative feelings during the exam.

The ETDRS chart has several advantages. It is self-illuminated with high contrast and is on wheels, allowing it to be moved closer than 2 m if necessary. Also, the chart has a wide spectrum of visual acuity values, ranging from a "Snellen 200 ft" equivalent to a 10 ft equivalent. Since the testing distance is always recorded as the numerator of the Snellen fraction, this chart gives an acuity range from 10/200 (20/400) to 10/10 (20/20). If the chart is moved closer, the test distance is again recorded as the numerator. It is best not to convert the acuity to the 20 ft equivalent when recording vision so that the examiner may always know the test distance for subsequent evaluations. "Counting fingers" vision for measurement is generally not used during a low vision evaluation. The fingers subtend approximately the same visual angle as a 200 ft Snellen figure. Therefore, a patient should be able to read the top line of the ETDRS chart at a closer distance. Recording visual acuity as "3/200" instead of counting fingers at 3 ft is much more accurate, which is important in determining those optical devices that may be appropriate.

Determination of eccentric view, if suspected, can be done or confirmed during initial acuity testing. The easiest method is called the clock-face method. Patients are asked to keep their head still and to face straight ahead. The examiner then asks the patient to imagine that the eye chart is at the center of a clock. Patients are asked to move their eye in various positions of the clock until the top line becomes the clearest and most complete. Typically, but not always, a patient with acquired macular disease will attempt to place the image on the temporal retina where there is the most retina available, that is, the right eye will eccentrically view toward the right (3 o'clock) and the left eye will view toward the left (9 o'clock). This position should be demonstrated to the patient several times and recorded next to visual acuity. The knowledge of the exact location of the eccentric view will become useful for the remainder of the evaluation with devices. Further discussion of scotoma location is present later in this chapter.

Manifest refraction in a trial frame is generally the rule. In this case, the examiner can observe the patient's eyes, particularly to reinforce the eccentric view. A phoropter does not allow a patient's eyes to be observed and the use of an eccentric view by the patient becomes quite difficult. In addition, the lens increments may be too small for a patient to determine any subjective difference, that is, a patient with 20/200 vision will not appreciate a difference of ± 0.25 D. The examiner cannot easily make large increments of change in the phoropter for patients with poorer vision. Generally, a patient whose vision is less than 20/100 will appreciate 0.50 D lens changes. For vision between 20/100 and 20/200, the examiner should use 0.75 to 1.50 D changes. If a patient's vision is 20/200 to 20/400, 1.50 to 2.00 D lens increments should be used. This technique is called lens bracketing and is the most time efficient and effective. Likewise, when measuring astigmatic corrections, a higher powered Jackson Cross Cylinder (0.75–2.00 D) is employed to ensure that the patient appreciates the lens changes for power and axis refinements. To ensure that large refractive errors are not missed, keratometry, retinoscopy, and/or autorefraction offer a starting point. A scrupulous refraction is crucial before low vision devices are demonstrated. Spectacles should always be prescribed using polycarbonate lenses even if there seems to be a minimal increase in visual acuity; they serve as a important source of protection, particularly when the patient is engaged in activities where there may be hanging branches, flying objects, chemicals, or any other obstacle in their paths, or simply unfamiliar terrain.

Depending on the patient's expression of initial goals, either a brief or extensive telescopic evaluation is performed next. Improvement of distance vision may have not initially been an expressed goal since a patient may be mostly focused upon reading concerns. In any event, a brief introduction of a 3× or 4× powered telescope in the trial frame will demonstrate not only the device to the patient but also the possibility of enhancing distance vision. Vision should generally improve proportionately with the power of the scope. For example, if a patient has best-corrected vision of 20/200, vision should improve to 20/50 with a 4× telescope. Exceptions to this rule may be a large or irregular central scotoma or the coexistence of other media opacities. Generally speaking, most distance activities usually require a visual acuity of 20/30 to 20/50. It is rare that an individual would need to be corrected to 20/20 or better with a telescope. The aim should be to prescribe the lowest-powered telescope to achieve the required vision. The reason for this dynamic is that as a telescope's power becomes greater, the field of view becomes smaller and it becomes more difficult to use effectively. If visual acuity is nearly equal between the two eyes, the examiner may choose to prescribe a binocular system which will give a much larger field of view for activities such as watching television, going to shows, etc. Another alternative for increased visual field may be a contact lens telescope (CLT). In this case, a contact lens (high minus power) is used as the ocular in conjunction with a high plus lens as the objective in a spectacle (1). As vision approaches 20/400 and worse, standard telescopic devices may not be useful; a CLT as well as more advanced technological electronic devices should be considered.

The driving issue is one that remains controversial and requires special mention. Driving is an important component of everyday life for most patients. The inability to drive has psychological implications in terms of limited independence. The subject must be treated with extreme care and sensitivity. Driving remains an instrumental activity of daily living and should be routinely addressed during the case history and discussion of goals and expectations. Individuals with age-related macular degeneration do drive although their driving exposure is low by tending to avoid challenging and hazardous situations such as driving at night and in inclement weather (2).

Visually impaired people are permitted to use bioptic telescopes for driving in more than 40 states when visual acuity falls below the state's legal limit. The term bioptic simply implies two (bi-) optical centers. This form of a telescope is mounted several millimeters above the distance optical center (Fig. 30.2). Therefore, a patient looks through his/her natural prescription through the carrier lens housing the telescope. When a sharper acuity is needed for viewing street signs, etc., the patient lowers the chin and spots through the scope. This manner of use is similar to the fashion in which a driver would use the rearview mirror; the telescope is used only approximately 10–15% of the time while driving. This point is an extremely important one and often confused because it is thought that since there is a reduced field through the telescope, one could not possibly drive safely. Again, the driver is primarily looking

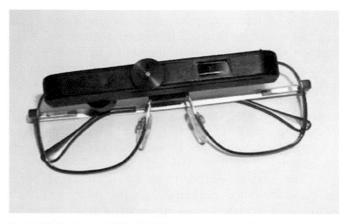

Figure 30.2 Ocutech VES-K™ bioptic telescope. *Source*: Photo courtesy of Henry Greene, OD and Ocutech.

through the carrier lens, not the telescopic device. Bioptic telescopes do meet the self-reported driving needs of the majority of visually impaired drivers and have been found to be a useful device for resolving details such as road signs, etc. (3).

Although visual acuity is a fundamental part of safe driving, several studies have demonstrated that peripheral field (or vision) appears to play a more critical role in driving than visual acuity (4–6). All states allowing bioptic telescopes have a minimum visual field requirement without the telescope (usually between 120° and 140°). Other requirements include maximum acuity without the telescope (usually 20/200) and minimum visual acuity with the telescope (20/40–20/60). Certainly, there are issues that go beyond visual acuity and peripheral field in determining whether any given driver will drive safely, particularly one with a visual impairment. Factors such as age, experience, visual attention and processing, reaction times, and cognitive deficits, all inarguably affect an individual's ability to drive safely and led to the development of a software called the Useful Field of View test (Visual Awareness, Inc., Birmingham, Alabama, USA). This test requires higher-order processing skills, and not only does it determine a conventional visual field, but also allows for the assessment of the visual field area over which rapid stimuli are flashed, that is, a car or other object moved into a cluttered background. Simulating the "real" driving experience with this test, an association has been shown between elderly drivers who have reductions in their useful field of view and crash involvement (7–9). This test is invariably more important in determining driving safety than traditional assessments of visual acuity and peripheral field. Other forms of simulated driving should be done when there are questions of safety.

Most drivers with visual impairment do limit driving exposure and tend to avoid challenging driving situations, that is, driving at night, on interstates, during inclement weather, etc. There has been no association found between drivers with macular degeneration and increased accident rates/fatalities; however, driving exposure is taken into account (10). One study has demonstrated that, although patients with macular degeneration performed more poorly on driver simulator and on-the-road tests compared with a control group, this did not translate into an increased risk of real-world accidents (11). Hence, it still remains unclear whether reduced exposure decreases a driver's risk or whether any association exists between increased injurious accidents and visual impairment secondary to macular degeneration. The decision to prescribe a telescopic device for a patient to legally maintain a driver's license is a joint decision best left to doctors, patient, and family; the decision should be made on an individual basis.

The next procedure to be done, following refraction and distance evaluation, is the near evaluation. Near visual acuity is most appropriately measured and evaluated with continuous-text reading cards. These cards will test a patient's functional ability to read versus the ability to read a line of numbers or letters. The Minnesota Read (MNRead™) and Sloan make continuous-text reading cards. "M" notation is generally used for recording near acuity. This notation uses the metric system, is standardized, and does not require a fixed testing distance. To begin the near evaluation, a reading lens addition should always be in place when testing patients above 50 years of age and test distance must be appropriate for the power of the add. For example, the test distance for a +2.50 D add should be 40 cm or 16 in. (100/2.50 = 40 cm; 40/2.50 = 16 in.), and the test distance for a +4.00 D add should be 25 cm or 10 in. (100/4.00 = 25; 40/4.00 = 10 in). Distance and near visual acuities (with standard +2.50 D add) should be approximately the same so that if a patient's best-corrected vision is 20/200 in the distance, the near vision with standard add should also be 20/200. Pupil size, asymmetry, significant media opacities, and large central scotomas may create disparities; however, large differences between distance and near acuities should alert the examiner to an inaccurate manifest refraction.

Once initial near acuity has been determined, the examiner increases the power of the add until the appropriate acuity is obtained. The approximate add it will take for any given patient to read newspaper size print (1 M or 20/50) can be predicted by calculating the reciprocal of the distance or near acuity. For example, if a patient's vision is 20/200, it will take at least a +10.00 D add (200/20 = 10) for the patient to read newspaper size print. This value may be modified depending upon the patient's initial expression of goals for reading. If a patient wishes to read the stock pages, then more plus may be needed, and if a patient only wishes to read large-print text, then less plus is needed.

Binocular adds are typically prescribed when the acuity is equal or near equal between the two eyes. Base-in prism is always required in binocular adds greater than +6.00 D because fusional vergence is exhausted and the eyes drift toward an exophoric posture. The amount of prescribed prism is two prism diopters more than the amount of plus. For example, if the examiner wishes to prescribe a +8.00 D add for both eyes (OU), the prescribed prism should be 10 prism diopters base-in total, split equally between the two eyes. Glasses should be prescribed in a half-eye frame size due to the thickness and heaviness of the lenses. Since the nasal edge of the standard lens becomes quite thick with increased prism, adds greater than +12.00 D should be prescribed monocularly with the eye not being used either occluded or the lens frosted to avoid diplopia. Recent advances using diffractive optics have greatly reduced the unsightly appearance of these half-eyes (Fig. 30.3). If a patient has one eye that is considerably better, the high add is prescribed monocularly. However, there may still be a "ghost" image or halo around letters or words coming from the poorer eye. In this instance, the lens of the poorer eye can be frosted (or occluded).

For higher adds, most patients continually need reinforcement regarding the appropriate and close working distance. Most people are able to conceptualize

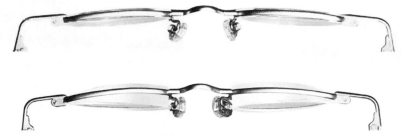

Figure 30.3 NOVES™ prismatic half-eyes (*top*) compared with that of standard thickness (*bottom*). *Source*: Photo courtesy of Eschenbach.

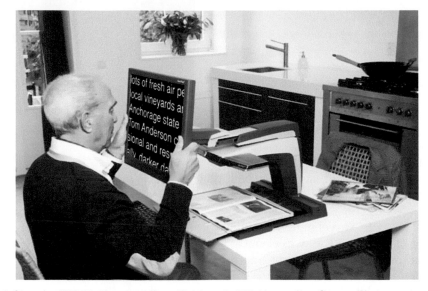

Figure 30.4 Clearview™ 517 video magnifier with integrated tiltable monitor. *Source*: Photo courtesy of Optelec.

inches rather than centimeters (see conversions on previous page). The patient should begin with larger text initially to become adjusted to the closer than usual reading distance and probably increased fatigue. If a patient has not yet accepted his/her visual loss, success with high adds and close reading distances is virtually impossible.

For those patients rejecting the close reading distance of high adds, other alternatives exist. Telemicroscopes (surgical loupes/telephoto lens) can be made with a specified reading distance. However, the patient must weigh the benefit of the increased distance versus the reduction in the field of view experienced. Although every attempt is made to prescribe a spectacle-borne reading device, electronic devices such as video magnifiers (CCTVs) are good alternatives to spectacles (Fig. 30.4). A patient can sit back at a comfortable distance and magnify the print large enough to read easily. A video magnifier has not traditionally been a portable device and can cost several thousand dollars, but clearly can have a tremendous impact in allowing a patient to read (or work) again. There have been major recent advances here as well in portable versions of the reading machines (Figs. 30.5, 30.6) allowing the devices to be carried to and from home, school, or work. Handheld or stand magnifiers can also increase the working distances and are typically prescribed in conjunction with spectacles. These devices are more useful for spot reading

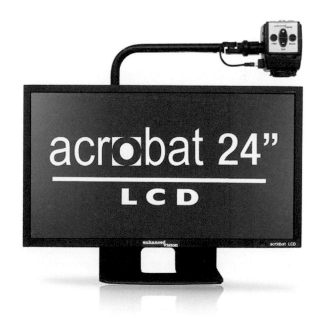

Figure 30.5 The Acrobat™. *Source*: Photo courtesy of Enhanced Vision.

rather than extended reading. However, for those patients rejecting spectacles, these devices are quite effective although the reading field of view is reduced.

Contrast enhancement and glare reduction provide the final steps to the low vision evaluation. Patients

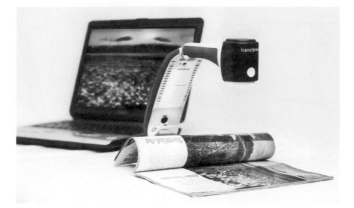

Figure 30.6 The Transformer™. *Source*: Photo courtesy of Enhanced Vision.

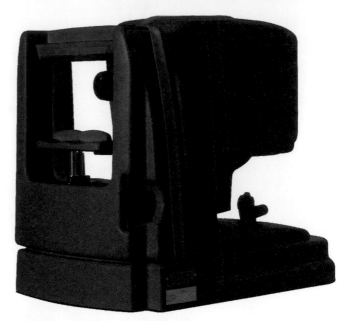

Figure 30.7 Nidek MP-1™ Microperimeter. *Source*: Photo courtesy of Nidek Incorporated.

with macular degeneration often experience a loss of contrast. Contrast enhancement lenses shield the eyes from very short wavelengths of light. These shorter wavelengths consist of high-energy visible blue light and can cause loss of contrast as well as glare, which reduces the eye's overall function. The Corning® GlareControl™ family of lenses consists of seven filters which selectively block specific wavelengths of blue light while transmitting light at other wavelengths. There are six graduated filter levels, each numbered to block below the corresponding wavelength (CPF® 450, 511, 527, 527×, 550, and 550× D). The filters range in color from yellow 450 to deep red 550. The seventh filter is called the GlareCutter™ lens and is for patients with initial to moderate light sensitivity. The lens color is more cosmetically appealing because it has more of a brownish hue rather than orange/red. All of the filters are photochromatic easing the transition between different light levels. These lenses are incredibly helpful to patients with macular degeneration. In addition to providing benefits of protection from ultraviolet (UV) light, they also provide contrast enhancement as well as glare reduction. Although the full range of filters are suitable for many ocular pathologies, usually the CPF 511 and 527 lenses work best in patients with moderate to advanced macular degeneration. Since the lenses are glass (and not high-impact polycarbonate plastic), they are best prescribed in the clip-on variety. These filters are now available in plastic also, yet are still photochromatic (Chadwick Optical, Inc., White River Junction, Vermont, USA) providing a nice alternative for prescription sun wear.

Visual Field Testing/Scotoma Plotting

There are many ways to obtain the location of the scotoma and to determine the preferred retinal locus (PRL). The scanning laser ophthalmoscope (SLO) macular perimetry (the gold standard) and the Nidek Microperimeter (Fig. 30.7) allow for the characterization of central field defects, that is, macular scotomata (12,13). The presence or absence of macular scotomata and their characteristics are extremely important indicators of reading success and speed with low vision devices as well as performance with activities of daily living (14). The confocal SLO has graphic capabilities which allow a retinal map of the scotomata to be drawn by determining the retinal location of visual stimuli directly on the retina. Thus, the patient can see the stimuli and the investigator can view the stimuli on the retina. From these capabilities, a preferred retinal locus (PRL) can be identified and both relative and dense scotomata can be mapped (15).

Patients with macular scotomata do not often perceive black spots. Rather they say that letters or words are missing in their central vision while reading or they simply have difficulties in functioning. The presence of these scotomata can decrease many areas of visual performance although the specific relationships between macular scotoma characteristics and visual performance have not been identified (16). Therefore, it becomes useful to be able to map out the scotomata and to know the exact location of preferred retinal loci in order to begin the rehabilitative process. Traditional approaches attempt to determine a direction of the eccentric view and then to basically repeat this direction to the patient during training, etc. Many times this technique is effective, but often patients do not respond as well as predicted to the devices, training, visual performance task, and/or during activities of daily living. The SLO can essentially determine the characteristics of the scotomata and their relationship to the PRL. Once the PRL is identified, the rehabilitative team can instruct and train the patient on better use of the PRL. Nilsson et al. (17) have also shown that using the eccentric view demonstrated in the SLO, patients with macular degeneration and large absolute central scotomata can be successfully trained and reading speeds increased by them using a new and more favorable retinal locus.

Studies with the SLO have shown that there are different shapes and patterns of scotomata from a round scotoma centered on a nonfunctioning fovea to a ring scotoma surrounding a functioning fovea to highly complex amoeboid shapes (14). While the majority of patients do have dense scotomata, it was found that if the scotomata are complex and surround the PRL by more than two of its borders, these patients have the most difficulties in performing visual tasks when compared with those with less encumbered PRL (14). This knowledge will aid in the prediction of patient success.

Visual Rehabilitation Considerations

Low vision rehabilitation is a necessary adjunct to the low vision evaluation and optical treatment for low vision. Visual rehabilitation specialists include a wide variety of professions: occupational therapists, certified low vision therapists, visual rehabilitation therapists, and teachers of students with visual impairments to name a few. They will evaluate patients regarding their abilities to perform their simple activities of daily living (ADLs) or their more complex instrumental activities of daily living (IADLs) necessary for independent living. ADLs consist of basic self-care of the body such as feeding and grooming and IADLs include more complex activities both in the community and home required for independent living, such as cooking, writing, and reading (18). Any low vision patient experiencing difficulties in the performance of ADLs or IADLs is a candidate for visual rehabilitation.

Low vision ADL and IADL assessments are done to determine the patient's reason for seeking intervention and to define what functional performance areas are being impacted by the visual impairment. A rehabilitation specialist can obtain this information through an interview process with the patient or perform a standardized assessment such as the Canadian Occupational Performance Measure (19). The information gleaned from the assessment used will assist the rehabilitation specialist and the patient to establish reasonable and attainable functional goals.

The rehabilitation specialists will train the patient in the maximal use of his/her remaining vision to facilitate the attainment of the patient's goals. This entails visual field defect awareness, training in the use of the PRL, and scanning training. When a maximal use of vision is achieved, the optical aids prescribed by the low vision practitioner and any adaptive techniques requiring vision are incorporated into the training and are better utilized by the patient. It is important to have information about visual field and scotoma location to begin the training. If the visual field information is not obtained through the low vision evaluation, then the therapist can perform his/her own non-diagnostic testing. The Amsler Grid chart, the California Central Visual Field Test, and the clock face are examples of nondiagnostic tests that provide the therapist with information regarding the patient's visual field and the scotoma location (20). Once the scotoma is located, the therapist can train the patient in scotoma awareness and the determination of the PRL location.

A reading evaluation is an essential aspect of the low vision evaluation to assess the patient's performance in functional communication but can also be a very useful tool in verifying the location of the scotoma (18). There are many standardized reading assessments: the MNRead, the Visual Skills for Reading Test and the Smith–Kettlewell Read Test to name a few (20). These tests offer varying font sizes and will assess the reading speed and accuracy. The MNRead is in a sentence format thereby it has a contextual component; the patient can sometimes figure out the next word or their errors intellectually based on the sentence content. The Visual Skills for Reading Test and the Smith–Kettlewell Read Test are noncontextual. None of the above tests assess reading comprehension. The Morgan Low Vision Reading Comprehension Test will assess the patient's grade reading level but does not assess reading speed and should be used in conjunction with other assessments (20). If the therapist is unable to access standardized tests then other methods can be employed to provide the information. For example, the therapist can have the patient read aloud, time the patient for one minute, and then count the number of words read to attain a reading speed. A therapist can often determine the patient's scotoma location by the errors given while the patient is reading. A patient who misses the endings of words has a scotoma more to the right or a patient who has difficulties returning to the start of the next line has a scotoma more toward the left. The object of therapy is to get patients to become aware of their scotoma location and efficiently use their PRL to diminish their reading errors, increase their reading speed, and improve their comprehension.

An assessment of the patient's environment is also critical. An understanding of the lighting, contrast, pattern, and the organization of the patient's ADL and IADL working areas and pathways is necessary for patient safety and efficiency of performance. This can initially be performed via the interview process to determine the patient's perceived areas of difficulty. A visit to the patient's home will complete the home assessment and allow the rehabilitation specialist to make recommendations based on the actual findings and performance observance.

The use of a PRL is not only for reading but it is carried over into any ADL for which the patient will be using vision. The therapist and the patient must determine whether vision will be used for an ADL or if a modification or adaptive equipment requiring another sense will be utilized. There are many modifications that use other senses. An example of a home modification that is frequently employed utilizing touch is the marking of appliance dials. Any type of marking that leaves a palpable mark is appropriate, from Velcro to raised fabric paint. A talking watch is an example of an auditory piece of adaptive equipment. Simplicity in the modification or the adaptive equipment makes utilization easier for most patients. For example, an oven dial that is marked every 50° will make it more difficult for the patient to discern which marking is 350°. Mark only the

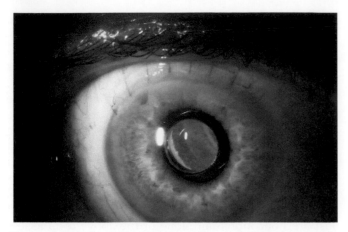

Figure 30.8 Implantable Miniature Telescope (IMT)™ Telescope prosthesis for end-stage age-related macular degeneration, 6-weeks post implantation. *Source*: Photo courtesy of VisionCare Inc./James Gilman, CRA.

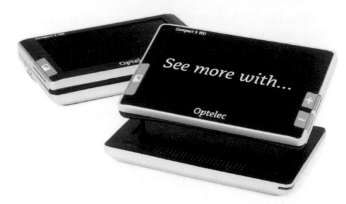

Figure 30.9 The Compact HD™. *Source*: Photo courtesy of Optelec.

temperatures the patient uses. Training of the patient with the modification or the adaptive equipment, including magnification is a must. There are many other non-optical large print adaptive devices which might be considered such as books, check registers, clocks, watches, playing cards, etc.

IMPROVEMENTS
New Technologies

1. The Implantable Miniature Telescope (by Dr Isaac Lipshitz) is a new technology that received FDA approval in July 2010. It is a visual prosthetic used to treat end-stage macular degeneration that is implanted into the lens capsule after cataract extraction (Fig. 30.8). The patient must have stable end-stage macular degeneration with a visual acuity of 10/160–20/800 in both eyes and be phakic. The prosthetic provides the patient with 3x hands-free magnification. Results from a multicenter clinical trial showed at least a 2 line improvement in visual acuity and an improvement in quality of life (21).

2. Many electronic video magnifiers (formerly called CCTVs) use flat panel LCD screens and folding armature that facilitate increased portability. Many offer diverse camera options such as near, distance, a true mirror image, multiple color options for enhanced contrast, and up to 82x magnification with differing screen sizes. Examples of such electronic magnifiers are Enhanced Vision, Inc's (Huntington Beach, California, USA) Acrobat LCD and Transformer (Figs. 30.5, 30.6) as well as Freedom Scientific's (St Petersburg, Florida, USA) Onyx Deskset XL video-magnifying systems. Many of these devices can be adapted for attachment to computers and can use a split screen view to allow reading and computer work simultaneously.

3. Improvements in technology have made portable electronic magnifiers more affordable and diverse than ever before. They are lightweight sometimes

offering more options in distance viewing. Optelec (Vista, California, USA) has a new Compact 5 HD electronic magnifier with a 5 in. HD screen that offers up to 18x magnification, can view objects up to a distance of 4 ft away, and is still small enough for a purse (Fig. 30.9).

SUMMARY POINTS

- Patient success with low vision devices is dependent upon a number of factors including age, physical and mental status, level and stability of visual acuity, patient's dependency on others, and the interval since visual loss.
- Resistance to low vision devices and thus limited success tend to be seen in those patients who have not yet accepted or mourned their visual loss. Generally speaking, the more profound the visual loss, the more difficult finding a means of enhancing vision becomes.
- Non-optical devices may be the only mechanism acceptable by the patient to regain a small degree of independence.
- The role of vocational rehabilitation, occupational therapy and orientation/mobility training for activities of daily living etc. should always be considered for patients with advanced macular degeneration.
- Support groups may also provide comfort and new friendships in helping to cope with the visual impairment.
- Sometimes it is best to wait for a low vision consultation and allow the patient to seek this care voluntarily after it has been suggested.
- Success with visual rehabilitation is always based on identification and satisfaction of the visual requirements and goals of the patient.
- There are exciting new applications and devices emerging in the field of low vision/visual rehabilitation. Much of the novelty utilizes the latest technology and will no doubt be of great benefit to many visually impaired patients suffering from macular degeneration.

COMPANY WEB SITES OF LOW VISION PRODUCTS FOR FURTHER INFORMATION

- Enhanced Vision Systems: www.enhancedvision.com
- Optelec: www.optelec.com
- Ocutech, Inc.: www.ocutech.com
- Designs for Vision: www.designsforvision.com
- Corning Medical Optics: www.corning.com
- Vision Technology, Inc.: www.visiontechnology.com
- Chadwick Optical: www.chadwickoptical.com
- Eschenbach: www.eschenbach.com
- Freedom Scientific: www.freedomscientific.com

REFERENCES

1. Lavinsky J, Tomasetto G, Soares E. Use of a contact lens telescopic system in low vision patients. Int J Rehabil Res 2001; 24: 337–40.
2. DeCarlo DK, Scilley K, Wells J, et al. Driving habits and health-related quality of life in patients with age-related maculopathy. Optom Vis Sci 2003; 80: 207–13.
3. Bowers AR, Apfelbaum DH, Peli E. Bioptic telescopes meet the needs of drivers with moderate visual acuity loss. Invest Ophthalmol Vis Sci 2005; 46: 66–74.
4. Kelleher DK. Driving with low vision. J Vis Impair Blind 1968; 11: 345–50.
5. Lovsund P, Hedin A. Effect on driving performance of visual field defect. In: Gale A, Freeman MH, Haslegrave CM, et al. eds. Vision in Vehicles. Amsterdam: Elsevier, 1989: 323–9.
6. Wood JM, Dique T, Troutbeck R. The effect of artificial visual impairment on functional visual fields and driving performance. Clin Vis Sci 1993; 8: 563–75.
7. Owsley C, Ball K, Sloane ME, et al. Visual/cognitive correlates of vehicle accidents in older drivers. Psychol Aging 1991; 6: 403–15.
8. Owsley C, McGwin G Jr, Ball K. Vision impairment, eye disease, and injurious motor vehicle crashes in the elderly. Ophthalmic Epidemiol 1998; 5: 101–13.
9. Owsley C, Ball K, McGwin G Jr, et al. Visual processing impairment and risk of motor vehicle crash among older adults. JAMA 1998; 279: 1083–8.
10. McCloskey LW, Koepsell TD, Wolf ME, Buchner DM. Motor vehicle collision injuries and sensory impairments of older drivers. Age Aging 1994; 23: 267–72.
11. Szlyk JP, Pizzimenti CE, Fishman GA, et al. A comparison of driving in older subjects with an without age-related macular degeneration. Arch Ophthalmol 1995; 113: 1033–40.
12. Chen FK, Patel PJ, Webster AR, et al. Nidek MP-1 is able to detect subtle decline in function in inherited and age-related macular disease with stable visual acuity. Retina 2011; 31: 371–9.
13. Chen FK, Patel PJ, Xing W, et al. Teste-rest variability of microperimetry using the Nidek MP-1 in patients with macular disease. Invest Ophthalmol Vis Sci 2009; 50: 364–71.
14. Fletcher DC, Schuchard RA, Livingston CL, et al. Scanning laser ophthalmoscope macular perimetry and applications for low vision rehabilitation clinicians. Ophthalmol Clin North Am 1994; 7: 257–65.
15. Schuchard RA, Fletcher DC, Maino J. A scanning laser ophthalmoscope (SLO) low-vision rehabilitation system. Clin Eye Vis Care 1994; 6: 101–7.
16. Fletcher DC, Schuchard RA. Preferred retinal loci relationship to macular scotomas in a low-vision population. Ophthalmology 1997; 104: 632–8.
17. Nilsson UL, Frennesson C, Nilsson SEG. Patients with AMD and a large absolute central scotoma can be trained successfully to use eccentric viewing, as demonstrated in a scanning laser opthalmoscope. Vis Res 2003; 43: 1777–87.
18. American Occupational Therapy Association. Occupational therapy practice framework: domain and process. 2nd edn. Am J Occup Ther 2008; 62: 625–83.
19. Gilbert MP, Baker SS. Evaluation and intervention for basic and instrumental activities of daily living. In: Warren M, Barstow EA, eds. Occupational Therapy Intervention for Adults with Low Vision. Bethesda, MD: AOTA Press, 2011: 227–67.
20. Barstow EA, Crossland MD. Intervention and rehabilitation for reading and writing. In: Warren M, Barstow EA, eds. Occupational Therapy Intervention for Adults with Low Vision. Bethesda, MD: AOTA Press, 2011: 105–51.
21. Bansal AS, Baker P, Haller JA. An implantable visual prosthetic for end-stage macular degeneration. Expert Rev Ophthalmol 2011; 6: 142–5.

31

Visual prosthesis for age-related macular degeneration: A challenging and important application

Bruno Diniz, James D. Weiland, and Mark S. Humayun

INTRODUCTION

The World Health Organization estimates that 5% of the global burden of blindness is caused by age-related macular degeneration (AMD) (1). AMD is estimated to affect more than 8 million people in the United States; and as the population over the age of 85 increases, the prevalence of AMD is expected to increase accordingly (2,3). Although treatment for geographic atrophy (GA) remains of limited or no benefit, there have been considerable improvements in the management of neovascular AMD to limit further visual loss. However no known treatment has been shown to restore useful vision once photoreceptors have been damaged severely, as in end-stage AMD. An emerging modality of treatment has been visual restoration through the use of visual prostheses (4).

The idea of electrically stimulating the nervous system to restore vision was first reported by Foerster in 1929 when he noted that stimulating the visual cortex of a human brain caused his subject to "see" small spots of light. Subsequently, Brindley implanted an 80-electrode device chronically onto the visual cortex of a blind patient and confirmed both the potential of electrical stimulation to restore vision and some of the barriers to implementation of a suitable device (5,6).

Technological advances, coupled with scientific investigations, have transformed the focus of the field; previous investigators asked whether it was possible to create visual perceptions through electrical stimulation; later researchers asked how those perceptions can be optimized for maximum benefit. Current questions being considered are related to the quality of images created by stimulation of many small areas of neuronal tissue and to the mechanical and electrical biocompatibility of microelectronic implants.

These implants are currently under evaluation for use in patients with either light perception or no light perception vision caused by outer retina degeneration (7). The challenge for these prostheses is even greater in patients with AMD, whose central visual acuity is often reduced only to the 20/400 level while their peripheral vision is spared. The prosthesis must be capable of improving this vision to justify the risk of implantation.

Whether useful vision can be rendered via artificial visual prostheses depends upon establishing a definition of useful vision based on the minimum number of pixels required for human beings to accomplish activities of daily living. A number of studies have tested humans with normal visual function by pixelating their vision via a portable simulator. These studies indicated that 625 electrodes implanted in a 1 cm² area near the foveal representation in the visual cortex could produce an image corresponding to a visual acuity of approximately 20/30 (8,9). Other studies showed that, theoretically, some reading ability could be restored with a 60-electrode retinal prosthesis. Subjects with a simulated prosthesis were able to read slowly, at an average speed of 20–35 words/ min, compared with an average adult's reading speed of 250 words/min (10). Daily activities, such as face recognition, have also been simulated. Subjects could correctly identify a face 50% of the time, even with a relatively low-resolution array (16 x 16), with 30% of the simulated pixels turned off. When the array density was increased to 25 x 25, recognition scores increased to 92%, again with 30% of the pixels turned off (11).

THE VISUAL SYSTEM IN AMD

In an emmetropic eye, the light stimulus that enters the eye is focused by the cornea and lens on the photoreceptors of the retina. Electrical signals from these photoreceptors are processed by the retinal neurons and sent via the optic nerve to the lateral geniculate nucleus (12); from there, 20–30% of the fibers connect to the superior colliculus, and the remaining fibers synapse in the visual cortex (13).

In AMD, morphometric analysis has shown a pronounced decrease in the number of macular photoreceptors remaining, with less than 20% preservation of rods and cones (14). Changes in individual cell structure and a significant rewiring process also occur (15). Despite the considerable loss of outer retinal cells and retinal remodeling, the inner retina retains enough structure to be a viable substrate for a visual prosthesis (16). Results to date have shown that electrical stimulation of localized areas of the retina elicits visual perceptions that spatially correspond to the stimulated region (4). However, in order for retinal prostheses to provide useful vision in AMD, not only does the resolution have to be improved but the prosthetic vision has to also work in tandem with the normal peripheral vision.

TYPES OF VISUAL PROSTHESIS

The term visual prosthesis refers to any device capable of eliciting visual percepts in an individual through electrical stimulation of any part of the visual system. Such electrically elicited percepts have been termed phosphenes.

Visual prostheses can use either a nonretinal or a retinal approach. Retinal approaches are aimed at eye pathologies in which at least part of the intraocular visual pathway remains intact, as in AMD. A nonretinal approach is warranted when the optic nerve is nearly completely damaged and/or the eye itself is disfigured or degenerated.

Recent advances in miniaturized electronic components have enabled the microfabrication of extremely dense integrated circuits that match the small sizes required for implantation in the human body. However, these devices must be packaged in such a way that they can last for decades in the body without corrosion or infection. Moreover, these devices must have an adequate and reliable power supply.

Nonretinal Approaches
Cortical Prosthesis

Cortical stimulation is still the only hope of providing vision to patients with pathologies such as glaucoma, optic nerve atrophy, or damage to the lateral geniculate.

One current model of an intracortical prosthesis is the Utah Electrode Array. This device consists of multiple silicon spikes arranged in a square grid (17). At the tip of each spike is a platinum electrode. Studies of the Utah Electrode Array in primates demonstrated that microstimulation of the primary visual cortex via a high-density array of penetrating microelectrodes is capable of evoking visual perceptions. The cortical visual prosthesis has an advantage over other approaches in that it bypasses all diseased visual pathway neurons rostral to the primary visual cortex. But the device has a number of limitations, such as induced cortical histological changes and surgical complications; increased risk to the patient from brain surgery; and loss of retinal, geniculate, and collicular visual processing.

Optic Nerve Prosthesis

Some investigators have targeted the optic nerve as a potential site for the implementation of a visual prosthesis (18,19). Veraart and colleagues attempted this method, employing the concept of a spiral nerve cuff electrode (20). Two patients who were implanted with an optic nerve prosthesis were able to detect light and perform simple visually guided tasks (21). Essentially, the electrode cuff is surgically implanted circumferentially on the external surface of the optic nerve. By controlling the stimulation parameters, the investigators were able to vary the position of the phosphenes and thus convey information about the surrounding environment.

The optic nerve is an appealing site for implementation of a visual prosthesis as the entire visual field is represented in a small area. This area can be reached surgically and presents a viable anatomic location for an implant; however, several hurdles must be overcome before initializing this approach. One important obstacle is the location of the macular nerve fibers, which lie most centrally within the optic nerve, surrounded by the more peripheral fibers.

Since the cuff electrode will necessarily stimulate both the central macular fibers and the overlying peripheral fibers, use of this approach, especially for AMD, will be dramatically limited (22).

Retinal Approaches (Fig. 31.1)
Epiretinal Prostheses
Approved Clinical Device

The epiretinal implants studied to date consist of implanted and external components. The external system uses a camera to capture an image, a wearable computer to process the image, and a wireless transmitter to send both data and power to the implant. The implant's electronics receive data and power wirelessly and produce a stimulus output based on the received data. Its protective packaging enables it to function electronically in a wet environment; and a grid of microelectrodes on the epiretinal surface (nerve fiber layer) applies the stimulus directly to the retina. The designs for these implants are eventually intended to yield a fully intraocular device; but thus far some of the components are extraocular. In the future, with the exponential increase of the power processing and miniaturization of the microelectronic components, creation of a fully intraocular prosthesis may be possible.

Humayun et al. pioneered the development of an intraocular retinal prosthesis and its implantation in patients (23,24). Early studies involved the temporary placement of a stimulating array in the eye in an operating room setting. During short periods of electrical

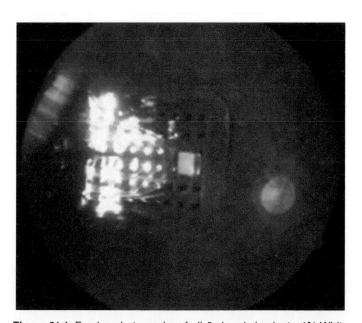

Figure 31.1 Fundus photographs of all 6 chronic implants. (**A**) White arrow showing Artificial Silicon Retina (Optobionics). *Source*: Photograph courtesy of Dr John Pollack. (**B**) Argus I (Second Sight Medical Products, Inc.). *Source*: Photograph courtesy of Second Sight Medical Products, Inc.). (**C**) Active Subretinal Device (Retina Implant, GmbH). *Source*: Photograph courtesy of Prof. Eberhart Zrenner. (**D**) Epi-Ret 25 electrode device. *Source*: Photograph courtesy of Prof. Peter Walter. (**E**) Forty-nine electrode epiretinal device (Intelligent Medical Implants). *Source*: Photograph courtesy of Prof. Gisbert Richard. (**F**) Argus II (Second Sight Medical Products, Inc.). *Source*: Photograph courtesy of Second Sight Medical Products, Inc. *Source*: From Ref. 4.

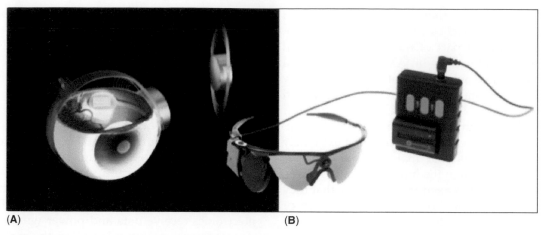

(A)   (B)

Figure 31.2 A schematic representation of the Argus II implant in the eye. (**A**) A 60-electrode array on the surface of the retina. (**B**) The external components (glasses with camera and video processing unit). *Source*: Photograph courtesy of Second Sight Medical Products, Inc.

stimulation, patients were able to identify crude forms such as letters or a box shape. The position of the percept reported by the patient was consistent with the location of the stimulus probe on the retina. Further, the patients reported no persistence of the image pursuant to stimulation (24).

Based on these encouraging results, a trial began in 2002 at the Doheny Eye Institute, Los Angeles, as part of a Food and Drug Administration investigational device exemption study. Six patients have received implants, each including a 16-electrode Argus I device (Second Sight Medical Products, Inc., Sylmar, California, USA). During the follow-up period, objective (electrically evoked responses recorded from the visual cortex) and subjective evidence of visual perceptions using psychophysical tests have been obtained. Patients reported visual percepts in locations consistent with the implanted electrodes, the ability to discriminate between percepts created by different electrodes based on the locations of the percepts, the ability to discern brighter or dimmer percepts with varying levels of current, and the ability to distinguish the direction of motion of objects (25).

These preliminary patient tests were most encouraging because they provided further evidence of the plasticity/learning curve of the visual pathway and demonstrated that epiretinal stimulation can be conducted in a retinotopic manner. The Argus I study was primarily a limited safety study, but two subjects implanted in 2004 remain active in the clinical trial at the time of writing of this manuscript (8 years later).

The Argus II improved on the Argus I by moving all of the implanted electronics into the orbit, increasing the number of electrodes, and increasing the visual field covered by the stimulating array. It consists of a 60-channel, surgically implanted, stimulating microelectrode array, an inductive coil link used to transmit power and data to the internal portion of the implant, an external video processing unit, and a miniature camera mounted on a pair of glasses (Fig. 31.2). The video processing unit digitizes the signal in real-time, applies a series of image processing filters, downsamples the image to a 6 x 10 pixilated grid, and creates a series of stimulus pulses based on pixel gray scale values and look-up tables

customized for each subject. The stimulus pulses are delivered to the microelectrode array via the inductive coil link and the application-specific circuitry.

The Second Sight Argus II Clinical Trial is a prospective, single-arm, nonrandomized trial with three years of follow-up per subject (www.clinicaltrials.gov, NCT00407602). Only individuals with severe-to-profound outer retinal degeneration (e.g., retinitis pigmentosa (RP), choroideremia, and Leber's congenital amaurosis) were enrolled at 10 clinical centers. This trial has the longest follow-up data (up to five years) with 30 patients implanted to date (7), As of this writing, this is the only retinal implant to receive a CE Mark in Europe in 2011, making it the first commercially available retinal implant in the world. The Argus II is currently being evaluated by the Food and Drug Administration for approval in the United States.

The implanted electronic components of this epiretinal prosthesis are sutured to the episclera under the rectus muscles. A ribbon cable enters the eye via a pars plana incision and is tacked to the retinal surface. The median implant surgery time was four hours and four minutes (range, 1 hour 53 minutes to 8 hours 32 minutes) for the clinical trial patients. During the implantation procedure, 67% of the subjects had their natural lens removed, leaving them aphakic. The width of the sclerotomy where the cable was inserted averaged 5.0 ± 0.5 mm. Most subjects had an allograft (either Tutoplast Sclera® or Tutoplast Pericardium®) placed over the extraocular portion of the device (under the conjunctiva) at the end of the surgery.

There were 17 serious adverse events. The vast majority of these occurred within the first six months after implantation. Conjunctival erosion and dehiscence over the extraocular implant, when combined, were the most common occurrences and were treated in all but one subject with additional sutures, placement of additional tissue (conjunctiva or sclera), or both. Culture-negative presumed endophthalmitis occurred and resolved in three subjects. None of the cases of endophthalmitis were associated with observed, pre-existing, conjunctival erosion or hypotony. All cases were treated with intravitreal vancomycin and ceftazidime, topical, and systemic antibiotics Three subjects experienced hypotony requiring surgical intervention. Two cases of retinal detachment requiring surgical intervention occurred during the five to six months after implantation. The first of these had a rhegmatogenous detachment associated with choroidal effusion; this is one of the three subjects described with hypotony above. At approximately five months after surgery, a second subject incurred blunt trauma to the implanted eye, resulting in a retinal detachment that was repaired successfully. Two subjects required the array to be retacked to the retina shortly after the implant surgery.

Of the electrodes that were enabled at the time of implantation, 94.4% remained enabled and functional throughout the study. All subjects (100%) were able to perceive light when their systems were stimulated (thresholds were measurable on at least one electrode). An average of 55.5% of all enabled electrodes across subjects had measurable thresholds of less than a charge density of $1.0 \ mC/cm^2$.

Subjects performed statistically better with the system *on* versus *off* in the following tasks: object localization (96% of subjects), motion discrimination (57%), and discrimination of oriented gratings (23%). Object localization tests used a target consisting of a 7-cm white square on a black LCD screen at a 30-cm distance. Both motion detection and object orientation were evaluated using a target of a white bar moving across a black LCD screen. Subjects' mean performance on orientation and mobility tasks was also significantly better when the system was on.

In terms of visual acuity, seven subjects have been able to score reliably on the scale (with visual acuity between 2.9 and 1.6 logMAR) with the system on. The best result to date is 1.8 logMAR (Snellen equivalent, 20/1262). The tests were performed without magnification or zoom, and none of the subjects has been able to reliably score on the visual acuity scale in either eye with the system off (7). However, recent testing with 8x zoom, has shown that the best visual acuity obtained can be as good as 20/200. There was a substantial increase in visual acuity from the Argus I (16-electrode implant) to the Argus II (60-electrode implant). The best performing Argus I subject had a visual acuity of 20/4000 (26).

This epiretinal prosthesis system was reliable over the long term (45.6 subject-years to date in this study) and provided benefit to implanted subjects during this period. On an average, prosthesis subjects have improved visual acuity from light perception to at least hand movements, with some improving to at least counting fingers (27). These visual acuity data combined with the safety and performance results to date demonstrate the ability of this retinal implant to provide meaningful visual perception and usefulness to subjects who have become blind as a result of end-stage outer retinal degenerations.

Investigational Devices

The remaining retinal prostheses discussed in this chapter are investigational in nature, with varying degrees of follow-up. Epi-Ret® (EpiRet, Gießen, Germany) is a 25-electrode epiretinal device and the data were recently presented on its clinical trial (28). This implant is designed to fit entirely inside the eye yet has a provision for external power via an inductive wireless link. Six legally blind patients with RP were included in the study, and all subjects reported visual percepts when stimulated by the implant. Activation of the implant to record visual sensations was performed during three sessions around postoperative days 7, 14, and 27, and the implant was removed at day 28 (28). Although the idea of a totally intraocular implant is one that all groups have imagined, engineering challenges abound. Provision of a protective barrier to prevent corrosion of the electronics becomes more difficult at higher densities, as does power delivery to the device. Because of these technical limitations, such a device is not realizable as of the writing of this chapter.

A third epiretinal implant is a 49-electrode epiretinal device from Intelligent Medical Implants (Intelligent Retinal Implant System, IMI, Bonn, Germany). The electronics of this implant is located in the same location as the Argus II implant (29). This device is currently under clinical investigation in a multicenter trial. The main findings of the trial until now are low thresholds to elicit visual perceptions, including form vision, and that the implant is reasonably well tolerated by the eye. To our knowledge, no camera was used in the functional testing and the device was activated only in the clinic. Most implants were removed after a few months (30).

General Advantages and Disadvantages of the Epiretinal Prosthesis

The epiretinal implant design has some advantages. First, the implant's contact with the aqueous humor in the posterior pole after the pars plana vitrectomy used for placement allows optimal heat dissipation, resulting in less thermal damage to the tissue and the possibility of using higher currents.

A second advantage is that the implantable part of the device can be small if all the microprocessing and image capture are placed outside the eye. In addition, all the wearable components can be easily upgraded along with upgrades in software. The epiretinal approach also leads to less tissue damage than the subretinal approach, since it doesn't disturb the normal contact between the retina and the retinal pigment epithelium/Bruch's membrane complex and choroid. Thus it is less likely to induce an inflammatory reaction or proliferative vitreoretinopathy.

However some disadvantages are also present, such as the challenge of fixating such a device to the inner surface of the retina without causing damage to the underlying tissue. Also, some groups have reported that epiretinal stimulation can result in unwanted stimulation of retinal ganglion cell (RGC) axons resulting in suboptimal, larger, and ill-defined percepts (31,32). One possible approach to overcoming RGC axonal stimulation would be through the use of different stimulation pulses. Past experiments by Greenberg (33) and later by Jensen (34) and Freeman (35) have found that although the stimulating electrodes are physically in closer proximity to the RGC axons and RGC bodies, varying the pulse width of the stimulating current to which the electrodes can be "tuned" selectively stimulates the retinal bipolar cells rather than RGCs. The RGCs responded to shorter pulse durations, while deeper retinal neural layers responded to longer pulse durations.

Subretinal Prosthesis: An Experimental Medical Device

The subretinal prosthesis is intended to replace the degenerated outer retinal layers, capturing the light stimuli and electrically stimulating the ganglion cell layer and bipolar cells. As of this writing, all types of subretinal prosthesis remain investigational, with follow-up in patients limited to less than one year.

Optobionics, Inc. implanted the artificial silicon retina (ASR, Glen Ellyn, IL) microchip in 10 patients in a single-center study and then in 20 subjects in a multi-center study. The implants, which are 3 mm in diameter with 3500 electrodes, deliver current to the retina when light is incident on the implant. The group reported in 2004 (36) that all six of their implanted patients had subjective improvements in vision. Three of six had improved ETDRS scores, while one in six had an enlarged visual field postoperatively. However, the improved vision included areas of the visual field far from the implant location. The authors concluded that the subretinal ASR implant was not directly mediating artificial vision (i.e., electrical stimulation of retinal neurons triggering visual perception); rather its effect in the subretinal space was through an "indirect effect," possibly through release of growth factors that improved the health of the retina (37).

The implantation can be done through a pars plana vitrectomy and retinotomy (*ab interno*) or through a transscleral approach (*ab externo*). This kind of array architecture is very appealing because the camera is in the eye; but considerable technological challenges need to be overcome. The first is the capability of the microphotodiodes alone to supply enough energy for retinal stimulation. The solar cells used today do not have the capacity to generate the amount of electrical energy required to stimulate the inner retinal layers; so the subretinal prosthesis now in clinical trials still relies on an extraocular power source.

Based on the inability of the passive ASR chip to directly elicit light perceptions through electrical stimulation with ambient light, other groups developing a subretinal device have abandoned the idea of using microphotodiodes alone. Instead, these researchers include electronics for powering a subretinal "controlled/active" implant.

Zrenner et al. developed a subretinal prosthesis consisting of a microphotodiode array powered by either a laser or telemetry for the replacement of degenerated photoreceptors in outer retinopathies (38–40). The initial Retina Implant (Reutlingen, Germany) AG Clinical Trial was a prospective, open-label, functional, placebo-controlled (i.e., system "on" *vs.* "off") acute trial approved for 14 subjects. The study duration was 126 days, including implantation and explantation of the device (41). Of all subjects who received the implant, data from only the last three subjects were reported in detail (two men, age range 38–44 years). Patients 1 and 2 were blind as a result of RP and patient 3 from choroideremia. Patients underwent psychophysical testing about one week after the device was implanted. The maximum visual acuity of the best subject was 20/1000 (logMAR = 1.69) (38).

This latest rendition of a subretinal prosthesis overcomes the issue of being underpowered by including a power source behind the ear with cables running into the eye to the subretinal chip. It continues to have the advantage of being in close proximity to the remaining bipolar cells and thus, theoretically, there is no need to mechanically fixate the implant in the eye wall. The disadvantages include the limited space for the chip in the subretinal space and the increased likelihood of thermal injury to the neural tissue. Also, with the lack of energy the actual microphotodiodes have to create a visual percept that the extraocular components are a necessity. There are surgical implantation problems, such as the likelihood of a massive choroidal hemorrhage or a retinal detachment and retinal incarceration, because of the transscleral and transchoroidal insertion.

Transchoroidal Prosthesis: An Experimental Medical Device

As with the subretinal prostheses, transchoroidal prostheses are an investigational device. Investigators from Japan have recently collaborated on a relatively new approach to artificial vision that they term suprachoroidal transretinal stimulation. They have hypothesized that placing a stimulating electrode in the suprachoroidal space or in the fenestrated sclera along with a ground electrode in the vitreous cavity, may allow for a less-invasive method to achieve functional percepts.

In 2011, Fujikado et al. reported their results with a semichronic, suprachoroidal implantation in two patients with RP (42). The visual acuity of their patients before implantation was light perception. The 49-electrode array (5.7 × 4.6 X 0, 5 mm) was placed in the suprachoroidal space without causing retinal detachment or vitreous hemorrhage, and the internal devices of the implant were placed under the skin on the temporal side of the head. The implants remained functional during the four weeks of the study. The implants were surgically removed after five weeks in their first patient and after seven weeks in their second patient.

Phosphenes were elicited by currents delivered through six electrodes in patient 1 and through four electrodes in patient 2. The success of discriminating two bars was better than that of chance alone in both patients. In patient 2, the success of a grasping task was better than the chance level, and the success rate of identifying a white bar on a touch panel increased with repeated testing (42). An Australian group is also investigating the feasibility of a suprachoroidal placement of the electrode array (43).

The advantages to such an approach are several: the surgery is less complicated; the electrodes are less invasive to the retina and more stably positioned; and the electrodes are relatively easy to remove or replace if damaged (44).

However, a significant shortcoming of this approach is the fact that the electrodes are further from the target neurons, thus requiring higher currents. In turn, these result in a greater current spread which limits resolution (44). Animal studies have already shown the ability to evoke cortical potentials using suprachoroidal stimulation of the outer nuclear layer, outer plexiform layer, and inner nuclear layer (45–50). What is required is to improve the resolution provided by such an approach.

CONCLUSION

Once the photoreceptors are lost, there is currently no known cure for either neovascular or non-neovascular AMD. With ongoing advances in the technology of array production, surgical techniques, and our increasing understanding of the visual nervous system's response to chronic stimulation, there has been significant advancement toward the possibility of restoring some vision to patients suffering from end-stage AMD.

Although significant advances have been made, the field of artificial vision is still relatively young. The complex nature of eye diseases requires sophisticated systems developed over time to achieve optimal treatment results. This is true for refractive surgery, retinal surgery, and cataract surgery. Visual prostheses are following a similar pathway; to achieve their full potential, we must allow time, not only for clinical and biological testing, but also for engineering and technical advances.

The visual prostheses, especially the retinal ones, have achieved significant developments in recent years. We see continued improvement in visual acuity with increasing numbers and densities of electrodes. Even though the resulting visual acuity is still poor relative to normal vision, these subjects can read letters using their implants. Perhaps more importantly, blind patients can use these devices for mobility and orientation.

Thus, some of the expectations surrounding artificial vision have begun to be fulfilled. The challenge is how to continue to improve the resolution such that not only those who are completely blind but also patients who are legally blind (20/200) can benefit through the use of retinal prostheses in their activities of daily living. This is especially true for patients with AMD as well as the fact that the retinal prostheses have to work in tandem with normal peripheral vision. The development of retinal prostheses to generate artificial vision for the blind is indeed a complex, long-term, expensive, and interdisciplinary undertaking. However, the payoff from developing such technology is also undoubtedly tremendous from both an economic and a humanitarian standpoint.

SUMMARY POINTS

- An emerging modality of treatment has been visual restoration through the use of visual prostheses.

- Despite the considerable loss of outer retinal cells and retinal remodeling in AMD, the inner retina retains enough structure to be a viable substrate for a visual prosthesis.
- Visual prostheses can use either a nonretinal or a retinal approach. Retinal approaches are aimed at eye pathologies in which at least part of the intraocular visual pathway remains intact, as in AMD.
- Nonretinal approaches (cortical and optic nerve) have shown limitations in the ability to precisely stimulate certain areas and translate the retinotopic distribution of visual perception.
- The Argus II epiretinal prosthesis (approved clinical device) subjects have improved visual acuity from light perception to at least hand movements, with some improving to at least counting fingers.
- Experimental retinal approaches include epiretinal (Epi-Ret), subretinal (Artificial silicone retina and Retina Implant AG), and transchoroidal prosthesis.

REFERENCES

1. Vision2020: right to sight. blindness and visual impairment: global facts. [Available from: http://www.vision2020.org/main.cfm?type=FACTS] (Accessed February 6, 2012).
2. Bressler NM, Bressler SB, Congdon NG, et al. Potential public health impact of age-related eye disease study results: AREDS report no. 11. Arch Ophthalmol 2003; 121: 1621–4.
3. Age-Related Eye Disease Study Research Group. A randomized, placebo-controlled, clinical trial of high-dose supplementation with vitamins C and E, beta carotene, and zinc for age-related macular degeneration and vision loss: AREDS report no. 8. Arch Ophthalmol 2001; 119: 1417–36.
4. Weiland JD, Choa AK, Humayun MS. Retinal prostheses: current clinical results and future needs. Ophthalmology 2011; 118: 2227–37.
5. Foerster O. Beitrage zur Pathophysiologie der Sehbahn und der Sehsphare. J Psychol Neurol Lpz 1929; 39: 463–85.
6. Brindley GS, Lewin WS. The sensations produced by electrical stimulation of the visual cortex. J Physiol 1968; 196: 479–93.
7. Humayun MS, Dorn JD, da Cruz L, et al. Interim results from the international trial of second sight's visual prosthesis. Ophthalmology 2012; 119: 779–88.
8. Cha K, Horch K, Normann RA. Simulation of a phosphene-based visual field: visual acuity in a pixelized vision system. Ann Biomed Eng 1992; 20: 439–49.
9. Cha K, Horch KW, Normann RA, et al. Reading speed with a pixelized vision system. J Opt Soc Am A 1992; 9: 673–7.
10. Fornos AP, Sommerhalder J, Pelizzone M. Reading with a simulated 60-channel implant. Front Neurosci 2011; 5: 57.
11. Thompson RW, Barnett GD, Humayun MS, et al. Facial recognition using simulated prosthetic pixelized vision. Invest Ophthalmol Vis Sci 2003; 44: 5035–42.
12. Fernandes RA, Diniz B, Ribeiro R, et al. Artificial vision through neuronal stimulation. Neurosci Lett 2012; 519: 122–8.

13. Levine MD. Vision in Man and Machine. New York: McGraw-Hill Publishing Company, 1985: 322–6.

14. Medeiros NE, Curcio CA. Preservation of ganglion cell layer neurons in age-related macular degeneration. Invest Ophthalmol Vis Sci 2001; 42: 795–803.

15. Marc RE Jones BW, Watt CB, et al. Neural remodeling in retinal degeneration. Prog Retin Eye Res 2003; 22: 607–55.

16. Kim SY, Sadda S, Pearlman J, et al. Morphometric analysis of the macula in eyes with disciform age-related macular degeneration. Retina 2002; 22: 471–7.

17. Maynard EM, Nordhausen CT, Normann RA. The utah intracortical electrode array: a recording structure for potential brain-computer interfaces. Electroencephalogr Clin Neurophysiol 1997; 102: 228–39.

18. Shandurina AN. Restoration of visual and auditory function using electrostimulation. Russian Fiziol Cheloveka 1995; 21: 25–9.

19. Shandurina AN, Panin AV, Sologubova EK, et al. Results of the use of therapeutic periorbital electrostimulation in neurological patients with partial atrophy of the optic nerves. Neurosci Behav Physiol 1996; 26: 137–42.

20. Veraart C, Raftopoulos C, Mortimer JT, et al. Visual sensations produced by optic nerve stimulation using an implanted self-sizing spiral cuff electrode. Brain Res 1998; 813: 181–6.

21. Brelén ME, Vince V, Gérard B, et al. Measurement of evoked potentials after electrical stimulation of the human optic nerve. Invest Ophthalmol Vis Sci 2010; 51: 5351–5.

22. Branner A, Normann RA. A multielectrode array for intrafascicular recording and stimulation in sciatic nerve of cats. Brain Res Bull 2000; 51: 293–306.

23. Humayun MS, de Juan E Jr, Dagnelie G, et al. Visual perception elicited by electrical stimulation of retina in blind humans. Arch Ophthalmol 1996; 114: 40–6.

24. Humayun MS, de Juan E Jr, Weiland JD, et al. Pattern electrical stimulation of the human retina. Vision Res 1999; 39: 2569–76.

25. Humayun MS, Weiland JD, Fujii GY, et al. Visual perception in a blind subject with a chronic microelectronic retinal prosthesis. Vision Res 2003; 43: 2573–81.

26. Caspi A, Dorn JD, McClure KH, et al. Feasibility study of a retinal prosthesis: spatial vision with a 16-electrode implant. Arch Ophthalmol 2009; 127: 398–401.

27. Bach M, Wilke M, Wilhelm B, et al. Basic quantitative assessment of visual performance in patients with very low vision. Invest Ophthalmol Vis Sci 2010; 51: 1255–60.

28. Klauke S, Goertz M, Rein S, et al. Stimulation with a wireless intraocular epiretinal implant elicits visual percepts in blind humans. Invest Ophthalmol Vis Sci 2011; 52: 449–55.

29. Keseru M, Feucht M, Bornfeld N, et al. Acute electrical stimulation of the human retina with an epiretinal electrode array. Acta Ophthalmol 2012; 90: e1–8.

30. Richard G. Long-term stability of stimulation thresholds obtained from a human patient with a prototype of an epiretinal retina prosthesis. Invest Ophthalmol Vis Sci 2009; 15: E-Abstract 4580.

31. Greenberg RJ, Velte TJ, Humayun MS, et al. A computational model of electrical stimulation of the retinal ganglion cell. IEEE Trans Biomed Eng 1999; 46: 505–14.

32. Lakhanpal R, Yanai D, Weiland JD, et al. Advances in the development of visual prostheses. Curr Opin Ophthalmol 2003; 14: 122–7.

33. Greenberg R. Analysis of electrical stimulation of the vertebrate retina- work towards a retinal prosthesis [dissertation]. Baltimore: The Johns Hopkins University, 1998.

34. Jensen RJ, Rizzo JF 3rd. Activation of ganglion cells in wild-type and rd1 mouse retinas with monophasic and biphasic current pulses. J Neural Eng 2009; 6: 035004.

35. Freeman DK, Eddington DK, Rizzo JF 3rd, et al. Selective activation of neuronal targets with sinusoidal electric stimulation. J Neurophysiol 2010; 104: 2778–91.

36. Chow AY, Chow VY, Packo KH, et al. The artificial silicon retina microchip for the treatment of vision loss from retinitis pigmentosa. Arch Ophthalmol 2004; 122: 460–9.

37. Ciavatta VT, Kim M, Wong P, et al. Retinal expression of Fgf2 in RCS rats with subretinal microphotodiode array. Invest Ophthalmol Vis Sci 2009; 50: 4523–30.

38. Zrenner E, Miliczek KD, Gabel VP, et al. The development of subretinal microphotodiodes for replacement of degenerated photoreceptors. Ophthalmic Res 1997; 29: 269–80.

39. Zrenner E, Bartz-Schmidt KU, Benav H, et al. Subretinal electronic chips allow blind patients to read letters and combine them to words. Proc Biol Sci 2011; 278: 1489–97.

40. Besch D, Sachs H, Szurman P, et al. Extraocular surgery for implantation of an active subretinal visual prosthesis with external connections: feasibility and outcome in seven patients. Br J Ophthalmol 2008; 92: 1361–8.

41. Zrenner E. Details on the technology of the subretinal implant, clinical study design, results and spontaneous reports of patients including nine movie clips on performance. Electron Suppl Mater Proc Biol Sci 2011; 278: 1489.

42. Fujikado T, Kamei M, Sakaguchi H, et al. Testing of semichronically implanted retinal prosthesis by suprachoroidal-transretinal stimulation in patients with retinitis pigmentosa. Invest Ophthalmol Vis Sci 2011; 52: 4726–33.

43. Shivdasani MN, Luu CD, Cicione R, et al. Evaluation of stimulus parameters and electrode geometry for an effective suprachoroidal retinal prosthesis. J Neural Eng 2010; 7: 036008.

44. Morimoto T, Miyoshi T, Fujikado T, et al. Electrical stimulation enhances the survival of axotomized retinal ganglion cells in vivo. Neuroreport 2002; 13: 227–30.

45. Nakauchi K, Fujikado T, Kanda H, et al. Transretinal electrical stimulation by an intrascleral multichannel electrode array in rabbit eyes. Graefes Arch Clin Exp Ophthalmol 2005; 243: 169–74.

46. Kanda H, Morimoto T, Fujikado T, et al. Electrophysiological studies of the feasibility of suprachoroidal-transretinal stimulation for artificial vision in normal and RCS rats. Invest Ophthalmol Vis Sci 2004; 45: 560–6.

47. Nakauchi K, Fujikado T, Kanda H, et al. Threshold suprachoroidal–transretinal stimulation current resulting in retinal damage in rabbits. J Neural Eng 2007; 4: S50–7.

48. Wong YT, Chen SC, Kerdraon YA, et al. Efficacy of suprachoroidal, bipolar, electrical stimulation in a vision prosthesis. Conf Proc IEEE Eng Med Biol Soc 2008; 2008: 1789–92.

49. Wong YT, Chen SC, Seo JM, et al. Focal activation of the feline retina via a suprachoroidal electrode array. Vis Res 2009; 49: 825–33.

50. Sakaguchi H, Fujikado T, Fang X. Transretinal electrical stimulation with a suprachoroidal multichannel electrode in rabbit eyes. Jpn J Ophthalmol 2004; 48: 256–61.

32

Clinical research trials

A. Frances Walonker, Kenneth R. Diddie, and Marcia Niec

INTRODUCTION
Historical Review

Age-related macular degeneration (AMD) is an important public health problem. Of the estimated 34.8 million people in the United States who were 65 years of age or older in 2002, approximately 1.6 million had some form of visual impairment. Approximately 600,000 of these will have experienced a rapid, devastating loss of vision due to choroidal neovascularization (CNV), "wet AMD," whereas the remaining 1.0 million may experience a slow, progressive retinal atrophy and possibly a severe visual handicap "dry AMD" (1). Most may have difficulty performing routine visual tasks, such as driving, reading printed material, or recognizing the faces of their friends.

As the U.S. population continues to age, more and more persons will become visually impaired from AMD; more, in fact, than from any other eye disease. The Eye Disease Prevalence Research Group predicted that the number of persons with AMD will increase by 50% by 2020 (2). In AMD with CNV, some of the worst losses of vision can occur. Because a large number of individuals have AMD complicated by CNV, effective treatment of even a fraction of all cases can lead to significant savings to society and can decrease the number of people requiring Social Security and other disability payments (not to mention the effects on patients' dignity and independence), with savings far outweighing the costs of clinical research, management, and treatment.

Treatments studied have included laser photocoagulation, photodynamic therapy, submacular surgery, radiation, medications such as interferon, thalidomide, corticosteroids, and anti-vascular endothelial growth factor drugs, as well as various oral supplements that are believed to be preventive. Because of randomized clinical trials, two drugs, ranibizumab (Lucentis®) and aflibercept (Eylea®) have been approved by the Food and Drug Administration (FDA) for the treatment of wet AMD. The Comparison of AMD Treatments Trial (CATT) study showed that Lucentis and bevacizumab (Avastin®) are quite comparable in their effect on AMD with CNV. At the present time a number of randomized clinical research trials are looking at therapies for macular degeneration. Basic scientists are working hand in hand with clinicians to find a cure for this blinding disease.

Clinical Relevance

Prior to the Macular Photocoagulation Study (MPS), there was no proven treatment for AMD with CNV. The use of low vision aids and mobility training were recommended but little could be done other than observe the natural history of AMD with CNV. The MPS, a randomized, multicenter trial, showed that laser photocoagulation of AMD with CNV prevented the most severe types of vision loss, compared with no treatment. The study was also important as a natural history study of macular degeneration (3). Since the 1980s, this randomized controlled clinical trial has served as a benchmark for AMD research, with other treatments evaluated in the same way.

CLINICAL RESEARCH METHODOLOGY

The path a new idea takes from the patient's problem to the basic research laboratory to the clinical research center and ultimately back to the treatment of the patient in the clinical setting is extensive and expensive. The final research question can be answered and practice guidelines established, but the cost in terms of time, commitment, and dollars is very high.

The pathway from the patient and back again to the patient starts when the ophthalmologist sees a patient with a disease that either has no cure or will benefit from an improved treatment. Case-series studies, in which an investigator has noted some interesting or intriguing observation, frequently lead to the generation of a hypothesis that will subsequently be investigated. The ophthalmologist then teams up with the basic scientist to address the hypothesis. Together, they design appropriate laboratory experiments to address the hypothesis. Results from these basic science studies lead to preliminary clinical investigations of a possible new diagnostic technique, a treatment, a drug, or even a drug delivery device. A small group of carefully selected patients participate in a pilot study to study the safety of these new treatments. In addition, for drug therapies, the dose levels that may be most effective are also studied. If successful, such a pilot study generates a single-center clinical trial to further evaluate the tolerability, safety, and efficacy of the treatments.

Subsequently a full-scale, multicenter, randomized clinical research trial is initiated to recruit enough patients to test the safety and the efficacy of the new procedure, operation, test, drug or device. These new approaches are also tested for their effects on the quality of life of patients with the initial disease. The order of the research steps is outlined in Table 32.1.

The randomized clinical research trial is the gold standard, or reference, in medicine, as it provides the

Table 32.1 Development Phases of a Clinical Trial

Phase I	Actions of drugs etc. in humans: determining safety and side effects of dose levels; early evidence of efficacy: may include normal subjects as well as patients; all subjects receive study product; 5–15 patients (pilot study); can be multi- or single center
Phase II	Evaluate efficacy/tolerability of drug etc. for a particular indication in patients with the disease under consideration looking at side effects and short-term risks; all study subjects get study product; can be multicenter or single center
Phase III	Expanded trials after preliminary evidence suggests efficacy; additional evidence of overall risk/benefit; may be randomized against standard of care for this disease, observation or a placebo; results submitted for approval pre-marketing
Phase IV	Post marketing to delineate additional information about the risks and benefits and the optimal use of the product

greatest justification for concluding causality and is subject to the least number of problems or biases. Clinical trials are the best type of study to use when the objective is to establish efficacy of a treatment or a procedure. Clinical trials in which patients are randomly assigned to different treatment arms are the strongest design of all.

These innovative approaches to clinical practice are then presented and taught to other ophthalmologists through continuing medical education courses, publications in peer review journals, and presentations at national and international scientific meetings. Finally, the new techniques, medications, or test materials are available to all patients under standard practice guidelines for diagnosis and treatment for disease.

Design of a Clinical Research Trial

The initial step in determining whether a research proposal will fulfill all the ethical and investigational guidelines necessary to protect human subjects involved in a clinical research trial, is to go through a formal decision making process. After all the data from previous observational, basic laboratory (in vitro and animal studies), case report studies, phase I and phase II studies have been analyzed, a protocol is created under which the trial will be conducted. This protocol is developed outlining every detail of the research study so that all personnel—investigator, coordinator, photographer, vision specialist—every participant in the study, is aware of the protocol detail and is able to follow this protocol for the length of the trial, maintaining standardization of evaluation, testing, surgery, and all other procedures. The steps that are involved in the development of a clinical trial are as follows.

The Rationale

The ophthalmologist will team up with a basic science researcher or will work in his/her own laboratory to design a series of experiments that may address a specific disease entity for which there may be no adequate treatment. The results of these experiments, done again and again and replicated in other laboratories, may suggest an intervention or therapy that would be tested on some laboratory animal under the strict guidelines of a research laboratory. The results serve as the basis for a limited trial on a small group of carefully selected patients. If these patients react well to the therapy or tolerate the therapy with minimal side effects, clinical research proceeds to the next phase: a single or two- to three-center clinical study of the therapy in patients with a specific disease.

This is the initial stage of the clinical research trial. All the data from prior studies are then analyzed along with any new information, and the rationale for conducting this particular study is outlined. Then, one enumerates the objectives of the study, the safety signals and efficacy endpoints of the treatment, the design of the experimental plan, the number of enrolled subjects required to prove the hypothesis and most importantly, whether the research study will benefit the population at large.

THE PROTOCOL
The protocol for the study will include the following:

Background

- The background of the disease to be studied and the results of all previous related research, both basic science and clinical.
- All information to support the justification of this research project and the impact it will have on the population in general and the population with this specific disease entity.
- The expected benefits to be obtained from the study.
- All the information about the study product, be it drug, device, surgery, or the delivery system, with all the risks and adverse events noted during the prior uses of the product.

Objectives

- The primary objectives of the study, for example, could be to halt the progression of the disease.
- The secondary objectives could be to improve visual acuity by greater than 3 lines of vision on the Early Treatment of Diabetic Retinopathy Study (ETDRS) chart

Study Design

- Description of the study includes:
- Type of study: randomized/open label/multi-dose

- Rationale answers why: Why that treatment? Why that dose? Why that duration?
- Outcome measures: primary measures, safety and tolerability; secondary measures, for example, the change in visual acuity/leakage
- Safety plan: unmasking/laboratory values/detailed adverse event evaluations

- Compliance: good clinical practice/FDA guidelines/IRB guidelines.

Material and Methods

- Subject selection criteria with the inclusion and exclusion criteria with justification for both
- Justification for or against inclusion/exclusion of vulnerable subjects
- Treatment assignment: randomized/stratified
- Study treatment details: formulation/dose/storage
- Excluded therapies
- Study assessments: visual acuity/photography/quality of life instruments/early exit criteria
- Discontinuation: subject/study
- Statistical methods: sample size/safety analysis/efficacy analysis
- Data quality assurance: Data and Safety Monitoring Committee (DMC) to periodically review the data for important patient safety issues/monitoring of the data

Safety Assessment

- Adverse event reporting. Serious adverse events that require hospital/surgical intervention or result in death are immediately reported to the IRB and the sponsor
- All adverse events are followed until resolution or stability
- All subjects are contacted after study completion if adverse events have occurred
- Medical condition confounders are identified
- Laboratory assessments are reviewed

The Informed Consent

Before any research trial that includes human subjects can be instituted, an Institutional Review Board (IRB) must approve all the components of the trial. The responsibility of an IRB is to establish the requirements and procedures for requests for the performance of human research, development, demonstration, or other activities involving patients or patient products, in addition to the usual scope of established and accepted methods. The IRB monitors approved research in accordance with the requirements of the Office of Human Research Protection (OHRP) from research risks, the regulations of the FDA, National Institutes of Health and the Department of Health and Human Services. The IRB uses a group process to review research protocols and related material, for example, informed consent documents and investigator brochures, to ensure the following:

- Risks to human subjects are minimized by using procedures that are consistent with sound research design and that do not unnecessarily expose subjects to risk. Whenever appropriate, such procedures already will have been performed on subjects for diagnostic or therapeutic purposes.
- Risks to subjects are reasonable in relation to the anticipated benefits (if any) to the subjects and the importance of the knowledge that may be expected from the result.
- The selection of the subjects is equitable, that is, the study subjects are of both genders and from different racial/ethnic groups, and no age limitations exist other than those associated with a disease entity. This will decrease the risk of bias in patient selection.
- Informed consent will be sought from each prospective subject or the subject's legally authorized representative and will be documented in accordance with and to the extent required by informed consent regulations. Provisions to prevent the suggestion of coercion are documented.
- Where appropriate, the research plan makes adequate provision for monitoring the data collected to ensure the safety of subjects either by using a Data Safety Monitoring Board that looks at the data to note any untoward adverse events or even unexpected improvement which may determine that the study should end.
- Adequate provisions are in place to protect the privacy of the subjects and to maintain confidentiality of the data.
- Appropriate additional safeguards have been included in the study to protect the rights and the welfare of subjects who are members of a vulnerable group (e.g., children, prisoners etc.).

The IRB has the authority to disapprove, modify, or approve studies based on consideration of human subject protection aspects. It also has the authority to suspend or terminate a study, to place restrictions on a study, and to require progress reports and oversee the conduct of the study and the study investigators.

The informed consent should be signed by the patient before entering into a clinical research trial. The informed consent will include the length of patient's participation, the alternatives to this treatment modality, the risks involved in this trial, and a statement allowing the patients to withdraw from the trial at any time without consequence.

Data Collection

It is imperative that the collection of the research data, based on the design of the study, is accurate and complete. All research trials have case report forms on which data are recorded. These forms do not contain any patient identifying information other than a unique identifying code number and/or a combination of the patient's initials. These forms are sent to the sponsor and, therefore, can only contain this unique identifying information. The types of data collected include the following:

- Results of laboratory testing
- Quality-of-life questionnaires
- Clinical evaluations
- Eligibility criteria
- Medications, medical history, and surgical history
- Detailed ophthalmic history including prior treatment details of the disease entity

- Adverse events, both serious and non-serious
- The study product
- Investigator signatures

All data have to be checked and corrected before they are sent to the sponsor and this is done by the representatives of the sponsor. These monitors' responsibilities include: ensuring the data are correct and legible; verifying the patients have met the enrolment criteria and received the correct treatment to which they were assigned. The clinical chart where the investigator notes the clinical examinations is known as the source document. The data on the case report forms are matched to the source documents. This crosscheck of data verifies accuracy.

All data and investigational study products are stored in a secured area with access to the area only by the study staff, investigator, and coordinator.

The principal investigator of the clinical research study is responsible for the conduct of the study, the accuracy of the data collection and the conduct of the study staff and the safety of the study subjects at all times.

Settings for Research Trials

Advancing medical knowledge—through screening, treatment, surgical, and pharmaceutical intervention—has prolonged the life of many people with disabling chronic disease conditions and increased the number of survivors of traumatic injury. It is estimated that the number of people over 65 years of age will grow to 23% of the population by 2040 (4). Caring for these people, including those with visual disorders, is costly. Health expenditures in the United States neared $2.6 trillion in 2010, over 10 times the amount spent in 1980 (5), and can be expected to continue to increase in the future.

With such huge expenditures anticipated for health care, and in response to continued pressure by government regulatory agencies to drive down costs, evaluation of cost in conducting research is suggested. Researchers must include cost research objectives, such as costs associated with screening programs, alternative treatments and procedures, and use of new technology and implementation of new regulatory measures associated with programs and trials. The results obtained from various including cost analysis in research help health care decision makers weigh the costs and consequences of competing treatment alternatives. Cost information provides additional data that can supplement clinical judgment when making therapeutic choices. Therefore, clinicians and researchers at major academic institutions need to focus on advancing the care and prevention of eye disease. Efforts should be based on rigorous clinical methods, i.e., randomized controlled clinical trials and analysis of economic and humanistic outcomes. With research of this nature, the results can be applied directly to the patient, where they will accomplish the greatest good. This is especially true when these outcomes may mean the difference between sight and blindness, and when they impact on the outcome measures of quality of life and ultimately, life expectancy.

Limitations of Randomized Clinical Trials

The cost of developing the necessary infrastructure to support the scientific and clinical activities involved in conducting major national and international clinical research makes it prohibitive except for large academic ophthalmology centers unless under the sponsorship of industry. There are obvious downsides to this type of sponsorship that is somewhat obviated by the inclusion in the project of an independent clinical research organization.

Most major academic ophthalmology centers involved in clinical and basic science research are referral centers for patients with complicated disease who have not responded to standard therapy or who have a disease with no known cure. However, because of the nature of this population, that is, those with severe disease as well as those with rare and complicated disease, the numbers of patients who would be eligible to enter a clinical research trial would be limited, making recruitment difficult. This places a potential for selection bias on these clinical research studies, such that when the studies are completed, they may not translate to the population in general.

On the other hand, a more common disease entity, such as macular degeneration, with its potential for marked vision loss if untreated, offers access to more subjects for inclusion in a clinical trial. These patients are seen routinely in the private practice ophthalmologists' offices, which are now actively involved in clinical research. The disadvantage to academic institutions that have invested in the development of an infrastructure to rigorously support all basic and clinical research is that, frequently, their access to large numbers of this patient population is limited. The disadvantage to the patient may be that the strict protocol that is the hallmark of academic institutional research, both in university settings and in the private practice settings that have developed clinical research expertise, may not be adhered to so rigorously in a community where that infrastructure is not present.

Another limitation is access to the underserved; those people who have no access to healthcare providers, either because of lack of insurance or distance from those same providers. These patients are likely to postpone needed care until their conditions have escalated in severity. This group would have no representation in the clinical research arena; the subsequent lack of diversity in the research population may result in possible bias and hence limited applicability to those excluded groups.

The tremendous increases in new technology have not been accompanied by changes in the clinical evaluation of new approaches. As a result, new approaches may become "standard practice" despite an actual harmful side effect. Researchers may have difficulty obtaining approval to perform properly designed clinical trials from the human subjects committees that oversee the ethics of research because of the presumed standard of practice that is present in the field. For example, in the case of the use of intravitreal triamcinolone for diabetic macular edema, many practitioners were using this new treatment instead of laser photocoagulation. The Diabetic Retinopathy

Clinical Research Network showed that intravitreal was no better than laser and in fact caused more harm by inducing cataracts and elevated intraocular pressure in a significant proportion of triamcinolone-treated patients (6).

RESEARCH STAFF AND DOCUMENTATION

The goal of all clinical research is to provide information that will help the practitioner treat his or her patients more effectively. The clinical trial provides the best means to objectively quantify and compare the benefits and risks of new or alternative treatments to establish treatments for disease, especially when the difference between a new or old treatment is not clear or when a large number of factors may influence the course of the disease or the outcomes of the treatment (4). To ensure that the treatment groups are compared objectively, standardized methods of gathering data, training and certifying the personnel who collect the data, and treating patients either surgically or pharmaceutically are imperative. Continuous monitoring of adherence to the protocol, uniform data accumulation, and routine re-certification of personnel will eliminate any concerns of bias or ambiguity when the data are presented. All data accumulated on a case report form, the form that is submitted to a central data collection agency, must be documented in the patient file and these two documents must be reconciled at all times. All clinical research studies are monitored at regular intervals to ensure that all information are recorded on all the legal documents and that no data are missing or unsubstantiated. The success of all clinical research is totally dependent on this accurate and standardized collection of data, and strict adherence to the protocols.

SUMMARY POINTS

- Macular Photocoagulation Study was the first clinical study to look at macular degeneration.
- The aging population is 34.8 million with 1.2 million having some form of visual impairment.
- Clinical research is the best means to quantify and objectively compare the benefits and risks of new or alternative treatments for disease or injury especially when:
  ° The difference between a new or old treatment is not clear;
  ° The disease naturally follows a chronic, variable, and erratic course;
  ° A large number of factors, known or unknown, may influence both the course of the disease and the outcome of the treatment.

- A well-designed and conducted randomized clinical trial incorporates the following:
  ° High ethical standards—of paramount importance are patient welfare, informed consent, adherence to protocol, and careful data monitoring.
  ° Control groups that are matched to the treatment groups for the baseline characteristics.
  ° Random assignment of patients to both study and control groups when comparability of results among groups is essential.
  ° Masking to minimize bias of both the examiner and the patient, if possible.
  ° Enrollment of an adequate number of patients enrolled in the trial for the results to be statistically significant.
  ° Completeness of patient follow-up.
  ° Use of statistical methods for study design and data analysis.
  ° Continuous monitoring of adherence to protocol and accumulation of data by the Data Safety Monitoring Committee, the study Advisory Committee, the Executive Committee and the Steering Committee to ensure the safety of the subjects involved in the trial (7).

REFERENCES

1. Administration on Aging (AoA). A Profile of Older Americans. US: Department of Health and Human Services, 2000.
2. The Eye Diseases Prevalence Research Group. Prevalence of age related macular degeneration in the United States. Arch Ophthalmol 2004; 122: 564–72.
3. Photocoagulation Study Group. Argon laser photocoagulation for senile macular degeneration. results of a randomized clinical trial. Arch Ophthalmol 1982; 100: 912–18.
4. Walonker AF, Sturrock D. The Ryan Leopold Beckman Center for Clinical Research. Masters Thesis School of Public Health, UCLA, 1999.
5. Centers for Medicare and Medicaid Services. Office of the Actuary, National Health Statistics Group. National Health Care Expenditures Data, 2012.
6. Diabetic Retinopathy Clinical Research Network. A randomized trial comparing intravitreal triamcinolone acetonide and focal/grid photocoagulation for diabetic macular edema. Ophthalmology 2008; 1159: 1447–9, 1449. e1–10.
7. Clinical Trials Supported by The National Eye Institute. US: Department of Health and Human Services, 1987.

Index

T - #0233 - 191219 - C69 - 279/216/19 - PB - 9780367380663